# PEDIATRIC INTENSIVE CARE

**Haresh Kirpalani, BM, FRCP(UK), MSc (clin epi)**
Professor of Pediatrics University of Pennsylvania
Staff Neonatologist Children's Hospital of Philadelphia
Philadelphia, Pennsylvania and Department of Clinical
Epidemiology McMaster University Hamilton, Ontario

**Lennox H. Huang, MD, FAAP**
Associate Clinical Chair and Assistant Professor
Department of Pediatrics, McMaster University
Interim Chief of Pediatrics McMaster Children's Hospital
Hamilton, Ontario

Associate Editors:
**Mark Duffet, BSc(Pharm), ACPR, RPh**
Clinical Assistant Professor Division of Pediatric Critical
Care, Department of Pediatrics Staff Pharmacist, Pediatric
Critical Care Unit McMaster Children's Hospital
Hamilton, Ontario

**Michael Michenko, RN, BScN**
Education and Development Clinician Clinical Practice and
Education Hamilton Health Sciences Corporation
Hamilton, Ontario

2009
**PEOPLE'S MEDICAL PUBLISHING HOUSE – USA**
SHELTON, CONNECTICUT

**People's Medical Publishing House**
2 Enterprise Drive, Suite 509
Shelton, CT 06484
Tel: 203-402-0646
Fax: 203-402-0854
E-mail: info@pmph-usa.com

 PEOPLE'S MEDICAL PUBLISHING HOUSE

PMPH

ISBN 978-1-60795-010-3

Printed in China by People's Medical Publishing House of China
Copyeditor/Typesetter: Macmillan Publishing Solutions; Cover Designer: Mary McKeon

**Sales and Distribution**

*Canada*
**McGraw-Hill Ryerson Education**
Customer Care
300 Water St
Whitby, Ontario L1N 9B6
Canada
Tel: 1-800-565-5758
Fax: 1-800-463-5885
www.mcgrawhill.ca

*Foreign Rights*
**John Scott & Company**
International Publisher's Agency
P.O. Box 878
Kimberton, PA 19442
USA
Tel: 610-827-1640
Fax: 610-827-1671

*Japan*
**United Publishers Services Limited**
1-32-5 Higashi-Shinagawa
Shinagawa-ku, Tokyo
140-0002
Japan
Tel: 03-5479-7251
Fax: 03-5479-7307
Email: kakimoto@ups.co.jp

*United Kingdom, Europe, Middle East, Africa*
**McGraw-Hill Education**
Shoppenhangers Road
Maidenhead
Berkshire, SL6 2QL
England
Tel: 44-0-1628-502500
Fax: 44-0-1628-635895
www.mcgraw-hill.co.uk

*Singapore, Thailand, Philippines, Indonesia, Vietnam, Pacific Rim, Korea*
**McGraw-Hill Education**
60 Tuas Basin Link
Singapore 638775
Tel: 65-6863-1580
Fax: 65-6862-3354
www.mcgraw-hill.com.sg

*Australia, New Zealand*
**Elsevier Australia**
Locked Bag 7500
Chatswood DC NSW 2067
Australia
Tel: +61 (2) 9422-8500
Fax: +61 (2) 9422-8562
www.elsevier.com.au

*Brazil*
**Tecmedd Importadora e Distribuidora de Livros Ltda.**
Avenida Maurilio Biagi 2850
City Ribeirao, Rebeirao,
Preto SP
Brazil
CEP: 14021-000
Tel: 0800-992236
Fax: 16-3993-9000
Email: tecmedd@tecmedd.com.br

*India, Bangladesh, Pakistan, Sri Lanka, Malaysia*
CBS Publishers
4819/X1 Prahlad Street 24
Ansari Road, Darya, New
Delhi-110002
India
Tel: 91-11-23266861/67
Fax: 91-11-23266818
Email:cbspubs@vsnl.com

*People's Republic of China*
**PMPH**
Bldg 3, 3rd District
Fangqunyuan, Fangzhuang
Beijing 100078
P.R. China
Tel: 8610-67653342
Fax: 8610-67691034
www.pmph.com

# Contributors

**Section Editors**

Krishnapriya Anchala, MD, MS, FAAP
Assistant Professor
Division of Emergency Medicine, Department of Pediatrics
McMaster University
Medical Director, Pediatric Trauma
McMaster Children's Hospital
Hamilton, Ontario

Samra Sarigol Blanchard, MD, FAAP
Director, Pediatric Gastroenterology, Associate Professor
Division of Pediatric Gastroenterology, Department of Pediatrics
University of Maryland School of Medicine
Children's Hospital, University of Maryland Medical Center
Baltimore, Maryland

Diana Calligan, BA Sc. RD
Registered Dietitian
Pediatric Critical Care Unit, McMaster Children's Hospital
Hamilton, Ontario

Lisa Elden, MSc, MD, FRCS(C)
Associate Professor
Department of Otorhinolaryngology: Head and Neck Surgery
Associate Director of Pediatric Pediatric Airway Clinic
The Children's Hospital of Philadelphia
Philadelphia, Pennsylvania

Karen McAssey, MD, FRCPC
Pediatric Clerkship Director, Assistant Professor
Division of Endocrinology, Department of Pediatrics
McMaster University, McMaster Children's Hospital
Hamilton, Ontario

Paul M. Shore, MD, FAAP
Assistant Professor
Section of Critical Care Medicine, Department of Pediatrics
Drexel University College of Medicine
St. Christopher's Hospital for Children
Philadelphia, Pennsylvania

Peter Skippen, MBBS, FRCPC, FJFICM, MHA
Division Head, Associate Professor
Division of Pediatric Critical Care, Department of Pediatrics
University of British Columbia, BC Children's Hospital
Vancouver, British Columbia

Brigitte Strahm, MD
Centre for Pediatrics and Adolescent Medicine
University Hospital Freiburg
Departments of Pediatric Hematology and Oncology
Freiburg, Germany

## Contributors

Krishnapriya Anchala, MD, MS, FAAP
Assistant Professor
Division of Emergency Medicine, Department of Pediatrics
McMaster University
Medical Director, Pediatric Trauma
McMaster Children's Hospital
Hamilton, Ontario

Michael R Anderson MD FAAP
Associate Professor of Pediatrics
Division of Pharmacology and Critical Care, Department of Pediatrics
Rainbow Babies and Children's Hospital, Case Western Reserve
School of Medicine
Vice President and Associate Chief Medical Officer
University Hospitals
Cleveland, Ohio

Uma Athale, MD
Associate Professor
Division of Hematology and Oncology, Department of Pediatrics
McMaster University, McMaster Children's Hospital
Hamilton, Ontario

James Bain, MD FRCPC(S)
Department of Surgery, Division of Plastic Surgery
McMaster University, McMaster Children's Hospital
Hamilton, Ontario

Lara Bauman MSN, CNP
Department of Pediatric Gastroenterology
Rainbow Babies and Children's Hospital
Cleveland, Ohio

Samra Sarigol Blanchard MD, FAAP
Director, Pediatric Gastroenterology, Associate Professor
Division of Pediatric Gastroenterology, Department of Pediatrics
University of Maryland School of Medicine
Children's Hospital, University of Maryland Medical Center
Baltimore, Maryland

Diana Calligan, BA Sc. RD
Registered Dietitian
Pediatric Critical Care Unit, McMaster Children's Hospital
Hamilton, Ontario

Anthony K. C. Chan, MBBS, FRCPC
Division Chief & Professor
Division of Hematology and Oncology, Department of Pediatrics
McMaster University, McMaster Children's Hospital
Hamilton, Ontario

Catherine Chant-Gambacourt, RN BScN CCN(C) MN/APN (c)
Nurse Practitioner
Division of Pediatric Cardiology
McMaster Children's Hospital
Hamilton, Ontario

Karen Choong, M.B.BCh, FRCP(C)
Associate Professor
Division of Critical Care, Department of Pediatrics

McMaster University, McMaster Children's Hospital
Hamilton, Ontario

Arthur Cogswell    FRACP, FRCPC, FJFICM
Medical Director, ECLS Program
Division of Pediatric Critical Care, Department of Pediatrics
University of British Columbia, BC Children's Hospital
Vancouver, British Columbia

Dr. Anthony G. Crocco MD, FRCPC
Assistant Professor
Division of Pediatric Emergency Medicine, Department of Pediatrics
University of Calgary, Alberta Children's Hospital
Calgary, Alberta

John Crossley, MD, FRCPC
Assistant Professor
Division of Emergency Medicine
Department of Medicine
McMaster University, Hamilton Health Sciences Corporation
Hamilton, Ontario

Mark Duffet, BSc(Pharm), ACPR, RPh
Clinical Assistant Professor
Division of Pediatric Critical Care, Department of Pediatrics
Staff Pharmacist, Pediatric Critical Care Unit
McMaster Children's Hospital
Hamilton, Ontario

Walter Duncan, MD
Clinical Professor,
Division of Cardiology, Department of Pediatrics
University of British Columbia, BC Children's Hospital
Vancouver, British Columbia

Lisa Elden, MSc, MD, FRCS(C)
Associate Professor
Department of Otorhinolaryngology: Head and Neck Surgery
Associate Director of Pediatric Pediatric Airway Clinic
The Children's Hospital of Philadelphia
Philadelphia, Pennsylvania

Jonathan Gilleland, MD, FRCPC
Assistant Professor
Division of Pediatric Critical Care, Department of Pediatrics
McMaster University
Medical Site Director,
Ontario Critical Care Response Team Demonstration Project
McMaster Children's Hospital

Andrew Healey, BSc, MD, FRCPC
Department of Emergency Medicine
St. Joseph's Hospital
Critical Care Medicine Fellow, McMaster University
Hamilton, Ontario

Nancy Hemrica, RN, BScN
In-Hospital Organ and Tissue Donation Coordinator
Trillium Gift of Life
Hamilton, Ontario

Robert Hollenberg, MD FRCPCS
Associate Professor
Department of Surgery, Department of Pediatrics
McMaster University, McMaster Children's Hospital
Hamilton, Ontario

Lennox H. Huang, MD, FAAP
Associate Clinical Chair, Assistant Professor
Division of Critical Care, Department of Pediatrics
McMaster University
Interim Chief of Pediatrics
McMaster Children's Hospital
Hamilton, Ontario

C.Hui MD FRCPC
Director Paediatric Infectious Diseases training program, Assistant professor
Department of Pediatrics
University of Ottawa, Children's Hospital of Eastern Ontario
Ottawa, Ontario

Kevan Jacobson, MB BCh, FRCPC
Assistant Professor
Division of Gastroenterology, Department of Paediatrics
University of British Columbia, BC Children's Hospital
Vancouver, British Columbia

Paul F Kantor MBBCh, FRCPC
Associate Professor
Division of Pediatric Cardiology, Department of Pediatrics
University of Toronto, Hospital for Sick Children
Toronto, Ontario

Stephen Keeley, MBBS, FRACP, FRCP (Can), FJFICM
Clinical Associate Professor
Division of Pediatric Critical Care, Department of Pediatrics
University of British Columbia, BC Children's Hospital
Vancouver, British Columbia

Carolyn Kercsmar, MD
Co-Director, Professor of Pediatrics
Division of Pediatric Pulmonology, Department of Pediatrics
University of Cincinnati
Director, Asthma Center
Cincinnati Children's Hospital Medical Center
Cincinnati, Ohio

Aneal Khan, MD, MSC, FAAP, FRCPC, FCCMG
Assistant professor
Department of Medical Genetics
University of Calgary, Alberta Children's Hospital
Calgary, Alberta

Jennifer Kilgar, MD, FRCPC
Department of Emergency Medicine
London Health Sciences Corporation
University of Western Ontario
London, Ontario

Haresh Kirpalani, BM, FRCP(UK), MSc(clin epi)
Professor Pediatrics,

Division of Neonatology
Children's Hospital of Philadelphia
Pennsylvania School of Medicine
Philadelphia, Pennsylvania
and Department Clinical Epidemiology, McMaster Medical Center,
Hamilton, Ontario

Michael W. Konstan, M.D.
Professor of Pediatrics
Division of Pediatric Pulmonology, Department of Pediatrics
Case Western Reserve University School of Medicine
Director, the LeRoy W. Matthews Cystic Fibrosis Center
Rainbow Babies and Children's Hospital
Cleveland, Ohio

A. Desirée La Beaud, MD, MS
Fellow, Pediatric Infectious Diseases
Division of Pediatric Infectious Diseases & Rheumatology
Rainbow Babies and Children's Hospital
Case Western Reserve University School of Medicine
Cleveland, Ohio

Andrew Latchman, MD FRCPC
Assistant Professor
Division of General Pediatrics, Department of Pediatrics
McMaster University, McMaster Children's Hospital
Hamilton, Ontario

Robert Lloyd, MD, FRCPC
Associate Professor
Division of Pediatric Critical Care, Department of Pediatrics
McMaster University, McMaster Children's Hospital
Medical Director, Clinical Informatics, Hamilton Health Sciences Corporation
Hamilton, Ontario

Lia Lowrie, MD, FAAP
Interim Division Chief, Associate Professor
Division of Pediatric Pharmacology and Critical Care, Department of Pediatrics
Case Western Reserve University School of Medicine
Medical Director, Pediatric Intensive Care Unit
Rainbow Babies and Children's Hospital
Cleveland, Ohio

Seth Marks, MD, MSc, FRCPC
Assistant Professor
Division of Endocrinology, Department of Pediatrics
University of Alberta, Stollery Children's Hospital
Edmonton, Alberta

Karen McAssey, MD, FRCPC
Pediatric Clerkship Director, Assistant Professor
Division of Endocrinology, Department of Pediatrics
McMaster University, McMaster Children's Hospital
Hamilton, Ontario

Michael J. Michenko, RN, BScN
Education and Development Clinician
Clinical Practice and Education
Hamilton Health Sciences Corporation
Hamilton, Ontario

Tapas Mondal, MBBS, MD, MRCP, MRCPCH
Assistant Professor
Division of Cardiology, Department of Pediatrics
McMaster University, McMaster Children's Hospital
Hamilton, Ontario

David Munson, MD
Assistant Professor of Clinical Pediatrics
Division of Neonatology and Pediatric Advanced Care Team
Children's Hospital of Philadelphia
Pennsylvania School of Medicine
Philadelphia, Pennsylvania

Trisha Murthy, MD
Resident
Department of Pediatrics, McMaster University
McMaster Children's Hospital
Hamilton, Ontario

Kim Myers, MD
Fellow
Division of Cardiology, Department of Pediatrics
University of British Columbia, BC Children's Hospital
Vancouver, British Columbia

Jennifer Needle, MD, MPH
Assistant Professor
Division of Pediatric Critical Care, Department of Pediatrics
Oregon Health and Sciences University
Doernbecher Children's Hospital
Portland, Oregon

Raymond Nkwantabisa M.D.
Assistant Professor
Department of Pediatrics
Mount Sinai School of Medicine, Mount Sinai Medical Center
New York, New York

Allison Nykolaychuk, RRT
Education Coordinator,
Department of Respiratory Therapy
Atlantic Health Sciences Corporation
Saint John, New Brunswick

Isaac Odame, MB, CHB, MRCP (UK), FRCPath, FRCPCH
Associate Professor
Division of Hematology/Oncology, Department of Pediatrics
University of Toronto, Hospital for Sick Children
Toronto, Ontario

Alexander Pitfield, MD, FRCPC
Department of Pediatrics
University of British Columbia, BC Children's Hospital
Vancouver, British Columbia

Carol Portwine, MD, PhD
Associate Professor
Division of Hematology and Oncology, Department of Pediatrics
McMaster University, McMaster Children's Hospital
Hamilton, Ontario

Murray Potter, MD, FRCPC, FCCMG
Assistant professor, Pathology and Molecular Medicine
McMaster University
Head - Biochemical Genetics
Department of Laboratory Medicine, Hamilton Health Sciences Corporation
Hamilton, Ontario

Jim Potts, PhD
Clinical Epidemiologist
Division of Cardiology, Department of Pediatrics
University of British Columbia, BC Children's Hospital
Vancouver, British Columbia

Design Reddy, MD, FRCPC
Clinical Assistant Professor
Department of Anaesthesia,
McMaster University, McMaster Children's Hospital
Hamilton, Ontario

Kristie R. Ross, MD, FAAP
Instructor of Pediatrics
Division of Pediatric Pulmonology, Department of Pediatrics
Case Western Reserve University School of Medicine,
Rainbow Babies and Children's Hospital
Cleveland, Ohio

Shubhayan Sanatani, MD, FRCPC
Director of Cardiac Pacing and Electrophysiology
Division of Cardiology, Department of Pediatrics
University of British Columbia, BC Children's Hospital
Vancouver, British Columbia

Paul M. Shore, MD, FAAP
Assistant Professor
Section of Critical Care Medicine, Department of Pediatrics
Drexel University College of Medicine
St. Christopher's Hospital for Children
Philadelphia, Pennsylvania

Peter Skippen, MBBS, FRCPC, FJFICM, MHA
Division Head, Associate Professor
Division of Pediatric Critical Care, Department of Pediatrics
University of British Columbia, BC Children's Hospital
Vancouver, British Columbia

Paul G. Smith, DO, FAAP
Associate Professor of Pediatrics
Division of Pharmacology and Critical Care, Department of Pediatrics
Case Western Reserve University School of Medicine,
Rainbow Babies and Children's Hospital
Cleveland, Ohio

Neil Spenceley, MB ChB, MRCPCH
Fellow
Division of Pediatric Critical Care, Department of Pediatrics
University of British Columbia, BC Children's Hospital
Vancouver, British Columbia

Brigitte Strahm, MD
Centre for Pediatrics and Adolescent Medicine

Departments of Pediatric Hematology and Oncology
University Hospital Freiburg
Freiburg, Germany

Vandana Thapar MD
Fellow
Division of Pharmacology and Critical Care, Department of Pediatrics
Case Western Reserve University School of Medicine,
Rainbow Babies and Children's Hospital
Cleveland, Ohio

Philip Toltzis, MD, FAAP
Associate Professor
Division of Pharmacology and Critical Care, Department of Pediatrics
Case Western Reserve University School of Medicine,
Rainbow Babies and Children's Hospital
Cleveland, Ohio

Beth Vogt, MD, FAAP
Associate Professor
Division of Pediatric Nephrology, Department of Pediatrics
Case Western Reserve University School of Medicine,
Rainbow Babies and Children's Hospital
Cleveland, Ohio

Anupma Wadhwa, MD, MEd, FRCPC
Fellowship program director, Assistant Professor
Division of Pediatric Infectious Disease, Department of Pediatrics
University of Toronto, Hospital for Sick Children
Toronto, Ontario

J. Mark Walton, MD, FRCPC(S)
Assistant Dean, Post Graduate Medical Education
Associate Professor, Pediatrics and General Surgery
McMaster University, McMaster Children's Hospital
Hamilton, Ontario

Emad Zaki, MD, MSc, FAAP
Associate Professor
Department of Pediatrics, Division of Pediatric Nephrology
McMaster University, McMaster Children's Hospital
Hamilton, Ontario

# Preface

The world of the pediatric ICU is a daunting one when first entered. Any help is welcome! We hope this pocket manual will serve as an introduction for beginners and as an aid for those already immersed in the care of acutely ill children. However, some disclaimers are appropriate. First, it is not possible within the confines of a short text to be fully comprehensive. Second, given the relatively few trials done in the pediatric ICU as compared to the adult ICU, it is not possible to base these guidelines wholly on the highest level of evidence. Therefore the book takes an approach in which whatever evidence might exist at the level of randomized clinical trials is combined with sensible clinical guidelines from experienced clinicians. We are grateful for the contributions of our many friends, colleagues, and staff members of the ICUs and hospitals in which we have had the privilege to work. Most of all, this book would not be possible without all the children and families who have needed care all over the world.

—Haresh Kirpalani
and Lennox Huang

# Foreword

Pediatric critical care medicine is a relatively new speciality. It is, however, undergoing dramatic changes—changes spurred by an exponential rise in knowledge and therapeutic options for the critically ill or injured as well as by the recognition of the importance of team dynamics, ethical decision making, and family involvement in care. The delivery of pediatric critical care should ideally start from the first telephone contact to a practitioner and extend beyond the delivery of care within the walls of the intensive care unit. Adaptation of critical care expertise to environments outside the double doors of the intensive care unit, where resources may be limited and practitioners may have varying degrees of skill, expertise, and comfort in treating the critically ill child, poses tremendous challenges on many fronts.

One area of deficiency is the lack of easily available information for frontline caregivers (including emergency and critical care providers), early response and transport teams, and pediatric and critical care trainees. Ideally, all persons involved in the treatment of critically ill infants and children should have the basic knowledge and skills to be able to recognize critical illness and provide aggressive early cardiopulmonary resuscitation and monitoring as well as vital organ support and preservation. Pediatric and critical care trainees should not only learn the basic skills, but also be knowledgeable about the more complex aspects of critical care and organ support that are provided in tertiary critical care units.

Training in and acquisition of these critical care skills can be daunting, and the search for a quick, easy reference can leave one bewildered and confused. Any attempt to distill the salient information required for providing care into a concise form so that clinicians caring for the acutely ill and injured child can have it within easy reach is a laudable goal. This handbook is a brilliant attempt to do just that. It is a concise and useful guide for all aspects of care for the critically ill or injured child from initial recognition of critical illness through completion of the child's care in the ICU. The information and lessons presented here will help those who care for the critically ill and injured child and, if studied and kept close at hand, should bolster their confidence and lessen their anxiety.

This book is a welcome addition to the literature. It provides didactic and practical advice about many aspects of pediatric intensive care and highlights many of the salient points that are needed to provide timely and appropriate care. It is a reasonable compromise between voluminous and complex textbooks and didactic outlines without any explanation of the physiological rationale. It provides enough information for the "doers" who need a more efficient resource than one containing a detailed discussion of pathology and the physiological rationale for treatment, but also provides enough of that information to whet the appetite of the intellectually curious. The text should be within easy reach of all trainees and those who may encounter acutely ill or injured children in their practices.

—Niranjan Kissoon, MD,
British Columbia Children's Hospital

# Contents

# Chapter 1

# Introduction to Pediatric Critical Care

Lennox Huang
Haresh Kirpalani

This handbook is only a primer—it is meant as a survival guide for staff (and their patients) and an initiation to the practice of pediatric critical care. Reflecting the discipline as a whole, it can only dangle a few completed and explicit evidence-based guidelines. Thus far, relatively few randomized controlled trials have been performed in this discipline. Nonetheless, it does offer the trainee an evidence-based approach—and it makes explicit where evidence is lacking to date. Here we offer some more philosophical thoughts about the principles that underlie ICU care.

Intensive care can be defined as a service for patients who can benefit from more detailed observation and invasive treatment than can safely be provided in non-intensive care settings. Intensive care is a relatively young specialty that has roots in anesthesia with the worldwide development of advanced life support as a response to the polio epidemic of the 1930s. As the specialty continues to grow and evolve, a number of important themes have arisen.

## Teamwork

Multidisciplinary teamwork is crucial to daily ICU functioning. Studies in the ICU show that team structure, management, and rounding styles affect the ability of a unit to accomplish daily goals. Communication flow in the ICU is extremely complex and

*Table 1*

# Physician Management Index Attributes

- Acknowledged own mistakes
- Acknowledged team's perceptions/concerns
- Acted as role model for the team
- Communicated goals and expectations
- Emphasized team's progress/development
- Encouraged a safe learning environment
- Encouraged input from other team members
- Exemplified own expectations
- Focused on results
- Gauged the team performance
- Gave team members a sense of responsibility
- Managed conflict with other groups
- Managed conflict within the team
- Managed stress effectively
- Managed time effectively
- Set high standards
- Showed appreciation for team's work
- Showed cross-cultural sensitivity
- Showed self-confidence
- Triaged patient flow appropriately

involves multiple services and teams outside of the unit. These can be summarized in the following core set of principles:

- Members focus on the needs of the patients and families.
- Contributions of team members are recognized but not the primary goal.
- Mutual respect, understanding, and recognition are vital.
- Clear identification of a team leader provides structure.
- Closed-loop communication and inclusion of all team members keep information flowing appropriately.

The attending physician functions as the medical team leader in PICUs. The physician management index collates these principles into criteria that was correlated by Stockwell with the ability to achieve daily goals in the unit.

## Family-Centered Care

This term was coined by Helen Harrison, a parent whose child underwent critical care, and was set out in the first article in *Pediatrics* by a layperson. A natural extension of teamwork in the ICU is to include patients and families in decision making and daily care. Family-centered care is a philosophy practiced by many children's hospitals and PICUs that is now expanding to adult medicine. When a loved one is ill, families have identified the following needs:

- Proximity and availability of health care providers
- Assurance from caregivers
- Information about illness and treatment
- Support and comfort from the team
- The ability to partake in key medical decisions for the child

In practical terms, family-centered care is realized through a variety of practices, including the following:

- Open visiting hours
- Family presence at bedside during resuscitations
- Open bedside rounds with family presence
- Design of new units with input from family advisory committees
- Ability to have families room-in with patients
- Care by parents when transitioning out of the PICU

A growing body of evidence supports each of these practices. In a study of bedside rounds in a PICU, open bedside rounds were perceived positively by the MD, RN, and parents; confidentiality was not seen as a problem; and average rounding time decreased. Studies of family presence during resuscitation have shown no difference in patient outcomes. Litigations have not increased as a result of family presence, and overall families report a high satisfaction level when allowed to be present for at least some portion of a resuscitation.

## Rounding and Checklists

Although rounding is a part of daily ICU routines, format varies considerably and depends upon local needs and practices. Many rounds are conducted at the patient bedside with the entire multidisciplinary team, and in keeping with family-centered care, rounds increasingly include the family and patient. A major quality improvement measure is the introduction of daily goals forms and checklists. One example of a daily checklist used in adult ICUs is FAST-HUG, an acronym for feeding, analgesia, sedation, thromboembolic prophylaxis, head of bed elevation, ulcer prophylaxis, and glucose control. Studies of similar pediatric daily goals forms have shown improvement in communication after implementation.

## Scoring Systems

In general, scores are designed as an epidemiologic tool to aid research and quality assurance and should not affect immediate individual patient management. It could be questioned: Why should residents know about these? The answer lies in the resident appreciating the dynamic nature, and the limits of knowledge. Moreover, by the act of filling in the details of the scoring system, they instill a clinical sense of what is important in administering clinical care.

Scores can be used to compare populations between ICUs, assess whether individual hospital mortality is appropriate for the types of patients seen, or even provide an estimate of individual patient risk of mortality either pre-ICU admission or post-admission. Scores generally predict or measure illness severity based on physiologic and laboratory data; the most commonly used scores worldwide are PRISM III and PIM 2. Other validated scores are listed below:

> PRISM (Pediatric Risk of Mortality)
> P-MODS (Pediatric Multiple Organ Dysfunction Score)
> DORA (Dynamic Objective Risk Assessment)
> PELOD (Pediatric Logistic Organ Dysfunction)
> PIM (Pediatric Index of Mortality)

## ICU Admission Criteria

Deciding when a pediatric patient needs intensive care is the role of every pediatrician, but the decision will fall ultimately to the intensive care team. Intensive care units by definition should be one of the most heavily resourced areas within a hospital. It is neither practical nor appropriate to have every patient admitted into an intensive care unit. Various admission criteria have been developed to better define the types of patients who should be admitted into PICUs; these criteria will vary according to local resource availability. The AAP offers the following guideline to developing local admission and discharge policies.

# Respiratory System

Patients with severe or potentially life-threatening pulmonary or airway disease. Conditions include, but are not limited to:

1. Endotracheal intubation or potential need for emergency endotracheal intubation and mechanical ventilation, regardless of etiology
2. Rapidly progressive pulmonary, lower or upper airway, disease of high severity with risk of progression to respiratory failure and/or total obstruction
3. High supplemental oxygen requirement ($FIO_2 \geq 0.5$), regardless of etiology
4. Newly placed tracheostomy with or without the need for mechanical ventilation
5. Acute barotrauma compromising the upper or lower airway
6. Requirement for more frequent or continuous inhaled or nebulized medications than can be administered safely on the general pediatric patient care unit (according to institution guidelines)

# Cardiovascular

Patients with severe, life-threatening, or unstable cardiovascular disease. Conditions include, but are not limited to:

1. Shock
2. Postcardiopulmonary resuscitation
3. Life-threatening dysrhythmias
4. Unstable congestive heart failure, with or without need for mechanical ventilation
5. Congenital heart disease with unstable cardiorespiratory status
6. After high-risk cardiovascular and intrathoracic procedures
7. Need for monitoring of arterial, central venous, or pulmonary artery pressures
8. Need for temporary cardiac pacing

# Neurologic

Patients with actual or potential life-threatening or unstable neurologic disease. Conditions include, but are not limited to:

1. Seizures unresponsive to therapy or requiring continuous infusion of anticonvulsive agents

2. Acutely and severely altered sensorium where neurologic deterioration or depression is likely or unpredictable, or coma with the potential for airway compromise
3. After neurosurgical procedures requiring invasive monitoring or close observation
4. Acute inflammation or infections of the spinal cord, meninges, or brain with neurologic depression, metabolic and hormonal abnormalities, and respiratory or hemodynamic compromise or the possibility of increased intracranial pressure
5. Head trauma with increased intracranial pressure
6. Pre-operative neurosurgical conditions with neurologic deterioration
7. Progressive neuromuscular dysfunction with or without altered sensorium requiring cardiovascular monitoring and/or respiratory support
8. Spinal cord compression or impending compression
9. Placement of external ventricular drainage device

## Hematology/Oncology

Patients with life-threatening or unstable hematologic or oncologic disease or active life-threatening bleeding. Conditions include, but are not limited to:

1. Exchange transfusions
2. Plasmapheresis or leukopheresis with unstable clinical condition
3. Severe coagulopathy
4. Severe anemia resulting in hemodynamic and/or respiratory compromise
5. Severe complications of sickle cell crisis, such as neurologic changes, acute chest syndrome, or aplastic anemia with hemodynamic instability
6. Initiation of chemotherapy with anticipated tumor lysis syndrome
7. Tumors or masses compressing or threatening to compress vital vessels, organs, or airway

## Endocrine/Metabolic

Patients with life-threatening or unstable endocrine or metabolic disease. Conditions include, but are not limited to:

1. Severe diabetic ketoacidosis requiring therapy exceeding institutional patient care unit guidelines (if hemodynamic or neurologic compromise, see specific section)

2. Other severe electrolyte abnormalities, such as:

   a. Hyperkalemia, requiring cardiac monitoring and acute therapeutic intervention
   b. Severe hypo- or hypernatremia
   c. Hypo- or hypercalcemia
   d. Hypo- or hyperglycemia requiring intensive monitoring
   e. Severe metabolic acidosis requiring bicarbonate infusion, intensive monitoring, or complex intervention
   f. Complex intervention required to maintain fluid balance

3. Inborn errors of metabolism with acute deterioration requiring respiratory support, acute dialysis, hemoperfusion, management of intracranial hypertension, or inotropic support

## Gastrointestinal

Patients with life-threatening or unstable gastrointestinal disease. Conditions include, but are not limited to:

1. Severe acute gastrointestinal bleeding leading to hemodynamic or respiratory instability
2. After emergency endoscopy for removal of foreign bodies
3. Acute hepatic failure leading to coma, hemodynamic, or respiratory instability

## Surgical

Post-operative patients requiring frequent monitoring and potentially requiring intensive intervention. Conditions include, but are not limited to:

1. Cardiovascular surgery
2. Thoracic surgery
3. Neurosurgical procedures
4. Otolaryngologic surgery
5. Craniofacial surgery
6. Orthopedic and spine surgery
7. General surgery with hemodynamic or respiratory instability
8. Organ transplantation
9. Multiple trauma with or without cardiovascular instability
10. Major blood loss, either during surgery or during the post-operative period

## Renal System

Patients with life-threatening or unstable renal disease. Conditions include, but are not limited to:

1. Renal failure
2. Requirement for acute hemodialysis, peritoneal dialysis, or other continuous renal replacement therapies in the unstable patient
3. Acute rhabdomyolysis with renal insufficiency

## Multisystem and Other

Patients with life-threatening or unstable multisystem disease. Conditions include, but are not limited to:

1. Toxic ingestions and drug overdose with potential acute decompensation of major organ systems
2. Multiple organ dysfunction syndrome
3. Suspected or documented malignant hyperthermia
4. Electrical or other household or environmental (eg, lightning) injuries
5. Burns covering >10% of body surface (institutions with burn units only; institutions without such units will have transfer policy to cover such patients)

## Special Intensive Technologic Needs

Conditions that necessitate the application of special technologic needs, monitoring, complex intervention, or treatment including medications associated with the disease that exceed individual patient care unit policy limitations.

# Suggested Readings

American Academy of Pediatrics, Committee on Hospital Care and Section on Critical Care Medicine. Guidelines and levels of care for pediatric intensive care units. Pediatrics 1993;92:111–175.

Guidelines for developing admission and discharge policies for the pediatric intensive care unit. Pediatrics 1999 April;103(4):840–2.

Kleiber C, Davenport T, Freyenberger B. Open bedside rounds for families with children in pediatric intensive care units. Am J Crit Care 2006 Sep;15(5):492–6.

Lacroix J, Cotting J. Severity of illness and organ dysfunction scoring in children. Pediatr Crit Care Med 2005 May;6(3 Suppl):S126–34.

Latour JM, van Goudoever JB, Hazelzet JA. Parent satisfaction in the pediatric ICU. Pediatr Clin North Am 2008 June;55(3):779–90, xii–xiii.

Reader T, Flin R, Lauche K, Cuthbertson BH. Non-technical skills in the intensive care unit. Br J Anaesth 2006 May;96(5):551–9. Epub 2006 Mar 27.

Smith G, Nielsen M. ABC of intensive care. Criteria for admission. BMJ 1999 June 5;318(7197):1544–7.

Stockwell DC, Slonim AD, Pollack MM. Physician team management affects goal achievement in the intensive care unit. Pediatr Crit Care Med 2007 Nov;8(6):540–5.

Tsai E. Should family members be present during cardiopulmonary resuscitation? N Engl J Med 2002 Mar 28;346(13):1019–21.

# Chapter 2

# Rapid Response Systems/Medical Emergency Teams

Lennox Huang
Robert Lloyd
Jonathan Gilleland

- Rapid response systems (RRS) and medical emergency teams (MET) are a natural extension of critical care targeted at improving patient safety and quality of care. Although some practitioners use MET to refer only to the actual team, the terms are often used synonymously in the literature and for the purposes of this chapter we will use MET to refer to both the team and the surrounding system.
- A MET responds to a variety of medical crises and is proactive and preventative in practice. The general principle is to create a team of caregivers with trained expertise in assessment and management of critical illness, immediately available to all patients outside of critical care areas.
- The specific members of the team usually include a critical care physician and nurse, but this varies between institutions. In addition, the specific mechanism varies between individual institutions.
- The definition of a medical crisis is analogous to the physiologic definition of shock on a systems level. A crisis occurs when there is a mismatch between resources and demands for a particular patient problem.

# Key Principles

- Rapid response systems (RRS) is an early response system for any hospital crisis.
- The medical emergency teams (MET) is a multidisciplinary team closely linked with the intensive care unit (ICU).
- Natural extension of ICU care beyond the physical ICU—"ICU without walls."
- Bypasses traditional hierarchical model of medical care activation.
- May improve quality of care in the ICU and the rest of the hospital.

# Goals of MET

The general goal is to create a favorable balance between resource and demands for a specific crisis, thus improving quality of care and patient outcomes.

Specific goals include the following:

- Decrease number of cardiopulmonary resuscitation events
- Decrease "preventable" deaths—aiming for a goal of zero
- Decrease adverse events
- Identify safety issues at a systemic level
- Support ward teams
- Support families and health care teams in transitioning patients through chronic illness and end-of-life palliation
- Identify need for advance directives
- Outreach education for medical teams

## Efferent and Afferent Limbs

Afferent and efferent limbs of an RRS surround an acute event:

- Afferent limb—triggers and systems that activate the MET
- Efferent limb—pertains to the MET team itself, for example, training, composition, interventions taken, identification of system, or patient safety issues

## Team Composition

There are many possible members of the team.

Core team:

- Nursing staff form the core of emergency response teams and have the following characteristics:

  - Immediate responder
  - Must have critical care or emergency care experience
  - Advanced nurse specialists, nurse practitioners

- Supervising physician

  - Critical care fellows, attending acute care physicians
  - The supervising physician must be experienced in critical or emergency care
  - Depending on the model, physician may respond immediately in person, after initial nursing contact, or over the phone after nursing evaluation

- Optional members

  - Physician learners—for example, residents
  - Respiratory therapist
  - Pharmacist
  - Physician assistant

## MET Training

An initial training program followed by continued maintenance is required. Successful team education devotes equal amounts of time to both communication and clinical skills. There is no published consensus on what must be included in initial and ongoing training of METs. Most training programs consist of small-group sessions with simulation training and should include the following components:

- Resuscitation skills

  - Members should be certified in Pediatric Advanced Life Support (PALS) and should consider additional training in advanced trauma life support (ATLS) or advanced pediatric life support (APLS)

- Acute emergencies

  - Recognition and initial management of medical and surgical emergencies

- End-of-life care

  - Principles of palliative care, comfort measures, breaking bad news

- Intermediate or high-fidelity simulation

  - Role play and simulation may be useful in both evaluation and practical application of didactic knowledge

- Communication

  - Crew and crisis resource management
  - Interdisciplinary communication
  - Conflict resolution

## Medical Problems Addressed by MET

- Shock of any etiology and symptoms of shock

  - Altered mental status
  - Cardiac or pulmonary compromise

- Isolated respiratory compromise or deterioration
- Isolated cardiac compromise or deterioration
- Isolated neurologic compromise or deterioration
- Cardiac arrest

  - In many institutions, the MET is separate from the code team; however, there are some models where the MET serves a dual purpose.

- Conflict or disagreement with the management of an acutely ill patient
- End-of-life care

### Administrative Component

Implementation of a MET requires a significant culture shift in many institutions. Support for the team must come from all levels of hospital leadership and administration. Hospital-wide education and promotion are critical to an effective and sustainable team.

Maintenance of mortality and morbidity statistics in addition to other quality of care indices aids in monitoring team efficacy. Careful data collection can also provide a strong case for rational expenditure, or the need for additional support.

## Sample Guidelines for Activation/Team Consultation

Activation of the MET may be initiated by any health care professional including but not limited to nurses, respiratory therapists, residents, fellows, and staff physicians. Activation of the MET should not require approval from a supervisor as that will introduce systemic delays. Many centers allow students to activate the MET as well, and some centers allow patient families to activate the MET.

In a recent prospective before-and-after trial looking at the efficacy of a medical emergency team in a large tertiary

*Table 1*
**Sample Guidelines for Activation**

Nurse, physician, or family member worried about clinical state, cardiac, or respiratory arrest

| **Airway** | | | |
|---|---|---|---|

Threatened or obstructive symptoms: stridor, excessive secretions

| **Breathing** | | | |
|---|---|---|---|

Severe respiratory distress, apnea, tachypnea, or cyanosis

| Age | Respiratory rate/min | Hypoxemia | |
|---|---|---|---|
| Term–3 months | >60 | $SaO_2$ <90% in >40% $FiO_2$ | |
| 4–12 months | >50 | | |
| 1–4 years | >40 | $SaO_2$ <60% in >40% $FiO_2$ | |
| 5–12 years | >30 | (cyanotic heart disease) | |
| 12 years+ | >30 | | |

| **Circulation** | | | |
|---|---|---|---|
| Age | Bradycardia (beats/min) | Tachycardia (beats/min) | BP (systolic mm Hg) |
| Term–3 months | <100 | >180 | <50 |
| 4–12 months | <100 | >180 | <60 |
| 1–4 years | <90 | >160 | <70 |
| 5–12 years | <80 | >140 | <80 |
| 12 years | <60 | >130 | <90 |

| **Neurologic State** | | | |
|---|---|---|---|

Acute change in neurologic status or convulsion

pediatric hospital, the most common triggers of the MET in the pediatric population include:

| | |
|---|---|
| • Hypoxemia | 47% |
| • Respiratory distress | 39% |
| • Caregiver "worry" about the patient | 27% |
| • Airway threat | 27% |
| • Altered neurologic exam | 20% |
| • Tachycardia | 14% |
| • Tachypnea | 13% |

## Interventions Undertaken by Teams

- A rapid full assessment of the patient
- Advice and guidance to the primary medical team
- Perform acute cardiorespiratory interventions and continue care to ICU level care
- Able to provide critical care outside of the walls of the ICU for a limited period of time while awaiting transfer and definitive care in the ICU

Generally, the most common actions performed by the MET team include:

- Advice only
- Supplemental oxygen or increased oxygen administration
- Intravenous cannulation
- Fluid administration
- Basic airway support
- Bag-valve-mask ventilation

## Evidence for MET

Several large single-center prospective before-and-after trials in adults and one in children show a beneficial impact attributed to medical emergency teams. These include:

- Increased ICU admissions
- Decreased ICU stay
- Decreased ICU mortality
- Decreased hospital mortality
- Decreased ICU severity of illness
- Decrease respiratory arrest
- Decrease cardiac arrest

Several larger prospective cluster-randomized trials have been performed, the largest of which is the Medical Emergency Response Improvement Team (MERIT) study that included 23 hospitals in Australia. The results of these trials have failed to demonstrate efficacy of a MET; however, many authors cite the "Hawthorne effect," contamination and a dose-response effect as reasons for lack of statistical benefit.

# References

Braithwaite RS, DeVita MA, Mahidhara R, et al. The Medical Emergency Response Improvement Team (MERIT). Use of medical emergency team (MET) responses to detect medical errors. Qual Saf Health Care 2004; 13:255–9.

Tibballs J, Kinney S, Duke T, et al. Reduction of paediatric in-patient cardiac arrest and death with a medical emergency team: preliminary results. Arch Dis Child 2005;90:1148–52.

DeVita MA, Braithwaite RS, Mahidhara R, et al. The Medical Emergency Response Improvement Team (MERIT). Use of medical emergency team responses to reduce hospital cardiopulmonary arrests. Qual Saf Health Care 2004;13:251–4.

Galhotra S, DeVita MA, Simmons RL, et al. Members of the Medical Emergency Response Improvement Team (MERIT) Committee. Impact of patient monitoring on the diurnal pattern of medical emergency team activation. Crit Care Med 2006;34:1700–6.

Jones D, Bellomo R. Introduction of a rapid response system: why we are glad we MET. Crit Care 2006;10:121 [epub ahead of print].

# Chapter 3

# Pediatric Critical Care Transport

Jennifer Needle
Michael R Anderson

## Key Principles

- Interhospital transport teams consist of a variable makeup of highly skilled nurses, paramedics, pediatric and neonatal intensivists, pediatric emergency medicine specialists, and respiratory therapists.
- Studies show that morbidity and mortality are decreased when children are transported by intensive care and specialized personnel.
- Patient management decisions should balance risks of transport and risks of on-site management, against benefits of transport to a center for definitive care.

## Team Structure

- The AAP Section on Transport Medicine recommends that transport teams (apart from a driver or pilot) consist of a minimum of two caregivers: one nurse with a minimum of 5 years clinical experience, generally leading one of the following team models:

  1. nurse–nurse
  2. nurse–respiratory therapist
  3. nurse-respiratory therapist–physician
  4. nurse–physician
  5. nurse–emergency medical technician/paramedic

- Essential personnel also cover coordination, communication, and pretransport stabilization as well as interhospital transport roles.
- A medical director is a key role. She/he is usually a specialist in pediatric critical care, pediatric emergency medicine, or neonatology. This individual may also play the role of the medical control physician, responsible for communicating with the referring hospital.
- Such initial communication should suggest possible therapies necessary for stabilization and therapy prior to arrival of the transport team.
- The transport coordinator administers needs of the team: scheduling, equipment maintenance, and support for the medical director.
- Transport physicians are usually pediatric specialists with a minimum of 3 years of postgraduate training. These physicians must be proficient in endotracheal intubation, venous and arterial access, pneumothorax evacuation, and ventilator management.
- Use of resident and fellow trainees is controversial and may be dictated by regional guidelines and regulations.
- For teams made up solely of nurses, one registered nurse (RN) assumes the role of team leader, performing all of the above skills required of the physician. The nurses assume responsible for interacting with the child's family as well as staff from the referring hospital.

## Modes of Transport

Multiple factors impact choice of mode of transport, including:

- Acuity of illness
- Cost balanced against available resources including personnel and necessary equipment for transport and weather
- Geographic conditions impacting safety and time required for transport
- Current modes of medical transport are ground ambulance, rotary-wing aircraft (helicopter), or fixed wing (airplane). Rotary-wing aircraft provide transport in approximately one-half of the time required by ground modes, depending on geography.
- The decision on mode of transport is made by the medical transport physician in close consultation with the referring physician. The nature of the illness and the condition of the child are the major factors impacting the decision.

- The pilot of the aircraft is responsible for determining the safety of flight and typically should not be influenced by the diagnosis of the patient.
- The safety of the medical team and patient based on weather and flight conditions must be taken into consideration when a decision is made to fly a patient to an accepting facility.

In large rural areas, fixed-wing aircraft may be required to transport patients to a receiving hospital with the resources necessary to manage critically ill children. Most fixed-wing aircraft can cover greater than 250 kilometers (150 miles) and are able to fly in more inclement weather conditions than rotary-wing aircraft, but are more expensive and require an airport runway.

Equipment for the tram includes the following:

- Resuscitation medications, both at the referring hospital as well as in the transport vehicle. Epinephrine, amiodarone, lidocaine, atropine, and adenosine available in the appropriate doses in the event of arrhythmia or cardiac arrest.
- Defibrillators with the ability to deliver pediatric doses of energy (2 to 4 joules/kg) for patients who develop ventricular fibrillation or pulseless ventricular tachycardia in route (see Chapter 5, "Resuscitation" for further details).
- Fixed-wing aircraft, which are able to carry more passengers and equipment, facilitating patients requiring highly technical therapies for transport, such as extracorporeal membrane oxygenation (ECMO) or continuous renal replacement therapies.

## General Assessment and Stabilization for Transport (see Figure 1)

The transport team should immediately perform a rapid assessment of the child's clinical condition, with special attention to the ABCs (airway, breathing, circulation). The referring hospital is responsible for the collection of data, copying of labs and imaging for transfer to the accepting facility, and giving a report of the patient's history, physical treatments, and current condition. A detailed and systematic physical examination should be performed prior to departure, as physical examination may be difficult while in transport. Diagnosis is not the priority, but rather a focused assessment of immediate life-threatening components of the child's condition and any stabilization that needs to take place prior to departure.

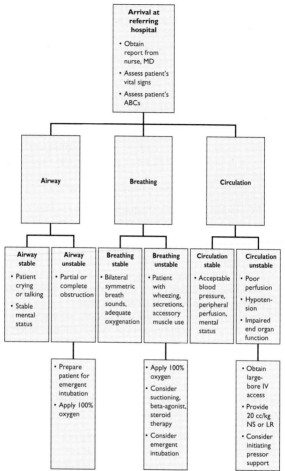

**Figure 1**    General assessment and stabilization for transport.

## Airway

The goal is to avoid the need for emergent airway stabilization during transport.

- Practical safety measures such as positioning, jaw-thrust, head-tilt, and chin-lift should be undertaken as necessary, often requiring a shoulder roll or oral airway.

- Whether or not to intubate the patient will depend on the patient's condition. Patients with clear respiratory failure, increased intracranial pressure, obtunded patients who may have lost airway protective reflexes, and patients in severe shock with potential for decompensation in route should be electively intubated.
- Intubation for transport should be performed by the most experienced person available, either from the transport team or from the referring hospital. The transport team will provide adequate sedation, and neuromuscular blockade as necessary, in order to ensure the safety of the endotracheal tube as well as the comfort of the patient.
- Place a gastric tube in any intubated patient for travel because gastric distention compromises ventilation and increases risk of emesis and aspiration.
- If the patient is already intubated, the team checks breath sounds, secures the endotracheal tube, and checks the chest x-ray for correct tube position prior to departure.

## Breathing

Regardless of the intubation status of the patient, frequent assessment of the breathing of the child is critical for the transport team. Pay special attention to breath sounds, respiratory effort and the use of accessory muscles, requirement of supplemental oxygen, and the patient's level of consciousness. Patients with hypoxia should receive 100% oxygen. Nonrebreathing masks provide the highest amount of oxygen with 80% to 95% delivered, followed by face tents, which can provide 40% to 50% oxygen for transport.

Patients with reactive airway disease will likely require continuous beta-agonist therapy in addition to oxygen. The goal of therapy should be to prevent the need for intubation, given the difficulty of mechanically ventilating these patients. Additional therapies should be considered, including magnesium, theophylline/aminophylline, and steroids.

Trauma victims should be assessed for the presence of life-threatening thoracic injuries such as pneumothorax (simple or tension), hemothorax, and/or cardiac tamponade. Care should be taken to treat these injuries prior to transport, where changes in cabin pressure could adversely affect the patient's condition.

## Circulation

Assessment of the child's circulatory status includes attention to vital signs such as heart rate and blood pressure, in addition to assessment of perfusion via capillary refill time, level of consciousness, and urine output. Ideally, intravenous access should be secured prior to the arrival of the transport team. In more critically ill patients, at least two IVs are necessary for infusing medications as well as backup in the event that one IV becomes nonfunctional in route.

Transport personnel should watch for early signs of shock and the need to initiate early therapies. Normal saline or lactated Ringer's, in boluses of 20 mL/kg, should be started immediately in patients with evidence of hypovolemic or distributive shock. Vital signs should be reassessed after the first fluid bolus and subsequent doses should be administered if there is evidence of persistent abnormalities. Patients in presumed cardiogenic shock should be given fluids to stabilize hypotension and tachycardia; however, subsequent fluids should be administered with caution because they may exacerbate the myocardial dysfunction (see Chapter 5, "Resuscitation").

An often forgotten cause of poor circulation in children, especially neonates, is hypothermia. Every attempt should be made to create a thermoneutral environment once initial stabilization occurs. In infants, hypothermia increases oxygen consumption, often leading to worsening cardiac performance and lactic acidosis. Transport isolettes are available for infants up to 5 kg; for larger children, warmed blankets are the most simple method to maintain thermoneutrality.

## Specific Conditions

Although a thorough review of all potential diagnoses faced by the transport team is well beyond the scope of this chapter, several key clinical caveats deserve attention.

## CNS

Critically ill children can present with a variety of central nervous system (CNS) problems: seizures are the most common, followed by trauma leading to subdural hematoma, epidural hematoma, and potentially increased intracranial pressure (ICP). If referring facilities have access to a computed tomography (CT) scanner, optimal management of the child with head trauma will include imaging prior to transport.

Children should not be transported until the seizure activity has been controlled. This may require intubation and sedation in a patient who cannot be managed with initial therapies of benzodiazepines. In a postictal patient with a stable airway, complete resolution of neurologic symptoms is not necessary for safe transport.

Attention to ABCs should be the first priority. IV access should be obtained and benzodiazepines should be administered within 10 minutes of the patient's arrival or initial seizure, if this occurs during transport. If a concern exists for meningitis as a possible cause of the child's seizures (eg, a child with fever, nuchal rigidity, or history of prior illness), transport personnel should ensure that the child receive antibiotics either before or during transport. Protection of team members should be assured by meticulous contact or droplet precautions (gowns, gloves, and appropriate barrier or N95 masks).

## Status Epilepticus (see Chapter 9, "Neurology")

Following hemodynamic stabilization, benzodiazepines should be administered to prevent initiation and inhibit the spread of epileptiform discharges. A rule of thumb is that a single dose of benzodiazepine should stop 75% of seizures within 10 minutes. Second- and third-line drugs are listed below, in the suggested approach to choice of drugs:

- Lorazepam IV is usually the first-line benzodiazepine, but diazepam or midazolam at appropriate doses may also be given.
- If IV access is not available, lorazepam or diazepam may be given rectally and midazolam may be given intramuscularly.
- Intravenous administration of benzodiazepines may cause apnea and intubation capabilities should be available when giving these medications to a seizing patient who may already have an inability to protect their airway.
- Patients with status epilepticus may require phenytoin or phenobarbital for seizure control. It is important to remember potential side effects of these medications when administering in a transport situation.

Although it is not the responsibility of the transport team to diagnose the cause of the seizures, history, physical exam, and basic lab data should be reviewed by the team prior to departure.

- In an infant or child with a history of water consumption in excess of any other form of hydration, hyponatremia should be considered. These patients will likely be refractory to therapy with benzodiazepines and should be treated with 3 to 5 mL/kg of 3% saline over 5 to 10 minutes, which should raise serum sodium by 3 to 5 meq/L and stop the seizures.

- Hypoglycemia can cause seizures when serum glucose falls below 2 mmol/L. In a seizing patient, glucose should be kept over 4 mmol/L with the use of dextrose in the IV fluids. In peripheral IVs, the maximum continuous dextrose to be administered is D12.5% to prevent vascular injury; however, in emergent conditions, dextrose should be given as needed to stop the seizures.
- In neonates with seizures, hypocalcemia should be suspected and additional information suggesting this diagnosis is the presence of a prolonged QTc interval on EKG. This can be treated with calcium gluconate for peripheral access or calcium chloride if central access is available.
- Clinical suspicion of meningitis should prompt antibiotics with or without a lumbar puncture (LP).

## Cardiovascular Lesions and CHF

The usual ABCs of resuscitation apply to all patients (see Chapter 4B); however, in newborns with a suspected ductal-dependent lesion, alternative management therapies can be life saving. In addition, for patients with known cardiovascular issues, knowledge of the patient's surgical history is important for appropriate management.

For congenital defects, these considerations are relevant:

- In normal infants, functional closure of the ductus arteriosus occurs at approximately 12 hours after birth with complete anatomic closure at 2 to 3 weeks.
- In children with limited pulmonary circulation, the ductus may be the only form of pulmonary blood flow and its closure can result in hypoxia, shock, and death.
- Medical personnel should have a high index of suspicion for a ductal-dependent lesion in a 2- to 4-week-old newborn presenting to an emergency department with hypoxia, poor perfusion, and potentially, shock.
- Differential diagnoses include critical aortic stenosis, coarctation of the aorta, hypoplastic left heart syndrome, and interrupted aortic arch.
- Lesions presenting with decompensation following closure of the ductus due to right outflow obstruction are tricuspid atresia with intact ventricular septum, pulmonary atresia with

intact ventricular septum, and critical pulmonic stenosis. The ductal dependence of patients with transposition of the great arteries will vary based on the degree of pulmonary vascular resistance—if PVR is high, blood shunts to the systemic circulation. Low PVR will result in increased pulmonary blood flow.

Confirmation of a ductal-dependent lesion requires echocardiography and possible cardiac catheterization. However, a simple bedside hyperoxia test may assist the appropriate interim management of a child. In a patient with a pulmonary etiology of hypoxia, providing 100% oxygen should increase the $PaO_2$ by at least 30 within 10 minutes. In children who do not appropriately increase arterial oxygenation, suspect a cardiac lesion.

The goal in stabilization of a patient with a ductal-dependent cardiac lesion is to maintain the patency of the ductus arteriosus. This is accomplished by limiting supplemental oxygen to maintain pulse oxygenation in the 80s and administering alprostadil (prostaglandin E1) 0.05 to 0.1 mcg/kg/minute. If the ductus arterious closure is the cause of the patient's decompensation, an increase in the patient's oxygen saturation should be evident approximately 10 to 15 minutes after the initial load. The major side effect of alprostadil is apnea and all patients requiring alprostadil should be placed on mechanical ventilation.

- Acyanotic congenital heart disease classically presents with signs and symptoms of congestive heart failure (CHF) rather than shock. This is due to the chronic development of pulmonary overcirculation due to outflow tract obstruction. Cardiac lesions that may present in this manner are aortic atresia, ventricular septal defect, AV malformation, AV canal, cor pulmonale as a result of bronchopulmonary dysplasia in premature infants, endocardial cushion defects, interrupted aortic arch, mitral valve atresia, and persistent patent ductus arteriosus.
- Signs and symptoms suggestive of a diagnosis of CHF from the history are poor feeding with or without cyanosis, diaphoresis with feeding, hepatomegaly, weight gain in excess of expectations, tachypnea, and tachycardia. Children are less likely than adult patients with CHF to present with jugular venous distention and edema.

The basics of management of children with CHF include oxygen, diuresis, and, if necessary, inotropic support. Furosemide (0.5 to 1 mg/kg) should be administered at the referring facility to children with evidence of poor perfusion, poor urine output, and hepatomegaly. Dopamine or milrinone should be considered in patients requiring increased inotropy.

Placement of a Foley catheter is important for the strict monitoring of urine output, achievement of thermoneutrality to decrease metabolic demands, and sufficient access to provide medications. Additional considerations should include maintenance of hematocrit above 40 g/dL for optimal oxygen delivery and appropriate provision of positive pressure to maintain the Qp:Qs below 1, thus decreasing pulmonary overcirculation.

## Shock (see Chapter 5, "Resuscitation")

Patients with shock will present with a spectrum of signs and symptoms, depending on the level of compensation. Clinical history will lend clues to the type of shock. History of trauma, vomiting or diarrhea, and poor oral intake should lead to the suspicion of hypovolemic shock. Exposure to elements to which the child is known to be allergic or a preceding infectious process suggests distributive shock due to anaphylaxis or sepsis. Children with known cardiac lesions leading to CHF, chest trauma leading to tension pneumothorax, or more subtly, preceding viral illness with development of signs of CHF and myocarditis, should raise concern for cardiogenic shock. Decompensated shock is not subtle and presents with hypotension, poor perfusion, and evidence of end organ dysfunction such as poor urine output and altered mental status.

Immediate management to improve outcomes in children with shock includes ABCs. Oxygen should be applied to improve already compromised tissue delivery. If the child is profoundly obtunded (Glasgow Coma Scale of <8), the patient should be promptly intubated. Large-bore IV access should be achieved within three attempts or 30 seconds and, if unsuccessful, an intraosseous line should be placed. The patient should receive immediate normal saline or lactated Ringer's bolus of 20 mL/kg with repeated assessments of blood pressure and perfusion. If perfusion and blood pressure are not improved after two boluses, vasopressor support should be initiated to obtain an improvement in peripheral perfusion and mean arterial pressure (MAP) appropriate for age.

Initial therapies may include dopamine or epinephrine to improve systemic vascular resistance. Caution should accompany the use of these medications in patients in whom cardiogenic shock is suspected as a result of their potential to exacerbate myocardial depression. In patients with obvious cardiogenic shock, milrinone may be the medication of choice, but careful attention should be paid to the patient's potential for worsening hypotension with the initiation of this medication. Adequate preload should be established prior to starting milrinone.

Communication between the transport team and the accepting facility is vital for reducing the morbidity and mortality in patients with cardiac issues, including shock. Cardiology including catheterization laboratory staff and cardiothoracic surgery should be informed of the potential need for intervention. Additionally, the pharmacy should be alerted to prepare necessary medications prior to the patient's arrival at the accepting facility.

## Respiratory

Transport personnel must be adept at recognizing and managing impending respiratory failure, performing intubation, initiating ventilator management, and troubleshooting problems with an intubated patient on mechanical ventilation.

**Intubation**    Indications for intubation include airway obstruction, failure of gas exchange due to secretions or infection, airway protection in patients with altered mental status, patients with shock or hemodynamic compromise who may deteriorate more slowly than children with isolated respiratory problems, and increased ICP that requires intubation for both airway protection as well as for management of head injury including sedation and hyperventilation.

Ideally, a child requiring transport should be intubated at the referring facility. Equipment and personnel are more readily available, and in addition to the stable environment of a hospital, the referring facility is free from the noise and movement that occur in a transport vehicle. In equivocal cases, it is better to err on the side of obtaining a secure airway prior to transport. Successful intubation requires careful preparation, from equipment to medications. The SOAP mnemonic ensures that everything necessary for intubation is present prior to starting.

Medications serve two purposes in patients requiring intubation: (1) safe induction and (2) maintenance of a secure airway for the duration of transport. Below is a list of some routinely used medications for intubation Figure 2 shows and approach to induction for intubation.

S is for suction—given the risk of emesis in patients with respiratory distress, who likely have not been nothing by mouth (NPO), a large-suction catheter as well as one that will fit deeply into the oropharynx needs to be on hand.

O is for oxygen—should be applied for at least 3 minutes prior to giving intubation medications, in an effort to eliminate nitrogen from alveoli. This will allow time for the intubation when oxygen is not being applied and a pulse oximeter should be attached to the patient and functioning well prior to initiation.

A is for airway equipment—mask, endotracheal tubes with stylets, laryngoscopes, $CO_2$ detectors, and equipment for emergency cricothyroidotomy/tracheostomy, if necessary.

P is for pharmacy—medications necessary to reduce the risk for aspiration, to adequately sedate the child to prevent trauma, and paralytics to allow for more rapid and safe intubation.

P is for personnel—nurses, respiratory therapists, and airway management specialists such as an anesthesiologist or ENT, if necessary.

Oxygen is one of the most vital "medications" for safe intubation. Preoxygenation with 100% oxygen for a minimum of 3 minutes prior to intubation helps to prevent significant desaturation during the time that the intubation is performed.

**Premedications**    Atropine is a vagolytic that is used to prevent the bradycardia associated with laryngoscopy. In addition, it decreases secretions, often voluminous in children with respiratory failure. This medication should be used with caution in patients with myocardial depression because it causes tachycardia. Lidocaine blunts the cough reflex and prevents the rise in intracranial pressure associated with endotracheal intubation. It should be administered in a dose of 1 to 2 mg/kg at least 2 to 3 minutes before intubation to achieve maximum effect.

**Sedatives/Induction Agents**    Benzodiazepines cause both anxiolysis and amnesia. Midazolam used at 0.1 to 0.2 mg/kg/dose produces sedation within 1 to 2 minutes and lasts for 1 to 2 hours. Midazolam infusions can help ensure security of an artificial airway while in transport. Benzodiazepines should be used cautiously in patients with hypotension or depressed cardiac function as it is a negative inotrope.

Barbiturates can be used to induce sedation and anesthesia. Among the barbiturates, thiopental is the most commonly used. Thiopental is the most efficacious sedative to use for intubation in a hypertensive isolated head trauma patient due to its decrease of cerebral metabolism and blunting of the hemodynamic response to intubation. Used at doses of 3 to 5 mg/kg, thiopental induces sedation within 1 to 2 minutes, but should be used with extreme caution in patients with hypotension or compromised cardiac function. In addition, thiopental causes histamine release and bronchospasm and is contraindicated in patient with reactive airway disease.

Etomidate has a pharmacodynamic profile similar to thiopental; however, it does not cause the same hemodynamic instability. Doses of 0.2 to 0.3 mg/kg can be used in head trauma patients with confidence because it reduces cerebral metabolism and blood flow without alteration of cerebral perfusion pressure. Etomidate is an ideal induction agent for the hemodynamically compromised head trauma patient.

Opioids such as morphine and fentanyl can be used for both induction as well as maintenance sedation in intubated patients. Opioids are excellent drugs for patients with significant pain who have exacerbated responses to noxious stimuli. Common adverse side effects of opioids include hypotension, nausea, and decreased GI tract motility.

Propofol is a rapid-acting sedative hypnotic, which reduces cerebral metabolism and blood flow similarly to etomidate and thiopental. However, propofol significantly reduces the MAP and should not be used for intubation or sedation in a hypotensive patient or a patient with new head trauma.

Ketamine is a dissociative anesthetic drug that can be used as an induction agent. It has a rapid onset of action with doses of 1 to 2 mg/kg but produces unpleasant emergence reactions that should caution its use in older children. The ideal patient for ketamine is asthmatics due to its bronchodilatory effects. It causes significant tachycardia and hypertension and should not be used in patients with increase ICP.

**Neuromuscular Blocking Agents**   Neuromuscular blockers (NMB) may be used to facilitate intubation and should be considered to ensure safety of the intubated patient during transport. Users should remember that these medications should only be used after the patient is given adequate sedation and analgesia.

1. Depolarizing NMB

Succinylcholine is the often used in acute situations because of its pharmacokinetic profile with onset of action within 30 to 60 seconds and a duration of 3 to 5 minutes. Succinylcholine may cause hyperkalemia and is therefore contraindicated for patients with neuromuscular disease due to increased neuromuscular junctions, patients with crush injuries or burns (who already likely have hyperkalemia), and should be used with extreme caution in patients with increased intracranial or ICP.

2. Nondepolarizing NMB

Rocuronium has a pharmacokinetic profile similar to succinylcholine and has replaced it in many centers as the neuromuscular blocker of choice for intubation. Paralytics with longer half-lives such as pancuronium or vecuronium should be used for maintaining airway security during the transport.

---

**D**isplacement

- Confirm appropriate placement of the endotracheal tube (ETT)—bilateral symmetric chest rise, observing water vapor in the ETT, appropriate color change in the $CO_2$ detector from purple to yellow

**O**bstruction

- Suction

**P**neumothorax

- Prepare for needle thoracostomy (see Chapter 22, "Procedures")

**E**quipment

- If patient is on ventilator, manually bag the patient to assess compliance, air entry, look for signs of improvement

---

## DOPE Mnemonic for Endotracheal Problems While in Transport

Note that physical examination of a child while in transport may be difficult: Suspected airway problems during land transportation should prompt the driver to pull over the vehicle until the resolution of the problem.

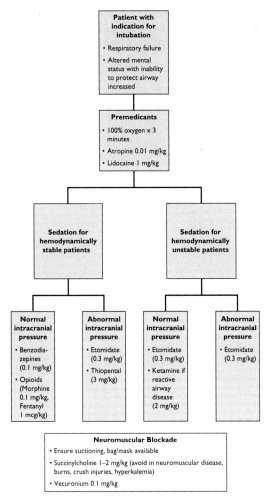

**Figure 2**    Induction approach to intubation.

Although it is rarely required, the most senior member of the transport team should be familiar with cricothyrotomy. This may be necessary for airway obstruction due to foreign body, severe orofacial injuries, or laryngeal fracture. There is no truly safe way to secure this airway and patients generally should not be transported with this device in place. The goal of an emergent cricothyrotomy is for oxygenation and a surgical tracheostomy should be established by surgical specialists as soon as possible.

Prior to departure from a referring facility, do the following:

- Check placement of all endotracheal tubes and intravenous lines.
- Attach patient to a functioning cardiorespiratory monitor to follow blood pressure, heart rate, and pulse oxygenation.
- 100% oxygen should be readily available throughout the transport, as well as IV fluids and medications for severe asthmatics such as salbutamol, magnesium, and terbutaline.

# Diabetic Ketoacidosis (see Chapter 16, "Endocrine")

Cerebral edema is the most dreaded outcome of both the disease process as well as the treatment of diabetic ketoacidosis (DKA). Cerebral edema results from shifts of fluid caused by rapid decreases in serum osmolality, whose major contributors are glucose and sodium. Cautious fluid replacement and insulin administration will reduce the likelihood of the development of cerebral edema. Commonly, patients with DKA will have received initial management prior to arrival of the transport team; however, it is a diagnosis that is occasionally missed and early recognition and therapy may be the responsibility of the transport team.

The initial transport management of DKA should consist of 10 mL/kg normal saline over the first hour, with more administered if the patient has hypotension, poor perfusion, or evidence of shock. Insulin should be initiated in a continuous manner of 0.05 to 0.1 units/kg/hour without the administration of a bolus dose. The goal in DKA is to decrease the glucose by 50 to 100 mg/dL/hour, thus slowly reducing the high osmolality inherent in DKA and reducing the risk for the development of cerebral edema. If fluid replacement and insulin reduce the glucose below 15 mmol/L, dextrose should be added to the IV fluids. Depending on the length of transport and the severity of illness, initiation of the insulin infusion may be delayed until the patient arrives at the receiving institution.

For further management of DKA see Chapter 16, "Endocrine."

## Adrenal Crisis

Patients presenting with shock, hypoglycemia, hyperkalemia, and hyponatremia should be presumed to have adrenal insufficiency because steroid therapy may be life saving. The initial treatment in these patients should follow the usual ABCs with the addition of glucose to fluids (10% dextrose) and stress dose hydrocortisone at a dose of 100 mg/m$^2$.

## Hypertensive Emergency (see Chapter 13, "Renal Failure")

Hypertensive emergency is defined as hypertension with the immediate threat to one or more organ systems, such as altered mental status, visual changes, headache, and oliguria. These patients require minute-to-minute titration of blood pressure to reverse signs and symptoms. For transport purposes, labetalol (alpha-/beta-blocker) or nicardipine (calcium channel blocker) are the safest and most effective continuous infusions as they do not require invasive arterial blood pressure monitoring for safe administration. This is in contrast to nitroprusside, which can cause large swings in blood pressure, making it less than optimal for a patient requiring transport to another facility.

## Conclusions

Safe and effective transport of the critically ill child to a specialized center has been proven to reduce morbidity and mortality. Understanding of common pediatric illnesses as well as their initial stabilization and management is a necessity for any medical practitioner responsible for either the inter- or intra hospital transport of a child. Together with pediatric subspecialists, the transport team is a vital link in the successful management of pediatric disease.

## Suggested Readings

Woodward, GA, ed. Guidelines for air and ground transport of neonatal and pediatric patients 3rd ed. American Academy of Pediatrics Section on Transport Medicine. American Academy of Pediatrics; 2007.

Johnson CM, Gonyea MT. Transport of the critically ill child. Mayo Clin Proc 1993;68:982–7.

Fiorito BA, Mirza F, Doran TM, Oberle AN, et al. Intraosseous access in the setting of pediatric critical care transport. Pediatr Crit Care Med 2005;6:50–3.

Woodward GA, Insoft RM, Pearson-Shaver AL, Jaimovich D, et al. The state of pediatric interfacility transport: consensus of the second National Pediatric and Neonatal Interfacility Transport Medicine Leadership Conference. Pediatr Emerg Care 2002;18:38–43.

Edge WE. Reduction in morbidity in interhospital transport by specialized pediatric staff. CCM 22;1994:1186–91.

Vos GD. Comparison of interhospital pediatric intensive care transport accompanied by a referring specialist or a specialist retrieval team. Intensive Care Med 2004;30:302–8.

# Chapter 4

# Monitoring in the ICU

## A. Noninvasive Monitoring

Allison Nykolaychuk

Respiratory monitoring of PICU patients begins with basic measures such as vital signs, including heart rate, blood pressure, temperature, respiratory rate along with work of breathing, and extends to more invasive measures such as central venous $PO_2$ and ventilatory waveforms.

Arterial blood gases are still the most accurate way of monitoring both oxygenation and ventilatory status; however, there are noninvasive ways of monitoring that can at least provide a trend.

### Vital Signs

Heart rates vary with age, activity level, and the child's condition. See Table 1 for normal heart rates.

Table 1
**Normal Heart Rates (Beats per Minute) by Age**

| Age | Awake Rate | Mean | Sleeping Rate |
|---|---|---|---|
| Newborn to 3 months | 85–205 | 140 | 80–160 |
| 3 months to 2 years | 100–190 | 130 | 75–160 |
| 2 years to 10 years | 60–140 | 80 | 60–90 |
| >10 years | 60–100 | 75 | 50–90 |

Adapted from Pediatric Advanced Life Support

*Table 2*
## Definition of Hypotension by Systolic Blood Pressure (mm Hg) by Age

| Age | Systolic Blood Pressure |
| --- | --- |
| Term neonates (0 to 28 days) | <60 |
| Infants (1 month to 12 months) | <70 |
| Children (1 to 10 years) | <70 + (2 × age in years) |
| Children (>10 years) | <90 |

Adapted from Pediatric Advanced Life Support

- Blood pressure also varies with age. Therefore, there is a large range of normal values for all age groups. See Table 2 for definitions of hypotension.
- Respiratory rates, as with the other vital signs, vary with age and condition of the child. See Table 3 for normal respiratory rates.
- A respiratory rate decrease from a fast rate to a normal rate can indicate an improvement in the child's condition. This would usually be accompanied by less work of breathing and a good level of consciousness.
- However, a decreasing respiratory rate may also be a sign of a child tiring and can indicate a worsening of the child's condition. In this case, other signs and symptoms may include a decreasing level of consciousness, shallow and/or irregular breathing, and an increase in work of breathing.
- Indications of an increased work of breathing include an irregular pattern, nasal flaring, tracheal tug, intercostal retractions (or indrawing), substernal retractions, and head bobbing.

*Table 3*
## Normal Respiratory Rates by Age

| Age | Breaths per Minute |
| --- | --- |
| Infants (<1 year) | 30–60 |
| Toddlers (1 to 3 years) | 24–40 |
| Preschoolers (4 to 5 years) | 22–34 |
| School age (6 to 12 years) | 18–30 |
| Adolescents (13 to 18 years) | 12–16 |

Adapted from Pediatric Advanced Life Support

# Monitoring Oxygen

## Noninvasive Pulse Oximetry

- This is the mainstay of monitoring a patient's oxygenation status; requires no calibration and gives a continuous, noninvasive reading.
- Utilizes the principle that saturated hemoglobin and desaturated hemoglobin absorb different frequencies of light.
- A red and an infra-red light are shined through the tissue. The monitor then reads the difference between the absorption rates and determines the amount of hemoglobin that is saturated with oxygen.
- The comparison of pulse oximetry ($SpO_2$) and the partial pressure of oxygen in a patient's blood are based on the oxygen-disassociation curve. See Figure 1.

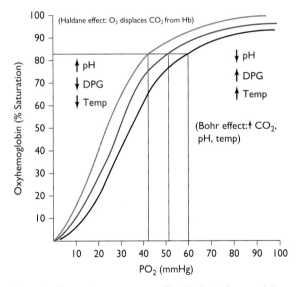

**Figure 1** Oxygen-disassociation curve. The blue line is the normal dissociation curve. The gray line indicates a left shift of the curve commonly caused by an increase in pH, decrease in either $CO_2$, temperature, or 2,3-DPG. When a left shift occurs, hemoglobin has more affinity to oxygen and is less likely to release it. Right shifts (indicated by the black line) commonly occur with decreases in pH, increases in either $CO_2$, temperature, or 2,3-DPG. In this case, hemoglobin more readily releases oxygen.

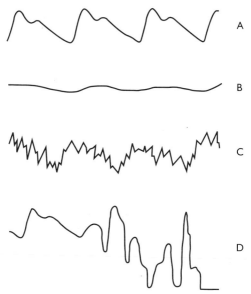

**Figure 2**   Common waveforms on a pulse oximeter. A: Normal waveform. B: low perfusion. C: Normal waveform with noise interference. D: Motion artifact.

- In order of importance, motion, poor skin perfusion, ambient light, and skin pigmentation may reduce saturations and interfere with accuracy.
- Dyshemoglobin anemias, such as carbon monoxide poisoning, methemoglobinemia, or sickle cell, cause inaccurate $SpO_2$ readings that may be artificially high or low.
- Pulse oximetry is also unreliable with saturations below 70%.
- Ensure a good perfusion wave form is present and the heart rate measured on the saturation monitor matches the patient's heart rate. Common $SpO_2$ waveforms are shown in Figure 2.

## Transcutaneous Monitoring

- Transcutaneous oxygen and carbon dioxide electrodes allow continuous indirect estimation of $PaCO_2$ and $PaO_2$ on young infants and some pediatric patients.
- Transcutaneous $PO_2$ ($tcPO_2$) measures the $PO_2$ of the skin; this is close to $PaO_2$ because of local cutaneous vasodilation caused by heating from the probe. In most instances when the

$PaO_2$ is <100 mm Hg, the $tcPO_2$ will be within 10 mm Hg of the $PaO_2$.
- Ease of use means pulse oximetry has largely supplanted the use of transcutaneous monitoring in most patient populations.

## Central Mixed Venous $PO_2$

- Normally, 20–25% of the oxygen delivered to the tissues is utilized.
- Oxyhemoglobin saturation of mixed venous blood ($ScvO_2$) is a measure of oxygen content of blood returning from the tissues, or "oxygen sufficiency" at tissue level.
- If a central venous catheter is in place for measuring CVP, it may be used for sampling venous saturation. The laboratory must be specifically asked to record this by co-oximeter function, rather than obtaining values by calculation.
- As a guide, for a normal arterial $PaO_2$, the expected venous $PO_2$ is 40 mm Hg.
- Bear in mind that cvp monitoring has its own risks and consider the risk benefit ratio carefully before insertion of a cvp line.

## Monitoring Carbon Dioxide

The $PaCO_2$ level from an indwelling arterial catheter provides the most accurate method of determining adequacy of alveolar ventilation.

Two other methods are used with different frequency in different units:

1. End-tidal $CO_2$ estimation (capnography see Figure 3)

   - It is relatively inexpensive, portable, noninvasive, and easy to use.
   - Mainstream units place the analyzer right at the endotracheal tube; this adds weight to the endotracheal tube and may cause instability, though the newer monitor adaptors are lightweight and add very little deadspace.
   - Mainstream units have the advantage of having very fast response times.
   - Side stream units continuously withdraw a small sample. The adapter is generally lighter, but the sample takes away from the tidal volume delivered to the patient.
   - Side stream units can also have the advantage of attaching a special set of nasal cannulae to monitor the non-intubated child.

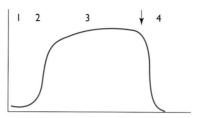

**Figure 3**  Normal capnography. The arrow indicates the etCO$_2$ value. 1. No CO$_2$, late inspiration. 2. Ascending limb, CO$_2$ from major airways. 3. Plateau, CO$_2$ from smaller airways. 4. Start of inspiration.

- etCO$_2$ monitors can display waveforms, the normal waveform having a steep portion at the beginning of exhalation, followed by a slowly increasing plateau. The end of the plateau is the end-tidal CO$_2$.
- Changes in the size or shape of the graph give indications of patient problems. Increases in etCO$_2$ are shown by a taller graph (within the same scale). Hypoventilation may show as a taller graph with fewer waveforms (higher etCO$_2$ with a low respiratory rate).
- Hyperventilation will result in more waveforms but with lower etCO$_2$ values. Figure 4 gives examples of other problems.
- Alveolar CO$_2$ approximates PaCO$_2$; therefore, a sample of end-tidal CO$_2$ gives a good estimate of PaCO$_2$, in some patient populations. Under normal physiological conditions, PaCO$_2$ is 2–5 mm Hg greater than the etCO$_2$.
- Any changes in the ventilation-perfusion ratio (V/Q ratio) will change the difference one way or the other in the pressure end-tidal CO$_2$ gradient. For this reason, it is important to monitor baseline arterial CO$_2$ (PaCO$_2$) once etCO$_2$ monitoring begins to determine the gradient.
- Other sources of inaccuracy could be infancy, and very fast respiriatory rates (not achieving alveolar plateau).

2. Transcutaneous CO$_2$ monitoring

- Provides continuous, noninvasive monitoring. TcPCO$_2$ is always greater than PaCO$_2$. It often provides a fairly linear relationship between TcPCO$_2$ and PaCO$_2$; therefore, it can be used to determine a trend.
- Accurate transcutaneous CO$_2$ monitoring relies on the monitor's ability to "arterialize" the skin by heating the skin to increase perfusion and therefore does not always work in older patients.

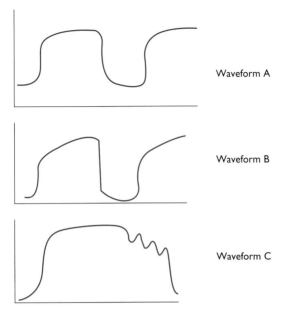

**Figure 4** Three capnographs. Waveform A: Baseline is not returning to zero, indicative of rebreathing. Waveform B: Shows an increase in the slope of the plateau. This is indicative of obstructive disease such as asthma. Due to bronchospasm, the alveoli have different time constants and those emptying more slowly increase the plateau. Waveform C: Demonstrates cardiogenic oscillations caused by heart's beating interfering with the capnograph.

## Monitoring Mechanically Ventilated Patients

### Pulmonary Physiology

- **Compliance** (unit of volume divided by unit of pressure required to move that volume) reflects how easily the lung and chest wall inflates with pressure. Most ventilators will perform this calculation for the clinician.
- **Dynamic compliance** is measured during delivery of flow to the patient; it includes not only the compliance, but also airway resistance.
- **Static compliance** is measured in "no-flow" situations, that is, during a breath hold. Static compliance reflects the pulmonary and chest wall compliance, without being affected by airway resistance.

- **Pulmonary resistance** is resistance to gas flow in the airways, resulting in friction (pressure per unit flow rate). Most ventilators can calculate and display patient resistance.
- **Time constants** are the product of compliance and resistance.

  - They indicate how quickly or slowly the lungs will inflate or deflate. A child with Acute Respiratory Distress Syndrome (ARDS) has a very "fast" expiratory time constant, meaning the patient exhales to equilibrium low lung volume very quickly. Children with asthma have air-trapping and a "long" time constant.
  - One time constant is needed to equilibrate 63% of the gas and five times the time constant for 95% of the gas.
  - A corollary is that very fast respiratory rates can be used with children with ARDS, whereas children with asthma have higher airway resistance. If there is a high airway resistance, the care-give should give the child a shorter expiratory times, to avoid exacerbating gas trapping.

- The respiratory equation of motion indicates that all these variables are highly interdependent—changing one variable will perforce alter the others:

$$P_{respsytem} = 1/ C_{RS} \times volume + R_{RS} \times flow$$

This states that the amount of pressure generated, in the respiratory system (ie patient and ventilator) to deliver a tidal volume, is equal to the pressure necessary to move a volume against the reciprocal of compliance of respiratory system, plus the pressure necessary to move the associated flow through the respiratory resistance (here, ventilator circuit and lung resistances).

## Ventilator Waveforms

- Although utility is untested, the use of ventilator waveforms has allowed the clinician to fine-tune the ventilatory parameters to suit each child.
- Waveforms give a visual indication of the child's resistance and compliance and whether changes have improved or worsened ventilation.
- The typical waveforms are pressure-time, flow-time, volume-time, flow-volume loops, and pressure-volume loops. Pressure-volume loops are sometimes referred as the compliance curve (compliance equals volume over pressure).
- The shape of each waveform will vary with the mode of ventilation.

## Pressure-Time Waveforms

- In pressure modes (ie, pressure control, pressure support), the pressure-time waveform is square. See Figure 5 below.
- In volume modes, the pressures continue to rise throughout the breath. This can lead to high airway pressures being delivered. These high airway pressures are not necessarily transferred to the alveoli. Plateau pressures are a better indication of pressures in the lungs. See Figure 6 below.

## Dysynchrony

- Abnormalities in a pressure-time waveform can be indicative of child-ventilator dysynchrony.
- Spikes on the pressure waveform at the end of inspiration usually demonstrate a child trying to exhale before the ventilator has finished delivering the breath. Quite often the child may look restless and appear to be "fighting" the ventilator. See Figure 7.
- Decreasing the set inspiratory time may allow the ventilator to cycle into expiration at the same time as the child, decreasing the dysynchrony or fighting of the ventilator.

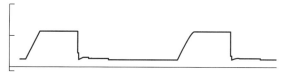

**Figure 5** This waveform is a pressure-time waveform, during a pressure mode. Note that the peak pressures remain constant from breath to breath. Baseline pressures do not return to zero due to the addition of PEEP. Waveform taken from the Servo' ventilator, manufactured by MAQUET Critical Care AB.

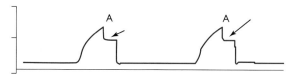

**Figure 6** Shows a pressure-time waveform during a volume mode. Note the pressures continuing to rise throughout inspiration. The points labeled A are the peak airway pressures. The flattened areas indicated by the arrows are the plateau pressures, created by an inspiratory breath hold. Waveform taken from the Servo' ventilator, manufactured by MAQUET Critical Care AB.

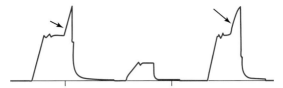

**Figure 7**   Above is a pressure-time waveform in a pressure mode. Note the abrupt increase in pressure at the end of the mandatory breaths, as indicated by the arrows. Caused by the patient exhaling before the end of the ventilator breath.

- In volume modes, pressures will vary breath to breath based on the lung characteristics. If a child is synchronized with the ventilator, the pressure waveform will be smooth and remain fairly consistent breath to breath.

## Assessing Sensitivity

- Ventilators capable of synchronizing ventilation with the patient's effort use either a negative pressure drop, or an inspiratory flow created by the patient, to detect "patient effort." If the sensitivity criteria are met, the ventilator responds with an assisted or supported breath.
- If the child has to create a large pressure drop to meet the ventilator's criteria, the pressure-time waveform will dip below baseline. Increasing the sensitivity will decrease the child's work of breathing.
- A leak around the endotracheal tube (ETT) will also result in a flow and/or pressure drop, causing the ventilator criteria to be met prematurely, and resulting in a breath being delivered. This is "auto-" or "self-cycling."

## Slope of Inspiration

- High initial flows can cause turbulence in patients with high airway resistance, seen as a pressure overshoot on the pressure waveform. Increasing the rise time decreases the turbulence, potentially improving ventilation.
- This is especially important in the infant with a small ETT, or the child with high airway resistance.

Figure 8 demonstrates the change in flow and pressure waveforms as a result of changing the slope or rise time.

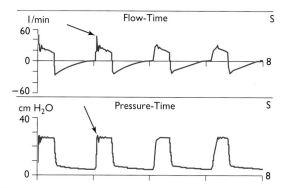

**Figure 8** The two time waveforms are flow and pressure by time. The arrow on the pressure waveform shows the flow and pressure overshoots due to a high initial flow causing resistance and back pressure.

## Flow-Time Waveforms

### Inspiratory Times (Ti)

- Clinical determination of Ti can be made by checking saturations, blood gases, and the child's comfort. Assessment of ventilator graphics can also be of help.
- As the patient's lung compliance worsens, pressures equilibrate toward set peak pressures faster, flows drop sooner, and volume delivery is decreased. If the inspiratory time is too short to allow the pressures to equilibrate completely with the targeted peak pressures, the volume delivered will be lower than it should be for any given pressure level.
- Setting the inspiratory time longer than necessary to equilibrate pressures results in no further volume delivery. A period of "no-flow" ensues, where the ventilator holds the pressure (akin to a patient holding their breath). See Figure 9.

### Assessing Expiratory Flows

- The expiratory flow pattern should return to zero before the start of the next breath. This indicates the patient has finished exhaling. If expiratory flow does not return to zero, then air trapping is present and being caused by the ventilator parameter settings. See Figure 10.

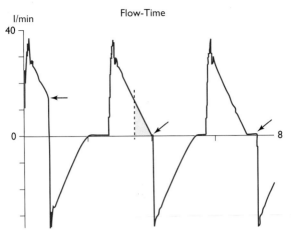

**Figure 9**  The diagram shows flow on the y-axis, by time on the x-axis. For each breath, the area under the waveform represents delivered volume. In the first breath, a very short inspiratory time is present and pressures cannot equilibrate. The end of the breath terminates abruptly. In the second breath, there is enough time to equilibrate the pressure, and additional volume is delivered (represented by the blue triangle). In the third breath, increasing the inspiratory time further as in the third waveform shows no additional delivery of volume and results in a breath hold. The arrows indicate when each breath is terminated.

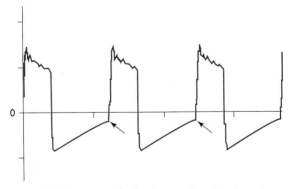

**Figure 10**  The arrows on the flow-time waveform show the expiratory flow not returning to zero before the next inspiration.

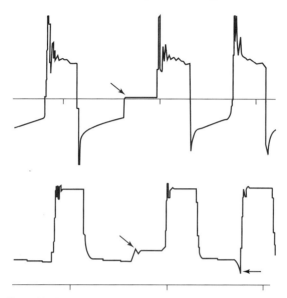

**Figure 11**   An expiratory hold has been activated at the blue arrows on the flow-time and pressure-time waveforms. The rise in baseline pressure demonstrates the auto-PEEP. The black arrow shows the patient attempting to breath and has dropped the pressure from the auto-PEEP level to the setting on the ventilator.

- Air trapping can lead to auto-PEEP, which can then lead to child-ventilator dysynchrony.
- Auto-PEEP (or inadvertent PEEP) can increase work of breathing if a ventilator's sensitivity is set to pressure sensing. The child has to overcome the additional pressure in their lungs plus the set value in order to cycle the ventilator. See Figure 11.

## Volume-Time Waveforms

- Volume-time waveforms can show the consistency or otherwise of the delivery of tidal volumes. In volume modes, the volume waveform remains generally unchanged between breaths, but care must be taken in in-homogeneity as volume delivery will be to areas of least resistance.
- In pressure modes, as lung characteristics change so do volumes. When ventilating in a pressure mode, if the child's lung disease worsens, this would be seen as decreasing tidal volumes.

- Leaks will cause abnormalities on volume-time waveforms. The waveform will show a certain amount of gas being delivered to the patient. The expiratory phase of the waveform will show only the volume being exhaled through the ETT; therefore, if there is a leak around the ETT, less volume will be measured. Most ventilators will show an inspiratory and an expiratory tidal volume and large discrepancies between the two volumes may indicate a leaks.

## Flow-Volume Loop

- Flow-volume loops have traditionally been used with spirometry and are now available with most ventilator waveform packages.
- It is important to note that, depending on mode of ventilation, the ventilator settings will control the inspiratory portion of the flow-volume loop. For instance, inspiratory flow patterns are determined by the ventilator and the mode of ventilation. Many ventilators have a pressure mode that uses a decelerating flow waveform that can be seen on the flow-volume loop, as can a constant inspiratory flow delivered in some volume modes.
- The expiratory phase of the loop is determined by the child and may be useful in determining the expiratory airway resistance and possibly the effectiveness of bronchodilators.
- If the expiratory phase is concave, there is a likelihood of increased airway resistance. With improvement, the flow decay is more linear. See Figure 12.

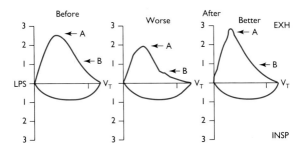

**Figure 12**   On these flow-volume loops, the inspiratory phase is below the VT line and the expiratory phase is above the line. The first flow-volume loop is pre-bronchodilator. The second loop shows worsening airway resistance, with the third loop showing improvement. Point A indicates peak expiratory flow and point B indicates changes in the expiratory phase due to airway resistance.

## Pressure-Volume Loop

- Pressure-volume curves are also known as compliance curves as the most common use of the curve is to determine or estimate a patient's compliance.
- There are two portions of the loop or curve. The first is the inspiratory curve, which starts at zero and is the lower curve. The second phase of the curve is the expiratory phase and is the upper curve on the graph. The difference in the curves is a result of hysteresis. The lung must generate a high pressure to open alveoli; once open the pressures are lower (as on expiration), so that at any given pressure, the volume is greater on expiration. See Figure 13.
- Measuring the slope of a pressure-volume loop determines the patient's dynamic compliance. Changes in compliance can be seen by comparing one loop to another to determine if the slope has decreased (compliance worsening) or increased (compliance improved).

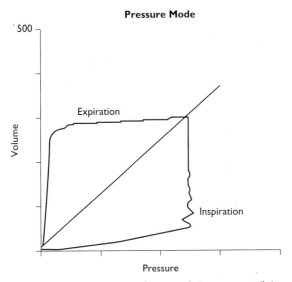

**Figure 13**   This shows a pressure-volume curve during pressure ventilation. The straight line in the middle of the curve is the slope or compliance. Note the inspiratory portion of this curve is controlled by the ventilator settings.

## Work of Breathing

- Other uses of the pressure-volume curve include evaluating work of breathing during breaths.
- Work is the product of pressure and volume. Work can be performed by either the ventilator or the patient.
- As the patient will generate a negative pressure to draw in volume, spontaneous breaths are on the left of the pressure axis.
- Assisted or supported breaths will have the patient work to the left and then the ventilator work to the right. See Figure 14.

## Over-distention

- When in volume modes, over-distention will show as a flattening or "beaking" on the pressure-volume curve. As the ventilator attempts to deliver the set volume, pressures continue to rise but with little volume delivery.

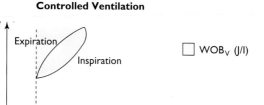

**Controlled Ventilation**

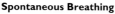

**Spontaneous Breathing**

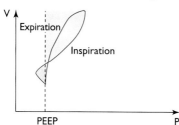

**Figure 14**   The top waveform is a mandatory breath in which all work is performed by the ventilator. The bottom loop is an assisted or supported breath, where the patient has created an effort and the ventilator has responded. The colored area to the left of the line marking PEEP is patient work. The colored area to the right is ventilator work. Graph from Siemens-Elema AB, Electromedical Systems Division.

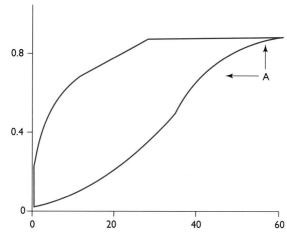

**Figure 15**  Point A is at the area of flattening or "beaking." As pressures increase, there is no addition of volume.

- This does not show in pressure modes as the ventilator limits the amount of pressure delivered. See Figure 15.
- Over-distention can be caused by too much volume being delivered or too high of a PEEP setting.
- Ventilator waveforms are useful potential tools for ventilation, although they have not been compared in randomized trails to confer benefit. They allow the clinician to fine-tune the ventilator settings to best match the patient.

## References

Ralston M, Hazinski MF, Zaritsky AL, Schexnayder SM, Kleinman ME, editors. Pediatric advanced life support. Dallas, Texas: American Heart Association; 2006.

Siemens Medical Solutions. etCO$_2$ + respiratory mechanics reference handbook. Sweden: Siemens Medical Solutions; 2002.

McFayden, JG. Respiratory gas analysis in theatre. Practical Procedures. 2000;11: Article 7:1–2. www.nda.ox.ac.uk/wfsa/html/u11/u1107_01.htm (accessed February 24, 2008).

MAQUET Critical Care AB. Ventilation of neonates and pediatrics pocket guide. Sweden: MAQUET Critical Care AB; 2005.

Hess DR, Kacmarek RM. Essentials of mechanical ventilation. 2nd ed. New York, New York: The McGraw-Hill Companies; 2002.

Nilsestun, JO, Hargett K. Managing the patient-ventilator system using graphic analysis: An overview and introduction to Graphics Corner. Resp Care 1996;41:1105–22.

Puritan Bennett. Waveforms: The graphical presentation of ventilatory data. Pleaston, California: Puritan Bennett; 1991.

# B. Cardiovascular Monitoring

Haresh Kirpalani

Lennox Huang

## Key Principles

> - Cardiovascular monitoring is an essential component of critical care.
> - Both invasive and noninvasive techniques can be used to gather physiologic data.
> - Level of monitoring should correspond to severity of illness.
> - Risks of invasive monitoring should be balanced against benefits for the patient.

## Blood Pressure

### Why Monitor?

Blood pressure is the easiest parameter, along with heart rate (discussed in Chapters 5 and 8), to gauge CVS functioning. All patients in an ICU setting should have at least intermittent BP measures. It is generally accepted that a combination of this value and capillary filling and heart rate enables the clinician to gauge how effective peripheral perfusion is maintained. However, capillary filling is assessed poorly and inconsistently. This makes understanding the limitations of BP measures critical. If used as a screen for hypertension in children, solitary measures of BP are not useful. However, in critical care the BP is more usually targeted at detecting hypotension. The accuracy of the measure used will vary by route measurement (noninvasive or invasive). Accordingly, higher accuracy comes with a cost in the complication rate (see below). Always consider whether the risk:benefit ratio justifies arterial cannulation.

### Normal Ranges (Figures 1–3)

BP is a physiological variable that normally fluctuates rapidly throughout the day and is very responsive to external stimuli. In the ICU setting, most attention is directed at evidence of hypotension rather than hypertension. In hypertension, causes such as pain and anxiety with an inadequate sedation-analgesia level are considered. Other causes include central nervous and renal issues. (See Chapter 13, "Nephrology.") Hypotension will prompt considerations of the causes of

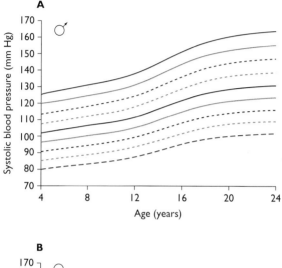

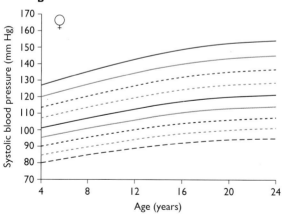

**Figure 1** Systolic blood pressure centiles in male (A) and female (B) participants. The centiles are spaced two-thirds of a standard deviation score apart. Systolic pressure rises progressively with age, but rises more steeply in puberty, particularly in boys.

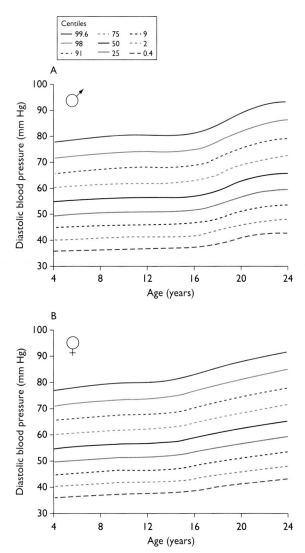

**Figure 2** Diastolic blood pressure centiles in male (A) and female (B) participants. The centiles are spaced two-thirds of a standard deviation score apart. Diastolic pressure rises slowly in childhood, but as with systolic pressure, rises more steeply in puberty.

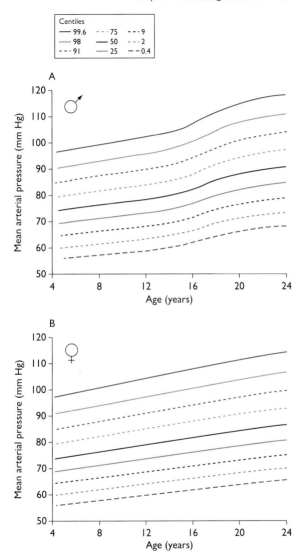

**Figure 3** Mean arterial pressure centiles in male (A) and female (B) participants. The centiles are spaced two-thirds of a standard deviation score apart. Mean arterial pressure rises progressively with age.

shock. (See Chapter 5, "Resuscitation."). Normal ranges for BP in children outside the neonatal period are based on large population studies. BP tends to rise with age, and is strongly correlated with weight; it is higher in boys than in girls. The question of what is normal is interwoven with a rising obesity rate, and is so far unresolved. The curves given are firstly those used in the United Kingdom drawn from 22,000 children in population surveys and only depicted by age. Adjusted curves for height and weight are also given, derived from the US normative data.

## Noninvasive Blood Pressure Monitoring

- Usually performed by oscillometry
- Has inherent errors in very small newborns but correlates in general well with invasive intra-arterial monitoring
- Is usually intermittent, and thus gives "snapshots"

Recent promise is shown in the technique of a photoplethys-mographic device on a finger giving a beat-to-beat BP, termed the Finapres method. It has been evaluated in children between 6 and 16 years of age, and is now validated in younger children. In some instances for near critical-care situations, longer periods of recording might be needed without so-called "white coat hypertension" being ruled in. In these circumstances, ambulatory BP monitoring can be considered; these rely on oscillometry as well. One should note that lower-extremity BPs are normally lower than upper-extremity BPs on oscillometric measurement.

## Invasive Blood Pressure Monitoring

Such monitoring is obtained via cannulation of arterial vessels. (See Chapter 22, "Procedures.") Common indications include shock, hypertensive emergencies, inotrope infusions, and the need for frequent blood sampling. Assessment of the arterial wave form is essential to accurate and precise monitoring and may yield clues to important physiologic changes. Under-damping or overshoot problems lead to an overestimation of systolic and underestimation of diastolic pressures. Overshoot can be identified by an exaggerated dicrotic notch and super-imposed oscillations on the square wave test. Over-damped arterial lines underestimate the systolic pressure. The mean arterial pressure is relatively unaffected in both under- and over-damped lines.

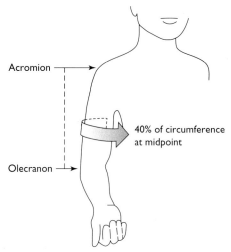

Bladder width should be 40% of the circumference of the arm.

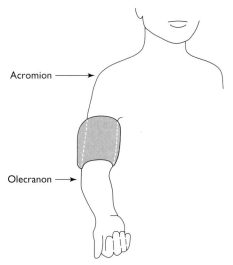

Cuff should cover 80–100% of circumference of the arm.

**Figure 4** Proper BP cuff size and placement.

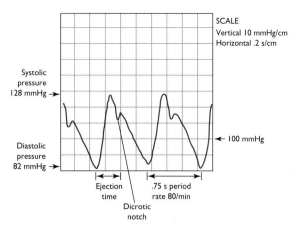

**Figure 5**    Normal arterial blood pressure tracing.

## Complications of Invasive Monitoring

These are common, up to 10% in a large series. This mandates attention to which patients really require an indwelling arterial measurement. Of these the vast majority was infection (61%), but this cannot be easily distinguished from thrombus (7.5%). Other complications included mechanical and vascular device malfunction. The highest predictor of complications was age at <4 months of age. Use of heparin and papavarin is unit dependent and increasingly uncommon.

### Troubleshooting an Arterial Line Problem

- Look at the patient to ensure that the pressure reading is not real.
- Examine for signs of local infection (erythema, pain).
- Consider using oscillometric measurement to correlate.
- Reposition arm in a slightly dorsiflexed position with an armboard in place.
- Ensure line is zeroed and flushed with no air in the tubing.
- Proper pressure tubing is essential to prevent under-damping of the line.
- Check level of transducer (should be at heart level).
- Determine appropriateness of frequency filter on monitor.
- Consider rewiring line if tracing is persistently damped, or poor waveform is seen.

# Cardiac Output Monitoring

**Which patients should be considered for monitoring?**
Patients in shock from any cause, and post-cardiac surgical patients with congenital heart disease.

**Why monitor?** Cardiac systolic function is considered to be the result of four interrelated variables: heart rate, preload, contractility, and afterload (or systemic vascular resistance).

Cardiac output is closely related to blood pressure as seen in the following equation:

Mean blood pressure = cardiac output $\times$ systemic vascular resistance

Because blood pressure in part reflects autonomic tone balancing vasoconstriction and vasodilatation, cardiac output measures might be a "purer" signal of cardiac function. Technically, CO can be measured; however, it is unclear whether this aids pediatric management due to a paucity of pediatric trials. This makes adult data important to consider. An important RCT that targeted high CO (as measured by thermodilution) in critically ill adult patients suggests that it worsens outcomes. This may be because clinicians are unable to properly interpret the relevant data. Furthermore, a recent consensus conference states: "We do not recommend routine measurement of CO for patients with shock." Meta-analysis of the efficacy and safety of the pulmonary artery catheter (to obtain CO by thermodilution measures) included 13 RCTs; and a total of 5,051 patients—concluding that such data did not confer benefit. The consensus does, however, state, "We suggest considering echocardiography or measurement of CO for diagnosis in patients with clinical evidence of ventricular failure and persistent shock despite adequate fluid resuscitation." A distinction is also sometimes made between "early" use of such invasive measures and "too-late" use. In synthesizing these data, a reasonable approach is to utilize noninvasive methods first and if these are failing to consider more invasive approaches, including CO determination, or CVP monitoring and superior vena cava saturation ($ScvO_2$) (see below). Never rely simply upon a "number" such as CO, BP, CVP, or $ScvO_2$ in isolation. Consider what other markers of tissue perfusion are available, for example, urine flow rates. (See Chapter 5, "Resuscitation.")

*Table I*

**Common Measured and Calculated Haemodynamic Variables**

| Parameter | Formula | Normal range | Units |
|---|---|---|---|
| Cardiac index | $CI = CO$/body surface area | 3.5–5.5 | l/min/m$^2$ |
| Stroke index | $SI = CI$/heart rate | 30–60 | ml/m$^2$ |
| Arterial oxygen content | $CaO_2 = (1.34 \times Hgb \times SaO_2) + (PaO_2 \times 0.03)$ | | ml/l |
| Oxygen delivery | $DO_2 = CI \times CaO_2$ | 570–670 | ml/min/m$^2$ |
| Fick principle | $CI = VO_2/(CaO_2 - CvO_2)$ | 160–180 (infant $VO_2$) | ml/min/m$^2$ |
| | | 100–130 (child $VO_2$) | ml/min/m$^2$ |
| Oxygen extraction ratio* | $OER = [SaO_2 - SvO_2]/SaO_2$ | 0.24–0.28 | ml/min/m$^2$ |
| Oxygen excess factor* | $\Omega = SaO_2/(SaO_2 - SvO_2)$ | 3.6–4.2 | |
| Systemic vascular resistance index | $SVRI = 79.9 \times (MAP - CVP)/CI$ | 800–1600 | dyn-s/cm$^5$/m$^2$ |
| Left ventricular stroke work index | $LVSWI = SI \times MAP \times 0.0136$ | 50–62 (adult) | g-m/m$^2$ |

CO, cardiac output; CI, cardiac index; CVP, central venous pressure (mm Hg); $CaO_2$, arterial oxygen content; $CvO_2$, mixed venous oxygen content; $DO_2$, oxygen delivery; Hgb, haemoglobin concentration (g/l); LVSWI, left ventricular stroke work index; MAP, mean arterial pressure (mm Hg); OER, oxygen extraction ratio; $PaO_2$, partial pressure of dissolved oxygen; $SaO_2$, arterial oxygen saturation; $SvO_2$, mixed venous oxygen saturation; SI, stroke index; SVRI, systemic vascular resistance index; $VO_2$, oxygen consumption; $\Omega$, oxygen excess, factor.

*The equations given for OER and $\Omega$ are only valid if the contribution from dissolved oxygen is minimal. If this is not the case, oxygen content ($CaO_2$, $CvO_2$) must be substituted for saturation ($SaO_2$, $SvO_2$).

## Normal Ranges

These depend upon the modality to be used to measure CO, and normal ranges need to be discussed with your local technical collaborators. However, for the most prevalent measures, these are tabulated as below drawn from Tibby.

Calculation of pulmonary to systemic blood flow ratio (Qp:Qs):

Qp:Qs = $(SaO_2 – SvO_2)$ / (sat pulm venous–$O_2$ sat PA)

$SaO_2$–arterial $O_2$ sat measured from ABG

$SvO_2$–mixed venous sat, may be taken from CVP line

Sat pulm venous–can't be measured but assume 100% with healthy lungs

Sat PA–can be measured from RA line or assumed to be $SaO_2$ in patients with pulm blood from aortic shunt (eg Norwood)

## Noninvasive Cardiac Output Monitoring

**Arterial Pulse *Pressure* Waveform Analysis**    The area under the systolic portion of the arterial pulse wave from the end of diastole to the end of systolic ejection can provide an estimate of cardiac output and offers the advantage of continuous beat-to-beat measurements. All these analyses, however, require a calibration from another measure of CO. The methodological characteristics of these tests (reproducibility, precision, etc.) are also not perfect as yet and thus has not been adopted as a standard of care.

**Esophageal Doppler-Measured CO**    Doppler ultrasound 2D echocardiography examines blood velocity to detect frequency shift of reflected ultrasound waves. This is usually measured in the aorta, from either the transthoracic or intraesophageal routes. It is thought that the transesophageal route is preferable due to minimizing the inaccuracy of the measure of the aortic cross-sectional area. When a 4 MHz probe is evaluated against the invasive gold standard of thermodilution, it has good measurement properties. In detecting stroke volume improvement following volume loading in children, it was superior to the use of CVP. Nonetheless, potential inaccuracy is possible as either load and/or contractility changes, altering the aortic annulus diameter requiring remeasurement.

**Bioimpedance**    Thoracic bioimpedance detects current when the chest wall impedance changes with blood volume and heart rate. This allows stroke volume to be calculated. To date, it has not gained much use in children, however.

# Invasive Cardiac Output Monitoring

**The Fick Principle**   This principle governs most invasive measures (see below) and measures the systemic oxygen consumption and the arteriovenous oxygen content difference to derive the cardiac output. The derivation usually involves measures of the oxygen content in arterial and mixed venous blood ($CaO_2$–$CvO_2$; see Table 1). If $CO_2$ is used instead of $O_2$ values, invasive determination is avoided by measuring the expired $CO_2$ to estimate a mixed venous $CO_2$ value. Portable metabolic monitors, therefore, now allow a noninvasive application for children. The utility and practicality of this noninvasive measure for children still has to be shown, however.

**Dilution Techniques**   After a central venous injection of either a dye (Indocyanine green, Evans blue) or other indicator (heat, lithium chloride) measuring time decay of the indicator with timed concentrations of indicator distal to the injection port, estimates blood flow. Full mixing of the indicator with blood, and minimal to no anatomical shunt or valve regurgitation, are required conditions. Most commonly, thermodilution injection is used into a pulmonary artery catheter with a dilution passage through the lungs. A modification allows thermodilution into large peripheral vessels (femoral or brachial artery) if injected volumes are at less than 10°C. This is often regarded as the gold standard for infants and children.

**Complications of Invasive Cardiac Output Monitoring**   Depending on the indicator, there may be some specific complications (eg, lithium toxicity with repeated examinations). Generally, complications involve catheterization of the vessel involved. As discussed with invasive BP monitoring and CVP monitoring, this entails risk of thrombosis. Accidental bleeding, puncture, and other iatrogenic compilations are discussed under procedures (see Chapter 22, "Procedures").

**Central Venous Catheterization and Monitoring**   In addition to providing measures of cardiac output, central venous catheterization allows for direct monitoring of Central Venous Pressure (CVP), which in turn reflects central filling pressures or preload. As with arterial pressure monitoring, patients in shock from any cause should be considered for monitoring.

**Why Monitor?**   As discussed under cardiac output, an adequate preload is necessary for effective cardiac function and cardiac output. Preload and mixed venous oxygen can be

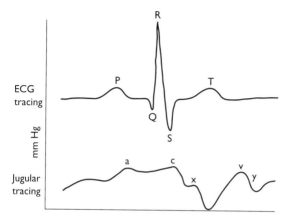

**Figure 6**   Central venous pressure waveform. A wave: Atrial contraction. Absent in atrial fibrillation; more pronounced in tricuspid stenosis, pulmonary stenosis, pulmonary hypertension, and complete heart block (cannon a wave). C wave: Bulging of tricuspid valve into the right atrium with ventricular contraction. X descent: Atrial relaxation. V wave: Increased atrial pressure before tricuspid valve opening; more pronounced in tricuspid regurgitation. Y descent: Atrial emptying, absent in tamponade.

assessed either via the central veins draining into the heart, or by a pulmonary capillary wedge pressure using a pulmonary artery catheter. However, the latter approach will not be further discussed in light of the meta-analysis discussed previously under CO. Because placement of the central venous catheter is usually aimed at either the right atrium or at the junction of the SVC and IVC, this measure of CVP can be coupled with the $ScvO_2$. The catheter incorporates an optic fiber that is connected to a continuous $O_2$ monitoring system (Edwards Lifesciences, Irvine, CA). Proponents point out benefits seen in a randomized controlled trial (RCT) in children. This compared the survival in severe sepsis using an "early" goal-directed therapy approach aimed at maintaining CVP. This pediatric trial protocol followed the "early" goal-directed therapy approach of the American College of Critical Care Medicine, which is summarized in a recent review of 11 adult, largely observational, studies. The potential for the full clinical use of the $ScvO_2$ is not defined, but a pediatric case report suggests it may be broader than just in sepsis.

## Invasive Measures

### Central Venous Catheterization of Large Central Veins
If only a central venous pressure is needed, the femoral vein is good enough to access the IVC and correlates well to SVC measures of CVP. To date, no studies are reported to assess the validity of using this route for also obtaining the $ScvO_2$.

### Complications of Invasive Monitoring
Overall, complication rates of all severity vary widely, but are in the range of <1%. Such complications are much higher in newborns, rising to 3% of which 1% was fatal.

(i) **Successful correct placement:** The difficulty of obtaining this without complication should not be minimized. To this end, 2D-ultrasound obtains higher success rates and is being increasingly used in the pediatric population. A meta-analysis of pediatric studies confirms a higher success rate when aiming at the cannulation of the internal jugular vein.

(ii) **Complications of upper body central vein placement versus right atrium:** Placing the catheter in central veins rather than in the right atrium minimizes arrhythmias, thrombosis, and perforation of the right atrium.

(iii) **Complications of upper body versus lower body central vein:** A prospective study showed a 3.7% complication rate for catheterization of the femoral vein compared with a rate of 7.3% for non-femoral access. Most would argue that the inferior vena cava route via the femoral vein is technically easier and safer. However, it is clearly operator-dependent and others prefer the subclavian route. In addition, appropriate-sized trials have not been done.

(iv) **Thrombosis:** Other than immediate trauma from placement, this is the most worrying complication overall, excluding the immediately traumatic. Perhaps the most comprehensive multi-center study to date, found that among 158 children, 21 (13%) had thrombo-embolic consequences. They found that the rate was increased with femoral CVL (32%) and subclavian CVL (27%), as compared to brachial CVL (12%) and jugular CVL (8%). This complication also probably underlies part of the next complication.

(v) **Catheter-related sepsis:** This rate is highly dependent upon center also, but studies estimate up to 13.8 per 1,000 catheter days. Consensus guidelines that have been drawn up to minimize infection should be adhered to.

# Suggested Readings

Andriessen P, Schraa O, Van Den Bosch-Ruis W, et al. Feasibility of noninvasive continuous finger arterial blood pressure measurements in very young children, aged 0–4 years. Pediatr Res 2008; 63:691–6.

Hanna B. Where do we go from here? Cardiac output determination in pediatrics. Crit Care Med 2008;36:1377–8.

Jackson LV, Thalange NKS, Cole TJ. Blood pressure centiles for Great Britain. Arch Dis Child 2007;92;1045–6.

King MA, Garrison, MM, Vavilala MS, et al. Complications associated with arterial catheterization in children. Pediatr Crit Care Med 2008 Jul;9(4):367–71.

Kobos AT, Menon K. A multidisciplinary survey on capillary refill time: Inconsistent performance and interpretation of a common clinical test. Pediatr Crit Care Med 2008;9:386–91.

Male C, Julian JA, Massicotte P, et al. Significant association with location of central venous line placement and risk of venous thrombosis in children. Thromb Haemost 2005;94:516–21.

National High Blood Pressure Education Program Working Group on High Blood Pressure in Children and Adolescents. The fourth report on the diagnosis, evaluation, and treatment of high blood pressure in children and adolescents. Pediatrics 2004 Aug;114(2 Suppl 4th Report):555–76.

O'Grady NP, Alexander M, Dellinger P, et al. Guidelines for the prevention of intravascular catheter related infections. Pediatrics 2002;110:E51.

Ronco R, Riquelme C. Cardiac output measurement in children: What is lacking? Pediatr Crit Care Med 2008;9:333–4.

Shah MR, Hasselblad V, Stevenson LW, et al. Impact of the pulmonary artery catheter in critically ill patients. JAMA 2005;294:1664–9.

Sheridan RL, Weber JM. Mechanical and infectious complications of central venous cannulation in children: Lessons learned from a 10-year experience placing more than 1000 catheters. J Burn Care Res 2006 Sep–Oct;27(5):713–8.

Skippen P, Kissoon N. Ultrasound Guidance for Central Vascular Access in the Pediatric Emergency Department. Pediatric Emergency Care 2007;23:203–207.

Spenceley N, Skippen P, Krahn G, Kissoon N. Continuous central venous saturation monitoring in pediatrics: A case report. Pediatr Crit Care Med 2008;9:e13–e16.

Stenzel J, Green T, Fuhrman B, et al. Percutaneous central venous catheterization in a pediatric intensive care unit: A survival analysis of complications. Crit Care Med 1989;17:984–8.

Tibby SM, Hatherill M, Marsh MJ. Clinicians' abilities to estimate cardiac index in ventilated children and infants. Arch Dis Child 1997;77:516–8.

Tibby SM, Hatherill M, Murdoch IA. Use of transesophageal Doppler ultrasonography in ventilated pediatric patients: Derivation of cardiac output. Crit Care Med 2000;28:2045–50.

Tibby SM, Murdoch IA. Monitoring cardiac function in intensive care. Arch Dis Child 2003;88:46–52.

Tibby SM, Murchoch IA. Measurement of cardiac output and tissue perfusion. Current Opinion in Pediatrics 2002;14:303–9.

# Chapter 5

# Resuscitation

## A. Airway Management

Haresh Kirpalani

### Key Principles

- Periods of hypoxemia during pre-intubation and intubation increase mortality.
- Of children with a respiratory arrest without a cardiac arrest, some 75% are discharged alive, 88% of whom achieve good outcome.
- The obvious lesson is to avoid hypoxemia, and that prompt and effective oxygenation could prevent cardiac arrest.

### Goals of Airway Management

- Recognizing and relief of obstruction
- Preventing gastric content aspiration
- Ensuring adequate gas exchange

### Anatomic Considerations in Children

- Large occiput in young children—may require shoulder roll to align airway planes
- Tongue relatively large to mandible <2 years of age—ensure not obstructing
- Infant epiglottis floppy and overlies the glottis
- To visualize the larynx, may need to lift the epiglottis directly with a straight blade

# Upper Airway Obstruction

Presentation: Noisy breathing, distress and "air hunger"—leading to hypoxemia.

- Explore if antecedent history or new episode—any prior neurologic symptoms? (Consider aspiration, or vocal cord paresis)
- Is there:

  - Any prior history of anaphylaxis?
  - Any relation to feeds? (Consider laryngo-tracheo-esophageal fistula)
  - History of being able to eat or drink—dysphagia? (Consider epiglottitis)
  - Any history of trauma?

Examine for evidence of:

- Pharyngeal-oral anatomical abnormality—Is there drolling? Is child able to phonate?
- If suspecting upper airway pathology do *not* fiddle with oral examinations—do not use tongue depressor or oral airway—unless experienced personnel available
- If child naturally has adopted "sniff position" sitting forward, do *not* to attempt to lie patient down—this may exacerbate obstruction
- Stridor? If inspiratory consider supraglottic obstruction; both inspiratory and expiratory suggest infraglottic pathology
- Chest movement: Is there any paradoxical movement?
- Are accessory muscles being used? Is there any cough?
- Are there signs of respiratory distress such as nasal flare, respiratory rate, low saturations and/or cyanosis, poor air entry?

Consider first whether the child is being adequately oxygenated. If yes: Consider whether there is a need for further investigation (lateral neck film epiglottis and foreign body) inspired and expired films (air-trapping). *Never leave* patient alone without health care attendant, or without a monitor. Having ensured that the upper airway is not threatened by likely laryngospasm (epiglottitis, etc) proceed with ABC. The initial steps of the A B of "ABC" are described below.

Clearing of airway

- First, visually ensure there is no foreign material—using gloved hand manually clear material.
- If needed, use suction catheter to clear mucous blood, etc.

## Differential Causes Upper Airway Obstruction

| Congenital | Acquired |
|---|---|
| *Mandibular hypoplasia* <br> Pierre-Robin Syndrome and variants <br> Treacher-Collins syndromes | *Infection Glottis* <br> Epiglottis <br> Retropharyngeal abscess <br> Anaphylactic edema or spasm <br> Lower tract: <br> croup <br> (Laryngotracheobronchitis) <br> tracheitis |
| *Macroglossia* <br> Beckwith-Wiedemann <br> Down Syndrome | |
| *Tracheal* <br> Sub-glottic stenosis <br> Laryngo-tracheo-malacia <br> Cysts or webs <br> Laryngo-tracheo-esophageal fistula | *Trauma* <br> Direct external <br> Foreign body aspiration <br> Postintubation <br> Burns <br> Acid ingestion |
| | *CNS* <br> Shock <br> Head injury <br> Drug overdose <br> Hypoxemia <br> Abnormal metabolic conditions <br> Raised intracranial pressure |

Positioning

- Ensure there is no obvious cervical spine injury. Look at spine. Has there been evident trauma?
- Perform a jaw lift-thrust (index or middle fingers under angle of jaw and push anteriorly—thumbs rest on cheeks of patient to keep head straight).

  - This moves the tongue anteriorly with the mandible, minimizing the tongue's ability to obstruct the airway. With the patient supine, the clinician stands at the head of the bed, placed the heels of both hands on the parieto-occipital areas on each side of the patient's head, grasps the angles of the mandible with the index and long fingers, and displaces the jaw anteriorly.

- Tilt head posteriorly and maintain position.

  - Do not "over" overextend—can distort or collapse the trachea especially of the neonate—place padding under the shoulders and head
  - "sniffing air" position ideal

- Lift mandible anteriorly using hand under chin or thumb inside of mouth to lift mandible forward

See diagrams (on page 78) for sniffing position that aligns the various axes of the mouth, phayrnx, and laryngeal opening.

# Oropharyngeal and Nasopharyngeal Airways

Oropharyngeal airway

This inserts to give a space between lips, teeth, tongue, and the glottis area. It overcomes trismus (clenched jaws, or masseter spasm) and allows room for gas or suctioning catheters.

- Place an oropharyngeal airway in place unless child is conscious. Estimate length by placing oral airway against side of the face with the flange at the corner of the child's mouth and the tip reaching the angle of the mandible or use distance from tip of nose to jaw angle.
- Never use if there is any question of basal skull fractures. Consider possible if:

  - Battle's sign (ecchymosis of the mastoid process of the temporal bone).
  - Raccoon eyes—is periorbital ecchymosis, ie, "black eyes"
  - Cerebrospinal fluid rhinorrhea
  - Cranial nerve palsy
  - Bleeding from the nose and ears

- If these procedures, together with an oxygen flow (see below), do not maintain an adequate oxygenation and/or respiratory airway, move toward assisted ventilation with mask and/or bag and mask ventilation.

Nasopharyngeal airway

- If child is conscious, continue to position the child in the "sniff posture" so that the airway is maintained; if more is needed for airway security, consider a nasopharyngeal airway ("nasal trumpet"). If needed consider 2% lidocaine gel for local anesthesia and a vasoconstrictor such as epinephrine, phenylephrine, or xylometazoline nasal spray to shrink nasal mucosa and reduce bleeding.

Oxygen equipment to maintain adequate oxygenation (definition: >90% saturation)

The various available options are in effect graded upward in terms of the degree of support required to maintain adequate oxygenation.

- If the patient breathes spontaneously, consider administering 100% blow-by oxygen
- If this is insufficient, further oxygen can be by two modes: Either low flow delivery (nasal cannulae, low-flow oxygen masks, which deliver oxygen at less than peak inspiratory flow rate) or, high flow with masks incorporating the Bernoulli effect
- Nasal cannulae: can deliver up to 50% $FiO_2$—up to flow of 1 L/min
- Low-flow face mask: can deliver up to 50% $FiO_2$—up to flows of 4–6 L/min
- Non-rebreathing masks: can deliver up to 100% $FiO_2$—flows 4–6 L/min
- High-flow Venturi masks: can deliver up to 50% $FiO_2$—up to flows of 8–12 L/min L/minute

# Bag-Valve-Mask Ventilation (BVM)

Familiarity with bag and mask ventilation is an essential technique. In a clinical trial, the use of BVM gave comparable gas exchange to a variety of other techniques.

Moreover, in a landmark RCT, survival with BVM versus endotracheal tube intubation (ETI) was comparable, when used in out-of-hospital pediatric arrest.

Although the necessary assistance is possible with one person alone, always obtain urgent help as tidal volume delivery is more efficient with a 2-person technique.

- Maintain the oral airway in place.
- Using left hand, perform the E-C clamp technique: Cover mouth and nose with mask and anchor with your little finger underneath the patient's chin.
- Spread the little, ring, and index fingers over the mandible from the angle of the jaw forward toward the chin as an "E."
- Then lift the jaw, pulling the face into the mask. Place the thumb and forefinger over the mask as a "C." Finally squeeze the mask onto the face forming a seal is between the mask and the face.
- Ensure your little finger does not occlude the soft tissues of the neck in young child, thereby creating an obstruction.
- Ensure mask seal okay. Place rim of the mask between lower lip and chin and keep mouth open.
- Listen and feel for leak under the cuff.

- Maintaining tidal volume: Appropriate tidal volume is that volume allowing the chest to visibly rise.
- Deliver breaths over 1–1.5 seconds.
- If excess pressures apparent, re-position mask and/or airway; re-check for obstruction
- Pass an nasogastric (NG) tube to avoid gastric dilation

## Masks

If in the field, use a mask with a one-way valve allowing protection from potential exposure. Ensure there is a good fitting mask.

In hospital, fit available systems with 100% oxygen and proceed. The possible choices of masks, in any given hospital, are likely to be site-specific, but invariably includes either:

- a self-refilling $O_2$ Bag and Valve Mask resuscitation bag (BVM) or
- an anesthesia bag (eg, Ayre's Bag, Jackson-Rees) (AB)

For either, the gas flow is directed to a mask or to an endotracheal device. It is important to understand that the use of either (especially perhaps self-inflating resuscitation bags) filled with oxygen as a source of oxygen for spontaneously breathing patients without active compression of the bag, and without a seal to the face or airway (so-called "blow-by") is not going to be sufficient to maintain oxygenation.

Given a minute volume of gas flow of two to three times the minute tidal volume delivered, a "non-rebreathing" state is achieved.

There are theoretical relative advantages to an anesthesia bag system (there is a tendency to over-ventilate more with the BVM as the bag is more resistant, and the standard BVM cannot maintain positive end expiratory pressure (PEEP) without an additional PEEP-valve while the A-bag outlet can be partially colluded to provide this PEEP).

However, inexperienced operators should always use the BVM.

Nonetheless, even this may have mechanical faults; although the BVM has few parts, even the simple spring loaded valve may get detached.

## Progression Toward Endotracheal Intubation

- Given adequate ventilation with a bag and mask and adequate oxygenation, you may be able to wait for potential recovery from the child depending on the clinical situation.

- If this seems unlikely from the child's course, it may be necessary to proceed to intubation. If there is partial obstruction, proceed quickly toward intubation as partial relived obstruction can deteriorate quickly.
- If the child is obtunded, it is possible that intubation is needed irrespective of underlying condition.
- Stabilization with bag and mask ventilation can proceed for some time, allowing time for the most experienced members of the team to be present, since a hurried but inexperienced intubation may be deleterious. Recall above findings of a large randomized, clinical trial (RCT) showing efficacy of BMV.

# Assessment to Predict the Difficult Intubation

Assessment of the airway ease for intubation enables a sensible triage decision by virtue of the team members to be present and your own skills.

| Question to pose | Underlying condition to be concerned about |
|---|---|
| Is the mouth able to be opened fully? | Micrognathia: eg, cri-du-chat, Di George Pierre Robin |
| | Mid-face hypoplasia: eg, Craniofacial dysostoses, Goldenhar syndromes |
| Are you likely to be able to visualize easily? | Macroglossia: eg, Beckwith-Wiedemann, Trisomy 21 |
| Is there a short neck or rigidity? | Rheumatoid arthritis, short-limbed dwarf syndromes, obesity |
| Is there need to limit neck movement? | Motor vehicle spinal disruptions, patients in halo traction; some patients with Down syndrome: also in Down with possible subluxation |
| Is there facial trauma, or smoke injury? | Hematomas to underlying soft tissue, obstruction, burns, angioedema |

These situations make for special consideration. In these circumstances, especial care must be taken to ensure:

- bag and mask ventilation is able to be achieved prior to any paralytic agent introduced
- more skilled assistance is available and/or informed as early as possible of impending airway crisis—if need be urgent consultation with anesthesia

Following assessment of these, and with appropriate skill levels present, proceed to the following:

Pre-Oxygenation

- In order to avoid hypoxemia, ensure that the patient is well oxygenated. Optimal oxygenation is 100% for several minutes to displace nitrogen and ensure lung reserve store of oxygen present.
- This means hyperventilate the child on bag and mask (24–60 min) for 20–30 s prior to attempted intubation.
- Recent experience suggests that a short period of time on noninvasive ventilation might improve oxygenation by optimal recruitment, before intubation.

Preparation and Equipment

A team should be assembled with some designated responsible for preparing equipment and some for positioning and ensuring patient's safety.

It is advised that an initial endotracheal airway is secured with an oral tube followed by a nasal placement after airway is secured and ventilation established.

The following should be ready to hand, and where appropriate attached to patient.

- Monitoring equipment: ECG; saturation pulse oximeter; end-tidal $CO_2$ monitors
- Drugs (see below)
- Airways: oral and nasopharyngeal
- Adhesive tapes skin protectors
- Suction: large-bore tracheal suction catheters and tonsil suction (Yankauer)
- Uncuffed and cuffed endotracheal tubes of varying sizes for children <10 years of age
- Stylets for endotracheal tube
- Bags for ventilation

- Laryngoscope blades:

    - Miller straight sizes 0, 1, 1.5, 2, 3, 4
    - McIntosh curved: 2, 3, 4
    - The choice of type of blade is by the operators comfort
    - Largely speaking, it is advisable to use straight (Miller) blades up to an age of about 4 years

- Magill forceps
- Some commonly used guidelines for size of ETT to insert:

    - Child's age in yrs/4 + 4–up to 10 years
    - For smaller infants:

        - If age <1 yr: use from 1, 2, 3, 4 mm ID
        - Preterms: 2.5 by the operator's comfort and the patient's anatomy
        - Term infants 3.0–3.5
        - Up to 6 months 3.5–4.0
        - 7–12 months 4.0

- Or, approximately: external diameter ETT = patient's little finger, or the size of nares
- Cuffed tubes may be used safely in children >1 yr of age, uncuffed tubes may also be used, however, in children up to 8 yr of age
- Cuff should be inflated to allow for a leak at 20 mm Hg; 25 mm Hg is capillary perfusion pressure and pressures above that may cause tissue damage leading to subglottic stenosis (see Chapter 7, "Otolaryngology")
- Should also have tubes 0.5 mm smaller and 0.5 mm larger prepared in case of size errors

Size of Blade Selection

Place the blade at the upper incisor teeth to the angle of the mandible; the correct size blade should be no more than 10 mm (1 cm) of the mandible angle.

| Age (yr) | Laryngoscope blade | ETT ID (mm) | Length oral (cm) |
|---|---|---|---|
| Prematures | 0 | 2.5–3.0 | 7–9 |
| Newborn | 0 | 3.5 | 9–11 |
| 1 | 1 | 4.0 | 12 |
| 2 | 2 | 4.5 | 13 |
| 4 | 2 | 5.0 | 14 |
| 6 | 2 | 5.5 | 15 |
| 8 | 2–3 | 6.0 | 16 |

Or, use the following approximate guides:

Medications to use for intubation

- Awake intubation is unacceptable for young children.
- Combinations of drugs vary considerably. The selection of medications should be guided by the clinical condition of the patient, medication availability, and the knowledge and skill of the clinicians. Generally, three classes of drugs are given: an antiparasympathetic agent to dry secretions, followed by an induction agent or agents (to blunt awareness, resistance, and pain), then a paralytic agent. Lidocaine may be added to attenuate the rise in intracranial pressure (ICP).

# Standard Rapid Sequence Intubation

For intubation in any situation where the status of prior water and food intake is unclear (nothing by mouth [NPO] status); and for situations of a narrow margin of safety tolerance of suboptimal oxygenation. In most other situations for intubation either a period of fast has been undertaken, or there is time to empty the stomach via a nasogastric tube. It is now the commonest mode of intubation in pediatrics nowadays, and is safe in the great majority.

RSI consists of five steps

1) Preoxygenation with spontaneous respiration
   Note, do *not* use bag-valve-mask ventilation
   (unless patient decompensates)
2) Premedication: atropine and/or lidocaine
   *Caveats:*
   Likely there are vagal responses independent of hypoxia in children, not prevented by atropine
   However most would use atropine for very young children (<1 yr) and in children with lots of secretions
   Lidocaine: given about 3 min before intubation for ICP precaution
3) Induction with sedative and/or analgesic agent(s) (see table for drug dosing and effects)
4) Followed quickly by a paralytic agent (do not wait until induction agent takes full effect)
5) Finally, endotracheal intubation

|  | Drug | Dose | Onset of action | Comments |
|---|---|---|---|---|
| Premed-ication | atropine | 0.02 mg/kg | 1–2 min | minimum 0.1, |
|  | lidocaine | 1.5–2 mg/kg | 2–5 min | maximum 1 mg |
| Sedatives | midazolam | 0.1–0.25 mg/kg | 1–2 min | ↓BP if hypovolemic, minimal effect on ICP |
|  | propofol | 1–2 mg/kg | <1 min | ↓ICP, ↓BP |
|  | thiopental | 2–5 mg/kg | <1 min | ↓ICP, ↓BP |
|  | etomidate | 0.2–0.4 mg/kg | 1 min | ↓ICP, minimal effect on BP. May cause adrenal suppression |
| Analgesics | morphine | 0.2 mg/kg | 2–5 min | Minimal effect on ICP, may ↓BP |
|  | fentanyl | 2–5 micro-gram/kg | 1 min | Minimal effect on ICP and BP |
|  | remifen-tanil | 2–4 micro-gram/kg | <1 min | Duration of action 3–10 min |
| Sedative/an algesic | ketamine | 1–2 mg/kg | 1–2 min | bronchodilation, ↑ICP, little effect on BP |
| Paralytics | rocuron-ium | 1 mg/kg | 45–90 s | Nondepolarizing agent. Duration of action: 30–60 min |
|  | vecuron-ium | 0.2 mg/kg | 0.5–2 min | Nondepolarizing agent. Duration of action 30–60 min |
|  | succiny lcholine | 1–2 mg/kg | 45–60 s | Depolarizing agent. Duration of action: <10 min Contraindicated in hyperkalemia, burns crush injuries, renal failure, increased ICP. Repeat doses not generally recommended |

# Special Situations Mandating Special Choices

## Raised ICP

- Attempt to blunt the cardiovascular system (CVS) responses with particular care in this situation.
- Intubation should be accompanied by end-tidal monitoring throughout to ensure no undue upward flux, which will increase ICP.
- Lidocaine + thiopental or etomidate + rocuronium or vecuronium.
- Avoid hyperventilation unless herniation suspected.
- If still not completely relaxed, add further 1 mg/kg IV thiopental.
- Avoid ketamine due to increased ICP and systemic hypertension.
- Avoid propofol as hypotension may compromise cerebral perfusion pressure (CPP), and may alter cerebral autoregulation.
- Be aware of the risk of increased ICP secondary to muscle fasciculation with succinylcholine.

## Asthma (see Chapter 6, "Pulmonary")

- A decision to intubate these patients is only made when tiring is apparent, and ideally should be early enough so a "semi-elective" procedure is performed.
- Timing is, therefore, a "last resort" but not "too late."
- This should always be done as a rapid sequence induction, with the proviso that patients may not have adequate oxygen reserves for 60 seconds.
- Combined agents of choice in asthma:

  - atropine + ketamine +/− midazolam + paralytic

## Positioning

- The intubator is at the head of the bed—remove headrests if needed.
- Place patients head in the "sniff position" (see below).
- Assistant restrains gently the shoulders and helps to position the shoulders and torso.
- In the below diagram, the effect of extending the head into the optimal "sniffing position" can be seen.
- By doing this, the alignment of the oral cavity, the pharyngeal cavity, and the opening of the larynx are brought optimally in-line for visualization.

This position can be achieved either with towels placed below the patient or by team members angling the child.

Head on Bed
Neutral Position

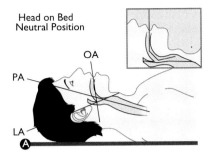

**Figure 1A:** Anatomic neutral position. The oral (OA), pharyngeal (PA), and laryngeal (LA) axes are at greater angles to one another.

**Figure 1B:** Head, still in neutral position, has been lifted by a pillow flexing the lower cervical spine and aligning the pharyngeal (PA) and laryngeal (LA) axes.

Head Elevated on Pad
Neutral Position

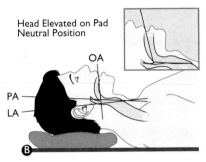

Head Elevated on Pad
Head Extended on Neck

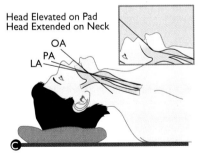

**Figure 1C:** The head has been extended on the cervical spine, aligning the oral axis (OA) with the pharyngeal (PA) and laryngeal (LA) axes, creating the optimum sniffing position for intubation.

From *Pediatric Airway Management* by Dave French

Sellick maneuver (or cricoid pressure) helps prevent regurgitation of stomach contents into the larynx during intubation and induction, and sometimes helps to align the larynx into a visual plane. In children, it limits gas insufflation into the stomach.

- An assistant locates the cricoid cartilage before induction (see diagram)
- Applies backward pressure with thumb and forefinger following induction of anesthesia
- Releases pressure after endotracheal intubation confirmed
- It is unhelpful to have too much or too little pressure
- Insertion of blade:

  - from the right corner
  - Control the tongue
  - If using the Miller: Lift epiglottis
  - If using Macintosh place into the vallecula, and then if needed, lift the epiglottis

## Depth of Insertion

Correct placement defined as tip of the ETT below the thoracic inlet and >0.5 cm above carina.

- Common formulae used are:

  - Depth of black mark on the ETT
  - 15 + age in yr divided by 2 for nasal tubes
  - Three times ID ETT for oral
  - 12 + age in yr divided by 2

An alternative method is to use the so-called Breslow formula, likely to be more accurate. In this measure, the child's length determines ETT.

It must be understood that:

*ALL THESE ARE ONLY GUIDELINES*

- Always confirm ETT placement:
- Firstly by clinical examination

  - Listen carefully for equality of breath sounds
  - Mist in tube
  - Equal chest rise

- Then by secondary confirmation (essential)

  - End-tidal $CO_2$–monitor or colorimetric device
  - $O_2$ saturations maintained

- Finally, in a hospital setting, CXR should be done to confirm depth of placement
- Newer modalities for confirmation of tube placement include bedside ultrasound
- DOPE pneumonic helps to troubleshoot problems while intubated

  D   displacement
  O   obstruction
  P   pneumothorax
  E   equipment failure

If visualization of cords is not possible:

- Are you overextended? Tilt the head back and forth.
- Was there right degree of cricoid pressure exerted? Add or diminish cricoid pressure.
- Was tongue obstructing view? Do you need a larger blade?
- Excess secretions? Suction with Yankauer.
- Sometimes the "BURP" maneuver—Backward, Upward, Rightward, Pressure—on glottis helps.

Restrict yourself to three failed attempts at maximum. Always recover the patient in between attempts and ensure there is no hypoxia.

## Other Airway Management Modalities

### Laryngeal Mask Airway (LMA)

These are a vital reserve for situations that ventilation is needed but there is no success, and no more expert intubator present. In general, LMAs are a temporizing solution before establishing a definitive airway.

---

**Table of LMA Sizes**

1: Neonates <5 kg, <4 mL air
1 1/2: Children 5–10 kg, <7 mL air
2: Children 10–20 kg, <10 mL air
2 1/2: Children 20–30 kg, <14 mL air
3: Children 30–50 kg, <20 mL air
4: Small/normal adults <30 mL air
5: Normal/large adults <40 mL air

---

ST if written on the tube stands for short

- Can either be of a type that enables assisted ventilation, or where they can be used as a guiding channel whereby to achieve a blind endotracheal intubation.
- They can be used for any age and are easy to place with little training.

Ketamine and lidocaine may be used to anesthetize the pharynx and oral cavity in cases where the patient is not fully sedated.

There are a couple of contraindications:

- A strong gag reflex is present.
- Foreign bodies are present.
- There is an airway obstruction.
- A high ventilation pressure is required.

## Heliox

In situations of increased airway resistance helium-oxygen mixtures may be of benefit.

- Helium is the second lightest element, thus helium-oxygen is less dense than room air.
- Density of fluids and gases affect viscosity: lower viscosity gases have less turbulent flow and promote laminar flow.
- Heliox also promotes elimination of carbon dioxide with increased diffusion.

Controversy continues on the use of Heliox but it may benefit individual patients with a variety of conditions causing upper and lower airway obstruction including croup, postintubation airway inflammation, bronchiolitis. Used as a co-intervention with albuterol a controlled study showed benefit in moderate pediatric asthma, although the controlled literature overall shows mixed results.

- Side effects: hypoxia, hypothermia (rare)

Practically: Helium-oxygen mixture, there are two commonly available proportions, there is no evidence to favor one mixture over the other—typically the choice is made based on the patient's $O_2$ requirements:

- 21% oxygen 79% helium (3 times less dense than air)
- 30% oxygen 70% helium (2.3 times less dense than air)

# Percutaneous Cricothyroidotomy

- The need for this procedure is extremely rare in pediatric critical care.
- Cricothyroidotomy is a temporary airway, often only able to provide some degree of oxygenation, but not adequate gas exchange for ventilation.
- Surgical consultation is essential to establish a permanent and secure artificial airway (tracheostomy).

## Indications

Where there is a critical need for airway management, failed attempts with all other modalities including nasotracheal/orotracheal intubation, LMA, bag-valve-mask ventilation, spontaneous ventilation

## Equipment

- Sterile prep, towels.
- Multiple large IV catheters (18 gauge or larger).
- 3–5 mL syringe.
- 8 mm tracheal tube adapter (from an endotracheal tube).

## Procedure

- Use as sterile technique as possible depending on the clinical situation.
- Ensure adequate analgesia or sedation if patient is conscious.
- Landmark and identify the cricothyroid membrane by palpating the thyroid notch and moving caudally to the space between the thyroid and cricoid cartilages (diagram 1).
- Stabilize trachea with nondominant hand.
- Introduce large IV catheter at a 45-degree angle to the trachea, aiming caudally.
- Aspirate air to confirm placement.
- Leave syringe connect, remove plunger.
- Connect 8 mm tracheal tube adapter to syringe barrel and attach to ventilation system.
- Patient will require high pressures to achieve some measure of ventilation.

## Complications

- Failure to obtain airway/misplacement of catheter.
- Hemorrhage.

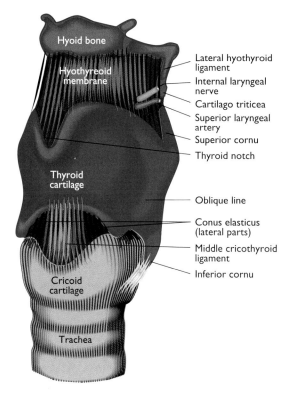

Hyoid bone

Hyothyreoid membrane

Lateral hyothyroid ligament

Internal laryngeal nerve

Cartilago triticea

Superior laryngeal artery

Superior cornu

Thyroid notch

Thyroid cartilage

Oblique line

Conus elasticus (lateral parts)

Middle cricothyroid ligament

Inferior cornu

Cricoid cartilage

Trachea

Diagram of cricothyroid membrane.

## References

Davis DP, Dunford JV, Poste JC, et al. The impact of hypoxia and hyper-ventilation on outcome after paramedic rapid sequence intubation of severely head-injured patients. J Trauma 2004;57:1–8; discussion 8–10.

Young KD, Seidel JS. Pediatric cardiopulmonary resuscitation: a collective review. Ann Emerg Med 1999;33:195–205.

Gausche M, Stratton SJ, Henderson FP, et al. Bag-valve-mask ventilation (BVM) for children in the prehospital setting. Acad Emerg Med 1996;3:404–5.

Rumball CJ, MacDonald D. The PTL, Combitube, laryngeal mask, and oral airway: a randomized prehospital comparative study of ventilatory device effectiveness and cost-effectiveness in 470 cases of cardiorespiratory arrest. Prehosp Emerg Care 1997;1:1–10.

Gausche M, Lewis RJ, Stratton SJ, et al. Effect of out-of-hospital pediatric endotracheal intubation on survival and neurological outcome: a controlled clinical trial. JAMA 2000;283:783–90.

Davidovic L, LaCovey D, Pitetti RD. Comparison of 1- versus 2-person bag-valve-mask techniques for manikin ventilation of infants and children. Ann Emerg Med 2005;46:37–42.

Airway maintenance techniques and assessment of ventilation in pediatric resuscitation. http://patients.uptodate.com/topic.asp?file=ped_res/2259 (last accessed August 7, 2008).

Carter BG, Fairbank B, Tibballs J, et al. Oxygen delivery using self-inflating resuscitation bags. Pediatr Crit Care Med 2005;6:125–8.

Mondolfi AA, et al. Comparison of self-inflating bags with anesthesia bags for bag-mask ventilation in the pediatric emergency department. Pediatr Emerg Care 1997;13:312–6.

Ainsworth SB, Humphreys R, Stewart L. The pressure is on! The danger of a broken blow off valve on a bag valve mask. Arch Dis Child Fetal Neonatal Ed 2006;91:F233.

Ehrlich PF, Seidman PS, Atallah O, et al. Endotracheal intubations in rural pediatric trauma patients. J Pediatr Surg 2004;39:1376–80.

Baillard C, et al. Noninvasive ventilation improves preoxygenation before intubation of hypoxic patients. Am J Respir Crit Care Med 2006;174:171–7.

Mellick LB, Edholm T, Corbett SW. Pediatric laryngoscope blade size selection using facial landmarks. Pediatr Emergency Care 2006;22:226–9.

Sagarin MJ, Chiang V, Sakles JC, et al. Rapid sequence intubation for pediatric emergency airway management. Pediatr Emerg Care 2002;18:417–23.

French D. Pediatric Airway Management. http://ems.aanet.org/info/PediatricAirways_06.ppt (last accessed August 7, 2008).

Moynihan RJ, Brock-Utne JG, Archer JH, et al. The effect of cricoid pressure on preventing gastric insufflation in infants and children. Anesthesiology 1993;78:652–6.

Phipps LM, et al. Prospective assessment of guidelines of determining appropriate depth of ETT placement in children. Pediatr Crit Care Med 2005;6:519–22.

Knill RL. Difficult laryngoscopy made easy with a "BURP". Can J Anesthesia 1993;40:279–82.

Bahk JH, Sung J, Jang IJ. A comparison of ketamine and lidocaine spray with propofol for the insertion of laryngeal mask airway in children: a double-blinded randomized trial. Anesth Analg 2002;95:1586–9.

Gupta VK, Cheifetz IM. Heliox administration in the pediatric intensive care unit: an evidence-based review. Pediatr Crit Care Med 2005;6:204–11.

Myers TR. Use of heliox in children. Respir Care 2006 Jun;51(6):619–31. Review.

Kim IK, Phrampus E, Venkataraman S, et al. Helium/oxygen-driven albuterol nebulization in the treatment of children with moderate to severe asthma exacerbations: a randomized, controlled trial. Pediatrics 2005;116:1127–33.

# B. Shock

Vandana Thapar
Michael R Anderson

## Definition

Shock is a clinical syndrome of circulatory dysfunction that results in a failure to deliver sufficient amount of oxygen and other nutrients to meet the metabolic demands of peripheral tissues. The definition of shock does not depend on an exact number for blood pressure (BP), but BP defines what phase of shock a patient is in: compensated, decompensated, or irreversible.

When perfusion falls below a critical level, compensatory mechanisms are activated. Such mechanisms include the release of antidiuretic hormone (ADH) and stimulation of the renin-aldosterone-angiotensin (RAA) system, which helps maintain systemic vascular resistance (SVR) and organ perfusion. During this phase of shock, children maintain a normal to elevated BP. Once these compensatory mechanisms are exhausted, *decompensated* shock can develop and BP can fall, sometimes rapidly. If a patient's shock progresses even further, *irreversible* shock can develop and the patient will die regardless of interventions undertaken.

Although pediatric shock can be caused by a multitude of etiologies (see below), the basic clinical findings in children with shock are quite similar.

- tachypnea with varying levels of respiratory distress
- tachycardia
- evidence of poor peripheral or end-organ perfusion

Early recognition of the signs of shock and aggressive resuscitation is central. An etiological diagnosis of shock is equally important, but may require a more thorough evaluation after initial resuscitation.

## Shock State: Signs and Symptoms

Signs and symptoms of shock reflect a hypoperfused state and attempt to compensate by shunting blood flow to maintain key organs. The initial exam requires a careful answer to the question "is this patient's cardiac output meeting his/her metabolic demands?"

1. Mental status: changes in mental status, ie, fussiness, irritability, agitation, lethargy and/or unconsciousness (poor CNS substrate delivery)
2. Respiratory: tachypnea, increased work of breathing, shallow breaths, decreased effort, grunting and/or crackles (evidence of lactic acidosis, pneumonia, and/or pulmonary edema)
3. Cardiovascular: tachycardia, thready or weak pulse, cyanosis, pulse pressure is dependent on etiology of shock, orthostatic changes, and possible difference in upper and lower extremity blood pressure (evidence of poor cardiac output)
4. Skin: temperature can be hyperthermic or hypothermic, capillary refill may be prolonged, color pale or plethoric extremities, and/or mottled extremities (evidence of poor skin perfusion)
5. Mucous membranes: may be dry, especially with hypovolemia
6. Urine: decreased urine output, increased specific gravity (determination of urine output may require several hours of observation and obviously diagnosis of shock does not require low urine output) (evidence of poor renal perfusion)

## Initial Management

### Treatment of Shock

**General Principles**   The basic tenets are to recognize shock, and to re-establish adequate end-organ perfusion as quickly as possible. The assessment of airway, breathing, and circulation are paramount. We discuss this approach as it relates to the balance of oxygen delivery and oxygen consumption.

Oxygen delivery ($DO_2$) equals the amount of oxygen delivered to the body:

$$DO_2 = \text{arterial oxygen content } (CaO_2) \times \text{cardiac output (CO)}$$

Recall that $CaO_2 = 1.36 \times Hgb \text{ (g/dL)} \times (\text{ % oxygen saturation} + PaO_2) \times 0.003$

If one uses the $DO_2$ equation as a guide to the initial resuscitation, then the goal of optimizing oxygen delivery becomes even clearer:

$SaO_2$: Ensure that a patient has an adequately saturated hemoglobin

Hgb: Ensure that a patient has an appropriate Hgb level

Preload: Ensure that a patient has an adequate filling pressure

Afterload: Ensure that a patient has an optimal blood pressure/SVR

Contractility: Ensure that a patient has adequate myocardial contractility

Figure 1 outlines the numerous factors contributing to normal oxygen delivery and consumption.

- An important aspect is to optimize $O_2$ consumption ($VO_2$) (see Figure 1) by minimizing variables increasing $VO_2$ (ie, shivering, pain, agitation, work of breathing) may allow a more balanced

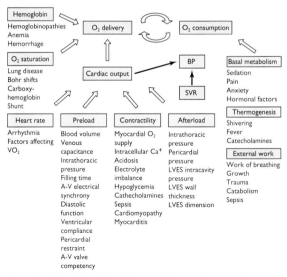

**Figure 1** Normal physiology of oxygen delivery and consumption.

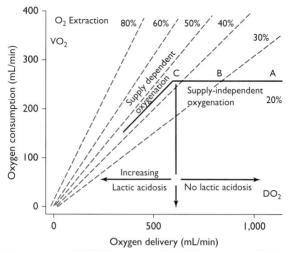

**Figure 2**   Oxygen delivery versus consumption.

DO$_2$ to VO$_2$ relationship. Examples of treating an increased O$_2$ consumptive state include sedation, mechanical ventilation, and fever control. When DO$_2$ falls below a critical level, profound tissue hypoperfusion ensues, lactic acidosis worsens, and SvO$_2$ falls to dangerous levels (Figure 2).

All this must be preceded with strict adherence to assessment and intervention of airway, breathing, and circulation.

**Assessment of ABCs**    This evaluation should take less than 30 seconds.

General appearance: What is the general color of patient? Is patient awake and responsive, responding to voice or pain, or sleepy/lethargic and nonresponsive? Are there any movement of extremities, what is muscle tone?

Airway: Is it clear? If it is clear, will the patient be able to maintain a clear airway, does the patient need to be intubated to protect airway?

Breathing: Are there breath sounds? Or any respiratory effort? Evaluate RR, depth of breathing—shallow? Is patient tachypneic? Are there any respiratory sounds, wheezing, stridor? Evaluate if sounds of tidal volume (inspiratory and expiratory volume) are adequate, and obtain pulse oximetry.

Circulation: What is the heart rate and are the pulses present? Obtain skin temperature, capillary refill, color of extremities (pink, pale, blue, or mottled), blood pressure, later identify urine output.

## Therapy and ICU Monitoring of Shock Patient

### IV Access Options/Monitoring of Shock Patient

| Line | Location | Benefits | Risks |
|------|----------|----------|-------|
| Peripheral IV | Anywhere | Infuse volume and medications | Phlebitis, pain, and hematoma |
| Arterial line | Radial, axillary, femoral, posterior tibial, and dorsalis pedis arteries | Continuous BP monitor, checking frequent labs | Infection, hematoma/ thrombosis, and ischemia |
| Central line | Femoral, subclavian, and internal jugular veins | Multiple ports can infuse multiple drugs, measures filling pressure and venous saturation | Infection, pain, hematoma, thrombosis ischemia, artery puncture, and pneumothorax or hemothorax in subclavian or internal jugular |
| Pulmonary artery catheter | Pulmonary artery through femoral, subclavian, or internal jugular veins | Measures cardiac output and pulmonary artery occlusion pressure | Infection, pain, hematoma, thrombosis, ischemia, arterial puncture, pneumothorax, hemothorax, arrhythmia, valve, arterial, or ventricular wall puncture |

1) Fluid resuscitation:

Regardless of underlying insult causing shock, patients usually have a relative hypovolemia. Aggressive fluid resuscitation with crystalloids of colloids (20 mL/kg/bolus at a time) with frequent re-assessment of the clinical status of the patient is quite important. Up to 60 mL/kg/her and possibly higher as needed.

The American Heart Association and PALS Group recommend boluses until perfusion improves or new physical signs supervene (eg, pulmonary crackles or a newly felt liver margin).

2) Vasoactive infusions:

Should be used in the context of abnormal hemodynamics after adequate fluid resuscitation. Choice of drug(s) is based on goal for that drug.

Figure 3 outlines the initial approach to shock management.

3) Classifications of shock

Once again, the initial resuscitation of the child in shock calls for a high index of suspicion and aggressive attention to augmenting $DO_2$ and optimizing $VO_2$. Once stabilized, assess the underlying nature of the shock state:

- Hypovolemic
- Cardiogenic
- Obstructive
- Distributive
- Dissociative
- Septic

1) Hypovolemic Shock

- *Etiology:* Hemorrhage (trauma, GI bleeding and postoperation), fluid and electrolyte loss (gastroenteritis, DIC), plasma loss (burns, nephritic syndrome), and endocrine.
- *Pathophysiology:* Loss or shift in the intravascular blood volume leading to decreased preload/venous return and cardiac output to the extent that effective tissue perfusion cannot be maintained. Due to decrease in cardiac output, the central and peripheral baroreceptors stimulate the release of catecholamines. Because of the homeostatic mechanisms,

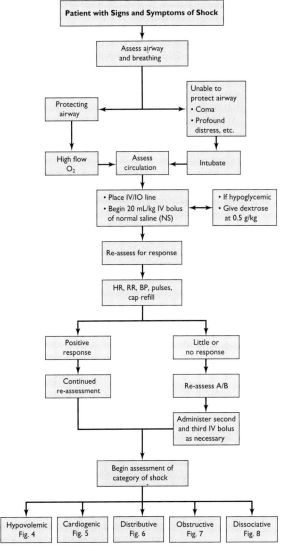

**Figure 3** Initial approach to shock management.

hypotension may not be present but rather peripheral vaso-constriction and tachycardia.

- *Signs and symptoms in early compensated states:*

  - Persistent tachycardia (consider the normal ranges for age) is the most reliable clinical indicator of early compensated hypovolemic shock.
  - Signs arising from cutaneous vasoconstriction with decrease in pulse pressure, poor skin perfusion: mottling of skin, prolonged capillary refill (<2 s), cool extremities, and decreased urine output.
  - Neurologic status may be normal and changes indicate worsening condition.
  - BP is not a reliable clinical indicator of early hypovolemic states. If continued loss of blood volume and fluid replacement is delayed, the body decompensates. The increase in vasoconstriction and hypovolemia creates ischemia and hypoxia, with anaerobic metabolism, creating acidosis and damages other vital organs. It is important to stress that only after the body's ability to compensate is hypotension seen.

- *Therapy* (Figure 4)

The most common cause of hypovolemic shock in children is gastroenteritis, although based on the history of the patient, other etiologies may need to be entertained.

2) Cardiogenic Shock

- *Etiology:* Cardiomyopathy secondary to infection, metabolic disorder, or genetic abnormality, and congenital heart disease are the most common. Diastolic dysfunction is another cause of cardiogenic shock. This is when the myocardial tissue cannot relax and fill, thus decreasing cardiac output.
- *Pathophysiology:* Cardiac abnormality is responsible for the failure of the cardiovascular system to meet the metabolic needs of the tissues. The body utilizes its compensatory mechanisms as in hypovolemic shock, although in cardiogenic shock the mechanisms can be harmful. When cardiac output decreases, contractility is poor, and SVR increases which increases the work of the heart secondary to increased afterload. When there is increased left ventricular pressure it builds up and creates pulmonary edema. This is clinically shown with dyspnea and crackles. Increased left ventricle diastolic pressure decreases myocardial perfusion pressure leading to subendocardial ischemia.

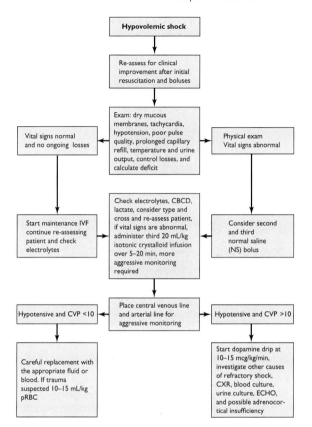

**Figure 4** Management of hypovolemic shock.

- *Signs and symptoms*

  1. Increased work of breathing
  2. Tachypnea with feeds
  3. Increased frequency of feeds but decreased volume
  4. Excessive sweating
  5. Upper respiratory infection symptoms (cough, rhinorrhea)
  6. Failure to gain weight

- *Physical exam*

  1. Tachycardia and tachypnea
  2. Gallop rhythm

3. Cold extremities with weak peripheral pulses
4. Wheezing and rales
5. Dyspnea and cough
6. Cyanosis
7. Diaphoresis
8. Hepatomegaly
9. Lethargic (Figure 5)

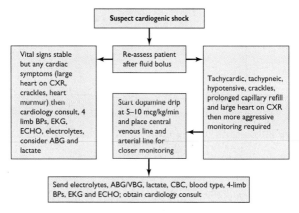

Figure 5   Management of cardiogenic shock.

3) Obstructive Shock

- *Etiology:* Pericardial tamponade, tension pneumothorax, pulmonary or systemic hypertension, pulmonary embolus, and congenital or acquired outflow obstructive lesions (valvular stenosis, coarctation of aorta and idiopathic hypertrophic subaortic sclerosis [IHSS]).

- *Pathophysiology:* There is inadequate cardiac output despite normal intravascular volume and myocardial function. This may be secondary to pulmonary or systemic circulation, or be cardiac in origin. Cardiac tamponade is cardiac compression secondary to accumulating pericardial contents.

    The symptoms in the beginning are nonspecific, but when cardiac output is compromised patient will present with tachycardia, hypotension, mottled skin, cool extremities, and oliguric. Depending on the etiology the patient may have chest pain, dyspnea, or tachypnea or desaturation disproportionate to presentation (see Figure 6).

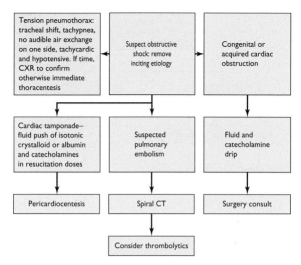

**Figure 6**  Management of obstructive shock.

4) Distributive Shock

- *Etiology:* Distributive shock may be anaphylaxis, adrenal insufficiency, anesthesia, spinal cord transaction (usually above T1), or vasodilator medications.
- *Pathophysiology:* Abnormal distribution of blood flow due to alteration in vasomotor tone. This creates inadequate tissue oxygenation (see Figure 7).

5) Dissociative Shock

- *Etiology:* Carbon monoxide, methemoglobinemia, and cyanide toxicity.
- *Pathophysiology:* This results from the inability of the body to use the oxygen which is bound in the blood. Cyanide inhibits the last step in oxidative phosphorylation which then prevents the aerobic use of oxygen. Methemoglobinemia is a state when iron is oxidized from $+2$ to the $+3$ state. In this form oxygen is not reversibly bound; thus oxygen delivery is compromised. Carbon monoxide reversibly binds to hemoglobin and has a stronger affinity for hemoglobin than oxygen. Most importantly, it causes a leftward shift in the oxyhemoglobin dissociation curve. This means, it increases the affinity of hemoglobin for oxygen which decreases the release of oxygen to the tissues (see Figure 8).

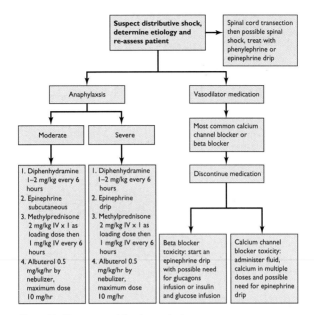

**Figure 7**   Management of distributive shock.

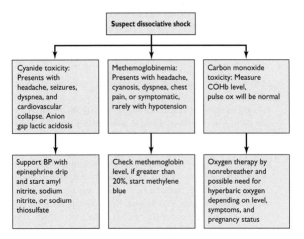

**Figure 8**   Management of dissociative shock.

6) Septic Shock (see Chapter 18, "Infection")

- *Pathophysiology/Definition*
- Infection: an inflammatory response with presence of microorganism in a host
- Bacteremia: bacteria in the blood may or may not be causing infection
- Sepsis: systemic inflammatory response syndrome with source of infection

Septic shock: sepsis and the inability of the body to meet the metabolic demands of the tissues, hypotension despite adequate fluid resuscitation.

Most children present with hypovolemia secondary to decreased intake, capillary leak, increased microvascular permeability, possible inappropriate polyuria. Increased fluid expenditures secondary to fever, diarrhea, increase respiration rate, and vomiting.

*Therapy*

- Identification and treatment of septic shock state
- Removal or treatment of microorganisms and antibiotic therapy

## Respiratory and Cardiovascular Support

**Complications of Shock** If left untreated or if the treated patient continues to progress in the shock state, other organ systems can be affected. Patients can develop multi-organ

Examples of MODS:

| System | Effect | Treatment |
|---|---|---|
| Respiratory | Increased work of breathing creating decreased lung function and muscle fatigue; acute respiratory distress syndrome (ARDS), pneumonia | Supplemental oxygen, if unable to protect airway; possible need for intubation |
| Cardiac | Myocardial dysfunction, decreased cardiac output, hypotension | Catecholamine drugs to increase contractility, increase cardiac output and sequential vascular response (SVR) |

*(continued)*

| System | Effect | Treatment |
|--------|--------|-----------|
| Renal | Prerenal azotemia creating acute tubular necrosis and cortical necrosis | Volume resuscitation, possible need for renal-dose dopamine and last hemodialysis |
| Hematology | Decreased hematocrit and disseminated intravascular coagulation (DIC) due to systemic inflammatory response | Transfuse blood, monitor prothrombin time (PT)/partial prothrombin time (PTT)/international normalized ratio (INR), platelets, possible need for fresh frozen plasma (FFP), cryoprecipitate, vitamin K and platelets |
| Hepatic | Decreased perfusion to liver causes hepatocellular damage | Monitor liver function tests (LFTs) and dose drugs metabolized by liver accordingly |
| Gastroenterology | Decreased perfusion to gastrointestinal (GI) tract induces stress ulcer, ileus, and bacterial translocation | Use proton pump inhibitors (PPIs) or histamine blockers, monitor electrolytes |
| Endocrine | Adrenal insufficiency | Adrenocorticotropic hormone (ACTH) stimulation test and treat with steroids |

dysfunction syndrome (MODS). These patients can have a very high mortality rate.

## References

Carcillo JA, Davis AL, Zaritsky A. Role of early fluid resuscitation in pediatric septic shock. JAMA 1991;266:1242–5.

American Academy of Pediatrics: American Academy of Emergency Physicians (APLS). The Pediatric Emergency Medicine Resource. 4th ed. Jones and Bartlett Publishers, Inc., 2005.

Shock Recognition and Management in: American Academy of Pediatrics, American Heart Association, Pediatric Advanced Life Support – Provider Manual. 2006:61–111.

Tobin JR, Wetzel RC. Shock and multi-organ system failure. In: Rogers MC, ed. Textbook of Pediatric Intensive Care. Baltimore, MD: Lippincott, William & Wilkins; 1996: 555–605.

# C. Cardiopulmonary Resuscitation

Andrew Healey

Lennox Huang

The resuscitation of a child in cardiac arrest is a rare occurrence even in the largest of centers. Consequently, considerable time must be devoted to maintaining competence in the individual skills of resuscitation (eg, bag-mask ventilation, intubation, electrical cardioversion/defibrillation) and the leadership of critical time-dependent resuscitations. There is excellent evidence to demonstrate rapid decline in psychomotor skill retention in skills and equally good evidence that demonstrates attrition in the rate of decline with practice. Frequent practice in a variety of forms (courses, mock resuscitations, simulation) is likely to improve outcome in pediatric resuscitation although this has not been demonstrated to date in the literature.

This chapter explores the key principles of resuscitating a child in cardiac arrest or precardiac arrest.

## Key Principles

- An effective, calm and well-organized Code Team Leader is crucial in the resuscitation of a critically ill patient.
- Code Team Leaders must acknowledge the abilities of their team and their own limitations.
- Clear, concise, and respectful communication is essential in the emotionally charged pediatric resuscitation room.
- Ensure team members complete assigned tasks and are given further tasks to perform.
- Early recognition of the critically ill child who is compromised but still compensating allows for far better outcomes than the eventual resuscitation of a child in cardiopulmonary failure.

- When individuals are uncertain about what the next step should be, an aggressive resuscitation approach should be taken until help arrives.
- Ensure effective chest compressions and ventilation prior to thinking about providing definitive management of the airway with endotracheal intubation.
- Electrical approaches to treating dysrhythmias is the fastest method of converting a child with a tachydysrhythmia and poor perfusion to a perfusing rhythm.
- Appropriate procedural sedation and analgesia must be provided for all children with awareness when performing invasive or painful procedures.
- Literature exists to support that inviting family to be present during a resuscitation is often helpful to the family in the grief process and most certainly is not harmful. This should be accomplished within an organized system to support both family and health care providers.

## Epidemiology

**Out-of-Hospital Pediatric Cardiac Arrest**    The most recent study of out-of-hospital pediatric cardiac arrest (OHCA) was a substudy of the Ontario Prehospital Advanced Life Support Study. The authors sought to determine the etiology of pediatric OHCA over an 11-yr period using the coroner's diagnosis to classify the cause of death (Table 1).

*Table 1*
**Major Causes of Pediatric Out-of-Hospital Cardiac Arrest by Coroner's Diagnosis**

| Major Causes of Cardiac Arrest | % Total |
| --- | --- |
| Natural death | 47.3 |
| Accidental death | 31.4 |
| Suicide | 6.6 |
| Homicide | 3.4 |
| Undetermined | 11.2 |

Adapted from Ong et al., 2006

- Approximately 43% of cardiac arrests were younger than 1 yr of age.
- The commonest causes of natural death were SIDS, cardiovascular, and respiratory causes, in that order.
- A great proportion of deaths were from nonnatural causes. From those accidental deaths, the largest majority by far were caused by drowning (27% of accidental deaths).
- Survival to hospital discharge was rare (1.9%).

## In-Hospital Pediatric Cardiac Arrest

The most recent study of in-hospital pediatric cardiac arrest comes from Helsinki, Finland, and identifies the etiology of cardiac arrest in this population (Tables 2 and 3).

*Table 2*
**Major Causes of In-Hospital Pediatric Cardiac Arrest in a Tertiary Care Institution with Pediatric Cardiac Surgery Service**

| Major Causes | % Total | % Survival at 1 year |
|---|---|---|
| Cardiovascular | 71.2 | 17.9 |
| Respiratory | 8.5 | 50.0 |
| Oncologic | 4.2 | 0 |
| Gastrointestinal | 3.4 | 0 |
| Congenital/chromosomal | 6 | 1 |
| CNS | 2.5 | 0 |
| Other | 5.1 | 0 |

Adapted from Suominen et al., 2005

*Table 3*
**Location of In-Hospital Pediatric Cardiac Arrest in a Tertiary Care Institution with Pediatric Cardiac Surgery Service**

| Location | % Total |
|---|---|
| PICU | 64 |
| OR | 26 |
| Ward | 10.2 |
| ER | 0.8 |
| Cardiac cath lab | 2.5 |

Adapted from Suominen et al., 2005

- Short duration of external chest compressions was the best positive prognostic indicator.
- Because of the cardiac surgery population, a high prevalence of cardiac causes of arrest is noted.

## Physiological Principles of Resuscitation

The etiology of pediatric cardiopulmonary arrest is normally the progression of respiratory failure or circulatory shock, as opposed to a primary cardiac insult. Several changes in the philosophy of resuscitation have been based on pathophysiological principles and animal studies that support them.

**Chest Compressions**    There is excellent evidence in the adult literature, likely extrapolatable to the pediatric literature, that chest compressions are performed poorly.

- In both the prehospital and in-hospital setting, we perform chest compressions poorly. Specifically, the chest compressions are of inadequate depth and inadequate rate.
- Often full chest recoil is not permitted by the rescuer as s/he "camps" on the chest preventing cardiac filling ("mechanical diastole"). This decreases effective cardiac output, decreases coronary perfusion pressure, and increases resting intrathoracic pressure. This will likely represent decrease in survival.
- Chest compressions produce flow in both the thoracic aorta and the pulmonary artery during the compression phase of CPR and retrograde flow occurs during decompression. Survival is decreased in slow chest compression groups in adult studies. At the same time, there is a plateau at which there is benefit. In dogs, coronary blood flow is reduced as chest compressions exceed 120 compression per minute. Recommended rates account for this therapeutic range.
- Coronary perfusion pressure increases with each subsequent chest compression and falls off rapidly with interruptions to continuous chest compressions. Consequently, more compressions and fewer interruptions result in better coronary perfusion pressure. There is directly proportional relationship between coronary perfusion pressure and survival in cardiac arrest.

---

**Effective Chest Compressions**

- Push hard, push fast
- Allow complete chest recoil
- Do not interrupt compressions

**Effects of Ventilation**   Aufderheide has written several provocative papers and editorials that question the value of ventilation during CPR. Given the etiology of cardiac arrest in children, it is difficult to extrapolate this to a pediatric population.

- It is clear that chest compressions are important.
- Over-ventilation is harmful in that it increases intrathoracic pressure, decreases coronary and cerebral perfusion pressure, and subsequently reduces survival.
- Where the etiology of cardiopulmonary arrest is hypoxic or primary respiratory arrest, ventilations are likely to be more beneficial earlier in the resuscitation; however, over-ventilation is still harmful.
- Relatively low-tidal volume, low rate of ventilation, and attention to avoiding hyperventilation are important during acute resuscitation of children (and adults).

## Prognostication in Pediatric Cardiac Arrest

There are no reliable predictors of outcome to assist in guiding termination of resuscitation efforts at this time. Initially, children who received two doses of epinephrine were considered to have a poor prognosis; however, recent reports of neurologically intact survival after prolonged in-hospital resuscitation have been reported. This is particularly true when access to extracorporeal membrane oxygenation is available during the cardiac arrest.

When considering terminating efforts of resuscitation, careful consideration must be made for situations where there is reasonable evidence of intact neurological survival despite prolonged resuscitation recurring or refractory VF or VT, drug toxicity, or primary hypothermia.

## Resuscitation Teams

Table 4 illustrates the roles of individuals during a cardiac arrest. They are arbitrarily assigned. The code team leader is the director of the play that is the resuscitation effort and must be in control at all times. He or she must know the expertise of those individuals on the team and assign roles appropriately. Effective communication is absolutely essential to both patient and rescuer safety as well as to the ultimate success of the resuscitation effort.

The roles of the individuals as outlined in Table 4 are one model for a resuscitation team.

*Table 4*
**Resuscitation Team Composition and Roles of Members**

| Individual | Role |
| --- | --- |
| Code Team Leader | Expert in resuscitation skill |
| | Expert in communication |
| | Directly responsible for all aspects of resuscitation |
| | Monitoring completion of his/her orders |
| | Monitoring effectiveness of interventions (eg, compressions) |
| Respiratory Therapist/ Anesthesia | Airway and breathing assessment |
| | Ventilation |
| | Intubation, as necessary |
| | Sedation |
| Nurse 1 | Intravenous therapy and drug administration |
| Nurse 2/or other delegate | Recording of resuscitation event |
| | Timing of medications and interventions |
| Social Work | Liaison with family and staff |
| | Organize family presence in room |
| | Postresuscitation support for team |
| Spiritual Care/Clergy | Liase with appropriate clergy for family |
| | Family support |
| Child Life Therapist | Assist with acutely ill children undergoing procedures |
| | Assist with communication with siblings |
| | Support siblings in presence during resuscitation |
| Learners | Presence |
| | . Assist with familiar procedures |
| | Active involvement where possible |

## Differential Diagnosis/Etiology

A useful way to approach the child in cardiac arrest is with the following potential etiologies in mind, commonly known as the 6 Hs and 6 Ts (Table 5).

*Table 5*
**6 Hs and 6 Ts**

| Condition | Diagnostic Clues | Management |
| --- | --- | --- |
| **H**ypovolemia | History of volume loss<br>Sinus tachycardia | Crystalloid infusion rapidly |
| **H**ypoxia | Low $SaO_2$<br>Bradydysrhythmias | |
| **H**ion (Acidosis) | DKA<br>Renal failure<br>Premorbid condition | Effective ventilation<br>Treat cause |
| **H**ypokalemia | ECG<br>• Flattened T waves<br>• Prominent U waves<br>• Wide QRS<br>• QT prolongs<br>• Wide complex tachycardia<br>History of vomiting, diuretic use | Rapid, controlled correction if cardiac arrest<br>Consider magnesium |
| **H**yperkalemia | ECG<br>• Peaked T waves<br>• Flattened p waves<br>• QRS widens<br>• Sine-wave pulseless arrest (PEA)<br>Renal failure<br>Medications<br>Poisoning | Nebulized salbutamol<br>Calcium chloride (if QRS wide)<br>Glucose + Insulin (ECG changes)<br>Sodium polystyrene sulfonate<br>Sodium bicarbonate (if acidotic)<br>Dialysis |
| **H**ypoglycemia | Diabetes mellitus<br>Altered LOC<br>Infection<br>Poisoning | Glucose<br>Glucagon |
| **H**ypothermia | Exposure history<br>Core body temperature | Not dead until warm and dead<br>Potential for excellent outcome |

*(continued)*

| Condition | Diagnostic Clues | Management |
|-----------|------------------|------------|
| **T**rauma | Trauma history<br>Signs of external trauma | Crystalloid infusion<br>Blood products (pRBCs)<br>Rule out obstructive shock (eg, tension pneumothorax, tamponade)<br>Early imaging or OR |
| **T**oxins | History, history, history!<br>Look for toxidromes<br>High degree of suspicion<br>Not responding to traditional measures | Empiric antidotes<br>Call for help early |
| **T**amponade | History (eg, postcardiac surgery)<br>Trauma<br>Sinus tachycardia<br>Distended neck veins<br>Low-voltage ECG | Pericardiocentesis |
| **T**ension pneumothorax | Trauma<br>Subcutaneous emphysema<br>Asymmetric breath sounds*<br>Tracheal deviation (late)* | Needle decompression |
| **T**hrombosis, Pulmonary Embolism | Hypercoagulable<br>Clotting disorder | Volume resuscitation |
| **T**hrombosis, Acute MI | Clinical history (eg, cocaine) | Call for help early<br>Aspirin |

*May not be present in children

# Clinical Features: The Rapid Cardiopulmonary Assessment

The assessment of any critically ill child must be a deliberate and systematic process with clear, concise decisions made at each step in the assessment. Clear communication of your interpretation of the assessment with team members facilitates team work in preparing for your next steps in management. Consider early use of the Broselow tape so that as treatment decisions are made, doses and sizes of equipment can be readily available. In a setting in which invasive monitors have already been placed (eg, arterial line), the data from these monitors should be correlated with the clinical status of the child and interpreted accordingly. This information can be exceptionally helpful in both assessment and monitoring the effectiveness of therapy (eg, arterial line to monitor effectiveness of chest compressions).

## General Appearance

- Color
- Mental status (appropriate for age?), responsiveness
- Tone, activity, movement

## Physical Examination of the ABCDEs *(perform rapidly)*

## Airway

- Decision: Clear? Maintainable? Critical action required?
- Trauma: Consider c-spine precautions.

## Breathing

- Work of breathing
- Respiratory rate, mechanics
- Stridor? Breath sounds/air entry?
- Pulse oximetry

## Circulation

- Obtain vitals (HR, BP, capillary refill time centrally)
- Brain perfusion: Observe mental status: Alert? Responds to verbal? Responds to pain? Unresponsive?
- Skin perfusion: Feel skin temperature, peripheral pulses, capillary refill

- Caution: Pulse check unreliable, when in doubt: poor perfusion, bradycardia: initiate effective chest compressions
- Kidney perfusion: Measure urine output—late marker
- Trauma: Control hemorrhage

## Disability

- Glasgow coma scale or modified assessment of level of consciousness
- Pupils—size? symmetry? reactivity?
- Moving all four limbs? Response in all four limbs?

## Exposure

- Rapid head-to-toe survey searching for limb or life-threatening injuries only
- Consider temperature control: watch out for iatrogenic hypothermia

After completing the rapid survey above in less than 60 s, a decision is made about the physiologic status:

- Stable
- Respiratory distress? Respiratory failure?
- Shock: compensated (maintaining blood pressure with poor perfusion)
- Shock: decompensated (no longer maintaining blood pressure)
- Cardiopulmonary failure and arrest

Treatment during the primary survey should be restricted to life threats as you encounter them while remembering, a rapid primary survey (Table 6) allows the general assessment of the patient.

*Table 6*
**Normal Ranges for Heart Rate and Minimum Acceptable Systolic Blood Pressure by Age**

| Minimum SBP | | Normal Ranges for HR | | |
|---|---|---|---|---|
| Age | SBP (5th percentile) | Age | Awake HR | Mean HR |
| 0–1 mo | 60 | 0–3 mo | 85–205 | 140 |
| 1 mo–1 yr | 70 | 3 mo–2 yr | 100–190 | 130 |
| 1–10 yr | 70 + (2 × Age) | 2 yr–10 yr | 60–140 | 80 |
| >10 yr | 90 | >10 yr | 60–100 | 75 |

Adapted from Gillette et al., 1989 and Hazinski et al., 2002

## Management and Treatment—The PALS Algorithms

- Cardiopulmonary arrest is the endpoint where the compensatory mechanisms of the child have failed.
- In 2005, the International Liasion Committee on Resuscitation, in cooperation with the American Heart Association and the Heart and Stroke Foundation of Canada undertook a complete review of the literature of resuscitation and published the Consensus on Science with Treatment Recommendations and the Guidelines for Emergency Cardiac Care.

## Key Messages of the 2005 Guidelines for Pediatric Advanced Life Support

- Treating the child in respiratory distress or failure results in far better outcomes than if that child is allowed to progress to cardiac arrest. Most children who survive from cardiac arrest are neurologically devastated though significant progress is being made in the use of advanced therapies (eg, ECMO) that have shown promising results.
- Early, effective bystander CPR improves outcomes.
- The ratio of chest compressions to ventilations has been changed to allow for more "time on the chest" fewer interruptions, more effective compressions (push hard and push fast), longer sustained coronary and cerebral perfusion, and the prevention of hyperventilation.
- Intubation is not associated with increased survival; a renewed emphasis on effective chest compressions results in a renewed focus on ventilation as opposed to definitive airway management until there is a response to initial resuscitative interventions.
- Hyperventilation results in poor outcomes for several reasons such as increased intrathoracic pressure, decreased venous return, decreased cerebral and coronary perfusion pressures, and decreased cardiac output. Ventilation rates are often much higher than those recommended.
- Rhythm and pulse checks are limited to every 2 min after 2 full min of high-quality CPR. The reason not to check a pulse after defibrillation (see algorithm below) is that despite obtaining a perfusing rhythm, most patients will not obtain a measurable cardiac output for some time. The resumption of high-quality chest compressions allows for continued circulation and maintenance of coronary artery perfusion.
- A one-shock protocol has been adopted while the principle of "stacked shocks" has been removed. Subsequent shocks were not felt to offer an advantage and the resumption of CPR was felt to be of greater benefit.

- For every second electricity is not being delivered, effective chest compressions must be provided.

## Postresuscitation Stabilization

After cardiac arrest, there are several issues of which the receiving physician must be aware (Tables 7 and 8). Assuming primary and secondary surveys have been undertaken, a systems-based approach is necessary to review the critically ill child who has survived resuscitation.

This is not an exhaustive discussion of postresuscitation support but provides basic initial parameters to the approach of the most critically ill children. There are common pitfalls in postresuscitation management and commonly encountered problems. These are listed in Table 9. Caution should be paid to avoid occurrences of these events and rapidly treat them should they occur.

*Table 7*
**Postresuscitation Stabilization**

| System | Assessment and Interventions |
|--------|------------------------------|
| Airway and Respiratory Systems | Supplemental oxygenation<br>Review need for intubation if not intubated<br>Sedation, analgesia<br>Consider neuromuscular blockade<br>Review tube position, CXR, ABG<br>Initial ventilator settings<br>$CO_2$ measurements<br>Orogastric or nasogastric tube |
| Cardiovascular System | Continuous cardiorespiratory monitoring<br>Consider central access if IO access was necessary or peripheral access is tenuous<br>Consider arterial line to monitor MAP and provide access for frequent sampling<br>Vasopressor support<br>Inotropic support<br>Imaging echocardiogram<br>Monitor markers of perfusion to guide resuscitation (eg, lactate) |
| Neurologic System | Do not provide routine hyperventilation in absence of obvious signs of impending cerebral herniation<br>Consider postresuscitation therapeutic hypothermia<br>Monitor temperature and avoid hyperthermia<br>Treat sources of fever as necessary |

| System | Assessment and Interventions |
|---|---|
| Renal System | Monitor urine output |
| Interhospital Transport | Consider need for transport |
| | Specialized transport team availability |
| | Mode of transportation |
| | Monitor exhaled $CO_2$ en route |

*Table 8*

## Differences in Adult, Child, and Infant Cardiopulmonary Resuscitation

| Maneuver | ADULT Adolescent and older | CHILD 1 year to adolescent | INFANT Under 1 year of age |
|---|---|---|---|
| **Airway** | Jaw thrust | | |
| **Breathing** Initial | 2 breaths at 1 s/breath | 2 effective breaths at 1 s/breath | |
| **Rescue breathing without chest compressions** | 10–12 breaths min | 12–20 breaths min | 12–20 breaths min |
| **Rescue breaths for CPR with advanced airway** | 8–10 breaths min | 8–10 breaths min | 8–10 breaths min |
| *Conscious* patient, **Foreign-body airway obstruction** | Heimlich maneuver (abdominal thrusts) | Back blows and chest thrusts | Back blows and chest thrusts |
| *Unconscious* patient, **Foreign-body airway obstruction** | Begin CPR sequence. After chest compressions, check airway for object. | | |
| **Circulation** Pulse check ($\leq 10$ s) | Carotid | | Brachial |
| **Compression** landmarks | Lower half of the sternum, between nipples | | Just below nipple line (lower half of the sternum) |

*(continued)*

| Maneuver | ADULT Adolescent and older | CHILD 1 year to adolescent | INFANT Under 1 year of age |
|---|---|---|---|
| **Compression** method *Push hard, push fast, allow complete recoil* | Heel of one hand, other hand on top | Heel of one hand or as for adults | 2 or 3 fingers; 2 person: thumbs encircling technique |
| **Compression** depth | 1.5 to 2 inches | Approximately one third to one half the depth of the chest | |
| **Compression** rate | Approximately 100/min | | |
| **Compression-ventilation ratio** | 30:2 (one or two rescuers) | 30:2 (single rescuer) 15:2 (2 rescuers) | |
| **Defibrillation** AED | Use adult pads Do not use child pads | Use AED after 5 cycles of CPR (out of hospital). Use pediatric system for child 1 to 8 years, if available. For sudden collapse out of hospital or in-hospital arrest, use AED as soon as possible | No recommendations |

*Source:* Adapted with permission from the 2005 AHA Guidelines for Cardiopulmonary Resuscitation and Emergency Cardiovascular Care, Part 3: Overview of CPR, p. IV-15.

*Table 9*
## Common Pitfalls in Postresuscitation Stabilization

- Endotracheal tube displacement—consider continuous end-tidal $CO_2$ monitoring
- Hypoglycemia—consider frequent monitoring of blood glucose
- Electrolyte abnormalities
- Iatrogenic hypothermia
- Hypotension—ensure adequate preload and vasopressor/inotropic therapy

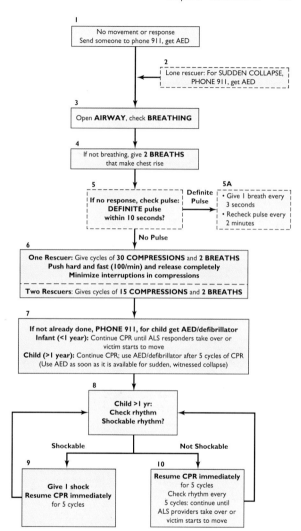

**Figure 9** Algorithim for first responders.
*Source:* 2005 AHA Guidelines, p. IV-158.

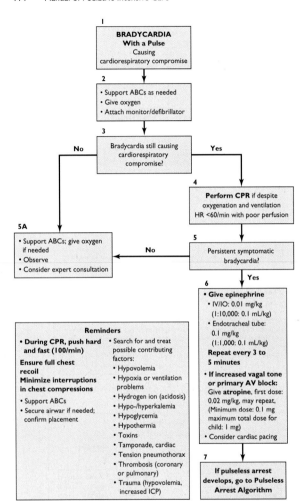

**Figure 10**  Algorithm for Bradycardia.
*Source:* 2005 AHA Guidelines, p. IV-176.

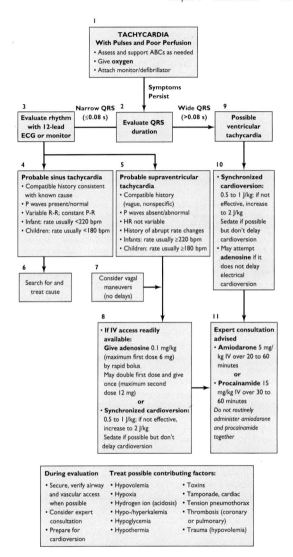

**Figure 11**   Algorithm for Tachycardia.

*Source:* 2005 AHA Guidelines, p. IV-178   •   For the treatment of a patient with poor perfusion and tachycardia is rapid electrical cardioversion. • Success of electrical cardioversion is high. Unless unconscious, appropriate procedural sedation and analgesia must be provided.

# References

Su E, Schmidt TA, Mann NC, Zechnich AD. A randomized controlled trial to assess decay in acquired knowledge among paramedics completing a pediatric resuscitation course. Acad Emerg Med 2000;7:779–86.

Young R, King L. An evaluation of knowledge and skill retention following an in-house advanced life support course. Nurs Crit Care 2000;5:7–14.

Schwid HA, Rooke GA, Ross BK, Sivarajan M. Use of a computerized advanced life support simulator improves retention of advanced cardiac life support guidelines better than a textbook review. Crit Care Med 1999;27:821–4.

Kaczorowski J, Levitt C, Hammond M, et al. Retention of neonatal resuscitation skills and knowledge: a randomized controlled trial. Fam Med 1998;30:705–11.

Kaye W, Mancini ME, Rallis SF. Advanced cardiac life support refresher course using standardized objective-based Mega Code testing. Crit Care Med 1987;15:55–60.

Boudreaux ED, Francis JL, Loyacano T. Family presence during invasive procedures and resuscitation in the emergency department: a critical review and suggestions for future research. Ann Emerg Med 2002;40:193–205.

Henderson DP, Knapp JF. Report of the National Consensus Conference on family presence during pediatric cardiopulmonary resuscitation and procedures. J Emerg Nurs 2006;32:23–9.

Ong MEH, Stiell I, Osmond MH, et al. Etiology of pediatric out-of-hospital cardiac arrest by coroner's diagnosis. Resuscitation 2006;68:335–42.

Suominen P, Olkkola KT, Voipio V, et al. Utstein style reporting of in-hospital pediatric cardiopulmonary resuscitation. Resuscitation 2000;45:17–25.

Wik L, Kramer-Johansen J, Myklebust H, et al. Quality of cardiopulmonary resuscitation during out-of-hospital cardiac arrest. JAMA 2005;293:299–304.

Abella BS, Alvardo JP, Myklebust H, et al. Quality of cardiopulmonary resuscitation during in-hospital cardiac arrest. JAMA 2005;293:305–10.

Aufderheide TP, Sigurdsson G, Pirrallo RG, et al. Hyperventilation-induced hypotension during CPR. Circulation 2004;109:1960–5.

Aufderheide TP, et al. Death by hyperventilation: a common and life-threatening problem during cardiopulmonary resuscitation. Crit Care Med 2004;32:S345–51.

Aufderheide TP. The problem with and benefit of ventilations: should our approach be the same in cardiac and respiratory arrest? Curr Opin Crit Care 2006;12:207–12.

Abella BS, Sandbo N, Vassilatos P, et al. Chest compression rates during cardiopulmonary resuscitation are suboptimal: a prospective study during in-hospital cardiac arrest. Circulation 2005;428–34.

Wolfe JA, Maier GW, Newton JR Jr, et al. Phsiologic determinants of coronary blood flow during external cardiac massage. J Thorac Cardiovasc Surg 1998;95:523–32.

Eftestol T, Sunde K, Steen PA. Effects of interrupting precordial compressions on calculated probability of defibrillation success during out-of-hospital cardiac arrest. Circulation 2002;105:2270–3.

Reis AG, Nadkarni V, Perondi MB, et al. A prospective investigation into the epidemiology of in-hospital pediatric cardiopulmonary resuscitation using the international Utstein reporting style. Pediatrics 2002;109:200–9.

Lopez-Herce J, Garcia C, Dominguez P, et al. Characteristics and outcome of cardiorespiratory arrest in children. Resuscitation 2004;63:311–20.

Duncan BW, Ibrahim AE, Hraska V, et al. Use of rapid-deployment extracorporeal membrane oxygenation for the resuscitation of pediatric patients with heart disease after cardiac arrest. J Thorac Cardiovasc Surg 1998;116-305–11.

del Nido PJ, Dalton HJ, Thompson AE. Extracorporeal membrane oxygenator rescue in children during cardiac arrest after cardiac surgery. Circulation 1992;86:II-300–4.

Gillette PC, Garson A Jr, Porter CJ, McNamara DG. Dysrhythmias. In: Adams FG, Emmanouilides GC, Reimenschenider TA, editors. Mossi Heart Disease in Infants, Children, and Adolescents. 4th ed. Baltimore, MD: Williams and Wilkins; 1989:725–41.

International Liason Committee on Resuscitation. 2005 International Consensus on Cardiopulmonary Resuscitation and Emergency Cardiovascular Care with Treatment Recommendations. Circulation 2005;112(suppl III).

2005 American Heart Association Guidelines for Cardiopulmonary Resuscitation and Emergency Cardiovascular Care. Circulation 2005;112(suppl IV).

# Chapter 6

# Pulmonary

## A. Cystic Fibrosis in the ICU

Kristie R Ross
Michael W Konstan

### Introduction

- Cystic fibrosis (CF) is the most common life shortening inherited disorder in Caucasians, affecting 1 in 3,000 to 4,000 live births.
- CF is characterized by a defect in the CF transmembrane conductance regulator (CFTR), a chloride channel located on the apical membrane of epithelial cells.
- Lack of functioning CFTR leads to impaired mucus clearance, chronic infection, chronic inflammation, and eventually bronchiectasis. Progression of lung disease due to this cycle of infection and inflammation remains the most common cause of morbidity and mortality. Other life-threatening pulmonary complications include massive hemoptysis and pneumothorax.

This chapter focuses on the ICU presentation, and only discusses the initial diagnosis in relation to this. Furthermore, treatment of a pulmonary exacerbation usually does not require an intensive care unit (ICU) setting. However, when exacerbations are severe and/or accompanied by other complications such as acute respiratory failure (ARF), massive hemoptysis, or pneumothorax, close monitoring and aggressive treatment in an ICU may be warranted.

### Exacerbation of Chronic Infection

- Exacerbations of chronic pulmonary infection with *Pseudomonas aeruginosa*, other gram-negative organisms and *Staphylococcus aureus* must be treated. Patients with exacerbations may present with worsening cough, increased sputum production, decline in pulmonary function (most frequently measured by $FEV_1$), dyspnea, and crackles on physical exam.

- The mainstays of therapy for exacerbations that have failed oral and inhaled antibiotics are intravenous antibiotics and intensification of airway clearance. Antibiotics should be directed against the pathogens isolated from sputum or oropharyngeal swabs.
- If no organisms are recovered, consider empiric anti-pseudomonal therapy.
- Bronchoalveolar lavage to detect pathogens should also be considered for patients refractory to therapy.
- Unlike treating acute pulmonary infections in non-CF patients where the goal of therapy is eradication of the pathogen, eradication of chronic infection in CF is uncommon.
- *Pseduomonas aeruginosa* and other gram-negative pathogens should be treated with combination therapy (most commonly with a β-lactam plus aminoglycoside) to improve efficacy and to decrease the emergence of resistant organisms. When available, in vitro susceptibility testing can guide antibiotic choices. Consult with CF physicians for guidance regarding antibiotic choice and dosing.
- Higher doses of antibiotics are used to treat CF patients because they have a higher volume of distribution and more rapid clearance for many drugs. Adhere to infection control practice guidelines described in the Cystic Fibrosis Foundation Consensus document. Some suggested guidelines are given below in Table 1.

*Table 1*
## Key Principles of Treating Exacerbations of Chronic Infection in CF

- Direct antibiotics against pathogens recovered in sputum.
- Use combination therapy for *Pseudomonas* and other gram-negative organisms.
- Assume all patients are infected with transmissible organisms; practice infection control.
- Goal of therapy is reduction of symptoms, not eradication of pathogens.
- Intensify airway clearance therapy with high-frequency chest wall oscillation, vibratory PEP, or percussion and drainage to at least three times a day.

- *Burkholderia cepacia* complex are gram-negative organisms that are often resistant to multiple classes of antibiotics. Infection with *B. cepacia* complex is sometimes associated with cepacia syndrome, which can result in sepsis and death. *B. cepacia* complex organisms are transmissible from person-to-person, so infection control must be practiced. Synergy testing at reference laboratories can guide antibiotic therapy directed against this pathogen; therapy generally includes meropenem in combination with another agent.

## Some Commonly Used Regimens

Although not meant to be an exhaustive list, some commonly used drugs and doses are listed below. Coexisting conditions such as renal insufficiency, liver disease, and other medications should be considered in determining appropriate dosing. The following dosing suggestions for intravenous antibiotics are for patients without clinically significant kidney or liver disease.

- Ceftazidine 150–200 mg/kg/day divided q8h, max 2 g/dose
- Colistin 5–7 mg/kg/day, divided q8h, max 100 mg/dose; requires close monitoring for renal and central nervous system (CNS) toxicities, consult practitioner experienced with using intravenous colistin prior to using
- Meropenem 120 mg/kg/day divided q8h, max 2 g/dose
- Piperacillin 400 mg/kg/day divided q6h, max 4 g/dose
- Tobramycin 10 mg/kg/day divided q8h or once daily; blood level monitoring is recommended for q8h dosing
- Vancomycin 40–45 mg/kg/day divided q8h in children (max 2 g/day), 1 g q12h in adults

# Respiratory Failure

- The unfavorable prognosis for CF patients requiring mechanical ventilation described more than 25 years ago led most CF practitioners to direct efforts at palliative care for end-stage lung disease. However, recent advances in care, including noninvasive positive pressure ventilation (NPPV) and lung transplantation, suggest that aggressive management may be appropriate in limited cases.
- The decision to initiate NPPV or invasive mechanical ventilation (IMV) for respiratory failure due to an exacerbation of

chronic infection is complicated. Under ideal conditions, it will involve joint discussions with the patient (if age appropriate), the primary CF physician and other CF team members, and the ICU physicians and staff. Patients suffering from progressive chronic respiratory failure often cannot be extubated once mechanical ventilation is instituted, thus prolonging end of life.

- The decision to initiate mechanical ventilation is more likely to be made for a patient experiencing ARF as opposed to slowly progressing chronic respiratory failure.

- Recent data demonstrates better outcomes for younger patients and for patients in whom respiratory failure is a result of a viral infection rather than an exacerbation of chronic bacterial infection.

- Some centers advocate mechanical ventilation as a bridge to transplant; the availability of organs and willingness of the transplant center to proceed with transplant in a patient requiring mechanical ventilation should be considered.

# Hemoptysis

- Hemoptysis is a common complication of CF. While it is most often present as blood-streaked sputum, life-threatening hemoptysis can occur in approximately 1% of CF patients per year. While the pathogenesis is not completely understood, massive hemoptysis in CF is usually the result of worsening infection and inflammation leading to erosion into the enlarged and tortuous systemic bronchial arteries.

- Massive hemoptysis, defined as >240 mL in a 24-hour period or several consecutive days of >100 mL/day, is a medical emergency and will most often require evaluation and treatment in an ICU setting.

- Emergent use of vasopressin should be considered prior to admission to the ICU. After initial stabilization of the patient, ensuring adequate airway, breathing, and circulation, the evaluation should be directed at determining the etiology and site of bleeding. The evaluation is outlined in Table 2. As with any patient presenting with massive hemoptysis, the possibility of a retained foreign body should be considered.

- CF patients are at risk for clotting dysfunction due to vitamin K deficiency and CF-related liver disease.

- Bronchoscopy is rarely indicated in the acute setting as localization of the source may be difficult to ascertain due to

*Table 2*
## Initial Evaluation of the CF Patient with Massive Hemoptysis

- Establish the bleeding is pulmonary in origin and not from the gastrointestinal (GI) tract or upper airway.
- Determine if drugs that exacerbate bleeding are being used.
- Obtain CBC, PTT, PT, liver function tests, type, and cross.
- Obtain CXR to evaluate for new lung disease, findings suggestive of fungal or atypical mycobacterial infection or retained foreign body.
- Obtain sputum culture and sensitivity.
- Bronchial artery angiography may be needed to determine the source of bleeding and to direct embolization.
- Bronchoscopy may be indicated to rule out retained foreign body, if the source of bleeding is in question, or if surgery is being considered as therapy.

CBC, complete blood count; PT, prothrombin time; PTT, partial prothrombin time; CXR, chest X-ray.

    movement of blood throughout the airways with cough and respiration.
- Angiography by experienced interventional radiologists is more likely to clearly define the source of bleeding and may be therapeutic if the involved vessels can be embolized.

The published recommendations for the treatment of massive hemoptysis in CF are based largely on expert opinion and are outlined in Table 3. Bronchial artery embolization has

*Table 3*
## Treatment of Massive Hemoptysis in CF

- Maintain an adequate airway, breathing, and circulation.
- Consider use of intravenous vasopressin to slow bleeding.
- Correct coagulation defects with vitamin K, fresh frozen plasma as needed.
- Replace acute blood loss if significant.
- Discontinue drugs that interfere with clotting.
- Treat underlying infection with IV antibiotics directed against pathogens identified by sputum culture.
- Local airway treatment for life-threatening bleeding may be considered including endobronchial/airway tamponade, topical therapy with alpha-agonists, selective intubation.
- Bronchial artery embolization may be needed if bleeding is not controlled with other measures.

a reported success rate of 75% to 93%, although it may require several procedures to attain success. Serious complications include organ infarction and death. If experienced interventional radiologists are not available, consideration for transfer to an institution with experience in this procedure should be considered. Rarely, bleeding will continue despite these therapies and local pulmonary resection may be indicated.

# Pneumothorax

- Pneumothoraces occur in CF as a result of rupture of blebs on the surface of the lung. The reported incidence of pneumothorax in CF is 1 in 100 to 167 per year and occurs more commonly in older patients with advanced lung disease.
- Presenting symptoms depend on the size of the air leak and may range from no symptoms, to mild to severe chest pain, to cardiac arrest due to tension pneumothorax. Additional presenting symptoms and signs include rapid onset of chest pain, tachypnea, tachycardia, dyspnea, decreased breath sounds, and excursion on the affected side. The chest radiograph is generally sufficient for diagnosis; inspiratory/expiratory films may aid in visualizing a small air collection.
- As with pneumothorax due to other diseases, therapy depends on the size and clinical presentation. Small (< 20%) or asymptomatic pneumothoraces can be managed conservatively with monitoring for expansion and resolution by repeat CXR. The use of 100% oxygen has not been established to be effective and should not be used in patients with advanced lung disease and carbon dioxide retention as the effect of oxygen may suppress the respiratory drive. Large, rapidly expanding pneumothoraces require chest-tube insertion (see Chapter 23, "Procedures"). Care should be taken to distinguish pneumothorax from bullous disease prior to consideration of chest tube placement. Chest tubes should be removed 12 to 24 hours after the air leak resolves. If the air collection is not improved 24 to 48 hours after chest tube insertion or recurs after chest tube removal, surgical intervention with chemical or surgical pleurodesis should be considered. Chemical pleurodesis is not as successful as surgical pleurodesis/partial pleurectomy, and should not be performed on patients who are lung transplant candidates.
- After resolution, patients should be counseled to refrain 2 to 4 weeks from activities that increase the risk of recurrence

*Table 4*
## Key Points in Evaluating and Treating Pneumothorax in CF Patients

- Maintain an adequate airway, breathing, and circulation
- CXR is the diagnostic modality of choice
- Small (<20%) asymptomatic pneumothoraces may be observed for expansion and resolution
- Avoid 100% oxygen in patients with evidence of $CO_2$ retention
- Chest tube placement is indicated in large or symptomatic pneumothoraces
- Surgical pleurodesis is indicated if the pneumothorax persists or recurs
- Chemical pleurodesis is an option for patients who are not surgical candidates
- Avoid air travel and pulmonary function testing for 4 weeks after resolution

CXR, chest X-ray.

including air travel and weight lifting/isometric exercise. Pulmonary function testing should also be avoided during this recovery period. Scuba diving is contraindicated in any CF patient who has had a pneumothorax, and in patients with moderate to severe lung disease.

# End-of-Life Care

- Despite attempts to predict mortality based on $FEV_1$ in CF, it is very difficult to accurately predict death in an individual CF patient. While discussions regarding end-of-life care are ideally held prior to admission to the hospital or ICU with respiratory failure, the difficulty in predicting mortality may preclude this.
- Decisions regarding resuscitation, continuation, or withdrawal of support and comfort measures should include the patient, the patient's family, and the CF and ICU teams.
- Standard care, including IV antibiotics and airway clearance (as tolerated), should be continued unless these therapies interfere with the patient's comfort.
- In patients in whom hypercapnia and depressed mental status predominate, few additional comfort measures will be necessary. However, some patients experience severe

hypoxemia and air hunger which must be addressed. Oxygen can aid in relieving dyspnea. While oxygen should be delivered cautiously, the terminal patient's comfort must be balanced with the clinician's hesitation to deliver enough oxygen to depress the respiratory drive. The other mainstay of treating dyspnea is intravenous morphine. Doses as low as 0.1 mg (total dose) may be effective in some patients; others will require doses up to 5 to 30 mg/h. There is little evidence for the use of nebulized opiates, although case reports suggest there may be a mild benefit.

- Consideration for where the patient will ultimately die depends on a number of factors, most importantly the patient's and family's wishes. Some may prefer the hospital ward (as opposed to the ICU) where they know the staff well due to frequent hospital stays; others may prefer a hospice setting or even at their home. As with any terminally ill patient, the family experiencing the loss of a loved one, particularly a child, will need support. Bereavement counseling and help with funeral arrangements should be considered, through institutional resources or hospice as appropriate. A sibling or other family member with CF will likely need additional emotional support.

## Unusual Presentations to the ICU

Although uncommon, children not yet diagnosed with CF may present to the ICU with life-threatening problems.

- Clinicians should have a high index of suspicion for CF in infants and young children who present with hyponatremic dehydration with altered mental status and seizures, or anasarca secondary to severe hypoproteinemia. Elevated concentrations of electrolytes in the sweat can result in hyponatremic hypochloremic dehydration with metabolic alkalosis. One study found the incidence of hyponatremic dehydration in newly diagnosed CF infants to be 16.5%; delayed diagnosis was identified as a risk factor.

- Less commonly, hyponatremic hypochloremic metabolic alkalosis progresses to severe hypoelectrolytemia with shock or mental status changes and seizures requiring management in the ICU. The diagnosis of cystic fibrosis should be entertained in these patients, particularly if the electrolyte abnormalities cannot be explained by GI losses.

- Many infants with pancreatic insufficiency maintain their weight by increasing caloric intake; however, severe untreated pancreatic insufficiency may manifest with profound hypoproteinemia leading to anasarca. Associated findings include anemia, acrodermatitis enteropathica, and failure to thrive. Infants and young children presenting with this constellation of findings should be tested for CF.

# References

Davis PB, Drumm M, Konstan MW. Cystic fibrosis: state of the art. Am J Respir Crit Care Med 1996;154:1229–56.

Orenstein DM, Rosenstein BJ, Stern RC. Cystic fibrosis medical care. Philadelphia: Lippincott Williams & Wilkins; 2000.

Gibson RL, Burns JL, Ramsey BW. State of the art: pathophysiology and management of pulmonary infections in cystic Fibrosis. Am J Respir Crit Care Med 2003;168:918–51.

Saminan L, Siegel J. Cystic Fibrosis Foundation Consensus Conference on infection control participants: infection control recommendations for patients with cystic fibrosis: microbiology, important pathogens, and infection control practices to prevent patient-to-patient transmission. Am J Infect Control 2003;31:S1–62.

Davis PB, di Sant'Agnese PA. Assisted ventilation for patients with cystic fibrosis. JAMA 1978;239:1851–4.

Berlinski A, Fan LF, Kozinetz CA, Oermann CM. Invasive mechanical ventilation for acute respiratory failure in children with cystic fibrosis: outcome analysis and case-control study. Pediatr Pulmonol 2002;34:297–303.

Sood N, Paradowski LJ, Yankaskas JR. Outcomes of intensive care unit care in adults with cystic fibrosis. Am J Respir Crit Care Med 2001;163:335–8.

Ellafi M, Visonneau C, Cost J, et al. One year outcome after severe pulmonary exacerbation in adults with cystic fibrosis. Am J Respir Crit Care Med 2005;171:158–64.

Schidlow DV, Taussig LM, Knowles MR. Cystic Fibrosis Foundation Consensus Conference report on pulmonary complications of cystic fibrosis. Pediatr Pulmonol 1993;15:187–98.

Flume PA, Yankaska JR, Ebeling M, et al. Massive hemoptysis in cystic fibrosis. Chest 2005;128:729–38.

Brinson GM, Noone PG, Mauro MA, et al. Bronchial artery embolization for the treatment of hemoptysis in patients with cystic fibrosis. Am J Respir Crit Care Med 1998;157:1951–8.

Spector ML, Stern RC. Pneumothorax in cystic fibrosis: a 26 year experience. Ann Thorac Surg 1989;47:204–7.

Flume PA. Pneumothorax in cystic fibrosis. Chest 2003;123:217–21.

Schluchter MD, Konstan MW, Davis PB. Jointly modeling the relationship between survival and pulmonary function in cystic fibrosis patients. Statist Med 2002;21:1271–87.

Robinson W. Palliative care in cystic fibrosis. J Palliative Med 2000;3:187–92.

Cohen SP, Dawson TC. Nebulized morphine as a treatment for dyspnea in a child with cystic fibrosis. Pediatrics 2002;110:e38.

Janahai IA, Maciewjewski SR, Teran JM, Oermann CM. Inhaled morphine to relieve dyspnea in advanced cystic fibrosis lung disease. Pediatr Pulmonol 2000;30:257–9.

Fustik S, Pop-Jordanova N, Slaveska N, et al. Metabolic alkalosis with hypoelectrolytemia in infants with cystic fibrosis. Pediatr Int 2002;44:289–92.

Whitehead FJ, Couper RT, Moore L, et al. Dehydration deaths in infants and young children. Am J Forensic Med Pathol 1996;17:73–8.

Muniz AE, Bartle S, Foster R. Edema, anemia, hypoproteinemia and acrodermatitis enteropathica: an uncommon initial presentation of cystic fibrosis. Ped Emerg Care 2004; 20:112–4.

Accurso FJ, Sontac MK, Wagener JS. Complications associated with symptomatic diagnosis in infants with cystic fibrosis. J Pediatr 2005;147:S37–41.

# B.  Bronchiolitis

## Lennox Huang

## Introduction

Bronchiolitis is an acute infection of the respiratory tract affecting upper and lower airways of young children and infants. In most countries there is a marked seasonal variation; for example, in North America and Europe this is almost exclusively a winter disease (November to March). While most cases of bronchiolitis are mild in nature, some children may have life-threatening presentations requiring intensive care unit (ICU) admission. Bronchiolitis may also have severe consequences in children with pre-existing comorbidities such as pulmonary hypertension, cardiac surgery, malignancies, and immunodeficiencies.

## Etiology

RSV is the most common etiologic agent for bronchiolitis. Rates of RSV disease have not decreased despite the introduction of RSV prophylaxis in high risk patients. There are indications that rates have increased and may reflect increasing survival in complex neonatal conditions, and increasing day care availability. Human metapneumovirus (hMPV) has recently been identified as an important etiologic agent; the exact frequency of hMPV infection causing bronchiolitis is unknown.

*Table 1*
### Etiologic Agents of Bronchiolitis

- RSV—respiratory syncytial virus
- Parainfluenza virus
- Adenovirus
- Influenza virus
- Mycoplasma pneumonia
- Human metapneumovirus (hMPV)

# Clinical Presentation

- Maximum age of presentation <1 year (Shay DS JAMA; 1999; 28: 1440–1446).
- Patients with bronchiolitis may present with a wide range of clinical symptoms. To some extent this varies by age, for example, newborns and infants, <6 months of age, often present with severe, life-threatening apnea, especially if prior history of apnea of prematurity.
- For older children a more classic presentation includes upper respiratory symptoms including nasal discharge combined with lower tract symptoms such as wheeze, cough, and lung hyperinflation.
- Radiograph findings may include hyperinflation, shifting/patchy atelectasis, and prominent bronchial markings.
- Fixed lobar infiltrates are more suggestive of bacterial pneumonia but may also be seen in some cases of viral bronchiolitis.
- Some 50% will have lower RT signs (JAMA Ibid).
- Patients requiring PICU admission usually present with the following:

  - Respiratory distress
  - Apnea
  - Shock
  - Multisystem organ failure

# Differential Diagnosis

- Asthma
- Pneumonia
- Foreign body
- Sepsis
- Congenital heart disease/congestive heart failure
- Differential diagnosis of apnea including the multiple causes of sudden infant death syndrome (SIDS)

## High-Risk Infants

Most infants have no high risk susceptibility, but the following are at especial risk:

- Preterms
- Chronic lung disease of prematurity (BPD)
- Cardiorespiratory disease
- Immunodeficiency

## Management

PICU management of a child with bronchiolitis is supportive in nature and is related to the severity of presentation. Close cardiorespiratory monitoring in addition to basic management of ABCs is essential. Patients frequently require supplemental oxygen, airway suctioning, chest physiotherapy, and nutritional support. Management varies a great deal between sites (Plint et al.), and many institutions have clear care paths for bronchiolitis.

### Prevention of Nosocomial Spread

This is by far the most important way in which successful prevention can be effected. All patients with clinical symptoms consistent with bronchiolitis should be placed in contact and or airborne precautions. Hand decontamination with proper handwashing or alcohol-based gels also aids in preventing spread of the infectious agent. These precautions are especially important in the ward where an infant is admitted with suspected RSV. There are implications also for sibling visiting during periods of high community prevalence.

As discussed above, there are a myriad of local approaches to bronchiolitis. However, recently, the AAP put out authoritative guidelines ranked by evidence base. We largely follow this approach.

### Bronchodilators

- Multiple meta-analyses and clinical guidelines recommend against the routine use of bronchodilators for bronchiolitis (AAP, Davison et al.).
- Bronchodilators may produce a temporary improvement in clinical symptoms, and may be trialed in a patient with significant respiratory distress, or in a patient with a possible diagnosis of asthma. Bronchodilators should be continued only if there is a documented response.
- Studies comparing nebulized epinephrine with nebulized salbutamol suggest greater clinical improvement with nebulized epinephrine but no difference in long-term outcome (Wainwright et al.).

### Steroids

This remains a controversial area. Although multiple trials have demonstrated no benefit to the administration of systemic or inhaled steroids for bronchiolitis, there is some contradictory data, suggesting that if early in the disease process there may be benefit (Schuh et al.). Nonetheless, the AAP guidelines reject the use of steroids. Steroids fail to produce any improvement in clinical score, length of stay, or admission rates. Systemic steroids should be considered only if a diagnosis of asthma is being entertained.

## Caffeine

Case reports suggest that intravenous caffeine may decrease RSV-associated apnea, especially in younger infants. Routine administration of caffeine is not recommended. A loading dose of intravenous caffeine may be considered as a rescue therapy prior to intubation for apnea.

## Heliox

Heliox (70% helium, 30% oxygen) administration has been demonstrated to lower clinical scores of respiratory distress with reduction of tachypnea, wheeze, and tachycardia. Addition of heliox in mechanically ventilated children does not appear to increase gas exchange. It is not clear whether heliox therapy affects rates of intubation, mechanical ventilation, or length of hospitalization.

## Noninvasive Positive Pressure Ventilation

Noninvasive positive pressure ventilation (NIPPV) includes a heterogeneous group of therapies including nasal or full-mask continuous positive airway pressure (CPAP), and bilevel positive airway pressure (BiPAP). Numerous studies have demonstrated improved ventilation and resolution of apnea with NIPPV. Patients on NIPPV require close monitoring and suctioning to ensure airway patency. NIPPV may decrease the need for intubation and invasive mechanical ventilation.

## Intubation and Mechanical Ventilation

Recurrent apnea, severe respiratory distress, failure of NPPV and decompensated shock are all indications for intubation. Patients with disease severity requiring intubation often remain intubated for over a week.

## Antibiotics

Routine or empiric antibiotics are not recommended for the treatment of viral bronchiolitis. Febrile infants younger than 60 days of age, however, are at risk for serious bacterial infections (SBI). Febrile infants who are RSV-positive are at lower risk than infants without RSV, but the rates of SBI remain significant and may warrant empiric therapy.

## ECMO

Extracorporeal membrane oxygenation (ECMO) has been successfully utilized to treat respiratory failure resulting from bronchiolitis when other modalities have been exhausted. Venovenous ECMO is most frequently used; however, full cardiac support may be required in cases of multisystem organ failure. Survival from ECMO for respiratory failure is high; one case series reported a 96% survival rate.

## Surfactant

Patients requiring mechanical ventilation who progress to ARDS may benefit from surfactant administration. For additional information on management of ARDS, see Chapter 6, "Pulmonary".

# References

American Academy of Pediatrics Diagnosis and management of bronchiolitis. Pediatrics 2006;118:1774–93.

Centers for Disease Control and Prevention. Respiratory syncytial virus activity—United States, 2003–2004. MMWR Morb Mortal Wkly Rep 2004;53:1159–60.

Davison C, Ventre KM, Luchetti M, et al. Efficacy of interventions for bronchiolitis in critically ill infants: a systematic review and meta-analysis. Pediatr Crit Care Med 2004;5:482–9.

Everard ML, Bara A, Kurian M, et al. Anticholinergic drugs for wheeze in children under the age of two years. Cochrane Database Syst Rev 2005; Jul 20;(3):CD001279.

Flores G, Horwitz RI. Efficacy of beta-2-agonists in bronchiolitis: a reappraisal and meta-analysis. Pediatrics 1997;100(2 Pt 1):233–9.

Gavin R, Anderson B, Percival T. Management of severe bronchiolitis: indications for ventilator support. N Z Med J 1996;109:137–9.

Kellner JD, Ohlsson A, Gadomski AM, Wang EE. Bronchodilators for bronchiolitis. Cochrane Database Syst Rev 2000;2:CD001266.

Khan JY, Kerr SJ, Tometzki A, et al. Role of ECMO in the treatment of respiratory syncytial virus bronchiolitis: a collaborative report. Arch Dis Child Fetal Neonatal Ed 1995;73:F91–4.

Levine DA, Platt SL, Dayan PS, et al. Risk of serious bacterial infection in young febrile infants with respiratory syncytial virus infections. Pediatrics 2004;113:1728–34.

Njoku DB, Kliegman RM. Atypical extrapulmonary presentations of severe respiratory syncytial virus infection requiring intensive care. Clin Pediatr (Phila) 1993;32:455–60.

Paret G, Dekel B, Vardi A, et al. Heliox in respiratory failure secondary to bronchiolitis: a new therapy. Pediatr Pulmonol 1996;22:322–3.

Plint AC, Johnson DW, Wiebe N, et al. Practice variation among pediatric emergency departments in the treatment of bronchiolitis. Acad Emerg Med 2004;11:353–60.

Schuh S, Coates AL, Binnie R, et al. Efficacy of oral dexamethasone in outpatients with acute bronchiolitis. J Pediatr 2002;140:27–32.

Schuh S, Johnson D, Canny G, et al. Efficacy of adding nebulized ipratropium bromide to nebulized albuterol therapy in acute bronchiolitis. Pediatrics 1992;90:920–3.

Stretton M, Ajizian SJ, Mitchell I, Newth CJ. Intensive care course and outcome of patients infected with respiratory syncytial virus. Pediatr Pulmonol 1992;13:143–50.

Tobias JD. Caffeine in the treatment of apnea associated with respiratory syncytial virus infection in neonates and infants. South Med J 2000;93:294–6.

Wainwright C, Altamirano L, Cheney M, et al. A multicenter, randomized, double-blind, controlled trial of nebulized epinephrine in infants with acute bronchiolitis. N Engl J Med 2003;349:27–35.

Williams JV, Harris PA, Tollefson SJ, et al. Human metapneumovirus and lower respiratory tract disease in otherwise healthy infants and children. N Engl J Med 2004;350:443–50.

Wohl ME, Chernick V. Treatment of acute bronchiolitis. N Engl J Med 2003;349:82–3.

# C. Severe Acute Asthma in the PICU

Kristie R Ross
Carolyn M Kercsmar

## Key Principles

> - Always consider nonasthma etiologies for wheezing.
> - Intubation and mechanical ventilation is a last-resort intervention.

## Epidemiology

Asthma is a chronic inflammatory disease of the airways characterized by episodic airflow obstruction that is at least partially reversible either spontaneously or with treatment. Acute asthma is common, with 5.4% of children reporting at least one asthma attack during 2004. While most children respond to standard therapy with systemic corticosteroids and low-to-moderate doses of inhaled bronchodilators either at home or in the acute care setting, some will require more intensive therapy. Severe acute asthma requires intensive care unit (ICU) admission with careful monitoring of vital signs, mental status, symptoms, and response to therapy. Risk factors for severe exacerbations are listed in Table 1.

*Table 1*
**Risk Factors for Severe Acute Asthma**

- Previous life-threatening acute exacerbation (rapid deterioration or respiratory failure)
- Food immediate hypersensitivity
- African American race
- Inability to perceive symptoms
- Recent change in controller medication use
- Recent treatment with systemic corticosteroids

Admission to the ICU should be considered if the child is not responding to standard emergency department or inpatient therapy. Maximal therapy given in an inpatient, non-ICU setting will vary among institutions, but generally includes oral or intravenous corticosteroid (1–2 mg/kg), nebulized bronchodilators (up to every 20 minutes for brief periods, usually 1 hour), and subcutaneous epinephrine. Findings that should prompt immediate consideration of transfer to an ICU are listed in Table 2.

# Pathophysiology

Airway inflammation is a key pathologic feature of asthma (see Table 3). Infiltration with lymphocytes and eosinophils, epithelial cell denudation, and thickening of the basement membrane are common findings. Acute bronchoconstriction can be triggered by many stimuli, including allergen-mediated histamine release from mast cells, viral pathogens, irritants, exercise, and cold air. These stimuli also increase airway edema and inflammation via action of leukotrienes and other

*Table 2*
**Guidelines for Admission to ICU**

- Failure to respond to standard inpatient therapy
- Decreased alertness
- Severe accessory muscle use (more than one site)
- Poor air exchange with biphasic wheeze
- Severe dyspnea (1–2 words)
- $PaCO_2 > 40$ mm Hg
- Severe hypoxemia ($O_2$ sat < 90% despite oxygen supplementation at a rate of 1–3 LPM by nasal canula or 30–35% $FiO_2$)

*Table 3*
**Pathophysiologic Features of Acute Asthma**

- Airway inflammation
- Bronchial smooth muscle constriction
- Mucous plugging
- Decreased lung compliance
- V/Q mismatch
- Air trapping

proinflammatory cytokines, proteases, and neurokinins. Airway edema, bronchoconstriction, inflammatory cell infiltrate, and mucous plugging all contribute to the airflow limitation that characterizes acute asthma.

## Clinical Presentation

Presenting complaints include cough, wheezing, chest tightness, and dyspnea. Physical examination findings include increased respiratory rate, cough, increased work of breathing with accessory muscle use, nasal flaring and grunting, prolonged expiratory phase, diminished air exchange, and wheezing (expiratory or biphasic). Rhonchi and rales may be present depending on the degree of mucous production and presence of inciting viral or bacterial lower respiratory tract infection. Cyanosis, depressed mental status, and apnea are late findings and indicate respiratory failure.

## Evaluation

Evaluation of the child admitted to the ICU for status asthmaticus should begin with attention to airway, breathing, and circulation as discussed elsewhere in this handbook. Initial therapy directed at stabilizing the patient (discussed later in the chapter) may be necessary before performing a complete evaluation. Once stabilized, evaluation should include a comprehensive history, physical examination, and radiologic and laboratory evaluation as summarized in Table 4.

*Table 4*
**Evaluation of the Child with Acute Asthma in the PICU**

| History. Complete medical history with focus on: |
| --- |
| • Identifying trigger |
| • Severity of chronic asthma |
| • History of previous severe exacerbations |
|    • ICU admissions |
|    • Use of noninvasive mechanical ventilation |
|    • Intubation |
|    • Hospitalizations/emergency department visits |
|    • History of exacerbations with rapid deterioration |

*(continued)*

- Medications
  - Preventative medication regimen
  - Frequency of rescue medication use
  - Adherence to therapy
- Presence of comorbid conditions
  - Allergy—food and inhalant
  - GERD
  - Sinopulmonary infections (viral/atypical bacterial, bacterial, TB)
  - Aspiration
  - Tracheo/bronchomalacia
- Questions addressing differential diagnosis (see Table 5)

## Physical Examination. Complete physical examination with focus on:

- Vital signs, if possible pulsus paradoxus
- Level of alertness
- Degree of dyspnea
- Accessory muscle use
- Air exchange
- Wheezing, cough, rales, focality of findings
- Cardiac examination

## Laboratory/Radiologic Evaluation

- Blood gas
  - Initial finding in acute asthma is respiratory alkalosis (hyperventilation)
  - Respiratory acidosis may indicate exhaustion, impending respiratory failure
  - Metabolic acidosis may develop due to increased work of breathing and lactate production
- Consider evaluation for infection
  - Viral antigen panel
  - CBC and differential
  - Mycoplasma/Chlamydia evaluation
- CXR
  - Typical findings include overinflation, peribronchial, and perihilar inflammatory changes
  - Look for pneumomediastinum/thorax, infection, focal air trapping, atelectasis
- Flexible bronchoscopy if indicated to rule out airway obstruction from retained foreign body or structural abnormality, evaluate for infection
- Peak flow monitoring: PEFR < 30% predicted associated with elevated $pCO_2$
- Pulmonary function testing may be useful in recovery phase

*Table 5*
**Differential Diagnosis of Acute Asthma**

- Foreign body aspiration
  - History of event often, but not always, elicited
  - Often, but not always, focal chest exam
- Vocal cord dysfunction
- Infection
- Acute hypersensitivity pneumonitis
- Anaphylaxis
- Tracheobronchomalacia
- Airway obstruction due to congenital anomaly
  - Endobronchial/intraluminal lesion
  - Extrinsic compression from thoracic lesion

# Differential Diagnosis

Severe acute asthma may be refractory to standard therapies due to severe underlying disease, comorbid conditions, or because the wheezing is not due to asthma. Therefore, consideration of other etiologies of wheezing must be considered even in the child with a known history of asthma.

# Management

Management of acute asthma in an inpatient setting requires a consistent approach with frequent examination and monitoring. Care paths and protocols have been shown to decrease length of stay, thus improving financial and clinical endpoints for hospitalized children with asthma.

## Pharmacotherapy

Standard initial therapy for severe acute asthma includes the use of inhaled beta-agonists and oral or intravenous corticosteroids. The addition of inhaled anticholinergics may yield small additional benefits with minimal adverse effects. Oxygen is recommended for most patients to maintain saturations above 90%. It may be reasonable to give $O_2$ to all acutely ill asthmatics, as it is a mild bronchodilator and might decrease work of breathing. Frequent reassessment is necessary as rapid deterioration is possible. A treatment algorithm is shown in Figure 1 and specific drugs are reviewed below.

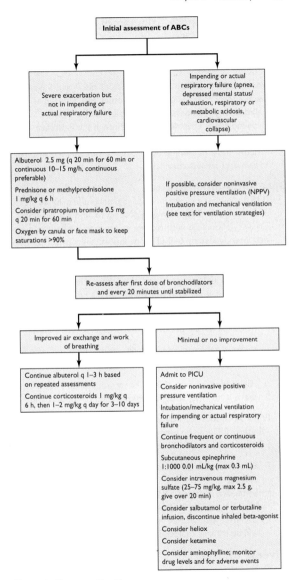

**Figure 1** Treatment Algorithm.

# Selective B2 agonists: Salbutamol, albuterol (racemic and levalbuterol)

## Mechanism

- Selective $\beta_2$-agonist, short-acting
- Racemic albuterol is a 50/50 mixture of the R and S isomers; Levalbuterol contains only the R-isomer and is dosed at one-half the standard doses of racemic albuterol
- Bronchodilator effect is mediated through the R-isomer
- Animal and in vitro studies have demonstrated bronchoconstrictive and proinflammatory effects mediated by the S-isomer; in vivo data are less convincing

## Dose and Administration

- 0.15 mg/kg/dose ( minimum of 2.5 mg) nebulized q 20 minutes x 3–6 doses, then 0.15–0.3 mg/kg/dose up to 10 mg q 1–4 hours
- Delivery should be with oxygen at appropriate flow rate for nebulizer (generally 6–8 LPM) to ensure appropriate particle size (0.8 to 3 μm)
- Delivery is better with mouthpiece rather than mask if age appropriate and patient is alert and cooperative
- May be given at increasing doses for severe cases

  - Continuous nebulized albuterol at rate of 0.3–0.5 mg/kg/h to a maximum of 15 mg/h, ideally given in large-volume nebulizer

    - Equal safety to intermittent dosing, some evidence for increased efficacy in severe exacerbations

  - Higher doses (up to 150 mg/h) recommended by some but there is no clear safety or efficacy data to support this

- IV administration for Salbutamol
- Albuterol MDI can be used at a dose of 4–8 puffs q 20 minutes x 3–6 doses then q 1–4 hours as needed.

  - Efficacy should be equal to nebulized form if technique is correct
  - Some data indicate MDI route superior for younger children
  - Must be given with age-appropriate valved holding device
  - Children with altered mental status or in severe distress will be unlikely to adequately perform correct technique

## Adverse Effects

- Tachycardia—especially in combination with other bronchodilators
- Tremor

- Nausea/vomiting
- Hypokalemia—especially when administered intravenously
- Hyperglycemia
- Increased V/Q mismatch ➜ worsening hypoxemia

# Epinephrine
## Mechanism
- Nonselective β-agonist

## Dose and Administration
- 0.01 mL/kg of 1:1000 solution, max 0.3 mL, given subcutaneously
- Unclear advantage over nebulized beta-agonists but may be useful in children uncooperative with nebulized medications or those with severe airway obstruction not responding to nebulized albuterol

## Adverse Effects
- Cardiovascular toxicities including tachycardia (common), and rarely arrhythmias, hypertension, hypotension, and myocardial ischemia
- Tremor
- Hypokalemia
- Hyperglycemia
- Worsening V/Q mismatch ➜ hypoxemia (may be less than with albuterol)

# Terbutaline
## Mechanism
- β-agonist

## Dose and Administration
- 5 μg/kg IV followed by a continuous infusion of 0.4 μg/kg/min
- The dose of the infusion is increased by 0.2 μg/kg/min every 10–15 minutes to a maximum of 12–16 μg/kg/min
- As with epinephrine, there is no clear evidence that intravenous terbutaline has any advantage over inhaled β-agonist but can be considered in severe cases

## Adverse Effects
- Tachycardia
- Nervousness
- Tremor

- Nausea
- Arrhythmias
- Paradoxical bronchospasm
- Cardiac toxicity

# Anticholinergics (most commonly ipratropium)
## Mechanism
- Bronchodilatation by decreasing parasympathetic cholinergic tone of airway smooth muscle

## Dose and Administration
- Ipratropium 250 to 500 micrograms nebulized
- Should be used in combination with β-agonist
- Repeated dosing (q 20 minutes x 2–3 doses, then q 2–4 hours) more likely to be beneficial than single dosing
- Many studies show modest improvement in pulmonary function data and symptom scores

## Adverse Effects
- Poorly absorbed across mucous membranes so there are minimal systemic anticholinergic effects
- Paradoxical bronchospasm reported ($<2\%$)

# Oral and Intravenous Corticosteroids
## Mechanism
- Decreased synthesis and release of NF-κB and other systemic inflammatory cytokines
- Inhibition of iNOS, cyclooxygenase, phospholipase $A_2$
- Increased β-adrenergic receptors

## Dose and Administration
- Dosing of steroids vary widely between institutions
- There is no advantage of higher doses or intravenous administration over oral administration
- Some theoretical advantage to methylprednisolone demonstrated in animal studies
- Lower doses start at 1 mg/kg/day but may be given up to 2 mg/kg q 6 hours
- Consider prophylaxis for gastritis in critically ill patients

## Adverse Effects
- Hyperglycemia
- Behavioral changes

- Short courses rarely result in significant systemic side effects
- Contraindicated in acute varicella infection, use with caution in patients with diseases likely to be exacerbated by steroids including diabetes mellitus, psychosis, hypertension, peptic ulcer disease

# Magnesium Sulfate
## Mechanism
- Calcium antagonist affecting smooth muscle calcium uptake → bronchodilatation
- Onset of action 20 minutes, persists for approximately 3 hours

## Dose and Administration
- 25–75 mg/kg (max 2.5 g) over 20 minutes (not as a rapid IV bolus)
- Consider for severe acute asthma not responding to inhaled bronchodilators and systemic corticosteroids

## Adverse Effects
- Flushing, hypotension, muscle weakness
- Contraindications: renal failure, heart block, history of cardiac ischemia, hypotension, myasthenia gravis, pregnancy

# Aminophylline
## Mechanism
- Bronchodilator
- Respiratory stimulant, increase in diaphragm contractility
- Anti-inflammatory
- Enhancement of steroid action

## Dose and Administration
- Not routinely recommended in National Heart Lung Blood Institute (NHLBI) guidelines due to narrow therapeutic index and lack of data showing benefit over selective β-agonists in mild to moderate exacerbations
- May have a role in the critically ill child not responding to aggressive therapy with systemic steroids, bronchodilators, anticholinergics and magnesium sulfate
- Loading dose of 6 mg/kg followed by continuous infusion based on age

  - 6 month–1 year    0.6–0.7 mg/kg/h
  - 1–9 years    1 mg/kg/h
  - 9–12 years    0.9 mg/kg/h
  - >12 years    0.7 mg/kg/h

- Blood level monitoring 30 minutes after loading dose and q12 hours during continuous infusion with target 10–20 mg/L, titrate to effect and adverse effect.

## Adverse Effects
- can occur at any blood level
- seizures
- arrhythmias
- headache
- nausea/vomiting
- tachycardia
- agitation
- tremor/nervousness
- multiple drug interactions—potential interactions with concurrent medications should be investigated prior to initiating therapy

# Heliox
## Mechanism
- Density is 1/7 that of air → improved flow through high-resistance airways
- $CO_2$ diffuses 4–5 times faster through helium than air
- A few small studies in children support its use early, to deliver bronchodilators or while intubated to improve gas flow and reduce barotrauma

## Dose and Administration
- Most useful when given as a helium-to-oxygen ratio of 80:20 (therefore not tolerated well in hypoxic patients)
- Can be given as 70:30 helium-to-oxygen
- Either formulation can be used to drive albuterol nebulization

## Adverse Effects
- No serious adverse effects, may not be tolerated in hypoxemic patients

# Ketamine
## Mechanism
- Bronchodilator (through effects on calcium influx and vagally mediated bronchoconstriction of airway smooth muscle)

## Dose and Administration
- Little evidence to support the routine use of ketamine in acute asthma; several case reports suggest it may reduce

the need for intubation/mechanical ventilation in impending respiratory failure
- IV bolus 0.2–1 mg/kg followed by continuous infusion 0.15–0.75 mg/kg/h

## Adverse Effects
- laryngospasm
- bronchorrhea
- dysphoria/hallucinations

## Inhalational Anesthetics
### Mechanism
- Bronchodilatory mechanism unknown

### Administration
- Case reports describe using halothane and isoflurane in mechanically ventilated children not responsive to standard therapies
- Pediatric anesthesiologists should manage these medications

### Adverse effects
- myocardial depression due to negative inotropic effects
- arrhythmias
- hypotension
- nephrotoxicity

## Noninvasive Positive Pressure Ventilation (NPPV)

Noninvasive positive pressure ventilation (NPPV) has been shown to be an effective therapy for acute respiratory failure in adults, but has not been adequately studied in children with acute asthma. Small studies do suggest that NPVV can be tolerated in children with severe acute asthma and can result in improved symptoms scores and gas exchange. The use of NPVV was significantly associated with decreased risk of intubation and mechanical ventilation in a retrospective cohort study of children treated for asthma in pediatric ICUs but the authors caution that this finding should be considered preliminary and that prospective studies are needed. Children may need anxiolytics to tolerate this therapy. Caution should be exercised in children with extensive mucous plugging as it may worsen air trapping.

## Mechanical Ventilation

Intubation and mechanical ventilation is a last-resort intervention. Absolute indications for intubation and mechanical ventilation are apnea, coma, and cardiovascular collapse. Relative indications include exhaustion, respiratory or metabolic acidosis, and depressed mental status.

If necessary, intubation should be performed by experienced personnel in a controlled environment. Children with respiratory failure due to status asthmaticus are likely to have significant air trapping and overinflation, complicating ventilator management. Permissive hypercapnia (or controlled hypoventilation) is a ventilator strategy advocated to minimize peak inspiratory pressure and is achieved by using low tidal volumes and longer expiratory time. Serial physical exams including evaluation of pulsus paradoxus can help guide the level of therapy needed. Ventilators that allow measurement of pulmonary mechanics can help determine appropriate settings; frequent assessment and adjustment may be necessary. Bronchodilators and corticosteroids should be continued in the asthmatic requiring mechanical ventilation. Rates of mechanical ventilation vary widely between centreers, many large high-volume centreers report very low rates of mechanical ventilation for status asthmaticus. See Chapter 6, "Pulmonary" for additional management.

## Disposition

ICU discharge criteria will vary among institutions, but most children should be stable while receiving bronchodilators every 2–3 hours, oral steroids and oxygen at a rate of less than 2 LPM by nasal canula or 35% by face mask. An exacerbation requiring treatment in the ICU represents a major failure of outpatient preventative therapy and should prompt evaluation by a specialist. Goals prior to discharge should include identifying the trigger for this and other severe exacerbations, assessing the child's and parent's understanding of the disease and adherence to preventative therapy, identifying barriers to care, and providing a written asthma action plan and outpatient follow-up.

## References

Expert Panel Report 3: Guidelines for the Diagnosis and Management of Asthma. National Heart Lung and Blood Institute. NIH publication 07-4051, 2007.

Expert Panel Report 2: Guidelines for the Diagnosis and Management of Asthma: Update on Selected Topics 2002 NIH publication no. 02–5074, 2003.

Bloom B, Dey AN. Summary Health Statistics for U.S. Children: National Health Interview Survey, 2004. National Center for Health Statistics. Vital Health Stat 2006;10:1–85.

Kercsmar CM. Asthma. In: Chernick V and Boat TF, editors. Kendig's disorders of the respiratory tract in children, 6th ed. Philadelphia, PA: Saunders; 1998:688–730.

Rodrigo GJ, Castro-Rodriguez JA. Anticholinergics in the treatment of children and adults with acute asthma: a systematic review with meta-analysis. Thorax 2005;60:740–6.

Ciccolella DE, Brennan K, Kelsen SG, Criner GJ. Dose-response characteristics of nebulized albuterol in the treatment of acutely ill, hospitalized asthmatics. J Asthma 1999;36:539–46.

Olshaker J, Jerrard D, Barish RA, et al. The efficacy and safety of a continuous albuterol protocol for the treatment of acute adult asthma attacks. Am J Emerg Med 1993;11:131–3.

Papo MC, Frank J, Thompson AE. A prospective, randomized study of continuous versus intermittent nebulized albuterol for severe status asthmaticu in children. Crit Care Med 1993;21:1479–86.

Carl JC, Myers TR, Kirchner HL, et al. Comparison of racemic albuterol and levalbuterol for the treatment of acute asthma. J Pediatr 2003;143:731–6.

Bolte RG. Emergency department management of pediatric asthma. Clin Ped Emerg Med 5:256–69.

Werner HA. Status asthmaticus in children. Chest 2001;19:1913–29.

Lin YZ, Hsieh KH, Chang LF, Chu CY. Terbutaline nebulization and epinephrine injection in treating acute asthmatic children. Pediatr Allergy Immunol 1996;7:95–9.

Craven D, Kercsmar CM, Myers TR, et al. Ipratropium bromide plus nebulized albuterol for the treatment of hospitalized children with acute asthma. J Pediatr 2001;138:51–8.

Gross NJ. Ipratroprium bromide. NEJM 1988;319:486.

Rachelefsky G. Treating exacerbations of asthma in children: the role of systemic corticosteroids. Pediatrics 2003;112:382–97.

Fiel S. Should corticosteroids be used in the treatment of acute, severe asthma? A case for the use of corticosteroids in acute, severe asthma. Pharmacotherapy 1985;5:327–31.

Ciarello L, Sauer A, Shannon M. Intravenous magnesium therapy for moderate to severe pediatric asthma: results of a randomized, placebo-controlled trial. J Pediatr 1996;129:809–14.

Cheuk DKL, Chau TCH, Lee SL. A meta-analysis on intravenous magnesium sulfate for treating acute asthma. Arch Dis Child 2005;90:74–7.

Wheeler DS, Jacobs BR, Kenreigh CA, et al. Theophylline versus terbutaline in treating critically ill children with status asthmaticus: a prospective, randomized, controlled trial. Pediatr Crit Care Med 2005;6:142–7.

Ream RS, Loftis LL, Albers GM, et al. Efficacy of IV theophylline in children with severe status asthmaticus. Chest 2001;119:1480–8.

Kass JE, Terregino CA. The effect of heliox in acute severe asthma: a randomized controlled trial. Chest 1999;116:296–300.

Carter ER, Webb CR, Moffitt DR. Evaluation of heliox in children hospitalized with acute severe asthma: a randomized crossover trial. Chest 1996;109:1256–61.

Kudukis TM, Manthous CA, Schmidt GA, et al. Inhaled helium-oxygen revisited: effect of inhaled helium oxygen during the treatment of status asthmaticus in children. J Pediatr 1997;130:217–24.

Abd-Allah SA, Rogers MS, Terry M, et al. Helium-oxygen therapy for pediatric acute severe asthma requiring mechanical ventilation. Pediatr Crit Care Med 2003;31:2052–8.

Gupta VK, Cheifetz IM. Heliox administration in the pediatric intensive care unit: an evidence based review. Pediatr Crit Care Med 2005;6:204–11.

Allen JY, Macias CG. The efficacy of ketamine in pediatric emergency department patients who present with acute severe asthma. Ann Emerg Med 2005;46:43–50.

Denmark TK, Crane HA, Brown L. Ketamine to avoid mechanical ventilation in severe pediatric asthma. J Emerg Med 2006;30:163–6.

Petrillo TM, Fortenberry JD, Linzer JF, et al. Emergency department use of ketamine in pediatric status asthmaticus. J Asthma 2001;38:657–64.

Ram FS, Wellington S, Rowe BH, Wedzicha JA. Non-invasive positive pressure ventilation for treatment of respiratory failure due to severe acute exacerbations of asthma. Cochrane Database Syst Rev 2005;1:CD004360.

Soroksky A, Stav D, Shpirer I. A pilot prospective, randomized, placebo-controlled trial of bilevel positive airway pressure in acute asthmatic attack. Chest 2003;123:1018–25.

Carroll CL, Schramm CM. Noninvasive positive pressure ventilation for the treatment of status asthmaticus in children. Ann Allergy Asthma Immunol 2006; 96:454–9.

Thill PJ, McGuire JK, Baden HP, et al. Noninvasive positive-pressure ventilation in children with lower airway obstruction. Pediatr Crit Care Med 2004; 5:337–42.

Akingbola OA, Simakajornboon N, Hadley Jr EF, et al. Noninvasive positive-pressure ventilation in pediatric status asthmaticus. Pediatr Crit Care Med 2002;3:181–4.

Bratton SL, Odetola FO, McCollegan J, et al. Regional variation in ICU care for pediatric patients with asthma. J Pediatr 2005:147–61.

Cohen NH, Eigen H, Shaughnessy TE. Status asthmaticus. Crit Care Clin 1997;13:459–76.

Dworkin G, Kattan M. Mechanical ventilation for status asthmaticus in children. J Pediatr 1989;114:545–9.

# D. Mechanical Ventilation of Pediatric Patients

Paul G Smith

## Introduction

- Mechanical ventilation is a hazardous life-saving modality. The full extent of its hazards has only recently been appreciated. Understanding respiratory pathophysiology and mechanical properties is necessary to match need with application and minimize iatrogenesis.
- As ventilators become more sophisticated, multiple modes enhance interactions between the machine and the patient.
- Basic concepts and physiology remain constant, and are necessary to aid to prioritize decision making.
- Both excess volume and excess pressure (volu-baro-trauma) are iatrogenic causes of Ventilator-Induced Lung Injury (VILI).

This chapter aims to review relevant physiology, and guide ventilator therapy and pitfalls.

## Nomenclature

### Respiratory Cycle

A respiratory cycle consists of a single lung inflation and exhalation. There are five variables that describe a single cycle of a mechanically ventilated breath.

1. Tidal volume
2. Pressure—Peak and PEEP
3. Time
4. Flow
5. Ratio of inspiratory to expiratory time

## Indications for Mechanical Ventilation

Mechanical ventilation is indicated for failure of any part of the respiratory system (from central and peripheral nervous system, to musculoskeletal, cardiovascular systems, upper airways, and lung parenchyma). Mechanical ventilation may also be indicated as adjuvant therapy of non-respiratory diseases (eg, pulmonary hypertension or various forms of shock). In both situations, early anticipatory use of mechanical ventilation must be combined with knowledge of respiratory physiology to deliver safe and optimal support. Direct selection of modes and settings is dictated by disease process. Recognize that the ventilator only supports while the process resolves; it does not treat lung disease. Termination of mechanical support should be accomplished at the earliest practical time that the disease process allows.

1. Respiratory failure—inadequate oxygenation, ventilation, or respiratory drive.
2. Pulmonary toilet—excessive secretions.
3. Airway protection—trauma (face, head, or neck), altered mental status, surgery. Consider intubation and mechanical ventilation if Glasgow Coma Scale is 8 or less. Goals are to match normal physiology and maximize patient comfort by enhancing patient/ventilator interactions.
4. Metabolic failure—Mechanical ventilation may be used to support critically ill patients when the lungs are not the major source of pathology, even in the context of near normal gas exchange (eg, shock, sepsis, or heart failure). Goals of therapy are to minimize oxygen consumption while maximizing oxygen delivery to tissues. Select a mode and settings that provide full support to minimize patient work-oxygen consumption. Initial settings might also need to provide extra positive end expiratory pressure (PEEP) to prevent alveolar collapse.
5. Controlled hyperventilation for specific diseases—In certain disease states one may need to alter arterial blood gases beyond physiological limits. Such diseases include:

   a. Cerebral edema—Hyperventilation can temporarily decrease intracranial pressure by decreasing the size of the cerebral vascular compartment. The safety of even brief periods of hyperventilation in cerebral edema has been recently questioned for the potential worsening of brain ischemia. Every effort should be made to avoid hypercarbia, but hyperventilation below normal $PaCO_2$ should be reserved for cerebral herniation (see Chapter 20, Head Injury for Additional Management).

b. Pulmonary hypertension—Both oxygen and hyperventilation are valuable means for treating pulmonary hypertensive crises.

c. Poisonings—Carbon dioxide and cyanide poisonings uncouple oxygen from hemoglobin causing tissue hypoxia. The goals of maximizing blood oxygen and minimizing oxygen consumption are provided by mechanical ventilation. Hyperventilation using an oxygen/carbon dioxide mixture shortens the elimination phase of carbon dioxide.

# Mechanical Determinants of Gas Exchange

The parameters selected in mechanical ventilators must take into account the mechanical characteristics of the patients. These relationships are summarized in the equation of motion of the respiratory system.

$$P_{mus} + P_{tr} = 1/C_{RS} \times \text{volume} + R_{RS} \times \text{flow}$$

This formula states that the amount of pressure generated (muscular or $P_{mus}$ added to transthoracic or $P_{tr}$ given by the ventilator) to deliver a tidal volume is equal to the pressure necessary to move the associated flow through the circuit and lung resistances ($R_{rs}$) plus the pressure necessary to move a volume against the reciprocal of compliance (elastance) of respiratory system. Accordingly, assuming a steady state:

1. The variables of pressure, flow, and volume are interrelated. Changing one must affect the others. If either more volume is to be delivered, or the rate of the volume delivery (flow) is to be increased, more pressure is required.

2. If a change in pressure is necessary to deliver a given tidal volume, this signifies there is a change in pulmonary mechanics [rule out: resistance problems of large airways (kinked endotracheal tube, mucous plugging), small airways (acute bronchospasm), or compliance (pneumothorax, pulmonary edema, or hemorrhage].

# Determinants of Carbon Dioxide ($CO_2$) Elimination

Carbon dioxide elimination from the lungs is directly related to minute ventilation.

$$\text{Minute ventilation} = \text{Respiratory Rate} \times \text{Alveolar Ventilation}$$

- For effective alveolar ventilation, gases must pass through a large, non-gas exchanging portion of the lung termed anatomic dead space. Dead space is a component of ventilation efficiency and normally accounts for at least one-third of the tidal volume. This percentage can be increased appreciably by certain diseases, long or voluminous ventilator circuits or by ill-advised ventilator management. Dead space can be either anatomic (eg., airways), or physiologic. Physiologic dead space signifies a virtual volume that represents both the anatomic dead space and the percentage of the tidal volume not participating in gas exchange, as occurs with gas trapping from hyperinflation of the lungs.
- End-tidal $CO_2$ monitors and real-time displays of mechanical parameters are excellent tools for determining physiologic dead space and seeing the real time effects of changes in ventilator settings.

## Hypercarbia

- First, always eliminate emergent problems such as mucous plugging, etc.
- Next, verify respiratory rate and tidal volume are adequate. If these are low, increasing either rate or tidal volume to physiologic limits is a reasonable first approach.
- If rate and tidal volume are within physiologic range, invariably dead space is abnormal. This is especially true if $CO_2$ rises when minute ventilation is increased (eg, with increased anatomic dead space such as long ET tubes).
- Alternatively, physiologic dead space might be increased: consider inspiratory time too short for diffusion of air to the alveoli; consider PEEP too low so that lung units are not well recruited; consider PEEP is excessive causing an increase in trapped gas.
- A common mistake is to simply increase the ventilatory rate or tidal volume resulting in worsening gas trapping and hypercarbia. Instead adjust settings to allow a longer expiratory time,

either by decreasing the respiratory rate or by shortening the inspiratory time.

- Gas trapping can also be a problem with excessive PEEP and an inadequate tidal volume combination, or excessive respiratory rates.

# Determinants of Arterial Oxygenation

Delivery of oxygen to the blood is dictated by the slow diffusion coefficient of oxygen, as compared to $CO_2$. The determinants of arterial oxygenation are $FiO_2$, ventilation, and blood flow.

Five basic processes can interfere with gas exchange causing hypoxemia. They can be differentiated in part by the response to therapy (Table 1).

- By far the most frequent of these is V/Q mismatch. Because the diffusion of oxygen is slow relative to the rate of blood flow, oxygen uptake into the blood depends on the ideal matching of blood flow (Q) to alveolar ventilation (V). In the normal adult lung, ventilation is about 4 L/min and blood flow about 5 L/min so a V/Q of about 0.8. If perfusion exceeds ventilation, there is a venous admixture. These conditions normally exist in the base of the lung where flow exceeds ventilation

*Table 1*
**Causes of Hypoxemia and Their Response to Therapy**

| | Increased ventilation | Increased $FiO_2$ | Mean airway pressure |
|---|---|---|---|
| Hypoventilation | ++++ | ++ | +/− |
| Low inspired $FiO_2$ | +/− | ++++ | 0 |
| Diffusion gradient | +/− | ++ | ++ |
| V/Q mismatch | +/− | +++ | +/− |
| Right-to-left shunt | 0 | 0 | 0 |

++++ = highly responsive;  ++ = partially responsive;
+/− = depends on multiple factors; 0 = no response

with a V/Q ratio of approximately 0.6. The ventilator effects on gas exchange are complex. Ventilation improves oxygenation by assuring oxygen reaches the alveoli and $CO_2$ is eliminated, but also by causing oxygen-dependent alveolar capillary dilation in pulmonary hypertension.

- Maximizing oxygen exposure to functioning alveolar surfaces and optimizing blood flow overcomes hypoxemia from many parenchymal lung diseases—a concept known as "Open the Lung."
- Oxygenation is most affected by 2 variables: inspired oxygen tension and mean airway pressure. Mean airway pressure ($P_{\overline{aw}}$) can be calculated by the formula

$$P_{\overline{aw}} = K \ (PIP\text{-}PEEP)(T_I/\,TCT) \ + \ PEEP$$

where $PIP_I$ the peak inspiratory pressure, PEEP the end expiratory pressure, $T_I$ the inspiratory Time, TCT the total cycle time, and K a constant adjusting the value for the shape of the pressure waveform. Think of $P_{\overline{aw}}$ as the area under the pressure waveform.

- In pressure control with a rapid rise in airway pressure, K approaches 1. In volume control with a gradual rise in airway pressure, K approaches 0.5. This formula predicts that the most efficient way to raise MAP is with PEEP. Increasing inspiratory time also increases $P_{\overline{aw}}$ without over-distension of the lung. Increasing the PIP yields very little increase in $P_{\overline{aw}}$ and entails a greater risk of lung damage.
- Remember that increasing $P_{\overline{aw}}$ can be either beneficial (by increasing recruitment of collapsed alveoli) or detrimental (by decreasing pulmonary capillary flow or restricting venous return impeding cardiac output).

## Variables on a Ventilator

Any conventional ventilatory mode can be described by specifying the four variables that need to be set for a ventilator respiratory cycle.

1. Triggering variable—This describes what initiates a ventilator inspiration. If the breath is initiated at a set time, the mode is referred to as a "control" mode. Other triggers are patient effort causing a drop in airway pressure, flow, or volume in which case the mode is an "assist" mode. Infrequently, the breath is initiated by the clinician (operator controlled).

2. Limiting variable—Unfortunately, there has been an overlapping of terminology in using the word control to describe the "limiting" variable. This variable is the set end-point the ventilator is programmed to reach. In **volume control** mode, a set tidal volume is delivered; if patient mechanics change, the ventilator needs adjustment of the pressure to guarantee the set volume. In **pressure control** mode, the peak pressure is set. If patient mechanics change, the volume delivered changes inversely to changes in resistance or elastance (worsening mechanics means less tidal volume delivery).

   In a few modes, time is the limiting variable as is the case in high-frequency ventilation.

3. Cycle variable—The cycle variable determines what "cycles" the ventilator from inspiration to expiration, and can be either time, volume, pressure, or flow.

4. Baseline—The baseline variable describes the characteristics of the expiratory phase and usually refers to PEEP but might describe a time-limited exhalation as is the case with APRV (described below).

## Basic Modes

**Pressure control ventilation** (PCV) delivers each breath to a pre-determined peak inspiratory pressure (PIP).

- Historically, regulating pressure was mechanically easier than regulating volume especially when delivering small volumes.
- Pressure control was used more frequently in neonatal ICUs for this reason. Tidal volumes for a 2 kg neonate might be as low as 10–20 mL per breath. This is more difficult to regulate than a peak inspiratory pressure of 20 or 25. VILI in that population had been more easily avoided when pressure gradients were limited.
- However, as ventilators became more sophisticated by means of electronic circuitry, volume-controlled ventilation is more common. VILI is caused by volume distension as well as excess pressures, hence the term barotrauma/volutrauma. An advantage is that the flow is delivered in a ramp decelerating waveform (Figure 1). This allows the pressure to build quickly and to be maintained at a constant level. This flow configuration can achieve a $P_{\overline{aw}}$ at a lower PIP and theoretically improve distribution of ventilation.

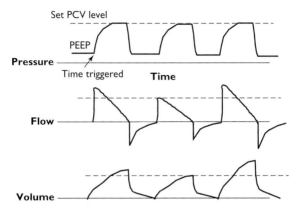

**Figure 1** Pressure Control Ventilation (PCV)—Time scale of PCV demonstrating the effects of changing mechanics on flow and volume. Pressure is held constant, but volume and flow are variable. Note the ramp deceleration waveform of flow as the set pressure is reached rapidly.

**Volume control** includes several modes wherein the ventilator delivers a constant volume with each breath. This might require adjustment of pressure in the face of changing mechanics.

- Modes that are volume controlled include Assist Control, IMV, or SIMV (see below).
- Advantages include the guarantee of constant minute ventilation, and control of tidal volume allowing reduction of volutrauma.
- Necessary in cerebral edema or pulmonary hypertension where hypercarbia might have deleterious effects.
- Beneficial in lung diseases characterized by rapidly changing pulmonary mechanics, such as asthma or congestive heart failure, to maintain constant tidal volume delivery as the disease progresses or resolves.
- Volume control also monitors changes in patient status breath to breath: if flow is kept constant, pressure has to change if patient mechanics changes. Because pressure alarms are more easily engineered, situations of worsening mechanics, accidental extubation, and plugs in ventilator tubing are rapidly noticed as compared to pressure control.

# Specific Modes

1. **Assist control**—ventilator breaths are time cycled and volume controlled, occurring at a regular interval, independent of patient effort.

- "Assist" signifies that in addition to a specified minimum number of breaths, a full breath is delivered with each patient effort (if of sufficient strength to trigger the ventilator).
- Theoretically, patient effort is minimized because each patient effort is fully supported.
- The primary disadvantage is the inability to use it as a weaning mode. No matter how few breaths are set, a full breath is delivered each time the patient makes a sufficient effort.

2. **Intermittent mandatory ventilation (IMV); Synchronized IMV**—In IMV or SIMV, volume controlled breaths are delivered at a set rate.

- Between breaths, flow is present allowing patient efforts to achieve extra ventilation though the valves and amount of flow can vary adding significant work to patient effort.
- The tidal volume achieved by patient effort between delivered breaths depends on muscle strength, drive, and the amount of flow available.
- In SIMV (synchronized IMV), patient effort can trigger a full breath within a discrete window of time shortly before a delivered breath was scheduled (Figure 2). However, a fully assisted breath is not available outside that window so that patient effort is not fully supported for any more breaths than are scheduled per minute. Minute ventilation is guaranteed but patient/ventilator dyssynchrony can still cause patient discomfort. SIMV may decrease patient work while delivering guaranteed minute ventilation. SIMV is a mode that allows easy transitioning from fully supported to fully independent breathing (weaning).

3. **Pressure support ventilation (PSV)** was designed to improve ventilator response to patient effort during spontaneous breathing. The patient determines the initiation and duration of the inspiration, and if the level of support is appropriate, the size of the tidal volume.

- Breaths are triggered either by a patient-induced drop in airway pressure or flow.
- The ventilator then generates sufficient flow to raise airway pressure to a preset level.

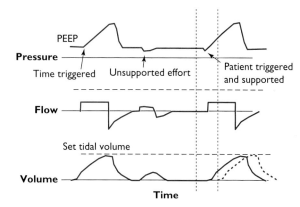

**Figure 2** Synchronized Intermittent Mandatory Ventilation (SIMV)—Breaths can either be time triggered or pateint effort triggered. The flow waveform is typically constant (square wave) as pressure and volume gradually increase. If a patient makes an effort (signified by a drop in airway pressure and inspiratory flow) outside a specifed window of time (vertical dashed lines), there is no mechanical support. If the effort comes within a specific window of time, they are able to initiate delivery of a complete breath. Tidal volumes of each delivered breath is constant.

- The greater the patient effort, the more flow the ventilator has to generate to maintain that pressure—so the tidal volume is determined by the pressure support level set, the magnitude, and the duration of patient effort.
- Tidal volumes vary from breath to breath instead of being ventilator controlled (Figure 3). They are either as a weaning mode or in combination with other modes such as SIMV to improve patient comfort.
- Despite goals of improving patient comfort, PSV may exacerbate distress (eg, the added work of the resistance of ventilator circuit, the time lag and effort needed to open the flow valves, and ability of the ventilator to deliver as much flow as the patient wants; respiratory distress can be excessive especially for infants treated on older model ventilators). PSV does not necessarily eliminate all work of breathing because patient effort and interaction with the ventilator are necessary. PSV is also inappropriate when there is diminished or absent central drive with depressed CNS function.

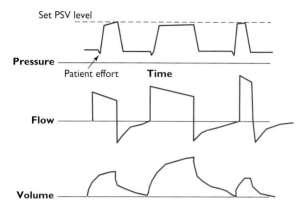

**Figure 3** Pressure support ventilation—Patient effort demonstrated by a drop in airway pressure initiates inspiratory flow assistance to whatever level necessary to maintain the PSV level set by the clinician. The interval between cycles, duration of inspiration, and tidal volume are determined by the patient's efforts.

- The first variable set is the triggering sensitivity. This usually is set as sensitive as possible without causing "auto-cycling" usually 1–3 cm $H_2O$ pressure.
- Auto-cycling occurs when the ventilator senses an effort that wasn't there and can be due to leaks from the circuit, or especially in young infants, movement of air in the ET tube with cardiac motion.
- The amount of patient effort required to trigger a breath is largely determined by setting the sensitivity of the ventilator to airway changes: the less sensitive, the greater the effort necessary to trigger the breath.
- The second setting determined is the amount of pressure to be maintained in the airways during inspiration. Sometimes the pressure support level is used only to overcome added resistance to breathing against ET tube resistance while another mode such as SIMV is being used for full support. This is empirically chosen to be somewhere between 5 and 8 cm $H_2O$ though external resistances can easily fall outside of this range. If the majority of the work of breathing is to be provided with PSV, pressures between 10 and 25 cm $H_2O$ above PEEP are often necessary (depends on the passive mechanics of respiratory system).

- Determine the PSV level necessary to minimize work by standing at the bedside and adjusting the pressure support level while monitoring for signs of distress.
- The patient determines breath termination. When patient effort decreases, to the point that flow necessary to maintain the preset airway pressure is less than a certain percentage of peak flow (often 75% of peak flow), the ventilator senses this as breath termination when supplemental flow from the ventilator ceases.
- Both the respiratory rate and tidal volumes vary between breaths in parallel with patient effort.
- Used in many settings either to deliver nearly full support, as a weaning mode (slowly adjusting the level of pressure support down) or simply to overcome ET tube resistance.

## Newer Modes

The development of microchips and improved electronic circuitry has allowed for the development of increasingly sophisticated modes. Theoretically they improve interactions with patients' efforts, while limiting injurious distending pressures and volumes. The following is a brief review of these modes, although they are not routine and have not yet established a role in pediatric respiratory failure. There is a serious paucity of randomized controlled clinical trial to evaluate any of these therapies. Even basic modes of ventilation suffer from this limitation.

### 1. Pressure-regulated volume control (PRVC)

PRVC aims to guarantee tidal volume and minute ventilation while simultaneously limiting the pressure at which the breath was delivered. These require feedback loop capability, to adjust flow rates throughout inspiration to keep airway pressure below a preset level, while responding to changes in patient mechanics. The ventilator delivers an initial small breath during which it calculates patient mechanics and derives an optimal flow rate to deliver the set volume within a pressure-limited parameter selected by the clinician. One potential advantage is that the decelerating ramp flow is maintained so mean airway pressure is augmented without increases in volume distension. Though this mode is being widely used, there is no evidence to suggest improved long-term outcomes. PRVC does not lend itself well as a weaning mode nor to use for patients with large air leaks from ET tubes or bronchopulmonary fistulas.

2. **Proportional assist ventilation or proportional pressure support** (the name depends on the ventilator brand) is where the ventilator guarantees the percentage of work in response to an individual's respiratory system mechanics (compliance/elastance and resistance). The pressure delivered varies from breath to breath, if there are changes in elastance, resistance, and flow demand from the patient. This requires constant monitoring of airway pressure and flow by the ventilator from which the ventilator derives the optimal flow to be generated. Usually this is set to overcome a set percentage of the work of breathing. For example, the pressure required to overcome 75% of the work created by an individual's respiratory system mechanics might be 15 cm $H_2O$. As the patient's disease or effort changes, the ventilator varies its output to maintain this proportion of the workload. To wean, the clinician decreases the delivered proportion of the work of breathing.

3. **Airway pressure release ventilation (APRV)**

APRV is essentially a high level of sustained airway pressure, around which a patient's spontaneous respiratory effort allows small changes in airway pressure and thus a reduced tidal volume (breathing against a high level of PEEP). This mode in effect elevates mean airway pressure without great increases in peak distending volume. Theoretically, APRV results in improved oxygenation through a maintained high mean airway pressure without increasing VILI from over distension. Enabling patients to breathe even against high airway pressure improves comfort and might enhance $CO_2$ elimination. To allow efficient $CO_2$ elimination, periodically this sustained pressure is "dumped" (pressure release), allowing alveoli to empty. Reports claim benefit in oxygenation, comfort, and cardiac output in select patients. Airway pressure release ventilation increases cardiac performance in patients with acute lung injury/adult respiratory distress syndrome. Large controlled studies showing changes in outcome with this mode are lacking. Only select ventilators are able to deliver this mode of ventilation.

4. **High-frequency oscillatory ventilation (HFOV)**

It has long been known that ventilation is possible to affect gas exchange with rapid vibrations with very adequate gas movement with the vibrations of, in essence, a large loud speaker; in the case of HFOV, gas movement is accomplished using a large diameter flexible piston (diaphragm) that oscillates toward and away from the airway perpendicular to a high bias flow of gas. Gas exchange is enhanced by the resulting turbulence and high flow of gas in the large airways as well as relative negative forces applied to the airways when the piston moves back. HFOV has for years been possible using only one FDA approved ventilator. Recently a ventilator more appropriate for larger patients has been marketed. There are some RCTs to evaluate HFOV, but these are mainly in newborns.

## Advantages of HFOV

- High mean pressure can be maintained constantly with little change in lung volume during the phases of the diaphragm movement.
- Smaller swings in lung volumes theoretically will cause less VILI while allowing high mean airway pressures.
- It works extremely well with small patients and low compliance lung diseases (eg, pneumonia, pulmonary edema).
- HFOV is effective in large bronchopulmonary fistulae because there is less gas flow through the disrupted lung unit, preserving healing.

HFOV is generally less effective in adults and high airway resistance diseases (asthma, bronchiolitis).

Setting up HFOV:

- First, set the mean airway pressure, usually 2–3 cm $H_2O$ pressure more than the mean airway pressure used on the conventional ventilator before changing modes.
- Rate (frequency) is initiated based on patient age; the younger the patient, the greater the rate. More rapid rates are appropriate in smaller children because the resonance frequency of the chest wall is greater.
- Select the driving pressure. The driving pressure is the pressure differential created by to-and-fro movement of the piston and is responsible for the to-and-fro movement of air in the airways. The greater the driving pressure, the more air that is moved into the airways with each oscillation. Because this pressure differential is attenuated with each change in airway caliber (from the ventilator tubing to the ET tube, trachea, and smaller airway) and because the ventilator rate is so rapid, the pressure differential the alveoli see is less than 10% of that created by the piston.

- The HFOV is simple to use. For oxygenation, one adjusts either the mean airway pressure or $FiO_2$. For changes in ventilation, the driving pressure is usually increased. While changes in rate can also change $CO_2$ elimination, this is usually discouraged because lower rates at the same driving pressure difference result in large volume swings in the lungs and attenuate the potential of beneficial effects inherent in HFOV.

# Noninvasive Mechanical Ventilation (NIMV)

Whenever practical, noninvasive ventilation offers some distinct advantages over endotracheal intubation and invasive ventilation. Rates of NIMV have increased in recent years with many practitioners utilizing it as a first step of respiratory support prior to intubation for mechanical ventilation.

Advantages of NIMV

- Eliminates need for endotracheal intubation and the risks associated with induction.
- May be started earlier in the disease process, potentially affecting the course of the disease.
- Less sedation is necessary, ventilator interactions with the patient are better and some complications are lessened.
- Can be used as an adjunct in extubation, allowing for shorter ICU stays and fewer ventilator dependent days.
- Can be used chronically and thus subsets of patients may be discharged home or to a chronic care facility on NIMV.
- Recently, noninvasive methods have become more successful with better interfaces (face and nasal masks) and ventilators sensitive to patient effort.
- There are 2 basic methods of NIMV.

**Continuous positive airway pressure (CPAP)** has only one level of pressure without inspiratory assistance.

- Useful in many settings, from central apnea of the newborn to obstructive sleep apnea.
- In severe asthma, CPAP can decrease work of breathing. In this case, small airway obstruction prevents complete equilibration of alveolar pressure with atmospheric pressure, analogous to intrinsic PEEP (positive pressure at the end of exhalation).

For inspiratory flow to be achieved without assistance, the patient must generate an additional negative pressure equal to this intrinsic PEEP before inspiratory flow is possible. CPAP provides this pressure so that work of breathing is decreased. CPAP can also improve V/Q mismatch by stenting areas of obstruction, allowing full expiration.

- CPAP is also useful in alveolar collapse (pulmonary edema) and elevated upper airway resistance resulting in increased work of breathing (obstructive sleep apnea, upper airway edema in infants).

**Bi-level positive airway pressure (BiPAP)** signifies additional pressure assistance during inspiration in addition to the constant positive pressure of CPAP.

- BiPAP offers all the advantages of CPAP and in addition decreases work of breathing where muscles may be tiring or inadequate for full lung expansion.
- BiPAP may be set to time cycle with a respiratory rate in cases where there is decreased respiratory drive.
- Useful where respiratory failure complicates terminal disease so invasive ventilation might not be reversible. This offers temporary help while a secondary disease is treated (eg, pneumonia complicating AIDS). Patients can interact with family and friends without the threat of death on a ventilator. Requires an interface between the patient's face and ventilator circuitry with very minimal pressure leak so that the ventilator can sense the effort necessary to trigger the inspiratory assist pressure. Such a tight seal between the mask and the patient's face can limit the number of hours a day that BiPAP can be used before skin breakdown is a problem.
- As survival with chronic conditions such as cystic fibrosis and neuro-degenerative diseases improves, NIMV is being used more frequently to prolong and improve quality of life with the gradual onset of respiratory insufficiency.
- When using either CPAP or BiPAP, patient acceptance is much better when very low levels of pressure are used initially (eg, 8 and 4 cm $H_2O$ for upper and lower pressures respectively) and then gradually increased (over minutes, not hours) to more effective levels. Ideally, the patient can communicate the levels of support that are most comfortable.

Limitations of NIMV

- Patient cooperation—young infants, toddlers, and young children are the most problematic age group for this reason.
- Feeding is problematic especially with high level BiPAP in acute respiratory disease. Air swallowing, emesis, and poor access to the upper airway combine to increase the risk of aspiration.
- Facial trauma and impaired levels of consciousness are also contraindications to NIMV.
- Respiratory compromise severe enough to prohibit periods of time without the face mask cannot be practically managed with NIMV because skin breakdown will be a limiting factor.

# Monitoring

In general, the continuous monitoring capability made possible by technological advances has proven much more useful than single point-in-time blood sampling. Continuous monitoring has helped shift the emphasis of ventilator strategies from the normalization of arterial blood gases to optimization of oxygen delivery and minimizing VILI and improved our understanding of respiratory physiology. **Arterial blood gas measurements** (ABGs) are the gold standard to which noninvasive modalities are compared and validated. They are invaluable for accurately assessing blood oxygen content, acid base status, and the lungs' capacity for gas exchange. Studies suggest frequent underutilization of the information available from the values and incomplete understanding of their limitations. The presence of an arterial catheter often leads to routine (unnecessary) blood gas analysis; blood gases should be restricted to assessment of clinical changes in the patient's condition.

---

Monitoring Modalities

1. Arterial blood gases
   ***Advantages/uses***
- Accurately determining and following the severity of lung disease and response to therapy. For example, various indices such as $PaO_2/FiO_2$ or Alveolar to arterial gradient are more exacting estimates of lung health than noninvasive monitoring

---

- Acid/base status
- Blood oxygen content and hemoglobinopathies
  **Disadvantages/limitations**
- Point-in-time measurement that can change rapidly with changes in $FiO_2$ or lung disease (5–20 min) so not useful for continuous monitoring
- Pain and potential of ischemia distal to site of arterial puncture

2. Pulse oximetry
   **Advantages/uses**
- Constant monitoring of blood oxygen saturation and early detector of respiratory compromise
- Nearly universal availability in developed countries
- Easy to use
- More useful than ABG for minute-to-minute adjustments in therapy
  **Disadvantages/limitations**
- In general read falsely high and so are inaccurate in hemoglobinopathies
- Less accurate at lower range than in normal range of blood oxygen saturation
- Can be difficult to use in low perfusion states

3. End tidal $CO_2$ ($ETCO_2$, capnometry, capnography)
   **Advantages/uses**
- Rapid indicator of changes in alveolar ventilation/dead space
- Useful for determining efficiency of ventilation (deadspace calculations)
- Sudden changes can be used to detect certain diseases such as pulmonary embolism, pneumothorax, dislodged, or malpositioned ET tube
  **Disadvantages/limitations**
- Inaccurate with large air leaks from ET tube or bronchopulmonary fistula
- Less accurate with small tidal volumes (neonates and infants) and rapid respiratory rates

Monitoring in the ICU often incorporates at least two of the modalities listed to overcome the respective limitations and disadvantages. Venous and capillary blood gases paired with pulse oximetry are also frequently used to assess ventilation and oxygenation, respectively. Central venous blood gases have the added advantage of estimating cardiac output and oxygen consumption via the $SVO_2$.

# Mechanics (See above under equation of motion)

Mechanical ventilation provides the positive pressure necessary to overcome opposing forces of elastance and resistance to allow gas exchange. Respiratory mechanics describes the physical characteristics of the respiratory system that impede lung inflation and deflation. Knowing which components are abnormal, directs medical and ventilatory therapy for specific diseases. Modern ventilators display parameters to allow continuous monitoring of respiratory mechanics.

The most basic displays show raw values of pressure, flow, and volume in a time scale. These allow derivation of total respiratory system resistance and dynamic compliance (during active inflation/deflation). The normal values of these parameters change with age (infants have higher airway resistance and lower respiratory system compliance). As noted above, the equation of motion of the respiratory system demonstrates the interdependence of the parameters of pressure, flow, and volume. For example, given a constant volume, increasing flow (delivering the breath in a shorter time) requires a greater pressure. Also, given constant volume and flow, a change mechanics will require an increase in delivery pressure.

During volume control, an increase in PIP can come from either a decrease in compliance or an increase in airway resistance. The first step should always be to check the patient for the following:

- Implies an increase in resistance or a decrease in compliance.
- First, examine the patient.
- Rule out mechanical problems with the circuitry such as mucous plugs, malpositioned or dislodged ET tube, or pneumothoraces prior to making ventilator adjustments.
- Patient effort or coughing is also frequent cause of sudden increases in PIP and might indicate a need for a change in support to improve patient comfort.

After examining these possibilities, consider whether there is a change in patient respiratory system resistance—or if there is a decrease in patient respiratory compliance.

- These two main causes can be differentiated using the ventilator derivation of dynamic compliance (Cdyn)—which is calculated by dividing the tidal volume delivered by the PIP-PEEP—to perform an end-inspiratory occlusion maneuver (occlude the airway at the moment inspiration complete). Occlusion stops flow, drops pressure from PIP until the pressure plateaus at a new lower level (the plateau pressure or Pplat).
- This initial pressure drop (Pinit = PIP − Pplat) is the pressure necessary to overcome airway resistance; a large pressure drop indicates a problem with airway resistance while a small pressure drop indicates a problem with compliance.
- Pplat can be used to calculate static compliance by the formula: Volume/Pplat − PEEP = Cstat.

## Using the flow waveform

- By convention inspiratory flow is above the zero line and expiratory flow below.
- Increases in airway resistance often manifest as a prolonged expiratory phase, usually with a concave shape. It is important to note if exhalation has stopped before the next breath is initiated by seeing the flow return to zero (Figure 4).
- If not, this indicates a degree of air trapping. Such trapping (breath stacking) causes lung hyperinflation, eventually decreasing compliance and requiring greater inspiratory pressure and increased work of breathing for the patient.
- This generates "intrinsic PEEP," ie, pressure in the alveoli at end exhalation greater than the set PEEP (Figure 4).

Strategies for improving breath stacking:

- Allow more time for exhalation.
- Shorten inspiratory time.
- Decrease rate.
- Decrease tidal volume.

Though these maneuvers might decrease minute ventilation, $CO_2$ elimination and mechanics parameters often improve because of more complete emptying of the lungs. Intrinsic PEEP might also indicate a need for more aggressive bronchodilator therapy or airway suctioning.

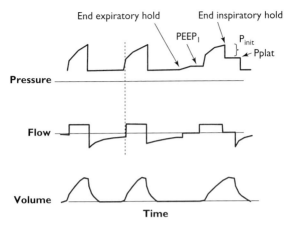

**Figure 4** Time scale waveforms of pressure, flow, and volume in a patient with small airway obstruction. In the first breath, note the prolonged and concave expiratory flow that continues even when the next breath is intiated by the ventilator. In the second breath, a dashed line has been drawn that shows that added pressure above PEEP has to be added before inspiratory flow is seen. This added pressure is refered to as intrinsic PEEP or $PEEP_i$ and represents the alveolar pressure still remaining at initiation of the next breath. $PEEP_i$ can be measured as the inspiratory pressure necessary for inspiratory flow to begin (where the dashed line meets the pressure waveform) or by an expiratory hold maneuver (first arrow). In this case, the ventilator closes stop all flow and the passive rise in pressure above PEEP is noted. The third breath further demonstrates the effects of increased airway resistance. In this breath, end-inspiratory hold maneuver has been performed. At this point, flow is stopped and the peak airway pressure (PIP) rapidly drops to a new, lower plateau (Pplat). The magnitude of the initial pressure drop from PIP to Pplat is termed Pinit and signifies the resistive pressure. A large Pinit signifies increased airway resistance.

# Manipulation of Ventilator Settings

## General Concepts

Historically, manipulation of settings emphasized normalization of blood gases and complete recruitment of all lung units. Modern management has now shifted to the following concepts:

1. Prevent VILI.
2. Facilitate patient comfort by minimizing work.
3. Enhance weaning from the ventilator.
4. Optimize oxygen transport (not the same as "normalization" of arterial blood gases).

Initial ventilator settings should take into account the condition necessitating mechanical assistance. For example, the need for simple airway protection should start with near physiologic parameters while shock and ARDS might be better served with initially greater mean airway pressures and tidal volumes until patient stability is assured and then gradual reduction.

1. **Normal lungs**—(eg, airway protection, postoperative patients, trauma): Initiate therapy with either SIMV or assist control with tidal volumes of 6–8 mL/kg and "physiologic PEEP" of 3–5 cm $H_2O$. $FiO_2$ is usually set at 1.0 and quickly weaned to something less than 0.5 to prevent oxygen-induced lung injury while following the pulse oximetry readings. It is important to guarantee both minute ventilation and patient comfort.

2. **Low compliance lungs**—Diseases characterized by low lung compliance (ARDS, pulmonary edema, etc.): Start with a volume control mode such as assist control or SIMV. Volume control mode guarantees minute ventilation in contrast to pressure control where minute ventilation will vary as the disease progresses or resolves. Furthermore, mechanical parameters are easier to follow and detect improvement or deterioration of the respiratory system. It is usual practice to initiate mechanical support on the "generous" side, and wean back rather than risk further patient instability through hypoxia, acidosis, or increased distress. Commonly tidal volumes of between 8 and 10 mL/kg, physiologic rates of 20–30 breaths per minute and at least 5 cm $H_2O$ of PEEP (to minimize progressive alveolar collapse) are chosen to assure initial stability. If the patient is making respiratory efforts, distress can be minimized with the addition of pressure support empirically chosen between 5 and 10 cm $H_2O$ pressure above PEEP.

3. The immediate goals after the initial setup are to try and reach lung protective settings as quickly as practical (see consensus statement of several critical care organizations).

4. Titrating increases in PEEP are used as necessary to achieve oxyhemoglobin saturation levels of at least 93% while weaning $FiO_2$ to less than 0.6. PEEP increases are usually made in increments of 2–3 cm $H_2O$ over a period of one or two hours until either oxygenation is improved or an adverse result is noted. These adverse events might include:

   a. Increase in PIP to 35 cm $H_2O$ (or plateau pressure over 30 cm $H_2O$). This is taken as indirect evidence of lung overdistension. When increased PIP is seen, first the patient should be evaluated for mechanical problems (mucous plugs, malpositioned ET tube, pneumothorax, intrinsic PEEP, etc.). Then the options are to lower the tidal volume to between 4 and 6 mL/kg and/or prolong the inspiratory time so that lung inflation is accomplished with less flow and pressure.

b. Hypotension suggests impedance to venous return. The first measure taken should always be to evaluate the patient for emergent causes such as pneumothorax. Once other reasons for hypotension have been eliminated, it is often reasonable to increase intravascular volume with fluid boluses. If hypotension resolves and oxygenation has not been adequately improved (oxygen saturation over 93% on less than 60% oxygen), further increases in PEEP can be attempted.

c. Hypercarbia that complicates increasing PEEP suggests gas trapping from excessive PEEP, and PEEP should be weaned.

d. PEEP approaching a level of 12–15 without improved oxygenation. It is useful at this point to obtain a chest radiograph to assess diaphragmatic position. If the diaphragms are above 9 posterior ribs, this suggests full lung recruitment has not been accomplished and further PEEP increases might be useful. If there is lung hyper-expansion below 9 ribs, this suggests too much PEEP is being used.

5. When PEEP is maximized without improvement in oxygenation, the choice should be made to try either other ventilator manipulations or alternative therapies. Other ventilator manipulations that increase mean airway pressure with no additional increase in volume distension include changing to a pressure-controlled mode or PRVC (see above). These modes typically use a ramp deceleration configuration of flow delivery with a higher mean airway pressure without adding to peak lung distension. Close monitoring of tidal volumes is necessary in the setting of changing mechanics, except with PRVC where tidal volume is controlled as well. Alternatively, increasing the inspiratory time will also increase mean airway pressure though it is important to assure exhalation time is not impinged on to the point that breath stacking is seen (Figure 4).

6. There are several alternatives to therapy in cases of hypoxia resistant to ventilator management. These are beyond the scope of this chapter but include prone positioning, nitric oxide, and lung recruitment maneuvers. Many clinicians when faced with high levels of PEEP and inadequate oxygenation

suggest early use of HFOV in an effort to prevent VILI. As will be covered in a subsequent chapter, nitric oxide, ECMO, and surfactant are also used in specific situations.

# Adjustment of Ventilation in Specific Diseases

## Asthma/bronchiolitis

When airway obstruction precipitates respiratory failure, the prominent patho physiologic defect is gas trapping from increased airway resistance, with hyperinflation. This results in increased work of breathing and flattening of the diaphragms placing them at a mechanical disadvantage. This culminates in the patient tiring and hypercarbia. Hypoxia results from concomitant V/Q mismatching, mucous plugging, and alveolar defects.

- Mechanical ventilation carries substantial risk of VILI; pneumothoraces, pneumomediastinum, and subcutaneous emphysema as air are forced into already distended lung parenchyma. Lung protective strategies were originally described in asthmatics and then later applied to patients with low compliance diseases such as ARDS.
- Historically, the major mortality and morbidity of mechanical ventilation in asthma was due to VILI. Lowering tidal volumes to physiologic or lower improves survival and shortens time of mechanical support.
- Lowering minute ventilation leads to elevated $PaCO_2$ levels and "**permissive hypercapnia**."
- There are relatively few known adverse effects of hypercarbia: Increased distress—may necessitate heavy sedation and at times neuromuscular blockade to prevent patient/ventilator dyssynchrony.

    1. Cerebral edema—usually this is insignificant if no pre-existing brain pathology and $PaCO_2$ levels are below 90 torr.
    2. If pre-existing pulmonary hypertension respiratory acidosis, hypercarbia is not recommended.

- Otherwise, $PaCO_2$ is often allowed to reach 80–90 torr despite pH levels of 7.20 or less. Some but not all centers use bicarbonate to combat this respiratory acidosis though there is no evidence that clinical outcomes are any different than with patients not treated with bicarbonate. Pharmacological approaches to improve airway relaxation should be aggressive.

- **Ventilator management:** concentrate on facilitating as complete exhalation as possible. Volume control modes prevent rapid changes in tidal volumes with rapidly changing lung mechanics.
- Close attention to the flow waveforms displayed on the ventilator screen allows early detection of incomplete lung emptying as marked by continued expiratory flow at the point of breath initiation (Figure 4). This display can then direct maneuvers to enhance lung emptying. These maneuvers include shortening inspiratory time, decreasing ventilatory rate, or lowering tidal volumes.
- Subsequently, less attention is given to $PaCO_2$ levels and more attention is given to lung mechanics.
- Use low tidal volumes, PIP less than 35 cm $H_2O$ and plateau pressures of less than 30 cm $H_2O$; usually low PEEPs. For additional guidance in asthma management, see Chapter 6C.

## Bronchopulmonary fistula (BPF)    The presence of a persistent BPF carries a significant risk of increased mortality and morbidity of prolonged mechanical ventilation.

- While defects in large airways often require surgical intervention, those in small distal airways require careful attention to ventilatory management to minimize continuous flow of air and delayed closure. When large volumes of air escape with each inhalation, gas exchange can be greatly compromised. Airflow will naturally follow the path of least resistance and so inflation of otherwise functional lung parenchyma is difficult.
- Several strategies exist for ventilatory management in such cases and these include positioning of the patient to compress the side with the leak, minimizing the suction on the chest tube and minimizing the tidal volume so that rapid rates with small tidal volumes are used.
- Pressure control might be advantageous because the high initial flow characteristic of the ramp decelerating waveform promotes distribution of the gas into the functioning parenchyma. When compared to the lung segment containing the fistula, normal lung is less compliant and so low constant flow tends to go the path of least resistance. The higher peak flow might distribute more to the normal lung.
- HFOV has been used with good success in persistent BPF. Because peak volume distension is lessened and constant flow is used for $CO_2$ elimination, gas exchange is enhanced at less

cost of air escape into the fistula and healing is not hindered to the same extent as with the tidal volume swings of conventional ventilation. The strategy with HOFV is to minimize the driving pressure and maximize the rate, further attenuating volume excursions of the lung.

**Congenital heart disease**   Children with congenital heart disease pose unique problems during ventilatory support because the interplay between the heart and lungs is both complex and dynamic. Obviously positive pressure surrounding heart chambers and blood vessels affects flow, but less obviously circulatory responses to blood gas tensions determine relative resistances. Furthermore, the relationships between intrathoracic pressure and systemic pressure determine preload and after-load. Combined with the abnormal communications or impedance to flow from septal or valvular defects, the problems can be quite complex. Many of the considerations are beyond the scope of this chapter and only general principles will be outlined. Mechanical ventilation affects both the right and left ventricles in addition to reducing metabolic demand, in most cases the net effect of cardiopulmonary interactions is positive with respect to cardiac output.

Effects of positive pressure ventilation on right ventricular function

- In the case of the right ventricle, the predominant effect is impairment of venous return that decreases preload. When the right ventricle is abnormally volume dependent, as is seen when hypovolemic shock, increased intrathoracic pressures can markedly diminish cardiac output.
- The effects of mechanical ventilation on right ventricular afterload are more complex. Assuming normal vascular reactivity of the pulmonary blood vessels, in general positive pressure ventilation will increase RV after-load.
- These detrimental effects on both preload and after-load of right sided chambers are exaggerated in cases where the right ventricular function is impaired or when pulmonary blood flow is only through passive pressure gradients from the systemic circulation as is the children who have undergone Glenn or Fontan procedures.
- Because the right ventricle is not contributing to pulsatile flow, cardiac output is dependent on the pressure-differential between the systemic circulation and the left atrium. Positive intrathoracic pressure diminishes this gradient both by impeding venous return and by compressing lung capillaries. Such

patient are best served by allowing spontaneous ventilation as soon as is practical and early extubation.

Pulmonary hypertensive crisis:

- In un-repaired septal defects or pulmonary venous congestion (mitral valve pathology or anomalous pulmonary venous return) the lungs see abnormally generous flow. Subsequent vascular remodeling leads to reactivity that limits pulmonary blood flow. This is especially true in patients with Down syndrome due to concomitant capillary hypoplasia.
- Pulmonary hypertensive crisis can almost totally prevent pulmonary blood flow and be fatal.
- Management includes sedation, neuromuscular blockade and generous oxygenation and adequate $CO_2$ removal or hyperventilation to maximize pulmonary capillary vasodilation. Oxygen should never be suddenly discontinued in such patients and hypoxia should prompt immediate attention.
- Recall that the pulmonary vascular resistance is lowest at normal lung volumes. Accordingly, hyperinflation increases vascular resistance due to compression and areas of collapse or atelectasis cause capillary narrowing. Therefore, increased mechanical ventilation can lower pulmonary vascular resistance by recruiting lung segments that are collapsed while in others positive pressure can be detrimental.

Effects of positive pressure ventilation on left ventricular function:

- Positive pressure in the thorax increases the pressure gradient between the intrathoracic aorta and the abdominal aorta, acting to reduce the after-load of the left ventricle. This reduction can be clinically significant and beneficial in the presence of left ventricular.
- Impedance to venous return is the major effect and other considerations are usually overshadowed by the interplay between the pressure differential between the inferior vena cava and the right-sided structures of the heart.

# References

Bernard GR, Artigas A, Brigham KL, et al. Report of the American-European consensus conference on ARDS: definitions, mechanisms, relevant outcomes and clinical trial coordination. The Consensus Committee. Intensive Care Med 1994;20(3):225–32.

Clark JG, Milberg JA, Steinberg KP, Hudson LD. Elevated lavage levels of N-terminal peptide of type III procollagen are associated with increased fatality in adult respiratory distress syndrome. Chest 1994;105(3 Suppl):126S–7S.

Dreyfuss D, Soler P, Saumon G. Mechanical ventilation-induced pulmonary edema. Interaction with previous lung alterations. Am J Respir Crit Care Med 1995;151(5):1568–75.

Gattinoni L, Presenti A, Torresin A, et al. Adult respiratory distress syndrome profiles by computed tomography. J Thorac Imaging 1986;1(3):25–30.

Murphy DB, Cregg N, Tremblay L, et al. Adverse ventilatory strategy causes pulmonary-to-systemic translocation of endotoxin. Am J Respir Crit Care Med 2000;162(1):27–33.

The Acute Respiratory Distress Syndrome Network Ventilation with lower tidal volumes compared with traditional tidal volumes for acute lung injury and the acute respiratory distress syndrome. N Engl J Med 2000;342:1301–8.

Gattinoni L, Tognoni G, Pesenti A, et al. Effect of prone positioning on the survival of patients with acute respiratory failure. N Engl J Med 2001;345:568–73 Abstract.

Guerin C, Gaillard S, Lemasson S et al. Effects of systematic prone positioning in hypoxemic acute respiratory failure: a randomized controlled trial. JAMA 2004;292:2379–87 Abstract.

Mancebo J, Fernandez R, Blanch L, et al. A multicenter trial of prolonged prone ventilation in severe acute respiratory distress syndrome. Am J Respir Crit Care Med 2006;173:1233–39 Abstract.

Guerin C, Badet M, Rosselli S, et al. Effects of prone position on alveolar recruitment and oxygenation in acute lung injury. Intensive Care Med 1999;25:1222–30 Abstract.

Meduri GU, Headley AS, Golden E, et al. Effect of prolonged methylprednisolone therapy in unresolving acute respiratory distress syndrome: a randomized controlled trial. Jama 1998;280(2):159–65.

Steinberg KP, Hudson LD, Goodman RB, et al. Efficacy and safety of corticosteroids for persistent acute respiratory distress syndrome. N Engl J Med 2006;354(16):1671–84.

Spragg RG, Lewis JF, Walmrath HD, et al. Effect of recombinant surfactant protein C-based surfactant on the acute respiratory distress syndrome. N Engl J Med 2004;351:884–92 Abstract.

Gregory TJ, Steinberg KP, Spragg R, et al. Bovine surfactant therapy for patients with acute respiratory distress syndrome. Am J Respir Crit Care Med 1997;155:1309–15 Abstract.

Anzueto A, Baughman RP, Guntupalli KK, et al. Aerosolized surfactant in adults with sepsis-induced acute respiratory distress syndrome: Exosurf Acute Respiratory Distress Syndrome Sepsis Study Group. N Engl J Med 1996;334:1417–21 Abstract.

Numa AH. Acute lung injury: outcomes and new therapies. Paediatr Respir Rev 2001;2(1):22–31.

Maruscak A, Lewis JF. Exogenous surfactant therapy for ARDS. Expert Opin Investig Drugs 2006;15(1):47–58.

Dellinger RP, Zimmerman JL, Taylor RW, et al. Effects of inhaled nitric oxide in patients with acute respiratory distress syndrome: results of a randomized phase II trial. Inhaled Nitric Oxide in ARDS Study Group. Crit Care Med 1998;26(1):15–23.

Lundin S, Mang H, Smithies M, Stenqvist O, Frostell C. Inhalation of nitric oxide in acute lung injury: results of a European multicentre study. The European Study Group of Inhaled Nitric Oxide. Intensive Care Med 1999;25(9):911–9.

Arnold JH, Anas NG, Luckett P, et al. High-frequency oscillatory ventilation in pediatric respiratory failure: a multicenter experience. Crit Care Med 2000;28(12):3913–9.

Finkielman JD, Gajic O, Farmer JC, Afessa B, Hubmayr RD. The initial Mayo Clinic experience using high-frequency oscillatory ventilation for adult patients: a retrospective study. BMC Emerg Med 2006;6:2.

Chan KP, Stewart TE. Clinical use of high-frequency oscillatory ventilation in adult patients with acute respiratory distress syndrome. Crit Care Med 2005;33(3 Suppl):S170–4.

Mehta S, Granton J, MacDonald RJ, et al. High-frequency oscillatory ventilation in adults: the Toronto experience. Chest 2004;126(2):518–27.

Pettignano R, Fortenberry JD, Heard ML, et al. Primary use of the venovenous approach for extracorporeal membrane oxygenation in pediatric acute respiratory failure. Pediatr Crit Care Med 2003;4(3):291–8.

Kreck TC, Shade ED, Lamm WJ, et al. Isocapnic hyperventilation increases carbon monoxide elimination and oxygen delivery. Am J Respir Crit Care Med 2001;163:458–62.

el-Khatib MF, Chatburn RL, Potts DL, et al. Mechanical ventilators optimized for pediatric use decrease work of breathing and oxygen consumption during pressure-support ventilation. Crit Care Med 1994;22:1942–8.

Kaplan LJ, Bailey H, Formosa V. Airway pressure release ventilation increases cardiac performance in patients with acute lung injury/adult respiratory distress syndrome. Crit Care Aug, 2001; 5.

Bryan AC. The oscillations of HFO. Am J Respir Crit Care Med 2001;163: 816–7.

International consensus conferences in intensive care medicine: Ventilator-associated Lung Injury in ARDS. This official conference report was cosponsored by the American Thoracic Society, The European Society of Intensive Care Medicine, and The Societe de Reanimation de Langue Francaise, and was approved by the ATS Board of Directors, July 1999. Am J Respir Crit Care Med 1999;160:2118–24.

Darioli R, Domenighetti G, Perret C. Mechanical ventilation in the treatment of acute respiratory insufficiency in asthma. Schweiz Med Wochenschr 1981;111:194–6.

Kempainen RR, Pierson DJ. Persistent air leaks in patients receiving mechanical ventilation. Semin Respir Crit Care Med 2001;22:675–84.

# E.  Acute Respiratory Distress Syndrome

## Raymond Nkwantabisa
## Paul G Smith

In 1994, the American-European Consensus Conference on acute respiratory distress syndrome (ARDS) developed uniform definitions to help improve the standardization of patient care, clinical research, and trials of potential therapies for the disease. These criteria were:

- Acute onset of development.
- Impaired oxygen regardless of the positive end-expiratory pressure (PEEP), with a $PaO_2/FiO_2 \leq 200$.
- Bilateral infiltrates on chest radiographs.
- Pulmonary artery occlusion pressure $<18$ mm Hg or the absence of the clinical evidence of left atrial hypertension.
- Lung disease fitting these criteria but with less severe presentation ($PaO_2/FiO_2$ between 200 and 300) were defined as acute lung injury (ALI).
- Note the change of terminology from previous ("adult" respiratory distress syndrome—signifying the awareness of common pathophysiology over age spectrum).

Here we will discuss causes and course of both ARDS and ALI together.

## Causes of ARDS

The causes of ARDS can be classified as either direct or indirect (eg, due to systemic inflammatory processes) insult to the lungs.

| Direct Causes of ARDS | Indirect Causes of ARDS |
|---|---|
| Aspiration | Sepsis |
| Pneumonia | Massive trauma |
| Near drowning | Pancreatitis |
| Toxic inhalation | Multiple transfusions |
| Pulmonary contusion | Burns |
| | Head injury |

# Key Principles

> - ARDS is defined by hypoxic respiratory failure with $PaO_2/FiO_2 \leq 200$, bilateral infiltrates on chest radiograph and absence of cardiac etiology
> - ARDS in children is still associated with a high mortality rate secondary to multiorgan failure
> - The goal of mechanical ventilation in patients with ARDS is not to maintain "normal blood gas values," but rather to optimize oxygen delivery and the protection of the lung from ventilator-induced lung injury (VILI).

## Clinical, Pathologic, and Radiographic Features

ARDS is often a progressive disease with distinct stages marked by specific clinical, radiologic, and histopathologic features. Whether due to indirect or direct injury, the sequence of events leading to ARDS is similar. All causes share capillary injury with endothelial cell damage and disruption of the alveolar epithelium as the inciting events.

Classic descriptions of ARDS outline three stages: the acute (or exudative), subacute, and proliferative. It is useful to think of the process as an initial breach of the vascular and airspace barrier, with subsequent acute inflammation, culminating in a pulmonary edema and potentially a chronic inflammation.

## Clinical Features of Acure Phase

- Rapid onset of respiratory failure with arterial hypoxemia refractory to treatment with supplemental oxygen.
- Bilateral infiltrates on CXR—homogeneous, patchy, or asymmetric—closely resemble those of cardiogenic pulmonary edema. Even when CXR suggests homogeneous infiltrates, there are marked in homogeneities in the distribution of lung involvement, with the greatest areas of consolidation occurring in the dependent lung regions.
- As a result, there is reduced lung volume available for gas exchange and reduced pulmonary compliance. The spared lung regions have normal to near-normal mechanical properties. There is thus preferential distribution of ventilator-generated volume and pressure so that the normal areas are more susceptible to VILI.

## Clinical Features of Chronic Phase (Fibrosing or Proliferative)

- ARDS and ALI may resolve completely or it may progress to fibrosing alveolitis with persistent hypoxemia, increased alveolar dead space and a further decrease in lung compliance.
- Chronic problems are often associated with additional insult such as a secondary pneumonia or sepsis ("second hit"). Prolonged exposure to inflammatory mediators is underlying probable cause.
- Proliferative phase (ie, fibrosing alveolitis) involves abundant collagen deposition, increased extracellular matrix deposition, alveolar, and interstitial scarring. Secondarily, capillary obliteration and disruption of acinar lung architecture. This leads to chronic pulmonary insufficiency, increased tissue elastance, and airway resistance. Some develop intractable respiratory failure and death.

# Ventilator-Induced Lung Injury (VILI)

- Substantial clinical and experimental evidence indicates that mechanical ventilation at high volumes and pressures can injure the lung.
- Cyclic opening and closing of atelectatic alveoli during mechanical ventilation causes lung injury independent of alveolar overdistention, secondary to exacerbated inflammation.
- CT scans of chest show that much of the lung is not able to be recruited by increasing pressure so the functioning lung is diminished in size (concept of the "baby lung"). Compliance of the respiratory system is linearly related to the dimensions of the "baby lung." This suggests that the aerated portions of the lungs in ARDS are not "stiff," but instead small with nearly normal intrinsic elasticity.
- Injurious ventilation strategies might promote bacterial translocation across the alveolar-capillary membrane, leading to bacteremia, systemic infection, and contributing to multiorgan failure.

# Resolution of Lung Injury

- For recovery of lung function, there has to be clearance of alveolar fluid, removal of soluble and insoluble proteins from alveoli, clearance of neutrophils from sites of inflammation, and the re-epithelialization of the denuded alveolar epithelium.

- Alveolar edema is signaled clinically by an improved oxygenation and liberation from mechanical ventilation.
- Removal of insoluble protein occurs much more slowly, but if impeded enables growth of fibrous tissue.

# Management of ARDS

## General

The major causes of mortality in ARDS are not respiratory failure, but the effects of the inciting event (sepsis, massive trauma, multiorgan failure, cerebral edema, and so on). Thus most patients die with, rather than of, ARDS. Hence:

1. First, manage the initiating insult.
2. Treat any source of infection or inflammation that is a continuing stimulus for systemic inflammation driving ARDS.
3. Maintain adequate nutrition by enteral feeding rather than parenteral nutrition, reducing risk of catheter-induced sepsis.
4. When the inciting cause of lung injury cannot be directly treated, such as aspiration or multiple transfusions, the emphasis should be directed toward optimizing supportive care of the patient.
5. The major goal is to optimize oxygen delivery to the tissues and prevent other end-organ dysfunction. This may entail aggressive support of cardiac function with inotropic agents.
6. The general goal of mechanical ventilation in patients with ARDS is not to maintain "normal blood gas values," but to optimize oxygen delivery and avoid VILI.

## Mechanical Ventilation

- Positive pressure ventilation is the mainstay of supportive. However, the ventilator does not cure lung disease; it only supports lung function and may exacerbate disease. Therefore minimizing the baro-volu-trauma is important.
- Goals to limit ventilator-induced lung damage of mechanical ventilation are to reach the following settings:

$FiO_2 < 0.6$

Tidal volumes of 4 to 6 mL/kg
Moderate to high levels of PEEP may be needed to achieve adequate oxygenation. There is no consensus regarding optimal levels of PEEP.

Peak inspiratory pressure (PIP) of < 35 cm $H_2O$ (if available for assessment on ventilator; this might be more exactly followed as an inspiratory plateau pressure of < 30 cm $H_2O$). See Chapter 6, "Pulmonary" for management strategies.

## Nonventilatory Therapies in ARDS

### Prone Positioning

- Shown in RCTs to improve arterial oxygenation by improving ventilation to the dorsal-dependent regions of the lung. The mechanisms accounting for this improvement are several: (1) placing the posterior segments of the lungs superiorly frees them from gravity compression, allowing positive pressure to inflate them; (2) it relieves the cardiac compression exerted on the lower lobes when patients are in the supine position; (3) it facilitates the drainage of secretions.
- Pragmatically: Common to use a protocol of 18 hours prone and 6 hours supine.
- The presence of catheters and monitors makes prone positioning of patients logistically difficult. But experienced nurses and therapists can manage the prone positioning of ventilated patients with an acceptably low rate of extubations, line disruptions, and other complications.
- Absolute contraindications to prone positioning include:

    - Spinal instability
    - Pelvic fractures
    - Increased intracranial pressure
    - Burns or open wounds on ventral body surface
    - Life-threatening circulatory shock

### Steroids

- Clinical trials have demonstrated no benefit for steroids in the prevention of the disease or treatment in the early stages.
- High-dose glucocorticoids may increase the incidence of infection, delay healing, and contribute to prolonged weakness in ventilated patients.
- Therefore, the routine use of glucocorticoids early in the course of ALI/ARDS is not recommended.
- However, there is a potential benefit of glucocorticoids in the treatment of late phase (fibrosing-alveolitis).
- Many centers initiate steroids if MV is still required after 7 to 10 days of illness.

## Surfactant

- In ARDS, surfactant production is diminished due to destruction of type II alveoli epithelial cells. Alveolar infiltration by proteinaceous fluid leads to inactivation of surfactant.
- The dramatic success of surfactant replacement therapy in premature infants with respiratory distress syndrome is not shown in adults with ALI or ARDS.
- However, recent studies in pediatric ARDS suggest the following benefits: improved oxygenation and ventilation, decreased ICU stay, decreased ventilator dependent days, and improved mortality. Questions remain about the optimal route or frequency of delivery and preparation of surfactant.

## Inhaled Nitric Oxide (iNO)

- iNO therapy causes selective pulmonary vasodilatation of pulmonary vessels that perfuse well-aerated lung units, and diverts blood from more poorly ventilated areas. This decreases pulmonary hypertension and intrapulmonary shunting. The systemic circulation remains unaffected.
- Randomized clinical trials show that iNO leads to a transient improvement in oxygenation for up to 72 hours, but no difference in ventilator-free days or mortality between the iNO treatment group and control group. Furthermore, the effect of iNO is heterogeneous among individual patients.
- There may be a role for iNO in patients with severe refractory hypoxemia; however its use should not be routine in ARDS.

## High-Frequency Oscillatory Ventilation (HFOV)

- This modality of ventilation employs high mean airway pressures to maintain an open lung and low tidal volumes at high frequencies that allow for adequate ventilation while at the same time preventing alveolar overdistension, minimizing VILI.
- It is indicated in ALI/ARDS when conventional ventilation (CV) fails. An earlier initiation of HFOV in ALI/ARDS may be associated with a lower mortality. An RCT comparing initial HFOV to CV in ALI/ARDS showed a nonsignificant trend toward a lower mortality rate in the HFOV group.

## Extracorporal Membranous Oxygenation (ECMO)

- ECMO provides gas exchange in severe ALI/ARDS and rests the lungs from MV.
- It can be provided by either venoarterial (VA) or venovenous (VV) access with an artificial membrane performing the gas

exchange function of the lung. In VA ECMO, blood is drained from the right atrium, circulates through a membrane oxygenator, and returned to the aortic arch via the common carotid artery. It provides both pulmonary and cardiovascular support for the patient. VA ECMO carries the risk associated with the cannulation and ligation of a carotid artery. Because blood is returned to the arterial circulation, there is a greater risk of embolic damage from either thrombi or air. VV ECMO provides gas exchange but no direct cardiac support. In VV ECMO, blood is drained from the right atrium or IVC and, after oxygenation by the oxygenator membrane, returned to the central venous circulation. VV ECMO has been shown to effectively provide adequate oxygenation for pediatric patients with severe acute respiratory failure. Potential advantages of VV ECMO include lack of carotid artery ligation, maintenance of pulsatile blood flow pattern, preservation of normal pulmonary blood flow with oxygenated blood, and preservation of normal cerebral blood flow velocities. Refer to Chapter 7, "Otolaryngology" for additional details.

# References

Bernard GR, Artigas A, Brigham KL, et al. Report of the American-European consensus conference on ARDS: definitions, mechanisms, relevant outcomes and clinical trial coordination. The Consensus Committee. Intensive Care Med 1994;20:225–32.

Pugin J, Verghese G, Widmer MC, Matthay MA. The alveolar space is the site of intense inflammatory and profibrotic reactions in the early phase of acute respiratory distress syndrome. Crit Care Med 1999;27:304–12.

Clark JG, Milberg JA, Steinberg KP, Hudson LD. Elevated lavage levels of N-terminal peptide of type III procollagen are associated with increased fatality in adult respiratory distress syndrome. Chest 1994;105(3 Suppl):126S–7S.

Baughman RP, Gunther KL, Rashkin MC, Keeton DA, Pattishall EN. Changes in the inflammatory response of the lung during acute respiratory distress syndrome: prognostic indicators. Am J Respir Crit Care Med 1996;154:76–81.

Laufe MD, Simon RH, Flint A, Keller JB. Adult respiratory distress syndrome in neutropenic patients. Am J Med 1986;80:1022–6.

Nelson S, Belknap SM, Carlson RW, et al. A randomized controlled trial of filgrastim as an adjunct to antibiotics for treatment of hospitalized patients with community-acquired pneumonia. CAP Study Group. J Infect Dis 1998;178:1075–80.

Pugin J, Ricou B, Steinberg KP, et al. Proinflammatory activity in bronchoalveolar lavage fluids from patients with ARDS, a prominent role for interleukin-1. Am J Respir Crit Care Med 1996;153(6 Pt 1):1850–6.

Dreyfuss D, Soler P, Saumon G. Mechanical ventilation-induced pulmonary edema. Interaction with previous lung alterations. Am J Respir Crit Care Med 1995;151:1568–75.

Gattinoni L, Presenti A, Torresin A, et al. Adult respiratory distress syndrome profiles by computed tomography. J Thorac Imaging 1986;1:25–30.

Murphy DB, Cregg N, Tremblay L, et al. Adverse ventilatory strategy causes pulmonary-to-systemic translocation of endotoxin. Am J Respir Crit Care Med 2000;162:27–33.

Meduri GU, Headley AS, Golden E, et al. Effect of prolonged methylprednisolone therapy in unresolving acute respiratory distress syndrome: a randomized controlled trial. JAMA 1998;280:159–65.

Steinberg KP, Hudson LD, Goodman RB, et al. Efficacy and safety of corticosteroids for persistent acute respiratory distress syndrome. N Engl J Med 2006;354:1671–84.

Numa AH. Acute lung injury: outcomes and new therapies. Paediatr Respir Rev 2001;2:22–31.

Maruscak A, Lewis JF. Exogenous surfactant therapy for ARDS. Expert Opin Investig Drugs 2006;15:47–58.

Dellinger RP, Zimmerman JL, Taylor RW, et al. Effects of inhaled nitric oxide in patients with acute respiratory distress syndrome: results of a randomized phase II trial. Inhaled Nitric Oxide in ARDS Study Group. Crit Care Med 1998;26:15–23.

Lundin S, Mang H, Smithies M, et al. Inhalation of nitric oxide in acute lung injury: results of a European multicentre study. The European Study Group of Inhaled Nitric Oxide. Intensive Care Med 1999;25:911–9.

Arnold JH, Anas NG, Luckett P, et al. High-frequency oscillatory ventilation in pediatric respiratory failure: a multicenter experience. Crit Care Med 2000;28:3913–9.

Finkielman JD, Gajic O, Farmer JC, et al. The initial Mayo Clinic experience using high-frequency oscillatory ventilation for adult patients: a retrospective study. BMC Emerg Med 2006;6:2.

Chan KP, Stewart TE. Clinical use of high-frequency oscillatory ventilation in adult patients with acute respiratory distress syndrome. Crit Care Med 2005;33(3 Suppl):S170–4.

Mehta S, Granton J, MacDonald RJ, et al. High-frequency oscillatory ventilation in adults: the Toronto experience. Chest 2004;126:518–27.

Pettignano R, Fortenberry JD, Heard ML, et al. Primary use of the venovenous approach for extracorporeal membrane oxygenation in pediatric acute respiratory failure. Pediatr Crit Care Med 2003;4:291–8.

# Chapter 7

# Otolaryngology

## A. General Approach to Upper Airway Problems

Lisa Elden

### Assessment

Observe patient to assess the status of the airway and need for airway intervention:

- General color (presence of cyanosis)
- Respiratory rate and effort
- Use of accessory respiratory muscles (including nasal flaring, suprasternal tracheal tug for upper respiratory problems and substernal retraction, intercostal retraction for lower respiratory problems)
- Oxygen saturation monitor
- Arterial blood gas as needed
- Presence and character of stridor (noisy breathing)

### Classification of Upper Airway Sounds

- Nasal sounds—snorting, snoring +/− paradoxical breathing pattern
- Stertor is noise coming from oral cavity/oropharynx—snoring, muffled voice (hot potato quality) that can be associated with dysphagia and drooling when severe.
- Stridor

    - Laryngeal

        - supraglottic—mostly heard on inspiration, usually loud high-pitched and crowing in quality, but voice normal.

- Glottic—two phases of stridor present (inspiration and expiration) but expiratory noise usually more difficult to hear and without stethoscope, voice normally hoarse or breathy.
- Subglottic—two phases of stridor present (inspiration and expiration) but usually both audible without stethoscope. Croupy cough very common, but voice usually close to normal.

- Tracheal—mostly heard on expiration, often associated with retained secretions in bronchi that may or may not clear with cough. May have prominent deep-pitched cough as well.

## Diagnostic Tests to Consider

a. Lateral and anterior/posterior radiographs of airway (thoracic inlet views)—useful to rule out retropharyngeal swelling, epiglottic and subglottic pathology.
b. Chest X-ray—useful to look for coexisting aspiration and lower tracheal pathology.
c. Flexible fiber-optic nasopharyngoscopy/laryngoscopy—gives direct view from level of nose to the glottic, but less useful for subglottic and tracheal pathology.
d. Airway fluoroscopy—useful to look at subglottis and trachea. Gives dynamic picture and may be one of the best ways to diagnose tracheomalacia.
e. Barium esophagram—useful to look for tracheoesophageal fistulas or clefts and to look for vascular webs of lower trachea and esophagus.
f. Echocardiogram—mostly helpful to rule out vascular malformations.
g. Diagnostic laryngoscopy and bronchoscopy—gold standard, allows whole airway to be viewed under direct vision. Requires use of rigid bronchoscopes and general anesthesia.
h. Gastrointestinal studies to look for reflux or abnormal swallow often useful as many patients with airway problems have coexisting gastroesophageal reflux disease (GERD) or abnormal oropharyngeal coordination.
i. Contrasted CT neck—necessary for identification and differentiation of neck masses, eg, abscesses, cysts, tumors—generally performed without sedation.

# Management

- In patients with upper airway obstruction and a threatened airway, avoid examination of oropharynx unless the team is prepared and able to intubate emergently.
- Avoid sedation in an un-intubated child with neck masses undergoing diagnostic procedures.
- After control of the airway is obtained, these patients are at risk for postobstructive pulmonary edema and should be closely monitored for increasing oxygen requirement or changes in lung compliance.

*If the patient is stable*

- Supplemental oxygen.
- Racemic epinephrine if acute laryngeal or tracheal swelling, but usually only effective for minutes to several hours after given. Repeat doses often needed so need to monitor heart rate.
- Systemic steroids (dexamethasone 0.5–1 mg/kg/dose) should be used if not contraindicated for diffuse upper or lower airway swelling.

*If the patient is unstable*

- Heliox is a blend of helium and oxygen that is less dense than room air. Heliox decreases the amount of turbulent flow and increases laminar flow in airways. Heliox has been found to be of benefit in both upper and lower airways disease.
- Oral/nasopharyngeal airway may be used for upper airway obstruction if tolerated but oral airways are contraindicated in conscious patients.

*Intubation*

- *Nasal* intubation over a flexible bronchoscope to provide direct vision during intubation—consider if oropharyngeal or oral swelling or masses present. The patient must sit up throughout procedure so usually not feasible in pediatric population except in cooperative older child or in an infant who can be restrained.
- *Oral* intubation with stylet and endotracheal tube that is one size smaller than standard for age to be used when there is diffuse laryngeal or tracheal airway swelling.

- Avoid paralyzing agents in patient with acute airway swelling.
- A rigid bronchoscope with a side vent for ventilating the patient may be used if unable to intubate with endotracheal tube.
- *Cricothyrotomy* or tracheotomy should only be considered as a last resort in the pediatric population as it is difficult to perform at the bedside (see Chapter 5, "Resuscitation").
- Once intubated, it is imperative that the child remains deeply sedated and restrained to avoid self-extubation while the airway is swollen. It is best to avoid paralyzing agents because the child will be able to protect his or her airway better if he or she self-extubates. Also, many of these patients require steroids and there is a high incidence of myopathy when steroids and paralyzing agents are used together.

# References

Myers TR. Use of heliox in children. Respir Care 2006;51:619–31.

Rutter MJ. Evaluation and management of upper airway disorders in children. Semin Pediatr Surg 2006;15:116–23.

# B.  Common Otolaryngology Problems in the Pediatric Intensive Care Unit (PICU)

Lisa Elden

## Nasal Obstruction

Most infants are obligate nasal breathers until about age 3–6 months so most have difficulty when the nose is blocked because of anatomic narrowing or inflammation. This is rarely an isolated problem after age 6 months because the infant no longer is an obligate nasal breather.

Signs and symptoms:

- Congested/snorting noises that come from nose/posterior nasopharynx
- Difficulty with feeding/failure to thrive because of nasal congestion
- If severe, paradoxical breathing pattern with dusky spells and desaturations with quiet breathing, but oxygen saturations and color normalize with crying

Diagnosis:

- Most newborn noses should accommodate a 3.5 mm endotracheal tube through each side
- Significant stenosis indicated by inability to pass a 6 or 8 French flexible suction catheter from anterior nasal opening into posterior nasopharynx
- Location of narrowing can be confirmed by

  i.  Flexible nasopharyngoscopy
  ii. Axial computed tomography of nose/nasopharynx

- For midline nasal masses, magnetic resonance imaging (MRI) should also be performed to rule out attachment to brain (more commonly associated with gliomas or encephaloceles but possible with dermoids)

Specific anatomic abnormalities that lead to obstructive symptoms:

- Anterior nasal piriform stenosis

- Bony narrowing at opening of nose
- If failure to thrive, or failure to maintain oxygen saturation, requires surgical repair

- Choanal stenosis/atresia

  - Unilateral

    - More common than bilateral
    - Rarely affects breathing significantly
    - Usually more of a social problem because of constant nasal discharge

  - Bilateral

    - Usually affects breathing significantly in newborns causing obstructive spells and oxygen desaturations
    - Often leads to failure to thrive and usually is diagnosed within a few days of birth

- Midline nasal masses: May have open sinus tract on nasal dorsum or mass under skin of dorsum and/or within nasal cavity. The mass in the nasal cavity can be midline within septum or may present as a pedunculated or broad-based lateral or superior nasal cavity mass.

  - Dermoids
  - Encephaloceles
  - Gliomas

- Lateral nasal masses: eg, nasolacrimal duct cysts—internal nasal exam reveals mass laterally along the floor of the nose under the inferior turbinate. It usually is associated with increased tearing from obstruction of the duct that drains into the nose.

Treatment for unilateral atresia/stenosis or bilateral stenosis:

- Primarily expectant management as symptoms usually improve by 3–6 months
- May need surgery later (3–5 years of age) if symptomatic rhinorrhea persists
- Saline drops/nasal aspirator
- Additional treatment depending on severity:

  - Home apnea monitor
  - Suction machine
  - Daily Decadron eye drops to control chronic congestion, must observe for systemic side effects

- Phenylephrine (Neo-Synephrine) or xylometazoline nasal (Otrivin) pediatric nasal drops for acute nasal inflammation (should not be used for more than a 3–5 day period)

Treatment of bilateral atresia/severe stenosis

- Requires surgical repair if atresia or significant stenosis
- Bilateral transnasal repair with stenting for 6 weeks to 3 months
- Tracheotomy done if other neurologic, congenital, or pulmonary problems
- Home apnea monitor and suction equipment required perioperatively
- CPR training for family and primary caregivers

Treatment of midline nasal masses:

- Surgical treatment required (otolaryngology +/− neurosurgery)

Treatment of lateral nasal masses:

- Surgical treatment—Aspiration/marsupialization cyst +/− lacrimal duct probing

# Oropharyngeal/Oral Cavity Obstruction

Etiologies of oral cavity airway obstruction can be grouped into the following categories:

1. Macroglossia
2. Pierre-Robin-like deformity (micrognathia, glossoptosis)
3. Adenotonsilar disease

1. Macroglossia
- May present with feeding or airway problems
- Feeding problems:

  - Are secondary to difficulty in handling the food or liquid during the oral or oropharyngeal stage of the swallow. This may lead to failure to thrive, periodic aspiration, and/or pneumonia.
  - Usually have more problems with liquid than with solids so thickening feeds and feeding in an upright position is helpful. Tongue reduction is rarely indicated for feeding difficulties.

- Airway problems:

  - Usually related to obstructive sleep syndrome, but rarely require treatment unless associated with an upper respiratory tract infection (URTI).

- In most cases, the child can breathe comfortably with the larger tongue during the daytime, but may have some obstructive symptoms at night when the muscles of the airway relax. However, most children compensate unless there is increased mucus from an URTI or unless the tonsils and adenoids are also hypertrophied.
- Usually can be treated acutely by addressing the URTI and by observing the patient in an ICU setting for signs of severe upper respiratory tract obstructive symptoms.
- Empiric antibiotics that cover the usual upper respiratory tract pathogens and systemic steroids are very effective if there is associated adenotonsillar hypertrophy or infection because the swollen lymph tissue responds well to these medications.
- It is best to avoid acute surgical management (tongue reduction or adenotonsillectomy) until the URTI has been fully treated given the increased risks of complications associated with intubation when the airway is acutely inflamed and with bleeding when the airway is inflamed.

Specific types of macroglossia:

- Diffuse tongue enlargement

  - Rarely needs tongue reduction
  - Down syndrome
  - Beckwith-Wiedemann syndrome

- Base of tongue enlargement

  - Usually requires elective tongue reduction.
  - Lingual thyroid: must establish presence of a normal thyroid before treatment. May be treated medically with thyroid hormone (reduces bulk) or with surgery.

- Midline dermoid of tongue—rare and usually treated with elective surgery.
- Midline teratoma of tongue—rare and usually treated with elective surgery.
- Other tongue masses

  - Lymphangiomas

    - May involve the tongue, the floor of mouth, and less often the oropharynx—usually present at birth and are distorting from a cosmetic point of view.
    - Most that are located in this area cause problems with feeding and upper airway obstructive syndrome at birth that may or may not require tracheotomy for airway

control until surgery performed or as a short-term measure perioperatively to ensure adequate airway control after surgery. They tend to grow at an unpredictable rate and rarely regress spontaneously.

- They usually become more problematic when the child develops an URTI because the involved areas swell. Antibiotics, steroids, and ICU observation usually help during an acute exacerbation, but the definitive treatment is surgical reduction. Alternatively, larger cysts may be controlled with scherotherapy by international radiologists. Many children require multiple surgeries over time, given the tendency for the lesions to grow.

- Hemangiomas

  - May involve the tongue, the floor of mouth, and less often the oropharynx.
  - Usually become apparent within 6 to 8 weeks of birth and peak in size about 6 to 12 months of age.
  - Most start to regress by 1 year of age and by 2 to 5 years of age, they have regressed significantly.
  - Although the airway can be problematic with URTI, it is best to treat acute exacerbations of swelling with antibiotics and steroids and avoid surgery all together.
  - Hemangiomas causing significant airway obstruction may be treated with a combination of intralesional steroid injection, laser ablation, surgical excision, and interferon alpha.

2. Pierre-Robin-like deformity

- Micrognathia, glossoptosis (posterior placement of tongue), and usually soft palate cleft.
- One-third have the isolated Pierre-Robin sequence.
- One-third have Sticklers syndrome (Pierre-Robin-like anomaly with connective tissue disorder that affects joints and the retina and can result in severe myopia).
- One-third associated with other congenital syndromes (chromosome abnormalities, etc.).
- Feeding-related problems are more likely to occur than airway problems. Liquids are more difficult than solids, placing the child at risk for recurrent aspiration pneumonitis and/or pneumonia.
- Airway-related problems occur because of difficulty in handling secretions and feeds.

Treatment

- Management is controversial; choice of treatment depends on severity of the problem and ability to feed/protect airway.
- Severity percent improves without needing surgery.
- Airway obstruction associated with isolated Pierre-Robin sequence or Sticklers syndrome usually improves within 1 to 5 years.
- In general, those with other neurologic or genetic abnormalities tend to require more invasive treatments.
- Mild forms—associated with noisy feeding and airway, but without failure to thrive, apneas, or aspirations.

  - Airway problem—position the child on the side.
  - Feeding problem—position the child upright for feeding and use a squeeze bottle and broad nipple to help with poor suck.

- Moderate forms—associated with some degree of failure to thrive, noisy airway but without significant apneas or aspirations.

  - Airway problems—treated by positioning the child on his/her side (prevents tongue/secretions from falling into oropharynx) and occasionally by using a nasopharyngeal airway (if tolerated) or a long pacifier with the tip cut off so child can breathe more easily. Often require home apnea monitor to watch for apneic spells.

- Severe forms—associated with documented failure to thrive, noisy airway with apnea or obstructive symptoms especially if retaining $CO_2$.

  - Tongue lip adhesion (TLA) has become a first line surgical procedure, which opens the airway by sewing the tongue to the lower lip. It is usually taken down by age 6–9 months.
  - If the TLA fails then tracheotomy, home monitoring, and CPR training are necessary. The average age for decannulation if a tracheotomy is required is 3 years.
  - In North America, approximately 10–20% receive tracheotomy to provide safe airway with home monitoring and CPR training for caregivers.
  - Feeding problems—usually can take some oral feeds, but may need supplemental NG. Many children with tracheotomy can tolerate thickened oral feeds.
  - However, if severe enough, require G-tube for at least supplemental feeds.

3. Adenotonsillar disease causing acute airway distress

- Usually occurs in otherwise healthy children with baseline large tonsils and adenoids that become more swollen after an URTI (viral or Strep A bacterial infections) and/or mononucleosis.
- Adenoids peak in size around age 2 to 5 years and tonsils peak in size around age 5 years.

History/Examination

- Obstructive problems with sleep because of larger tonsils and adenoids that become severely swollen due to overlying infection.
- Patient may have severe apnea, hypersomnolence, and change in mental status.
- The tonsils may be touching and this may pose some problems with intubation.
- Cor pulmonale must be considered if long history of severe sleep apnea syndrome.

Diagnosis

- Is usually evident because of large touching tonsils that may or may not have exudate.
- Monospot, EBV titres, and throat swabs are important to help guide treatment and need for antibiotics.

Treatment

- Antibiotics—penicillin or clindamycin to cover Strep A +/− oral anaerobic pathogens.
- Steroids (especially if the patient has mononucleosis).
- Avoid oversedation with pain medicine when acutely swollen.
- Rarely need intubation, but if necessary should avoid paralysis and have suction available to help reduce secretions and to increase visibility.
- If failed oral intubation, fiberoptic awake nasopharyngeal intubation more likely successful. Anesthesia and/or ENT back up should be available.

# Laryngeal Obstruction

Laryngeal obstruction may occur at the supraglottic, glottic, or subglottic level.

Supraglottic obstruction:

- Congenital laryngomalacia: most common airway-related problem in the newborn.
- More common in premature and neurologically compromised babies.
- High-pitched inspiratory stridor often associated with difficulty in handling upper airway secretions. High incidence of associated reflux, although the reflux is of variable clinical significance.
- Associated with soft compliant cartilages of the supraglottis including a long omega-shaped epiglottis and short aryepiglottic folds (laterally). The cartilage and soft tissues collapse into toward the glottis with inspiration and usually open easily with expiration.
- Only thought to be of clinical significance in about 10% to 15% of patients, mostly because of associated failure to thrive secondary to difficulty in handling feeds and upper airway secretions. Patients rarely have associated apnea spells when the child is asleep when the tissue is more compliant because of decreased muscle tone.
- Usually becomes obvious within a few weeks of birth and symptoms are most clinically significant within a few months of life. The stridor may get louder with time, but clinical improvement in feeding and airway issues usually markedly better by 3 to 6 months of age. Stridor usually is gone within a year.

Diagnosis:

- Based on clinical findings and confirmed by bedside flexible nasopharyngoscopy.
- 12% to 45% of patients have another airway anomaly that is mild and most often involves the vocal cords (weakness), the subglottis (stenosis or edema), or the trachea (tracheomalacia).
- It is important to look at lower airway with anterior-posterior (AP) and lateral soft tissue airway films for mild cases and direct laryngoscopy and bronchoscopy under general anesthetic for more severe cases to rule out a second possibly more significant lesion that may be present in 5% of patients.

Treatment:

- Mild cases: usually reassurance.
- Moderate cases (with associated feeding difficulties):

  - Rule out and treat GERD if present.
  - Occasionally NG feeds may be necessary.

- Severe cases (with associated feeding and airway difficulties):
  - Apnea monitor.
  - NG feeds.
  - Surgery: 5% to 10% require operative intervention.
  - Endoscopic supraglottoplasty to trim redundant tissue in cases in which there are no other congenital or neurological problems exist.
  - Tracheotomy +/− G-tube in cases in children who have other medical problems.
  - Other: supraglottic cysts—usually contain mucus and are treatable with endoscopic excision or marsupialization.

Glottic obstruction:

Unilateral vocal cord palsy

- Usually one vocal cord remains in the paramedian position and this produces an opening in the glottic airway that is present throughout respiration and phonation.
- Patients often have a weak, breathy voice, but the airway is rarely affected significantly.
- Newborn children and those with other neurologic problems are at greater risk for aspiration because the opposite vocal cord may not be able to compensate by closing the glottis to protect the airway.
- Glottic closure is only one of several mechanisms to protect the airway, so most children do not need any specific intervention.

Etiology

- Is variable. In the newborn, stretch injuries to the vagus nerve in the neck during difficult deliveries are not uncommon and most resolve spontaneously within 6 months to 1 year.
- May result from iatrogenic complication following cardiothoracic surgeries, eg, patent ductus arteriosus repair.
- Central causes are less common than in bilateral vocal cord palsy, but can occur secondary to brainstem pathology (such as with Arnold Chiari Malformations). MRI and CT are important studies to rule this out.
- Rarely occurs secondary to a primary muscle or neuromotor problems, but may be seen in children with mitochondrial abnormalities.

Diagnosis

- Definitive diagnosis is best made when the child is awake with flexible nasopharyngoscopy.

Treatment

- Usually supportive.
- May be necessary to thicken feeds to avoid aspiration.
- Occasionally, apnea monitor needed for first few months of life if prone to small aspirations.

## Bilateral vocal cord palsy

- Both vocal cords remain in paramedian position and fail to abduct which results in a severely compromised airway. The stridor is medium- to high-pitched in quality and present in both inspiratory and expiratory phases. The voice may be preserved as some degree of adduction may be possible, but it is usually weak.

### Etiology

- Is similar to that seen in unilateral vocal cord palsy; however, children with bilateral vocal cord palsy are less likely to recover and more often have had a more severe stretch injury or brainstem problem.

### Treatment

- Usually need some form of airway intervention, but it is very important to observe child for ability to compensate.
- In a minority of cases, the child can just be observed closely with apnea monitors.
- Approximately 50% to 60% improve spontaneously by 6 to 12 months.
- Intubation is usually easy as there is no fixed stenosis, but just immobile cords.
- A majority of patients (73%) require tracheotomy.
- If no signs of spontaneous improvement by 3 to 5 years of age, then the children usually undergo airway widening procedure (endoscopic or external approach to lateralize one vocal cord).

## Other glottic abnormalities

- Mucus or air containing supraglottic or glottic cysts that respond to endoscopic marsupialization.
- Laryngeal webs can occur anteriorly or posteriorly and partially fuse the vocal cords so the patient cannot completely abduct the cords. They usually present perinatally but can present later if mild. Most respond well to endoscopic lysis.

## Subglottic obstruction

## Subglottic hemangiomas

- Benign vascular tumor that usually present within weeks to a few months of birth when they undergo a period of rapid growth, then they slowly regress and are usually asymptomatic by age 2 years. Usually present with stridor and/or a history of recurrent croup in otherwise normal baby.

Diagnosis

- Made by history and usually confirmed by bronchoscopy.

Treatment

- Best to observe and/or use steroids to control airway exacerbations that can occur with URTIs. If more serious, then either endoscopic treatments to reduce bulk, open resection, or tracheotomy may be necessary.

Congenital subglottic stenosis

- Accounts for 5% to 10% of cases. The cricoid cartilage is the smallest point in the neonates airway. Can have congenital cartilaginous or mucosal narrowing without any previous airway trauma.
- Most commonly seen in children with Down syndrome. Usually not a big issue and just associated with increased frequency of croup, etc.
- Intervention is rarely required.
- It is important to treat gastroesophageal reflux to prevent exacerbation of the stenosis.

Acquired subglottic stenosis (Table 1)

- Usually a result of previous intubation injury and very common in children who had been premature or who have had previous subglottic hemangiomas. The subglottis is the smallest of part

*Table 1*
**Risk Factors for Acquired Subglottic Stenosis**

- Prolonged intubation >7–10 days.
- Multiple intubations during PICU stay.
- Oral intubation compared with nasal intubation because the tube is less secure.
- Increased tube size.
- Presence of infection, especially croup.
- GERD (especially in infants).

of the pediatric airway and is most vulnerable in developing fixed scarring.

- It is important to follow guidelines for recommended sizes of endotracheal tubes for pediatric patients carefully and to assess regularly to ensure that an air leak around the tube is measurable at 25 cm $H_2O$ cuff pressure.

Extubation failure with presumed subglottic stenosis

- Patients who fail extubation with upper airway symptoms should be presumed to have subglottic stenosis until proven otherwise.

  - Reintubate with an endotracheal tube that is one size smaller than the previous tube.
  - Give a 24 to 48 hour trial of high dose steroids to try to reduce swelling.
  - Ensure adequate sedation to prevent patient movement, which may exacerbate inflammation.
  - Ensure gastroesophageal reflux is well controlled.
  - Consider empiric antibiotic therapy if infection suspected.
  - Consider another trial of extubation after 24 to 48 hours if leak is present and patient meets other extubation criteria.

If attempted re-extubation unsuccessful,

- Refer to ENT for diagnostic laryngoscopy and bronchoscopy to be done in the operating room.
- Endoscopic laser or microscopic surgery may be helpful to remove obstructing airway granulomas that develop in response to intubation.
- If the airway is narrowed by more than 50%, then the chance that repeated attempts at extubation will be successful is small. In these cases, the child may require temporary tracheotomy.
- Alternatively, single-stage laryngotracheoplasty (SSLTP) may be considered to avoid tracheotomy. The SSLTP involves the use of local free cartilage grafts (often from the thyroid ala) placed in a vertical incision in the narrowed airway, allowing for airway expansion. It is only an option if the child has excellent pulmonary reserve. It is imperative that the patient's endotracheal tube remain in place during healing because reintubation in the acute stages after this operation can be very difficult.
- If the airway does not settle after these measures then a more definitive airway widening procedure may be done in the future in order to decannulate the patient (multistaged laryngotracheoplasty).

# Tracheal obstruction/abnormalities

Laryngotracheal clefts

- Split in posterior glottis between the arytenoid cartilages that can extend inferiorly along the whole length of the posterior trachea. The trachea and esophagus share a common lumen during embryogenesis and clefts result from failure of the tracheoesophageal septum to form between these two structures.
- Most are small and present later within the first few years of life. Patients have a history of recurrent aspiration or stridor. If they are larger and involve the trachea, then they are usually apparent at birth.
- Diagnosis—usually made with chest X-ray (signs of chronic aspiration), esophagram, and extent determined by direct bronchoscopy.
- Treatment—depends on severity. The smaller clefts can be repaired endoscopically, but more often require open procedures to repair. The larger clefts may require open repair, temporary tracheotomy, and G-tube/Nissen fundoplication as severe GERD may also be present.

Tracheomalacia

- Soft, compliant tracheal rings that rarely cause significant airway distress.
- The trachea is made up of incomplete horseshoe-shaped cartilages that support the airway and a vertically oriented posterior strip of muscle that allows for growth and expansion.
- Tracheomalacia occurs when the cartilage is weaker than normal and rarely results in clinical symptoms unless there is a coexisting tracheal abnormality such as a tracheoesophageal fistula or extrinsic compression from a vascular anomaly.
- Patients usually have expiratory stridor that presents within 6 months of birth and may also have recurrent bronchial infections.
- Diagnosis—usually made by chest X-ray, airway fluoroscopy, or direct exam with bronchoscopy. Bronchoscopy is important to ensure that the tracheal rings are not complete as the child's airway will fail to grow with time and his condition will deteriorate as he grows. An echocardiogram may be important to rule out an associated vascular anomaly that may be repairable.
- Treatment: primarily observation. Bronchodilators may worsen dynamic obstruction. In cases of severe acute obstruction, non-invasive positive pressure ventilation (NPPV), intubation, or tracheostomy may be required.

Other ENT Problems in the PICU
  Epistaxis

- Most cases of epistaxis in the PICU are benign and self-resolving. Nasal bleeding is usually due to dryness, nasogastric, (NG) or endotracheal tube (ETT) trauma. Important to rule out associated coagulopathy in the ICU setting by checking complete blood count (CBC), international normalized ratio (INR), partial prothrombin time (PTT).
- If a coagulopathy exists, treat the underlying coagulopathy and avoid further nasal trauma (including packing).
- Bedside use of humidifiers and twice daily application of Vaseline to the septal mucosa are helpful preventative measures.
- If bleeding is ongoing and packs are required, hemostasis may be achieved with the following protocol:

  - Soak cotton ball with topical thrombin or tranexamic acid with saline.
  - Evacuate the nose by having the patient blow or by gently suctioning out clots.
  - Apply cotton ball along the floor of the nose and squeeze soft part of nose for 5–10 minutes to occlude nostrils.
  - If still bleeding, apply absorbable packing coated with Vaseline or antibiotic ointment.
  - Useful absorbable thrombostatic materials include Gelfoam (spongy material that can be cut into strips and applied along the floor of the nose) or Surgicel (gauzy material that can be cut into long strips and applied along the floor of the nose).
  - Alternately, nonabsorbable Vaseline gauze can be applied to both the nasal cavities.

- If a coagulopathy is not present, try preventative treatment first and if not successful, proceed with packing using non-absorbable Vaseline gauze that is usually left in place for 48 hours.
- If nose continues to bleed heavily, posterior balloon packs using a Foley catheter coupled with Vaseline gauze anterior packs may be used.
- The patient should be treated with prophylactic antibiotic to cover *S. aureus* if bilateral packs are present or if packs stay longer than 24 to 48 hours as there is a risk of developing toxic shock syndrome due to retained packs.

Sinusitis

- Sinusitis is primarily an outpatient pediatric problem, unless intracranial/intraorbital abscesses or other complications co-exist. In these cases, broad spectrum antibiotics that cross the blood-brain barrier are indicated. Ophthalmology, otolaryn-gology, and neurosurgical physicians should be consulted when these complications have been diagnosed as it is imperative to promptly drain both the sinuses and the orbit or brain, if they are involved.
- In the PICU setting, acute sinusitis may manifest as fever without a source especially in immunocompromised patients. Nosocomial sinusitis is occasionally seen as a complication of prolonged nasotracheal intubation.

Diagnosis:

- Difficult diagnosis to make in the PICU especially if the patient is intubated. It is usually associated with tenderness over cheek or teeth pain and children may have associated periorbital erythema or cellulitis especially if the ethmoid sinuses involved. Without these symptoms and signs, the diagnosis may be difficult to establish.
- CT scans of the sinuses may aid in diagnosis; however, the CT can be misleading because the false positive rate of sinus CT is high and partial opacification of ethmoid or maxillary sinuses due to mucosal swelling and mucus retention is extremely common in the intubated patient regardless of whether infec-tion is also present.

Treatment:

- Empiric antibiotic coverage.
- Culture and drainage in the operating room is usually helpful if the patient is toxic or neutropenic.

# References

Tomaski SM, Zalzal GH, Saal HM. Airway obstruction in the Pierre Robin Sequence. Laryngooscope 1995;105:111–4.

Mancuso RF, Choi SS, Zalzal GH, Grundfast KM. Laryngomalacia. The search for the second lesion. Arch Otolaryngol Head Neck Surg 1996; 22:302–6.

Bower CM, Choi SS, Cotton RT. Arytenoidectomy in children. Ann Otol Rhinol Laryngol 1994;103:271–8.

Pransky SM, Canto C. Management of subglottic hemangioma. Curr Opin Otolaryngol Head Neck Surg 2004;12: 509–12.

# C. Tracheotomy

Lisa Elden

## Key Principles

- Tracheotomy may aid in the long-term management of a child with airway, lung, neuromuscular, or central nervous system (CNS) problems.
- Tracheostomy complication rates are higher in children than adults.
- Decision to undergo tracheostomy is complex and requires family consultation with a multidisciplinary team.

## Indications

The decision to proceed with a tracheostomy is complex and requires a detailed discussion with the family that touches on long-term implications. Morbidity and mortality related to tracheotomies in children is approximately twice that of the adult population with long-term mortality in infants ranging from 10 to 40%. However, the incidence of tracheotomy-related deaths is 0–3.4%. The overall complication rate for pediatric tracheotomies is 40%. Emergency tracheotomies are rarely necessary in children and unlike adults, transcutaneous placement of tracheotomies at the intensive care unit (ICU) bedside by Seldinger technique is not performed.

Characteristics of children requiring tracheotomy in the PICU

- Mean age 3.8 years; 50% <1 year old
- 60% have acute upper airway obstruction (croup, subglottic stenosis, etc.)
- 30% have a need for ongoing ventilatory support (lung-related problems)
- 10% have a need for chronic pulmonary toilet (cystic fibrosis)

Other indications include neurologic or neuromuscular diseases leading to inadequate ventilation or central respiratory drive.

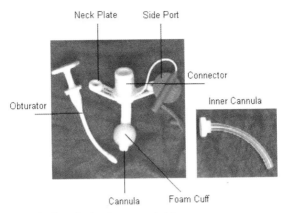

**Figure 1**    Example of tracheostomy tube kit.

Timing of tracheotomy versus continuing endotracheal intubation for mechanical ventilation is controversial in the pediatric population.

## Acute Complications

1. Accidental decannulation

   Ensure that the tracheotomy is adequately secured to the neck of the patient.

   It should be firmly tied with ties that allow only one finger-breadth in between ties and neck. Many surgeons also suture the tracheotomy plate to the patient's skin when first placed. The ties should always be changed by two people, one to hold the tracheotomy plate and one to change the ties.

   If the tracheotomy comes out, the physician can try to replace it through the stoma site, but if the site is new (within 3 days of surgery). The site may be difficult to identify and in that case the physician should re-intubate the patient orally. Usually most tracheotomy stomas are mature 5 to 7 days postoperatively.

   Children with tracheostomies should always have a replacement tracheostomy ready for use at the bedside.

2. Malposition of tracheotomy tube or plugging of tube

   Important to get a postoperative chest X-ray (CXR) to ensure the distal tip of the tube is not too low. In very small babies, the tube may be too long and this can result in a right main stem intubation.

The tracheotomy tube should be cleaned regularly with saline and suctioning to prevent tracheal tube plugging. Initially, frequent suctioning (every 30 minutes) may be needed.

3. Pneumomediastinum or pneumothorax

Pneumomediastinum occurs in 4% of cases and pneumothorax occurs in 1% of cases. In most instances, they do not require intervention, but should be followed with serial CXRs until sure they have stabilized.

4. Local stomal infection

Occurs in 8% of children and usually occurs several days after tracheotomy has been performed. Can be treated or prevented by increasing frequency of dressing changes and stoma cleaning. Rarely due to Candida, but should be considered in infant.

5. Local stomal bleeding

Usually minimal oozing from skin wound that responds to light packing, but given that the innominate artery can ride high near the stoma, ongoing bleeding or recurrent episodes of fresh stomal bleeding should be reported to the surgeon. Tracheoinnominate fistula is an extremely rare but often fatal complication; successful acute management has been reported in adults with digital pressure on the fistula and immediate extracorporeal life support or surgical repair.

## Long-Term Considerations

1. Phonation: In due course, with the assistance of play and speech therapists, the cuff can be deflated, and the patient encouraged to occlude the tube with a finger and to begin to phonate. Speech therapy is an essential part of long-term care for a patient with a tracheostomy.

2. Swallowing: Although swallowing is initially difficult with a tracheotomy tube in place, many children can swallow and feed normally with time. However, careful assessment of aspiration risk by a speech therapist is imperative before oral feeding starts.

3. Infection: Tracheostomies are frequently colonized by pseudomonas and staph species. Occasionally colonization may change into active disease requiring antimicrobial treatment.

4. Home care and equipment: At first, parents find this very difficult. Early intense training of family members is essential preparation for discharge. All household caregivers must learn to replace the outer cannula if decannulation occurs. Home

equipment should include saline, suction catheters, and a suction machine along with a spare tube with an obturator.

5. Decannulation: Tracheostomies are often temporary in children. If the underlying lung disease or airway obstruction has resolved, a trial of decannulation may be indicated. Decannulation often starts with downsizing of the tracheostomy with trials of plugging, followed by tube removal and/or a surgical procedure. Successful decannulation depends primarily on the underlying diagnosis.

# References

Lewis CW, Carron JD, Perkins JA, et al. Tracheotomy in pediatric patients: a national perspective. Arch Otolaryngol Head Neck Surg 2003;129: 523–9.

Thorp A, Hurt TL, Kim TY, Brown L. Tracheoinnominate artery fistula: a rare and often fatal complication of indwelling tracheostomy tubes. Pediatr Emerg Care 2005;21:763–6.

Alladi A, Rao S, Das K, et al. Pediatric tracheostomy: a 13-year experience. Pediatr Surg Int 2004;20:695–8.

# D. Upper Airway Infections

Lisa Elden

Lennox Huang

## Key Principles

- Epidemiology of infectious upper airway obstruction has changed; life-threatening cases are increasingly rare.
- Anesthesia and ears, nose, and throat (ENT) backup is needed for children with upper airway infections and a threatened airway.
- Most cases can be managed with a combination of systemic steroids and racemic epinephrine.

## Croup (laryngotracheobronchitis)

- The most common cause of stridor in infants.
- Most cases occur in children aged 6 months to 3 years.
- Usually caused by parainfluenza, but may also be caused by respiratory syncytial virus (RSV), influenza A, mycoplasma.
- Generally a mild, self-limited disease.

History

- Upper respiratory symptoms.
- Family members, close contacts with upper respiratory infections.
- Barking "seal-like" cough.

Diagnosis

- Generally made from history and physical examination.
- General appearance should be well.
- Child may have upper respiratory secretions and cough.
- Look for stridor at rest.
- Neck radiographs are generally unnecessary but if obtained, a classic steeple sign may be seen as anteroposterior (AP) and lateral views.

Treatment

- Systemic steroids are the mainstay for a child with croup, even well-appearing children benefit from a single dose

of dexamethasone, which may be administered orally, or intramuscularly.
- Prednisone has been less well studied in the setting of croup but appears to be effective as well.
- Inhaled steroids have shown benefit, but evidence suggests that they are less effective compared with systemic steroids.
- Racemic epinephrine for stridor at rest or significant respiratory distress.
- Rarely requires intubation and mechanical ventilation.

# Peritonsillar Abscess

- Usually associated with a preceding tonsillitis or upper respiratory tract infection (URTI). Usually occurs in teens and young adults, less often occurs in younger school age children.

Diagnosis:

> Swelling occurs lateral to the tonsil, and usually is unilateral resulting in asymmetric airway swelling with erythema of soft palate and lateral pharyngeal wall. The uvula may be deviated to the opposite side. The tonsil itself is rarely swollen.

Treatment:

> Normally, the airway is stable; IV antibiotics should be chosen to cover *Streptococcus* species and oral anaerobic pathogens (penicillin or clindamycin). Incision and drainage can often be done in the emergency department (ED) in older children.

> If the airway is significantly swollen, expect further swelling over the 12 to 24 hours postdrainage. Intensive care unit (ICU) observation may be necessary.

# Retropharyngeal Infection

- Usually associated with a preceding adenoiditis or URTI.

History:

> Usually occurs in younger children (age 2 to 3 years), but sometimes can be associated with trauma from a foreign body (fish bone or lacerated posterior pharynx from external trauma such as from a popsicle stick). Presentation may be similar to epiglottitis with increase temperature, dysphagia, and drooling; however,

there almost always is a several day history of a preceding URTI compared with epiglottitis that develops much more rapidly.

Examination:

Swelling and increased secretions are often present, but located behind the nose in the nasopharynx so it may be difficult to see signs on direct oral exam.

Diagnosis:

Usually made by history and confirmed by lateral soft tissue films of the neck. It is important to look for associated foreign body in reviewing the X-ray.

Alternatively, bedside flexible nasopharyngoscopy may confirm the diagnosis and rule out epiglottitis. The adenoids are usually inflamed and there may be a nasopharyngeal bulge present. Computed tomography (CT) of the head and neck soft tissues is helpful if concerned about degree of airway swelling or if patient fails to improve within 24 to 48 hours of treatment. However, it is not easy to differentiate between abscess and cellulitis even with CT in the early stages of the illness. Up to 25% to 50% of children with cellulitis and early abscesses can be treated medically without operative intervention if the airway is safe.

Treatment:

IV antibiotics to cover Strep A and oral anaerobic pathogens such as clindamycin or a combination drug such as ampicillin and sulbactam (Unasyn) to also include coverage of less common gram-negative aerobic pathogens such as *Haemophilus influenza*. One should have a low threshold in broadening antibiotic coverage in a patient who is quite ill or who fails to respond to antibiotics within 24 to 48 hours.

Surgical drainage for large abscesses.

If the airway has been assessed directly with nasopharyngoscopy and it appears to be safe, the child can be monitored in ICU or step down unit and white blood cell count, temperature and ability to drink followed to monitor improvement.

If the airway symptoms deteriorate after initial assessment or if the child does not improve within 24 to 48 hours, then the child should be taken to the operating room for intubation and possible incision and drainage of abscess.

# Epiglottitis/Supraglottitis

Although the rate of *H. influenza*–related epiglottitis has markedly decreased because of the HIB vaccine, it can still occur in nonvaccinated children and in teens/adults who have not been vaccinated. Also, supraglottitis may occur secondary to streptococcal or staphylococcal infections (although the latter more commonly causes a tracheitis with associated supraglottitis).

Supraglottitis should be suspected in a child who has become acutely ill over a period of 12 to 24 hours with high temperature, dysphagia, and drooling. Usually the child will sit in an upright position and there may be a characteristic muffled quality to the voice/speech. Do not examine oral cavity without clearance from ENT and anesthesia.

Diagnosis is confirmed with lateral soft tissue X-ray of the neck (classic thumbprint sign of swollen epiglottis) or by direct exam with bedside nasopharyngoscopy. If clinical suspicion of supraglottitis is high, then the patient should not leave the monitored setting for diagnostic purposes. A portable X-ray or nasopharyngoscopy exam can be done safely by the bedside in most instances.

Treatment:

If airway appears unstable, ENT and anesthesia should be consulted urgently so the patient may be intubated in the operating room with an endotracheal tube that has a stylet in place, and a rigid bronchoscope (to improve visualization) and/or tracheotomy should be set up to be used if routine intubation fails. Anesthesia is given by gas inhalational agents and not by paralyzing agents to try to preserve spontaneous respiration throughout induction as the child usually can protect the airway more effectively if he or she has not been paralyzed.

If airway appears stable, the child can be monitored in the ICU without intubation. However, if the child deteriorates and intubation seems eminent, then it should be done without paralyzing agents and hopefully with anesthesia and ENT physicians on hand.

Medical treatment:

In addition to intubation or airway observation, empiric antibiotics to cover *H. influenza*, streptococcal, and staphylococcal species (ceftriaxone or cefotaxime). Systemic steroids should be given to reduce the airway swelling and reduce the duration of time that the child requires intubation.

# Bacterial Tracheitis

With the decline of epiglottitis, bacterial tracheitis has now become one of the most common life-threatening upper airway infections. Patients may present with croup-like symptoms, respiratory distress, acute respiratory failure, or septic shock. Etiology is most often staph aureus with an increase in cases of MRSA in North America. Other organisms include *Moraxella catarrhalis*, group A strep, *Klebsiella*, and *H. influenza*. Bacterial tracheitis is often preceded by a benign viral infection, including croup.

Diagnosis

- Diagnosis is often made based on clinical presentation and cultures of tracheal secretions.
- Consider blood cultures if patient appears toxic.
- Neck radiographs are not necessary and do not show any specific abnormality.
- Laryngobronchoscopy provides the definitive diagnosis but is not always performed.

Treatment

- Airway management as outlined in the General Approach (Section A of this chapter) and Chapter 5, "Pulmonary".
- Intubation may be required.
- Empiric antibiotic therapy may start with a third- or fourth-generation cephalosporin or amoxicillin sulbactam. In confirmed cases of bacterial tracheitis in North America, vancomycin should be considered to treat potential community-acquired MRSA.

*Table 1*
## Infectious Causes of Upper Airway Obstruction

| | Age | Appearance | Examination | Radiograph | Organisms |
|---|---|---|---|---|---|
| Croup | 3 mo–3 yr | Well to moderately ill | Barky cough | Steeple sign (subglottic narrowing) | Parainfluenza, RSV, influenza, mycoplasma |

*(continued)*

| | Age | Appearance | Examination | Radiograph | Organisms |
|---|---|---|---|---|---|
| Epiglottitis | Historically 2–6 yr, now more often seen in adults and adolescents, mean age 11 yr | Toxic | Drooling, dysphonia, dysphagia | Thumb sign (swollen epiglottis) | *H. influenza, S. pneumoniae, Staphylococcus aureus* |
| Peritonsillar abscess | Older children and adolescents | Moderately ill | Uvula deviation, hot potato (muffled) voice | Normal | Group A strep, anaerobes |
| Bacterial tracheitis | Any age group, mean age 4 yr | Toxic | Dysphonia, nonspecific symptoms | Normal or subglottic narrowing | *S. aureus* (MRSA) *Haemophilus Spyogenes* |
| Retropharyngeal abscess | Over 6 yr of age | Toxic | Muffled voice | Thickened retropharyngeal space | *S. aureus, Streptococcus* species less often anaerobic bacteria |

# References

Hopkins A, Lahiri T, Salerno R, Heath B. Changing epidemiology of life-threatening upper airway infections: the reemergence of bacterial tracheitis. Pediatrics 2006;118:1418–21.

Rafei K, Lichenstein R. Airway infectious disease emergencies. Pediatr Clin North Am 2006;53:215–42.

Bjornson CL, Klassen TP, Williamson J, et al., and the Pediatric Emergency Research Canada Network. A randomized trial of a single dose of oral dexamethasone for mild croup. N Engl J Med 2004;351:1306–13.

# Chapter 8

# Cardiac

## A. Assessment of Patients with Suspected Heart Disease

Sandy Pitfield
Neil Spenceley
Stephen Keeley

### Key Principles

- Rapid clinical assessment is crucial to the management of children with suspected heart disease. Abnormalities of tissue perfusion, ventilation, and oxygenation need to be addressed aggressively. Such abnormalities are often addressed before a definitive clinical diagnosis is reached.
- Knowledge of the typical patterns of presentation of heart disease in children allows the clinician to institute appropriate therapies early.
- Neonates with cyanosis and those presenting with circulatory shock should have a prostaglandin infusion initiated urgently. Initiation of prostaglandin should not be delayed while awaiting diagnostic assessment.
- The vast majority of conditions can be adequately diagnosed by an echocardiogram performed by an experienced pediatric cardiac ultrasonographer, and this investigation should be performed urgently in an unstable child with suspected heart disease.

# Clinical Assessment

Initial clinical assessment of the child with suspected heart disease should focus on the need for resuscitative interventions (ABCs). Respiratory failure is commonly associated with severe heart disease, and requires intubation and mechanical ventilation. Circulatory shock requires administration of fluid boluses and initiation of inotropes. For children with circulatory shock of suspected cardiac etiology, concerns about potential fluid overload should not preclude aggressive fluid resuscitation.

Other components of the differential diagnosis (Tables 1 and 2) must be considered and ruled out. It is important to recognize that many of these children have coexisting conditions and/or cardiac lesions. The diagnoses listed represent only the most typical presentation pattern, and are not exclusive of other clinical findings.

Importantly, sepsis can mimic all presentations of cardiac disease at all ages, and early initiation of empiric antibiotic therapy until a diagnosis is reached is strongly recommended.

Clinical evaluation is primarily used to quantify the severity of cardiorespiratory dysfunction.

History: Historical data collection is dependent on age (Table 3).

*Table 1*
**Differential Diagnosis for Neonates Presenting with Suspected Heart Disease**

| Cardiac | |
|---|---|
| *Cyanosis* | *Circulatory shock* |
| • Cyanotic congenital heart diseases | • Left-sided obstruction |
| | • Arrhythmia |
| *Respiratory distress* | • Hypertrophic cardiomyopathy |
| • Left-sided obstruction | |
| **Noncardiac** | |
| *Cyanosis* | *Circulatory shock* |
| • PPHN | • Sepsis |
| • Pneumonia | • Metabolic disease |
| • TTN | |
| *Respiratory distress* | |
| • Pneumonia | |

*Table 2*
**Differential Diagnosis for Infants and Older Children Presenting with Suspected Heart Disease**

| Cardiac | |
|---|---|
| *Cyanosis* <br> • Eisenmenger's syndrome <br> • Shunt thrombosis/ stenosis <br> • Reduced pulmonary blood flow <br> *Respiratory distress* <br> • Volume overload (L → R shunting) <br> *Circulatory shock* <br> • Myocarditis <br> • Arrhythmia <br> • Endocarditis | *Failure to thrive/exercise intolerance* <br> • ALCAPA <br> • Hypertrophic cardiomyopathy <br> • Volume overload (L → R shunting) <br> • Decline in prosthetic function (valve, conduit, shunt, pacemaker) <br> • Complications of drug therapy |

| Noncardiac | |
|---|---|
| *Cyanosis* <br> • Pneumonia <br> • V/Q mismatch <br> *Respiratory distress* <br> • Pneumonia <br> • Sepsis <br> • Asthma | *Circulatory shock* <br> • Sepsis <br> *Failure to thrive/exercise intolerance* <br> • Anemia <br> • Malnutrition <br> • Malabsorption <br> • Metabolic disease |

*Table 3*
**Historical Data to Be Collected for Children with Suspected Heart Disease**

| Neonates | Infants and older children |
|---|---|
| Antenatal ultrasound reports <br> Infectious risk factors <br> Events of delivery <br> Course of life since birth <br> Initial management <br> Diagnostics performed | Family history of heart disease <br> History of heart disease or previous surgery <br> Symptoms of heart disease <br> Syncope <br> Current medications <br> Allergies <br> Other medical conditions |

**Physical Examination:** The primary focus of the physical exam concerns assessment of the triad of cardiovascular, respiratory, and central nervous system function. The focus in the newborn period is on assessing clinical signs and symptoms of the three most common presenting states: shock, hypoxemia, or cyanosis. The following parameters must be closely assessed:

- Heart rate and rhythm
- Blood pressure
- Pulse volume and quality
- Capillary refill time
- Hepatomegaly
- Skin temperature and color
- Respiratory effort and rate
- Oxygen saturation
- Urine output
- Level of consciousness

The same measures are followed during initial re-suscitative efforts and subsequent stabilization, with a goal of re-establishing all within their normal range.

The hyperoxia test is performed in addition to the usual physical examination for neonates with cyanosis. 100% oxygen is administered via head box or tight-fitting mask. For the noninvasive method, peripheral oxygen saturation is monitored. Significant increases in oxygen saturations are typically seen if the cyanosis results from respiratory disease, while lack of response suggests underlying cyanotic congenital heart disease. A more invasive method involves assessment of $PaO_2$ on arterial blood gas analysis. With pulmonary disease, $PaO_2$ usually rises to $>150$ mm Hg. In the case of cyanotic congenital heart disease, the $PaO_2$ typically does not exceed 100 mm Hg, and the rise is not more than 10 to 30 mm Hg.

In the older child with known cardiac disease, assessing for clinical signs and causes of congestive heart failure, ventricular dysfunction (right sided, left sided, or combined), or worsening cyanosis are the priority (Table 2).

## Laboratory Assessment

Laboratory assessment infrequently helps with the diagnosis. The primary objectives of laboratory assessment are:

- to guide ongoing resuscitative care and preoperative stabilization,

- to exclude noncardiac causes of the child's condition, and
- to detect and monitor organ injury secondary to the presenting cardiorespiratory failure

All children should have the following:

- CBC, differential
- Hematocrit in cyanosed children
- Blood cultures
- Blood glucose
- Serum electrolytes, BUN, creatinine, calcium, magnesium
- Arterial, venous, or capillary blood gas
- Serum lactate
- Coagulation studies (PT, PTT, fibrinogen)
- Liver function tests
- Liver enzymes
- Respiratory tract cultures/viral assays (for children with respiratory symptoms and/or fever)

Laboratory assessment of the adequacy of cardiac output in meeting the metabolic demands of the body includes:

- arterial blood gas (pH, serum bicarbonate),
- serum lactate, and
- mixed venous oxygen saturation (preferentially obtained from an intrathoracic central line—subclavian or internal jugular)

Chromosomal studies should be sent when indicated:

- Lesions commonly associated with chromosomal abnormality (AVSD (Trisomy 21); TOF, IAA, Truncus arteriosus (22q11 deletion))
- Dysmorphic features on clinical exam

More extensive bloodwork must be sent in the event that transplantation is being considered.

## Cardiac Diagnostic Assessment

CXR: Quick and easy to perform, the CXR aids the diagnosis in some cases. Specific areas of interest include cardiac size, pulmonary vascularity, and coexisting pulmonary disease. Lesion-specific findings (rib notching in coarctation, egg on a string in TGA, boot-shaped heart in TOF) can also be appreciated. Situs abnormalities of the major intra-abdominal organs can be appreciated.

Electrocardiography: Quick and easy to perform, the ECG can be diagnostic in some cases. Rhythm and conduction disturbances are easily appreciable. Ischemic changes can be appreciated in ALCAPA and Kawasaki disease, among others. Low voltages may be seen with myocarditis and pericardial effusions. Abnormalities of chamber size can be appreciated. Some structural heart diseases have typical features on ECG.

Echocardiography: It provides accurate anatomic diagnosis in most cases and is the preferred modality for diagnostic assessment. It also provides estimates of cardiac function and chamber pressures, and adequate information to plan surgical intervention in the majority of structural congenital heart diseases. It is inaccurate for assessment of diastolic function. Its ability to determine coronary anatomy and quantify valvular regurgitation is variable. Accurate diagnosis is usually available preoperatively for VSDs, AVSDs, TOF, IAA, HLHS, and coarctation.

Cardiac catheterization: As other noninvasive techniques become more sophisticated, cardiac catheterization is required less often. Currently, it is the only technique to give measures of absolute pressures in chambers and vessels, provide oxygen saturations, and offer pulmonary vascular resistance calculations, including the response of the pulmonary vasculature to pulmonary vasodilators. Its use is well established in angioplasty and stenting, valvuloplasty, device delivery such as to close ASDs and PDAs, and vascular communications such as Fontan fenestrations, and is expanding as new devices are developed, such as those for VSD closure and valvular implants. Tissue can be obtained for assessment in the case of suspected myocarditis or graft rejection.

CT angiography: This provides superb two-dimensional and three-dimensional imaging following a single breath-hold acquisition using iodinated contrast, but with the added risk over MRI of radiation exposure. CT angiography is usually more accessible than MR. Contraindications include those who have previously had contrast reactions.

Cardiac MRI: Image acquisition is triggered by the patient's ECG to minimize motion artifact and allow imaging of cardiovascular and mediastinal structures. It provides excellent anatomic detail and information about spatial relationships and qualitative and quantitative assessment of valve and ventricular function, including ventricular volume and mass, as well as intravascular flow dynamics, pressure gradients, and shunt calculation. Recent advances allow imaging of coronary arteries and myocardial viability. Techniques for determination of oxygen saturations are being developed. Imaging may be limited by an inability to gate in patients with irregular rhythms, to lie flat in those with failure, and patient claustrophobia. Contraindications are few and include pacemakers and retained wires, endovascular or intracardiac implants, and aneurysm clips exposed directly to the magnetic field.

## Noncardiac Assessment

Abdominal ultrasound: All children with complex congenital heart disease should have an abdominal ultrasound. Hepatic and splenic abnormalities (polysplenia, asplenia) can be suggestive of the heterotaxy syndrome. Renal abnormalities can complicate postoperative care.

Cranial ultrasound: All neonates with complex congenital heart disease should have a cranial ultrasound. It is essential to rule out significant intracranial hemorrhage prior to anticoagulation on bypass.

Near-infrared spectroscopy: It provides a numeric estimation of tissue oxygen content. The value expressed is a weighted average of arterial (25%) and venous (75%) oxygen saturation. Its role is not well established; however, trends tend to reflect changes in patient condition. Specifically, improvements in tissue perfusion are typically reflected by an increase in the NIRS value.

## Summary

Clinical assessment of the patient with suspected heart disease allows the physician to determine the rapidity with which further diagnostic assessment must occur. Initial resuscitative measures may include fluid resuscitation, initiation of prostaglandin infusion, intubation and mechanical ventilation, and initiation of inotropes.

Diagnostic assessment with echocardiography allows optimization of medical management and planning for surgical intervention. Additional diagnostic modalities may be used depending on the ability of the initial echocardiogram to accurately provide necessary information.

# Suggested Reading

Nichols DG, Ungerleider RM, Spevak PJ, et al. Critical Heart Disease in Infants and Children. 2nd ed. Philadelphia (PA): Mosby; c2006.

Nichols DG. Roger's Textbook of Pediatric Intensive Care. 4th ed. Philadelphia (PA): Lippincott Williams & Williams; c2008. Section IV, Cardiac Disease; p. 997–1196.

Chang AC, Hanley FL, Wernovsky G, Wessel DL. Pediatric Cardiac Intensive Care. Baltimore (MD): Williams & Wilkins; c1998.

Park MK. Pediatric Cardiology for Practitioners. 5th ed. Philadelphia (PA): Mosby; c2008.

# B. Pediatric Arrhythmias

Peter Skippen

Shubhayan Sanatani

Tapas Mondal

Catherine Chant-Gambacourt

Jim Potts

Paul F Kantor

## Key Principles

- Rhythm disturbances cause hemodynamic compromise in children due to rate abnormalities or loss of synchrony.
- The most common conditions predisposing to arrhythmias in children are congenital heart disease and postoperative cardiac surgery.
- Tachycardias are the most frequent rhythm disturbance in children.
- The most common mechanism of tachyarrhythmias in children are re-entrant tachycardias and enhanced automaticity.
- Cardiorespiratory collapse requires emergent cardioversion with or without IV/IO access.

## Generation of the Normal Electrocardiogram

The normal electrocardiogram represents the electrical waveform generated by spontaneous depolarization of cardiac myocytes. Myocytes in the nodal regions (sinus, atrioventricular) depolarize rapidly and hence function as pacemakers dictating the heart rates under physiological conditions. The sinus (sinoatrial) node triggers the sequence of events leading to a normal cardiac impulse. The electrical impulse spreads to the atria, resulting in the P wave on the surface electrocardiogram (ECG). (See Figure 1.) The wave of excitability then continues to the atrioventricular (AV) node where conduction is briefly delayed to allow for ventricular filling. This is seen as the PR interval on the ECG. Ventricular depolarization is

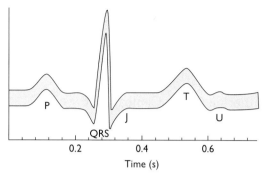

**Figure 1**    Normal electrocardiogram.

represented by the QRS complex. This is followed by ventricular repolarization, seen as the T wave on the surface ECG.

An appreciation of normal variation and differences in the pediatric ECG with age and maturation is essential for interpretation of pediatric rhythm disturbances (Tables 1 and 2). Moreover, when evaluating a child suspected of having structural heart disease, it is important to recognize the changes on ECG characteristic of various congenital cardiac lesions. In the intensive care unit (ICU), the ECG is used primarily to evaluate patients for rhythm disturbances,

*Table 1*
**Heart Rates and PR and QRS intervals According to Age**

| Age | HR | PR interval | QRS interval |
|---|---|---|---|
| 1–3 weeks | 100–180 | 0.07–0.14 | 0.03–0.07 |
| 1–6 months | 100–185 | 0.07–0.16 | 0.03–0.07 |
| 6–12 months | 100–170 | 0.08–0.16 | 0.03–0.08 |
| 1–3 years | 90–150 | 0.09–0.16 | 0.03–0.08 |
| 3–5 years | 70–140 | 0.09–0.16 | 0.03–0.08 |
| 5–8 years | 65–130 | 0.09–0.16 | 0.03–0.08 |
| 8–12 years | 60–110 | 0.09–0.16 | 0.03–0.09 |
| 12–16 years | 60–100 | 0.09–0.18 | 0.03–0.09 |

*Table 2*
**Features of Pediatric ECGs**

| |
|---|
| Sinus arrhythmia common |
| Wide range of normal rates |
| J point elevation is common |
| T waves inverted in right precordial leads until adolescence |
| Large mid-precordial voltages common in newborn |
| Right ventricular dominance in newborn, regresses over first few years of life |

myocardial ischemic changes, and changes secondary to systemic illness.

# Clinical Conditions Associated with Arrhythmias in Children

Arrhythmias occur under a wide variety of conditions in the ICU. The most common condition is in the post-operative cardiac patient. Table 3 lists common situations that predispose patients to arrhythmias.

*Table 3*
**Conditions Predisposing to Arrhythmias**

| **Structural** |
|---|
| Congenital heart disease |
| Postoperative cardiac surgery |
| Cardiomyopathies |
|         Hypertrophic cardiomyopathy |
|         Dilated cardiomyopathy |
|         Anthracycline toxicity |
|         Arrhythmogenic right ventricular cardiomyopathy |
| Myocarditis |
| **Primary Electrical Disease** |
| Wolff-Parkinson-White syndrome |
| Long QT syndrome |
| Catecholaminergic polymorphic ventricular tachycardia |

*(continued)*

| **Other Conditions** |
| --- |
| Electrolyte disturbances |
| Thyroid disease |
| Medication toxicity |
| Toxic ingestions |
| Cardiac contusion |

# Mechanisms of Arrhythmias

There are five common mechanisms responsible for arrhythmias in children:

1. re-entrant excitation
2. enhanced automaticity
3. failure of impulse propagation (conduction block)
4. failure of impulse generation
5. triggered activity

The first three are by far the most common encountered in the pediatric ICU.

# Hemodynamics and Arrhythmias

In children, heart rate rather than contractility plays a greater role in optimizing cardiac output. Therefore, rhythm disturbances that cause hemodynamic compromise in children are usually related to rate abnormalities or loss of synchrony. Cardiac output (heart rate × stroke volume) can be impaired if rate is too slow or too fast (not enough time for ventricular filling or myocardial ischemia). Tachyarrhythmias are the most frequently encountered arrhythmia causing hemodynamic compromise in children. The most obvious form of dyssynchrony is atrioventricular, which usually occurs when there is a long conduction time from the atria to ventricles (first-degree heart block) with atrial depolarization occurring prior to ventricular relaxation and opening of the AV valves. With complete AV dissociation, loss of atrial augmentation of ventricular filling occurs. Other forms of dyssynchrony can occur with regional wall motion abnormalities or conduction delays.

# Arrhythmia Diagnosis

To simplify cardiac assessment, rhythms can be initially classed into three categories: bradyarrhythmia, tachyarrhythmia, and collapse rhythms (electromechanical dissociation and asystole). Tachyarrhythmias can be further considered as wide complex versus narrow complex, stable or unstable.

A diagnosis of arrhythmias is made in the ICU primarily by clinical examination and a single ECG lead rhythm strip. A 12-lead ECG should be obtained whenever possible for additional diagnostic information. Preoperative and postoperative ECGs are especially useful for cardiac surgical patients. Ancillary information can be obtained from central line pressure waveform monitoring and, particularly in the post-operative patient, direct atrial and ventricular electrograms. Occasionally, an esophageal catheter can be placed to record atrial electrograms from the left atrium.

## A. Bradycardia and Block

**Sinus Bradycardia (Figure 2)**   The most common cause of bradycardia in children is hypoxemia, an ominous development that should be corrected urgently.

The lower limit of a normal heart rate in children is ill defined. Consideration of the clinical condition is required when assessing a low heart rate. A normal physiologic variation in impulse discharge from the sinoatrial node (SA node)

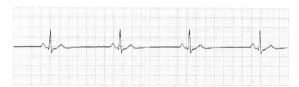

**Figure 2a**   Sinus bradycardia.

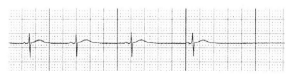

**Figure 2b**   Sinus bradycardia in a neonate with necrotizing enterocolitis (vagally mediated).

occurs with respiration. In addition, children on monitors are commonly noted to sustain very low heart rates. In such cases, one may see a junctional or ventricular escape rhythm. Transient junctional escape or Wenckebach conduction at the AV node (see below) is normal during sleep. Vagally mediated suppression of normal pacemaker activity is the usual cause of asymptomatic bradycardia. This does not require any intervention as long as the heart rate responds appropriately to their level of arousal. Clinical judgment as when to intervene is crucial and should be based on symptoms and not a specific rate. When evaluating a patient with bradycardia, a 12-lead ECG should be performed, with particular attention to the relationship of the "P" and "T" waves, and the QT interval.

Intervention should therefore be based on symptoms of low output, such as poor feeding, somnolence, postural hypotension, or syncope, and NOT on a specific rate. Conversely, even if the rate is in the normal reference range, it may be an inadequate chronotropic response; for example, this is seen in palliated complex congenital heart disease in the Fontan patients. Occasionally, a low ventricular rate is due to a rapid atrial rate or premature atrial complexes (PACs), which are not conducted to the ventricles. In severe cases of long QT syndrome, the subsequent sinus beat may fall into the abnormally long refractory period of the ventricle with resulting bradycardia. The most common noncardiac causes of sinus bradycardia is hypoxia and must be excluded. Other conditions to consider include hypothermia, hypothyroidism, raised intracranial pressure, and drug intoxication. Children who have undergone cardiac surgery have increased risk of sick sinus syndrome as a result of the atriotomy as well as direct injury to the SA node or arterial supply to SA node. Other rare causes of sinus bradycardia include sinus exit block or isomerism.

**Heart Block**    Atrioventricular block is a broad term referring to abnormalities in impulses from the atria reaching the ventricles and may be congenital or acquired. The most commonly encountered forms are benign variants related to changes in autonomic tone (specifically, an increase in vagal tone).

First-degree heart block occurs when the time from onset of atrial depolarization to ventricular depolarization is prolonged. All atrial impulses reach the ventricle. Therefore, the conduction delay may be the result of delay from sinus node to atrial tissue, delay within the atria, or delay within the AV

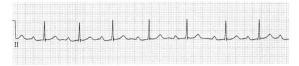

**Figure 3**   First-degree heart block.

node. First-degree heart block is usually benign and does not require intervention unless it results in dyssynchrony with atrial contraction occurring against a closed AV valve. However, evaluation for an acute underlying disease such as rheumatic fever is usually necessary (Figure 3).

Second-degree heart block can be subdivided into Mobitz type I AV block, also known as Wenckebach, and Mobitz type II AV block. In second-degree heart block, some impulses from the atrium do not reach the ventricle. In Wenckebach block (Figure 4), there is a gradual prolongation of the PR interval until one beat is not conducted to the ventricle. Wenckebach block is usually due to enhanced vagal tone and carries a better prognosis. In Mobitz type II block (Figure 5), there is usually conduction disease distal to the bundle of His. The PR interval is constant, usually prolonged, and there are atrial impulses that do not get conducted to the ventricle. The differentiation between these two types is not readily made in 2:1 block (two atrial impulses to one QRS complex), but an abnormal QRS generally accompanies Type II block. Type II block usually indicates structural heart disease or follows cardiac surgery and is an indication for pacemaker implantation.

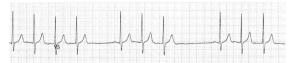

**Figure 4**   Mobitz type I (Wenckebach) heart block.

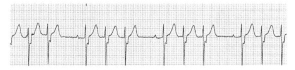

**Figure 5**   Mobitz type II heart block.

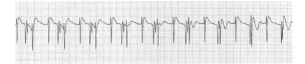

**Figure 6**   Wire study with third-degree heart block.

Third-degree heart block or complete heart block (Figure 6) may be congenital or acquired and occurs when no atrial impulses reach the ventricles. The ventricular rate is determined by an escape rhythm, either originating from the AV node (a junctional escape rhythm) or the ventricle. The most common cause seen in the PICU is postoperative heart block. The most common cause in newborns without congenital heart disease is due to maternal lupus antibodies. In lupus, treatment depends on the presence of symptoms, associated electrophysiological abnormalities, and the stability of the average escape rates. In the postoperative patients, it is typical to observe for a period of 7–10 days to allow sufficient time for AV node recovery before considering permanent pacemaker implantation.

## B. Tachycardia

When a tachycardia is recognized, the following considerations to diagnosis and management are suggested:

- Is the patient awake and have a palpable pulse?
- Is the rhythm regular or irregular?
- Is the QRS narrow or wide?
- Is there a P wave, and if so, is it regularly related to the QRS complex?

As with bradycardia, the upper range of normal varies widely and hence the tachycardia must be interpreted in the context it is occurring. For instance, a heart rate of 180 bpm in a crying neonate is not a cause for concern as compared to a heart rate of 140 bpm in a resting adolescent. The upper range of attainable sinus rhythm is age and circumstance dependent with the peak heart rate being approximately (220 − the age). It is customary to divide tachycardias into wide complex and narrow complex rhythms (Table 4). In addition, the origin of symptomatic tachycardia (sinus, supraventricular, or ventricular) must be determined because management varies.

*Table 4*

**Differential Diagnosis of Commonly Encountered Tachycardias**

| Narrow complex tachycardias |
| --- |

Automatic
  Sinus tachycardia
  Atrial ectopic tachycardia
  Junctional ectopic tachycardia
  Atrial fibrillation

Re-entrant
  Atrioventricular reciprocating tachycardia
    Wolff-Parkinson-White—orthodromic
    Concealed accessory pathway
    Permanent junctional reciprocating tachycardia
  Atrioventricular nodal re-entrant tachycardia
  Atrial flutter

| Wide complex tachycardias |
| --- |

Ventricular tachycardia

Ventricular fibrillation

Supraventricular tachycardias with abnormal conduction to the ventricles
  Supraventricular tachycardia with rate-related aberrancy or medication effect
  Supraventricular tachycardia with pre-existing bundle branch block
  Wolff-Parkinson-White—Antidromic tachycardia
  Atrial fibrillation or flutter with pre-existing bundle branch block or Wolff-Parkinson-White

Paced rhythms

## Narrow Complex Tachycardias

**Sinus Tachycardia (Figure 7)**    Sinus tachycardia is common and rates over 200 beats/min occur frequently in children up to 5 years of age. The causes are usually benign (crying, pain, anxiety). More serious conditions requiring specific treatment include fever, sepsis, hypovolemia, poisoning, and anemia. It is also possible for compromised stroke volume to be accompanied by sinus tachycardia, as seen in large pericardial effusions, cardiomyopathy, or myocarditis. Differentiating sinus tachycardia from

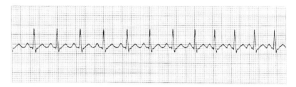

**Figure 7**   Sinus tachycardia.

an arrhythmia is critical for correct management. A decrease in heart rate should follow treatment of the common causes of ST. Persisting tachycardia after management of the obvious causes of sinus tachycardia should prompt consideration of the diagnosis of supraventricular tachycardia. Table 5 outlines differences between sinus and supraventricular tachycardia.

**Supraventricular Tachycardia**   The two main mechanisms of supraventricular tachycardia (SVT) in children are enhanced automaticity and re-entry (with or without an accessory pathway).

*Table 5*
**Differentiating between Sinus Tachycardia and Supraventricular Tachycardia in Infants**

| Sinus tachycardia | Supraventricular tachycardia |
|---|---|
| • History of a condition that causes volume loss, such as dehydration, fever, pain, anxiety | • Vague history; poor feeding, irritability, lethargy, tachypnea, sweating, pallor, or hypothermia |
| • Heart rate 160 to 220 bpm | • Heart rate >220 bpm |
| • P waves present with normal axis (may be difficult to see when rate >200 bpm) | • P waves are absent or abnormal in configuration if present |
| • Rate increase gradual; rate resolution gradual with calming or IV fluid, sedation, temperature therapy | • Usually fixed rate; abrupt onset and termination; respond to cardioversion |
| | • Ectopic tachycardias are catecholamine sensitive; rate may change |

The mechanism varies with age—typically SVT is accessory pathway mediated in the fetus and newborn, with a gradually increasing incidence of AV nodal mechanisms in the second decade.

## Re-entrant Tachycardia

The clinical features that would suggest re-entry tachycardia include:

- abrupt onset and termination with minimal beat-to-beat variation
- abrupt termination with electrical cardioversion or overdrive burst pacing
- ability to initiate and terminate with appropriately timed extra-stimuli
- predictable response to agents such as adenosine

A re-entrant tachycardia can be thought of as a circuit or loop, with certain electrophysiologic requirements (unidirectional block, dual pathways, and conduction delay in one pathway to allow recovery in the other). The electrical circuit may be large, such as with an accessory pathway (macro-re-entry) or small, such as within the AV node (micro-re-entry). Most children have a structurally normal heart but this arrhythmia is also common in Ebstein's abnormality and l-transposition of the great vessels. Common re-entrant arrhythmias are listed below.

**AV Reciprocating Tachycardia (AVRT) (Figure 8a and 8b)**     Pediatric SVT is most commonly caused by a re-entrant tachycardia via an accessory pathway or atrioventricular

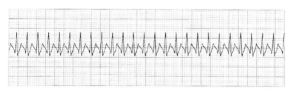

**Figure 8a**   Atrio-ventricular reciprocating tachycardia (AVRT).

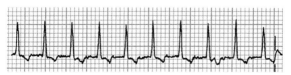

**Figure 8b**   AVRT.

reciprocating tachycardia (AVRT). It is a re-entrant tachycardia that employs the AV node and an accessory pathway between the atria and ventricles. When a concealed accessory pathway is involved, conduction is orthodromic or antegrade through the AV node from atrium to ventricle, via the His-Purkinje system to the ventricles. This results in a narrow complex QRS. Conduction is then retrograde from ventricle to atrium up the accessory pathway to the atria. The pathway is "concealed" because it is not apparent during sinus rhythm and does not conduct from atrium to ventricle. In AVRT or accessory pathway-mediated tachycardia, the RP interval is longer than 70 ms and atrial activation occurs after ventricular activation. The arrhythmia is paroxysmal and usually initiated by an atrial or ventricular ectopic beat.

Some patients with AVRT have a pathway that can conduct antegrade from atrium to ventricle. Therefore, during sinus rhythm the ventricle is "pre-excited" and Wolff-Parkinson-White syndrome (WPW) is present. However, one cannot differentiate this during SVT in most cases, but only when in sinus rhythm. In approximately 10% of cases of WPW, the AVRT will proceed from atrium to ventricle by the accessory pathway, with the AV node as the retrograde limb of the re-entrant circuit. This type of antidromic AVRT is characterized by a wide QRS during the tachycardia. Additionally, WPW carries a small risk of rapid conduction of atrial arrhythmias to the ventricles.

## Permanent Junctional Reciprocating Tachycardia (PJRT) (Figure 9)
PJRT is a rare tachycardia but can be an incessant tachycardia in children. It is a special form of re-entrant tachycardia with typical ECG features: long RP interval and negative P waves in leads II, III, and aVF. In all forms of pathway-mediated tachycardia (and AV node re-entry tachycardia), the rhythm is typically very regular. However, PJRT is often characterized by salvos of tachycardia with brief periods of sinus in between. The rate for PJRT is typically slower than other forms of AVRT since it is due to a slowly conducting accessory pathway. The incessant nature can lead to tachycardia-induced

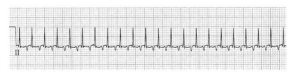

**Figure 9**   Permanent junctional reciprocating tachycardia (PJRT).

cardiomyopathy. It is not always easy to differentiate from ectopic atrial tachycardia.

**AV Nodal Re-entrant Tachycardia** The next most common form of SVT, AV nodal re-entrant tachycardia (AVNRT), is the most common cause of paroxysmal SVT in young adults and usually occurs in structurally normal hearts. It requires two distinct AV nodal inputs, a "slow" and a "fast" pathway. Usually, during SVT, the antegrade route is the slow pathway and the fast pathway is the retrograde limb with the atria and ventricles being activated simultaneously. The P waves are usually not visible, although in some patients, a notch after the QRS represents the retrograde atrial depolarization.

Differentiation of AVRT from AVNRT is not essential in the acute setting, as both respond well to maneuvers aimed at AV nodal conduction (eg, adenosine, vagal maneuvers) and terminating the re-entrant circuit (eg, cardioversion, overdrive pacing). For chronic management, AVRT may require more pathway specific therapies.

**Atrial Flutter (Figure 10)** Less than 10% of children with atrial flutter have a structurally normal heart. It is an uncommon arrhythmia in the perioperative period but may develop later in those with congenital heart disease. It is a form of intra-atrial re-entrant tachycardia with re-entry occurring in a macro-circuit around the atrial mass. Atrial distention and lines of conduction delay (eg, atriotomy scar) are precursors of this arrhythmia. The atrial rate may be as high as 500 bpm in infants, but usually around 250–300 bpm in older children. The ventricular rate response generally ranges from 120 to 150 bpm, depending on the degree of conduction block. Frequent atrial waves, with a "saw-tooth" pattern are typical of flutter in adults, but uncommon in children. Atrial flutter should be considered in the presence of an unexplained tachycardia without distinct "P" waves, or in patients with an elevated heart rate with little variation, as the second P wave may be hidden in the QRS complex

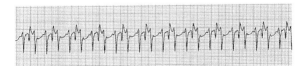

**Figure 10**  Wire study illustrating atrial flutter with 2:1 A-V block (large deflections represent atrial activity).

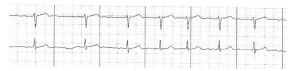

**Figure 11**   Atrial fibrillation.

or the T wave. Conduction of alternate or every third atrial beat to a QRS is common, and variable conduction block will give the ventricular response an irregular appearance. One-to-one (1:1) conduction may occur in neonates. Rapid conduction may result in aberrancy with a wider-than-expected QRS complex.

**Atrial Fibrillation (Figure 11)**   Atrial fibrillation is another form of intra-atrial re-entry characterized by fine irregular undulations of the baseline where the atrial activity is usually seen, with irregularly irregular ventricular activity resulting from random conduction of the atrial activity down to the ventricles. Atrial fibrillation is seen in the pediatric ICU setting in patients with dilated atria such as after prolonged AVRT, or in critically ill patients.

## Automatic Tachycardia

The second mechanism commonly encountered in the intensive care setting is enhanced automaticity. The ECG features that would suggest enhanced automaticity as the cause of tachycardia include:

- gradual onset with warming up (increase) and cooling down of the rate (over 10 to 20 cardiac cycles)
- a variable rate that changes with manipulation of autonomic tone or temperature
- unresponsiveness to electrical cardioversion or overdrive pacing maneuvers (although they may be transiently suppressed with overdrive pacing)
- minimal response to antiarrhythmics

The most common postoperative arrhythmias occurring as a result of enhanced automaticity in children are:

- junctional ectopic tachycardia
- atrial ectopic tachycardia
- accelerated junctional rhythm
- accelerated idioventricular rhythm

**Junctional Ectopic Tachycardia (JET) (Figure 12)** Junctional ectopic tachycardia (JET) is a narrow complex tachycardia caused by a focus of increased automaticity in the AV node or His bundle. It can occur as a congenital form in children with structurally normal hearts, but JET occurs most commonly in the postoperative setting following a cardiac repair in the vicinity of the AV node. Most commonly seen after repair of an AVSD, tetralogy of Fallot, arterial switch for TGA and TAPVR, JET contributes significantly to the morbidity and mortality in the pediatric cardiac ICU. The rhythm is usually incessant with AV dissociation, though retrograde conduction of P waves can occur. The rate range varies from 150 to 250 bpm, but is very dependent on the autonomic tone and external catecholamines. JET is typically very regular and difficult to treat. Intact AV conduction is present in about half of cases. The arrhythmia may slow briefly in response to adenosine, but will revert quickly to the initial rate.

**Atrial Ectopic Tachycardia (Figure 13)** Atrial ectopic tachycardia (AET) occurs when a non-sinus node focus within the atria has enhanced automaticity and becomes the pacemaker for the heart. AET can be incessant and can lead to tachycardia-induced cardiomyopathy. AET is relatively uncommon, though it is the most common incessant arrhythmia in children. The rate range is variable, reflecting normal maximum age-related sinus rates of up to 300/min in infants. It can occur in otherwise normal hearts as a chronic arrhythmia resulting in a cardiomyopathy, or as a transient disorder in the postoperative period following congenital heart surgery.

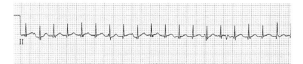

**Figure 12** Junctional ectopic tachycardia.

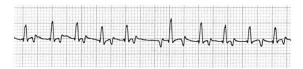

**Figure 13** Atrial ectopic tachycardia.

The diagnosis can be made by a surface ECG demonstrating a regular narrow QRS complex and an abnormal axis or morphology of the P wave, with rates excessive for age. It is characterized by a normal P-QRS sequence and a warming up and cooling down phenomenon. Occasionally, the focus will be near the sinus node and differentiation will be based on an elevated heart rate for the physiologic circumstance. AET is frequently accompanied by conduction block, most commonly first-degree AV block.

## Wide Complex Tachycardias

**Differentiating Wide Complex Tachyarrhythmias**    Tachycardia can also occur with a wide QRS complex. This can be due to aberrancy, medication effect, pre-existing conduction abnormalities, an antegrade conducting accessory pathway, or a paced rhythm with tracking of a supraventricular arrhythmia. Aberrancy is most commonly seen outside the ICU setting and occurs when the conduction tissue refractoriness limits the conduction velocity, resulting in a wide QRS. Usually, there is isolated right or left bundle branch block. Sodium and potassium channel blockers are the most commonly implicated medications.

The most important differential diagnosis is ventricular tachycardia. The rate and stability of the patient are not helpful in differentiating SVT with a wide QRS from VT. AV dissociation, structural heart disease, a complex QRS pattern, or a superior axis is much more likely to accompany VT. If the patient is stable, different maneuvers can be used in an attempt to accurately diagnose the tachyarrhythmia. These include vagal maneuvers or adenosine. In the unstable patient, or if the mechanism remains unclear, treatment for VT should be given.

**Ventricular Extrasystoles (Figure 14)**    A ventricular extrasystole is an impulse from a ventricular focus that is premature in relation to the prevailing rhythm. This

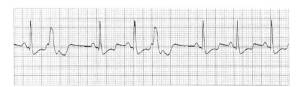

**Figure 14**    Premature ventricular complexes.

is manifest on the electrocardiogram as an atypical, usually wide QRS complex that is not preceded by a conducted P wave. The sinus node is not usually captured or reset by a PVC, yielding a pause, although if there is V-A conduction, the pause will not be fully compensatory. The repolarization that follows a PVC is also abnormal, reflecting the abnormal ventricular depolarization sequence. PVCs frequently occur in patterns alternating with one or more normal sinus beats; this is known as bigeminy, trigeminy, etc. This phenomenon is believed to be due to resetting of the ectopic focus during the pause following the PVC and is not significant prognostically. The differential diagnosis includes a premature atrial beat that is conducted aberrantly, due to the refractoriness of the conduction system. The only differentiating feature is the presence of a P wave that could reasonably have been conducted to the ventricles.

PVCs are common (up to 2% of normal children) and usually benign. However, PVCs that are polymorphic, are adrenergic, or occur in the setting of a prolonged QT interval may require further evaluation.

**Ventricular Tachycardia**  Ventricular tachycardia is a series of three or more ventricular depolarizations arising from below the bundle of His, at a rate exceeding the prevailing sinus rate. If the QRS morphology is uniform, the VT is considered monomorphic, as opposed to the polymorphic VT where the QRS complexes vary. VT associated with hemodynamic compromise or lasting more than 30 seconds is termed "sustained" VT, and increases the probability of an underlying cardiac abnormality.

ECG criteria for diagnosis of VT include:

- Atrioventricular (AV) dissociation is not essential but is present in the majority of children with VT
- QRS complex morphology is distinct from the normal sinus beat but may appear relatively narrow, especially in infants
- Intermittent fusion or capture beats

Ventricular tachycardia in the young most commonly occurs in a structurally normal heart and originates from the RV outflow tract or the LV apex. RVOT tachycardia has an LBBB morphology with a normal or inferior axis QRS. The second most common form is sometimes known as "Belhassen's tachycardia" and has a typical ECG pattern of RBBB and left axis deviation. These typically carry a favorable prognosis. Apart from these two distinct clinical entities, sustained VT in children most often develops as a result of:

- electrolyte or metabolic abnormalities
- drug or toxin exposure
- myocardial abnormalities, such as myocarditis, cardiomyopathy, congenital heart disease, or myocardial tumor
- prolonged QT

**Torsade de Pointes (Figure 15)**    This is a form of polymorphic VT developing in a patient with prolonged repolarization. It is characterized by changing polarity of the QRS around an isoelectric baseline, and often spontaneously terminates, or degenerates into ventricular fibrillation. Prolonged torsade de pointe is always poorly tolerated and should be cardioverted promptly.

There are multiple causes, both congenital and acquired. In the pediatric setting, acquired causes are more common and include electrolyte abnormalities (particularly hypocalcemia), cardiomyopathy, or medication effect. Congenital long QT syndrome is a heritable channelopathy in which the QT interval is prolonged and patients are prone to syncope and torsade under stress.

**Ventricular Fibrillation**    VF is a very rapid and irregular arrhythmia with low amplitude QRS complexes. Recent literature indicates that up to 20% of children who develop a

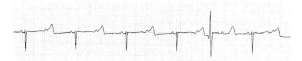

**Figure 15a**    Long QT syndrome with pseudo-block.

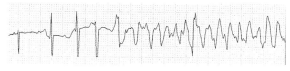

**Figure 15b**    Complicated with ventricular tachycardia (torsade de pointes).

cardiac arrest had VF as the cause for the arrest. Otherwise, it develops in response to severe global hypoxemia or degeneration of hemodynamically unstable VT or SVT. Most children who develop VF have a structurally abnormal heart, WPW syndrome, prolonged QT syndrome, or other channelopathy.

**Asystole**   Absence of a pulse may be asystole if there is no regular ECG activity or pulseless electrical activity. The cause of asystole in children is usually hypoxia related to a primary respiratory cause. PEA has many different considerations, depending on the clinical situation. Therapy should be aimed at identifying possible treatable causes while also performing acute resuscitation. PALS guidelines are a useful reference for resuscitation. (See Chapter 5, "Resuscitation.")

## An ICU Approach to the Acute Management of Arrhythmias

The initial approach to any child with an arrhythmia is determining cardiorespiratory stability. Patients with arrhythmias may appear stable but can deteriorate rapidly; hence, a functioning IV and monitoring in an intensive care setting is necessary. An understanding of the proarrhythmic properties of many of the antiarrhythmic agents is also essential. A hemodynamically unstable patient requires urgent attention to oxygenation, airway support, intravenous access, and initiation of PALS algorithms for resuscitation.

A. Bradyarrhythmia

  1. If clinically unstable,

   a. Support intravascular volume with 20 mL/kg bolus of 0.9% saline.
   b. Increase the heart rate by using (in ascending order):

   • atropine 20–40 mics/kg IV bolus
   • isoprenaline 0.01–0.1 mics/kg/min
   • temporary pacing, especially if postoperative with existing transcutaneous wires; otherwise, external pacing
   • if digitalis overdose, administer digibind

  2. If clinically stable, consider clinical context.

   • Discontinue medications that might be causing the bradycardia.
   • Have temporary pacemakers available.

B. Tachyarrhythmia: Consider cardiac echo to rule out structural abnormalities and function.

1. Regular 1:1 relationship of P with QRS and a long R-P (QRS-P >P-QRS interval)

   a. Sinus tachycardia (gradual "warming up" and "cooling down"; possible transient slowing with adenosine)

      • Treat underlying cause

   b. Sinus node re-entry tachycardia (abrupt onset and termination)

      • vagal maneuvers
      • adenosine, phenylephrine, edrophonium, esmolol, or IV verapamil (if >1 year of age)

   c. Atrial tachycardia (paroxysmal or incessant) may lead to tachycardia-induced cardiomyopathy if incessant

      • Trial of adenosine
      • Attempt overdrive pacing if temporary pacing wires present (postoperative patients)
      • If function normal, consider esmolol; if abnormal, consider rate control (eg, digoxin)
      • IV amiodarone most effective; add oral agent (class IC or III) for long-term control
      • May require radiofrequency ablation

2. Regular 1:1 relationship of P with QRS and a short R-P (QRS-P < P-QRS interval)

   a. AV reciprocating tachycardiac (AVRT)
   b. AV node re-entry tachycardia (AVNRT)

      • Vagal maneuvers
      • Adenosine, phenylephrine, edrophonium, or IV verapamil (if >1 year of age)
      • Atrial overdrive pacing may terminate if temporary pacing wires present (postoperative patients) or transesophageal pacing available.
      • If unstable and SVT is recurrent:

         • IV amiodarone
         • IV esmolol or procainamide
         • Consider radiofrequency ablation

      • If stable but SVT is recurrent:

         • as above

- if no delta wave with sinus beats, oral propranolol or oral digoxin
- oral propafenone, flecainide, sotalol, amiodarone

3. Nonsustained incessant tachycardia with long R-P

- If atrial tachycardia or PJRT with 1:1 P and QRS relationship, IV amiodarone for initial control.
- If P wave = QRS rate, and P waves negative in II, III, and aVF, likely PJRT, respond best to Class IC agents.

4. Regular R-R interval with VA dissociation, and QRS rate > atrial rate = JET

- Exclude residual outflow tract obstruction in postoperative patients.
- Normalize electrolytes, including Ca and Mg, treat fever, minimize catecholamines.
- IV Amiodarone.
- Cool to 33–35°C if rate uncontrolled.
- AV sequential pacing once rate controlled.
- Consider IV procainamide if rate still not controlled.
- May require radiofrequency ablation.

5. Irregularly irregular QRS rate with indistinct or sawtooth P waves = AF or flutter

- AIf AF of uncertain duration or >36 hours, cardiac echo to assess for atrial thrombus.

  - Consider anticoagulation.
  - Control ventricular rate with IV esmolol, verapamil, or diltiazem.
  - Synchronized DC conversion if no thrombus.

- If flutter, consider overdrive atrial pacing (temporary wires or esophageal lead).

  - Class IA (with calcium or beta-adrenergic blockers) IC, or III agents
  - Synchronized DC conversion

C. Wide complex tachyarrhythmia: a wide QRS tachycardia should be considered to be ventricular tachycardia (VT) until proven otherwise.

1. If unstable:

a. ABC—PALS algorithms
b. Electrical cardioversion: synchronized/unsynchronized

    c. Correct electrolyte abnormalities

    d. Trial of adenosine if diagnosis is in doubt (may convert some forms of VT)

    e. IV amiodarone

    f. Discontinue medications that may be contributing

    g. Specific therapies for intoxications, such as digibind

    h. ECMO if due to a reversible condition such as myocarditis

    i. Maintenance antiarrhythmic drug therapy will vary

    j. May need implantable ICD

  2. If prolonged QT interval:

    a. With incessant torsade de pointes:

      1. emergent asynchronous electrical cardioversion,

      2. magnesium

      3. isoprenaline

      4. correction of electrolyte abnormalities

      5. pacing

      6. consider lidocaine infusion if all else fails

      7. avoid Class Ia and III agents

    b. If torsade is not sustained, and in association with a prolonged QT syndrome:

      1. IV beta blocker

    c. If caused by a proarrhythmic agent:

      1. Pacing

      2. IV isoprenaline

  3. If stable:

    a. Remove aggravating actors such as electrolyte abnormalities, medications, etc.

    b. Attempt to make a diagnosis

    c. Initiate individualized drug trials to control the tachyarrhythmia (eg, beta blocker, sotalol, propafenone, Amiodarone)

D. Asystole

- Initiate CPR and PALS protocols
- Consider treatable causes during CPR:

  - Hypovolemia
  - Hypoxemia
  - Hypothermia

- Hyperkalemia/hypokalemia
- Tamponade
- Tension pneumothorax
- Toxins/drugs
- Thromboembolism

Table 6 outlines the standard classification of commonly used drugs used to treat arrhythmias. It provides a guide to the mechanism of action, but does not include digoxin or adenosine, and Amiodarone is somewhat of a misfit in Class 3.

*Table 6*
**Classification of Antiarrhythmic Agents**

| Class | Subclass | Drug | Pharmacologic effect |
|-------|----------|------|----------------------|
| I | | | Sodium channel blockers; depress rate of increase of action potential (slope 0) |
| | IA | Quinidine, Procainamide | Increased AP duration, and increased atrial and ventricular ERP; increased JT interval; vagolytic action |
| | | Disopyramide | |
| | IB | Lidocaine, Mexiletine | Unchanged QRS complex; decreased AP duration; increased ventricular ERP |
| | IC | Propafenone | Widening of QRS complex |
| | IC | Flecainide (Encainide) | Unchanged AP duration; increased atrial and ventricular ERP; unchanged JT interval |
| II | | Beta blockers | Beta-adrenergic receptor blocker |
| III | | Amiodarone | Increased AP duration (also IA actions on sodium channels; II and IV actions on SA and AV node) |
| | | Sotalol | Increased JT interval |
| IV | | Verapamil, Diltiazem | Ca++ channel blocker |

# Practical Considerations of Management

## a. Vagal Maneuvers

The vagal response slows AV node conduction, interrupting the AV node-dependent group of re-entry tachycardia. They are most effective shortly after initiation of the arrhythmia. If the child is <2 years of age and clinically stable, eliciting a diving reflex to treat the SVT can be attempted. EKG monitoring, suction, and other airway support should be in place. This is an elective procedure, and not recommended in an older child who has recently eaten.

- For infants, wrap the baby firmly in sheet or towel after connecting to an ECG, and then apply a bag of ice and water to the face using a wet cloth as an interface to avoid skin burns (duration 15 seconds), without obstructing respiration, although application over the lower third of the face is most effective. In neonates and small children, holding head down position sometimes produces an effective response.
- In older children, coughing, breath holding, bearing down (Valsalva maneuver), and standing on their head with support

Table 7

## Commonly Used Antiarrhythmics in PICU

| Medication | Mode of action | Dosage | Adverse & comments |
|---|---|---|---|
| Adenosine | Predominant effects in SA node, atrial myocytes, AV node through A1 receptors: increases Kout & hyperpolarizes cardiac cell membranes; also anti-adrenergic effect | 0.05–0.1 mg/kg per dose Need very rapid bolus Can increase up to 0.35/0.4 mg/kg | Transient bradycardia, asystole, PACs, PVCs, atrial fibrillation, rapid conduction of atrial arrhythmias, torsade Caution in asthmatics, transplant patients, unstable patients |

| Amiodarone | K channel blocker with minor Na channel blocking, beta-adrenergic blocking, and Ca channel blocking effects Lengthens action potential & refractory periods & decreases automaticity | IV: 5 mg/kg load over 5–10 min (may repeat up to total of 15 mg/kg) OR 25 mcg/kg/min × 4 hours, then 5–15 micrograms/kg/min as continuous infusion | Drug interactions, hypotension, proarrhythmia, bradycardia, AV block Other organ effects (skin, liver, thyroid) after prolonged use |
| --- | --- | --- | --- |
| Esmolol | Selective beta 1 blocker Decreases automaticity & AV nodal conduction | Load 500 micrograms/kg over 1 minute, infusion 50–500 micrograms/kg/min | Hypotension, bronchospasm, bradycardia hypotension, heart block, negative inotropy Caution in bronchospasm, diabetes |
| Lidocaine | Block fast sodium channel Action potential duration & refractoriness shortened in Purkinje & ventricular muscle | Load 1 milligram/kg, infusion 20–50 micrograms/kg/min | Seizures, apnea, proarrhythmia, hypotension |
| Procainamide | Block predominantly inactivated state of sodium channel Prolongs refractory periods in atrial & ventricular tissue | Load 10–15 milligrams/kg over 20 minutes, infusion 20–80 micrograms/kg/min | Negative inotrope, proarrhythmia, acceleration of ventricular response to atrial arrhythmias, bradycardia |

can be tried. Carotid sinus massage can be added to these measures. Eyeball pressure is not recommended. Gagging while being examined with a tongue depressor has also been described as a maneuver for SVT conversion.

Families of children who frequently present with sporadic SVT are often taught vagal maneuvers to facilitate home management. If symptoms of decreased cardiac output are apparent, pharmacologic and non-pharmacologic emergency treatments are required.

# b. Administering Adenosine (Figure 16)

The initial drug of choice to treat and diagnose presumed SVT is adenosine. Adenosine acts at specific receptors to cause a temporary block of conduction through the AV node, interrupting the re-entry circuit in AV nodal-dependent SVT. It can occasionally terminate other arrhythmias including certain forms of VT. It is also useful because all AV node-mediated ventricular activities will be temporarily suppressed, allowing accurate assessment of underlying atrial or spontaneous ventricular activity.

## Requirements

- continuous 3- or 12-lead rhythm strip recording
- free-flowing IV access, with as large a vein and IV as possible
- a stopcock attachment for a dual syringe bolus technique; alternatively, two syringes may be inserted into one injection hub

## Method of Administration

- 0.1 mg/kg initially, injected rapidly in IV line as close to the heart as possible, using a double-syringe method (3–5 mL of saline is injected immediately following medication). Both the adenosine and saline syringes are in the same injection port. The syringe emptied from adenosine should be held tight in

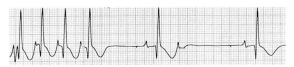

**Figure 16**   Adenosine termination of AVRT.

order to avoid backflow of saline with adenosine remaining in the tube and not being appropriately flushed in a timely fashion (its effect lasts only 10 seconds).

- If there is no response, the dose may be increased to 0.2 mg/kg, and subsequently 0.3 mg/kg; the theoretical maximum is 12 mg. It is important to realize that an arrhythmia may briefly be terminated by adenosine and then resume; this is not an adenosine failure, and likely indicates that further antiarrhythmic agents are required (see below).
- Adenosine is metabolized very rapidly by adenosine deaminase, which is abundant in red cells. Failure to note any EKG change may indicate an inadequate dose, inadequate or remote venous access, or inadequate bolus technique, in addition to an arrhythmia which is not responsive to adenosine.
- One should be prepared to cardiovert in the case that adenosine is proarrhythmic.

**Note:** Cardiorespiratory collapse requires emergent cardioversion, with or without IV/IO access.

## c. Failure to Convert to Sinus Rhythm

Re-examine the rhythm strips recorded. One of three possibilities may exist:

- Atrial-ventricular conduction was interrupted or delayed briefly, but the arrhythmia recurred almost immediately. In this case, the arrhythmia is likely a form of AV re-entry, but is recurrent and requires an alternative longer acting agent to suppress it.
- Atrial-ventricular conduction was interrupted or delayed, but the arrhythmia continued absolutely unchanged. In this case, the arrhythmia is independent of the AV node conduction pathway. Consider atrial flutter, or ventricular tachycardia, or more rarely a junctional ectopic tachycardia. Of note, some forms of VT do respond to adenosine.
- No effect was observed on atrial-ventricular conduction: Drug administration technique or dosage being delivered to the AV node is inadequate.

## References

Balaji S. Postoperative cardiac arrhythmias in children. 2001;3(5):385–392.

Chakrabarti S, Stuart AG. Understanding cardiac arrhythmias. Arch Dis Child 2005;90;1086–90.

Delaney JW, Moltedo JM, Dziura JD, et al. Early postoperative arrhythmias after pediatric cardiac surgery. J Thor Cardiovasc Surg 2006;131:1296–301.

Dodge-Khatami A, Miller OI, Anderson RH, et al. Surgical substrates of postoperative junctional ectopic tachycardia in congenital heart defects. J Thor Cardiovasc Surg 2002;123:624–30.

Doniger SJ, Sharieff GQ. Pediatric dysrhythmias. Pediatr Clin N Am 2006;53:85–105.

Hoffman TM, Wernovsky G, Wieand TS, et al. The incidence of arrhythmias in a pediatric cardiac intensive care unit. Pediatr Cardiol 2002;23(6):598–604.

Kothari DS, Skinner JR. Neonatal tachycardias: An update. Arch Dis Child Fetal Neonatal Ed 2006;91:136–44.

Manole MD, Saladino RA. Emergency department management of the pediatric patient with supraventricular tachycardia. Ped Emerg Care 2007;23:176–87.

Nichols DG, Ungerleider RM, Spevak PJ, et al. (editors). Critical heart disease in infants and children, 2nd ed. Location: Mosby Elsevier Publishing; year: pp.

Pediatric advanced life support. Circulation 2005;112:167–87.

Sen-Chowdhry S, McKenna WJ. Sudden cardiac death in the young: A strategy for prevention by targeted evaluation. Cardiology 2006;105:196–206.

Sharieff GQ. The pediatric ECG. Pediatr Clin N Am 2006;53:85–105.

# C. Heart Failure

Kim Myers
Walter Duncan
Tapas Mondal
Peter W Skippen

## Key Principles

- CHF occurs when hemodynamic demands exceed myocardial pump capacity.
- Cardiac output depends on preload, afterload, contractility, and heart rate.
- Acute management is aimed at restoring end-organ perfusion, maintaining oxygen delivery, restoring fluid balance, and preventing cardiorespiratory arrest and death.

## Introduction

Congestive heart failure (CHF) is a neurohumoral response that develops when the hemodynamic demands on the heart exceed the myocardial pump capacity. CHF encompasses conditions resulting in limitations to inflow or outflow. In volume overload lesions due to shunting, diastolic and systolic function are often preserved. In pressure overload lesions such as valvular stenosis, limitations in diastolic function are usually accompanied by systolic dysfunction. CHF does not always imply contractile dysfunction.

Most heart failure in children results from either structural heart disease, which produces either volume or pressure overload, or from functional heart disease, which may be due to either electrical disturbance such as incessant tachyarrhythmia, or myocardial disease. The most common causes of CHF are listed in Table 1.

*Table 1*
## Etiology of Pediatric Heart Failure

| Structural heart disease |
| --- |

- Volume overload lesions (ASD, VSD, AVSD, PDA, AVM, A-P window, aortic regurgitation)
- Pressure overload lesions (aortic stenosis, pulmonary stenosis, coarctation of the aorta, systemic hypertension)

| Functional heart disease |
| --- |

- Myocardial disease
  - Cardiomyopathy
  - Myocarditis
- Coronary artery disease
  - Anomalous origin of the coronary artery
  - Kawasaki disease with coronary artery involvement
- Rhythm and conduction disturbances (SVT, ventricular arrhythmias, bradycardia)
- Post-cardiopulmonary bypass
- Structurally normal heart
- Anemia
- AV fistula
- Hypoxia-ischemia
- Endocrinopathies
- Hypertension
- Sepsis
- Hypoglycemia
- Hypothyroidism
- Renal failure

# Pathophysiology

The heart has immediate and delayed responses to increased hemodynamic demands or diminished myocardial performance. The sympathetic nervous system (SNS) provides the rapid response reflexes. The renin-angiotensin-aldosterone system (RAAS) provides longer term mechanisms for expanding intravascular volume to improve preload. Sustained activation of both the SNS and RAAS exacerbates heart failure. Chronic volume overload occurs. Prolonged aldosterone exposure stimulates cardiac fibrosis, which results in myocardial damage. Chronic activation of the SNS impairs inotropic reserve through down-regulation of adrenergic receptors. Ventricular remodeling occurs, with diastolic and systolic dysfunction and increased myocardial oxygen consumption. In addition, vasopressin, endothelin, and peptide growth factors are released together with counter-regulatory natriuretic peptides. Ultimately, if the condition is untreated, blood flow is redistributed, resulting in the symptom complex of fatigue, weakness, and associated lactic acid and organ function impairment.

## Determinants of Cardiac Output

The main determinants of cardiac output and oxygen delivery are outlined in Figure 1. Infants are dependent on rate augmentation to improve their CO under conditions of stress. Stroke volume is dependent on loading conditions (preload and afterload) and myocardial contractility. Cardiac output is tightly coupled with oxygen consumption, as described by Fick. Oxygen consumption in the newborn reaches 6–8 mL/kg/min and decreases with age (adult 4–5 mL/kg/min).

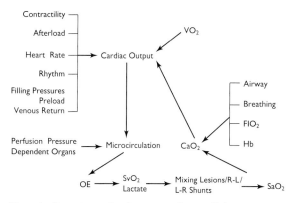

**Figure 1**   Determinants of cardiac output and oxygen Delivery.

$$Q = VO_2 \text{ (L/min)}/[a\text{–}v\ O_2 \text{ difference}] \text{ (Fick equation)}$$

Figure 2 graphically describes the cardiac function and venous return curves that are both plotted. The cardiac output curve depicts the change in stroke volume with increasing preload in a normal and a failing ventricle. The slope of the

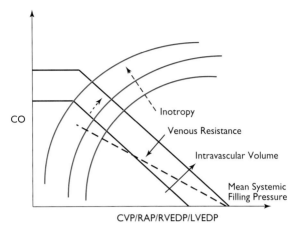

**Figure 2**  Veno-cardiac coupling.

curve represents contractility. With increased afterload or decreased inotropy, the curve shifts down and to the right. With decreased afterload or increased inotropy, the curve shifts up and to the left. Venous resistance and intravascular volume affect venous return curves. The intersection of the two curves gives the central venous pressure or right atrial pressure, at that specific degree of inotropy, vascular resistance and vascular fill.

## Preload

The Frank-Starling relationship describes the effect of changing preload on force of contraction. With increasing preload, there is greater overlap of actin and myosin filaments and an increased number of cross-bridging sites. Once maximal overlap is reached, further increases in sarcomere length result in reduced myocardial performance. Systemic venous return is a major determinant of preload. Volume-loading lesions such as left-to-right shunts and regurgitant lesions increase preload. Positive pressure ventilation, vasoactive medications, and changes in blood volume also affect preload. Tachycardia decreases ventricular filling time and loss of coordinated atrial contraction such as with atrioventricular dissociation both result in decreased preload.

## Afterload

Afterload is resistance to ejection from either the right or left ventricle. In children, it is important to think of afterload to each ventricle (unless univentricular). There are three major determinants of afterload. Peak arterial pressure can be elevated in diseases such as systemic hypertension, pulmonary artery stenosis, or coarctation of the aorta. Arterial compliance may be decreased when synthetic materials such as conduits are used to reconstruct the arteries or with long-standing hypertension and consequent loss of elastic tissue. Finally, changes in pulmonary or peripheral vascular resistance induced by neurohumoral mechanisms or pharmaceutical intervention directly affect afterload (eg, acidosis increases PVR). The effects of increased afterload can be acute or chronic. Acute effects of increased RV afterload include RV failure and low cardiac output syndrome; potential septal shifts with compromise to LV filling and mechanics. Chronic effects of increased afterload include ventricular hypertrophy.

## Contractility

Contractility in its purest form refers to the intensity of the force of contraction of heart muscle independent of preload and afterload. It is determined by the sensitivity of troponin to calcium and by the availability of calcium, which in turn is affected by circulating catecholamines and SNS tone. Myocardial sensitivity to the inotropic effects of calcium is age dependent as a result of immaturity of the sarcoplasmic reticulum of newborns. Pharmacologic measures can also augment or depress contractility.

## Heart Rate

Heart rate, in addition to preload, afterload, and contractility, is one of the major mechanisms of enhancing cardiac output, especially in young children. At excessive heart rates there is decreased diastolic filling time that results in decreased cardiac output.

# Presentation

Signs and symptoms at presentation are age dependent. Infants present with feeding difficulties and growth retardation, with tachypnea, tachycardia, and diaphoresis. The older child presents more like an adult with breathlessness and exertional dyspnea. Orthopnea, fatigue, and weakness are late symptoms.

# Physical Examination

## General Signs:

- Lethargy, irritable, anxious appearance, may be diaphoretic, feeding difficulties.

## Respiratory System:

- Dyspnea, tachypnea, and poor feeding are commonly seen with increased pulmonary blood flow in the setting of high-output cardiac failure. Children often require accessory muscle use with intercostals retractions, tracheal tug, and nasal flaring to maintain adequate ventilation.
- Wheeze and crackles may be evidence of cardiogenic edema.

## Cardiovascular System:

- Tachycardia: An increase in heart rate is one of the first hemodynamic responses to diminished cardiac output. It may also be the etiology for heart failure in the setting of tachyarrhythmia.
- Hypotension and poor peripheral perfusion: Weak peripheral pulses, low systolic blood pressure, skin mottling, and cool extremities.
- Gallop (S3/S4) may be audible when there is impaired ventricular filling.
- Active precordium, thrill, and ventricular heave may be palpable with structural lesions or ventricular enlargement; may see and feel displaced apical impulse with ventricular enlargement.
- Jugular venous distension is difficult to estimate in children, but elevated venous pressures are best reflected by hepatomegaly with ascites. Peripheral edema is uncommon in children.

## Gastrointestinal System:

- Hepatic and intestinal congestion

# Growth Retardation/Failure to Thrive:

- Despite adequate caloric intake
- High metabolic demands

## Heart Failure Classification

The New York Heart Association (NYHA) Classification is used in adult patients to assess functional limitation in patients with heart failure:

| | |
|---|---|
| Class I | Patients with no limitation of activities; they suffer no symptoms from ordinary activities (fatigue, palpitations, or dyspnea). |
| Class II | Patients with mild limitation of activity; they are comfortable at rest and with mild exertion. |
| Class III | Patients with marked limitation of activity; they are comfortable only at rest. |
| Class IV | Patients unable to carry out any physical activity without discomfort; symptoms of cardiac insufficiency at rest. |

The Ross Classification was developed for infants and young children and is based on clinical symptoms:

| | |
|---|---|
| Class I | Asymptomatic |
| Class II | Mild tachypnea or diaphoresis with feeding in infants; dyspnea on exertion in older children. |
| Class III | Marked tachypnea or diaphoresis with feeding in infants, prolonged feeding times with growth failure due to heart failure; in older children, marked dyspnea on exertion. |
| Class IV | Symptoms such as tachypnea, retractions, grunting, or diaphoresis at rest. |

## Investigations

Laboratory Studies: hemoglobin level appropriate for cardiac lesion, electrolyte and renal function, liver enzymes, coagulation profile, cardiac troponins, metabolic and infectious agent testing as indicated.

Chest Radiograph: pulmonary edema and effusion, cardiomegaly and chamber enlargement, lung volumes.

Echocardiogram: assessment of structural lesions, systolic and diastolic function, estimation of filling pressures, presence of pericardial effusion, pulmonary artery pressures.

Electrocardiogram: chamber enlargement and voltages, ventricular ectopy or arrhythmias.

Cardiac Catheterization: consideration in the setting of congenital heart lesions, cardiomyopathy and myocarditis. Endomyocardial biopsies may be useful to distinguish myocarditis from dilated cardiomyopathy although there is a low yield.

Cardiac MRI: may be useful to assess ventricular volumes and function as well as quantification of shunts and regurgitant fractions. Consider in the setting of single ventricle physiology, cardiomyopathies, and myocarditis.

## Resuscitation and Stabilization

Acute management should not be delayed for diagnosis and definitive management. The initial management of acute cardiac failure is aimed at restoring end-organ perfusion, maintaining oxygen delivery, restoring fluid balance, and preventing cardiorespiratory arrest and death. Investigations to determine the underlying cause and specific therapies can be performed after the patient is stabilized.

- ABCs

  - 100% oxygen by face mask to alleviate hypoxemia with bag mask ventilatory support as required.
  - Intubation as required for impending respiratory failure or airway compromise/provides a degree of cardiac support. The initial response to sedation for intubation and positive pressure ventilation could be worsening cardiac output or cardiovascular collapse.
  - May require volume resuscitation prior to, during, or after intubation prior to central venous pressure monitoring. Following the degree of hepatomegaly is a noninvasive way to assess the degree of venous fill.

- Consider the effect of therapeutic modalities on all aspects of cardiac output, including preload, afterload, contractility, and heart rate.

  - Preload augmentation: These children may have a depleted intravascularly circulating volume despite signs of pulmonary or peripheral congestion.

- Preload reduction: Diuretics are useful in the setting of high filling pressures and high output lesions with excessive pulmonary blood flow. Care is necessary to prevent a decrease in cardiac output with overdiuresis in the face of compensatory filling pressures. Loop diuretics such as furosemide are most commonly used.
- Afterload reduction: Peripheral vasodilatation is useful to decrease afterload and increase venous capacitance, which may also have the effect of reducing preload, all of which decrease myocardial work and improve blood flow. Milrinone, sodium nitroprusside, or nitroglycerine can all be used, depending on the clinical situation.
- Inotropes: May be required in acute heart failure with hypotension and/or hypoperfusion. A normal blood pressure does not give an indication of oxygen delivery and flow. Most inotropes increase contractility through increased intracellular levels of cyclic adenylate monophosphate (cAMP) (either increased production or decreased degradation), which augments cytoplasmic calcium at actin-myosin coupling, thus increasing contractility.

  - Epinephrine provides inotropic and chronotropic support. The receptor effects are dose dependent, with beta-agonist effects predominating at doses less than 0.1 mics/kg/min.
  - Norepinephrine also provides inotropic support but with predominant alpha-agonist effects, which increases peripheral vascular resistance and afterload.
  - Dobutamine has primarily a beta-adrenergic effect leading to inotropy but may result in hypotension due to beta-2 receptor stimulation with reflex tachycardia.
  - Dopamine has dopaminergic and beta-adrenergic effects, but at high dose it also has alpha-adrenergic response leading to peripheral vasoconstriction.
  - Milrinone is a phosphodiesterase III inhibitor. IV administration increases cardiac output and reduces cardiac filling pressures, pulmonary vascular resistance, and systemic vascular resistance. It has minimal effect on HR or BP.

- New agents:

  - Levosimendan sensitizes myofilaments to calcium, which increases inotropy without increasing intracellular calcium levels. This agent shows a lot of promise, but is currently not available in NA.

- Nesiritide is a recombinant B-type natriuretic peptide. Its endogenous counterpart is a neurohormone produced by the failing ventricle in response to volume expansion and pressure overload and counteracts maladaptive compensatory responses. It reduces preload and afterload and increases cardiac index without reflex tachycardia or direct inotropic effect. It results in diuresis and natriuresis and suppresses the RAAS and SNS. No pediatric data are yet available but adult studies have shown it to be effective in improving symptoms and hemodynamic abnormalities in acutely decompensated patients with CHF.

- Rate control: Excessive tachycardia may result in impaired ventricular filling and decreased cardiac output. Pharmacologic agents to lower heart rate and improve ventricular filling include beta blockade. However, these agents should be used with care and slowly uptitrated to avoid precipitous falls in cardiac output.

- Anticoagulation: Severely reduced systolic function and diastolic dysfunction are often associated with dilated chambers and sluggish blood flow, increasing the risk of intracardiac thrombus formation. This risk may be increased in the presence of atrial arrhythmias. Consideration of anticoagulation is recommended to decrease the risk of thromboembolism.

- Mechanical support:

  - Important option in treatment of acutely decompensated HF and low cardiac output unresponsive to pharmacologic therapy. Includes total heart-lung bypass (extracorporeal membrane oxygenation [ECMO]) or ventricular assist devices (VADs). Mechanical support maintains end-organ function and reduces myocardial oxygen demand during the period of cardiac recovery. It may also be used as a bridge to transplant.

## Longer-Term Support

**Digoxin**  Digoxin is commonly used to treat heart failure of various etiologies in children. There have been few pediatric studies in children, although adult studies show improvement in symptoms but not improved survival in heart failure. Higher doses offer no increase in efficacy but substantially greater risk of side effects and toxicity.

**Diuretics**   Adult heart failure guidelines recommend the use of diuretics as first-line agents in all patients with heart failure to maintain a euvolemic state. Loop diuretics such as furosemide are the most commonly used diuretics in heart failure.

**Aldosterone Antagonists**   Spironolactone has been shown to improve survival in adults with heart failure. Its beneficial effect is thought to be due to inhibition of myocardial fibrosis and promotion of nitric oxide release from vascular endothelium rather than its small diuretic effect.

**Angiotensin Converting Enzyme Inhibitors (ACEIs) and Angiotensin Receptor Blockers (ARBs)**   Angiotensin converting enzyme inhibitors (ACEIs) inhibit sodium and water retention and reduce venous tone, decreasing preload and pulmonary congestion. Reduction in preload and afterload decreases wall stress of the ventricle and myocardial oxygen demand. ACEIs limit ventricular remodeling and reduce sympathetic outflow. Multiple large RCTs in adults have demonstrated improved symptomatology and survival benefit with ACEI. Careful uptitration is required with adjustment of diuretics to manage initial hypotension. Adult studies have shown reduced risk of death or hospitalization with higher doses despite symptoms that are generally well tolerated. In fact, these studies suggest that target dose rather than symptomatology should be the clinical endpoint to achieve the benefit in outcome. Unfortunately, there are no trials in children defining target dosages, but studies have shown reduction in LV volume overload and hypertrophy in children with valvular insufficiency treated with ACEI. Adult studies have not demonstrated greater efficacy or safety with ARBs; however, they are indicated if patients are ACEI intolerant.

**Beta Blockers**   Multiple adult studies have shown a statistically significant reduction in mortality with metoprolol and carvedilol (34% reduction in mortality of mild to moderate CHF with metoprolol, 35% reduction in mortality in severe CHF with carvedilol). In pediatric patients with heart failure, metoprolol and carvedilol have been shown to improve ejection fraction and clinical status. A recent Cochrane review concluded that there was not enough data to recommend or discourage the use of beta blockers for heart failure in the pediatric population.

**Electrical Therapy**    Cardiac Resynchronization Therapy (CRT) has shown benefit in adult dilated cardiomyopathy with electromechanical dyssynchrony. It has been studied in children following cardiac surgery with some hemodynamic improvement in the early postoperative course. Conventional right ventricular pacing can induce abnormal ventricular interactions, compromising cardiac function. Several studies have demonstrated that some patients for heart transplant can be delisted due to improved left ventricular function with CRT.

# References

Frobel AK, Hulpke-Wette M, Schmidt KG, Läer S. Beta-blockers for congestive heart failure in children. Cochrane Database Syst Rev. 2009 Jan 21;(1):CD007037.

Moffett BS, Chang AC. Future pharmacologic agents for treatment of heart failure in children. Pediatr Cardiol 2006;27(5):533–51.

# D. Cardiomyopathy/Myocarditis

Kim Myers
Walter Duncan
Tapas Mondal
Peter W Skippen

## Key Principles

> - Cardiomyopathies are a heterogeneous group of myo-
>   cardial diseases with varied etiologies.
> - Cardiomyopathies may progress to heart failure or
>   sudden death.
> - Myocarditis is an inflammatory process of the myocar-
>   dium with varied causes.
> - For both myocarditis and cardiomyopathy, manage-
>   ment of heart failure and prevention of arrhythmias
>   are crucial. (See Section 8B (Pediatric Arrhythmia) and
>   Section 8C (Heart Failure).)

## Cardiomyopathies

Cardiomyopathies are defined by the American Heart Association as a "heterogeneous group of diseases of the myocardium associated with mechanical and/or electrical dysfunction
that usually exhibit inappropriate ventricular hypertrophy or
dilatation." The causes are varied and include those that are
genetic, toxic, infectious, and autoimmune in nature. It may
progress to heart failure or sudden cardiac death.

The consensus classification scheme (World Health Organization modified by American Health Association) dates from
2006, and agreed that cardiomyopathies be classified as primary,
including genetic and acquired subtypes, and secondary.

- Primary cardiomyopathies include hypertrophic cardiomyopathy, dilated cardiomyopathy, restrictive cardiomyopathy,
  arrhythmogenic right ventricular cardiomyopathy, ventricular
  non-compaction and ion channelopathies, as well as some

acquired causes including tachycardia-induced cardiomyopathy and inflammatory cardiomyopathy or myocarditis.

- Secondary cardiomyopathies reflected systemic disease (storage diseases, exposure to toxins such as anthracyclines, and neuromuscular disorders such as Duchenne-Becker muscular dystrophy).

Cardiomyopathies are further classified on the morphology of the affected ventricle.

- Dilated cardiomyopathy is characterized by a dilated ventricle with normal wall thickness and accompanied by impaired systolic function.
- Hypertrophic cardiomyopathy is characterized by a ventricle with thickening of walls and often hyperdynamic systolic function but "diastolic dysfunction."
- Arrhythmogenic right ventricular cardiomyopathy is characterized by thinning or aneurysmal changes of the right ventricular outflow tract and preserved ventricular function.
- Left ventricular non-compaction is characterized by a spongy appearance to the apical myocardium and abnormal systolic function.
- Restrictive cardiomyopathy is the exception, being characterized by altered hemodynamic profile rather than abnormal ventricular morphology.

## Hypertrophic Cardiomyopathy (HCM)

HCM occurs in 1:500 of the general population. It is the most common cause of sudden cardiac death in young people, especially athletes. It is transmitted as an autosomal dominant trait with phenotypic variability. Mutations in sarcomeric proteins, including troponin T, beta myosin heavy chain and myosin binding protein C, have been identified. There is a non-dilated left ventricle with asymmetric hypertrophy, often with obstruction of the left ventricular outflow tract at rest or with exercise. Some may progress to congestive heart failure. Mortality rates in children and adolescents are estimated at 1%. Higher risk (previous cardiac arrest, sustained ventricular tachycardia, abnormal blood pressure response to exercise, family history of HCM-related death, or documented genetic mutation consistent with HCM) confers an estimated annual mortality of 5%.

**Presentation**    Presentation may occur in neonates but is often delayed until adolescence. If left ventricular outflow tract obstruction is present, exercise may precipitate shortness of breath, chest pain, or palpitations. Malignant arrhythmia and sudden cardiac death may be the initial presentation even in the absence of left ventricular obstruction.

A loud systolic murmur of left ventricular outflow tract obstruction and bifid arterial pulse (two distinct impulses with each heartbeat) may be evident on physical examination.

**Investigations**    Chest radiograph: Often normal.

Electrocardiogram: May show left ventricular hypertrophy with a strain pattern and prominent septal Q waves (>3 mm deep or >0.04 seconds). Ventricular ectopy may be present.

Echocardiography: Shows the often asymmetric hypertrophy of the left ventricular posterior wall and septum, increased left atrial volume, and abnormal diastolic function indices.

Cardiac MRI: Cardiac MRI may identify areas of fibrosis and myocardial necrosis with delayed hyperenhancement.

## Management

- Reduce exertional symptoms including dyspnea, chest pain, and syncope, and decrease the risk of sudden cardiac death.
- Negative inotropic agents such as beta-adrenergic blockers are useful to reduce heart rate and improve ventricular filling in the setting of increased chamber stiffness.
- Verapamil may be used in the absence of outflow tract obstruction but has an increased mortality risk when obstruction is present.
- In severe obstruction, disopyramide in conjunction with beta blockade has shown some efficacy.
- Ventricular septal myomectomy has been used for symptomatic left ventricular outflow tract obstruction (unresponsive to medical therapy).
- In adults, percutaneous alcohol septal ablation will reduce the basal ventricular septal thickness and diminish outflow tract obstruction; but risks heart block and sudden death.
- Amiodarone reduces sudden cardiac death due to arrhythmia.
- Automatic implantable cardioverter-defibrillator (AICD) will give secondary prevention of sudden cardiac death (previous resuscitated sudden cardiac death) and should be considered for primary prevention in high-risk patients.

# Dilated Cardiomyopathy (DCM)

DCM is the most common form of cardiomyopathy, with an estimated annual incidence of 1.13 per 100,000 children. It is the most frequent indication for heart transplant in adults and children. It is the final common pathway of many varied disease processes. A familial etiology is found in 20–35% of cases. Familial causes include mutations in cytoskeletal proteins. Other etiologies include infectious agents resulting in myocarditis, toxins such as alcohol and cocaine, metals and chemotherapeutic agent toxicity, ischemic disease (anomalous left coronary artery from pulmonary trunk and Kawasaki disease) and systemic disorders, including collagen vascular diseases, neuromuscular disorders, and metabolic derangements (eg, selenium and carnitine deficiency). It is characterized by ventricular chamber enlargement with normal wall thickness and systolic dysfunction. Mortality in children ranges between 33 and 67% at 5 years.

**Presentation**   Symptoms: Congestive heart failure with fatigue, dyspnea and failure to thrive. Children may present with palpitations or arrhythmia. Sudden cardiac death is possible. Physical examination: Displaced apical impulse, muffled heart sounds, gallop and a soft systolic murmur of mitral regurgitation, pulses of low volume, and hepatomegaly.

**Investigations**   Chest radiograph: Cardiomegaly and pulmonary venous congestion.

Laboratory testing: May show elevated inflammatory markers and cardiac enzymes; increased ammonia and lactate levels and urinary ketones suggest carnitine deficiency.

Electrocardiogram: Nonspecific diffuse ST-T wave changes, chamber enlargement, and ventricular ectopy. Atrial and ventricular arrhythmias occur.

Echocardiogram documents ventricular dilatation and may show mitral regurgitation due to the distended annulus with poor coaptation of the leaflets. Systolic dysfunction is often significantly reduced. Intracardiac thrombus may be seen.

Endomyocardial biopsy is rarely useful but may postpone consideration for heart transplant if acute myocarditis is identified.

## Management

- Generally supportive (anticongestive medication) and used to control symptoms, limit progression of the disease process, and prevent complications such as thromboembolism.

- Angiotensin-converting enzyme inhibition (ACEI) is the cornerstone of treatment to control the activation of the renin-angiotensin-aldosterone system. Patients often cannot tolerate target doses of ACEI. Adult studies have shown a 12% reduction in mortality and hospitalization with the use of ACEI. Systolic hypotension that does not cause postural symptoms and mild renal impairment are not absolute contraindication to the use of target ACEI treatment.

- Spironolactone is an important adjunct in heart failure treatment, with a reported 30% reduction in risk of mortality in adult studies.

- Antiplatelet or anticoagulant therapy may be indicated, particularly if EF < 30%.

- Immunosuppressive therapy is of no proven benefit.

- L-carnitine is of no proven benefit but is used as part of a metabolic cocktail with co-enzyme Q in cases of suspected carnitine deficiency.

- Mechanical support with ECLS or ventricular assist devices may provide a bridge to recovery or heart transplant.

- Biventricular pacing has also been shown in adult studies to improve atrioventricular synchrony and cardiac output.

- Orthotopic heart transplant is considered for severe ventricular dysfunction with no improvement.

## Arrhythmogenic Right Ventricular Cardiomyopathy (ARVC)

ARVC carries an estimated prevalence of 1:5000 in the general population. It is the cause of up to 5% of sudden cardiac deaths in young adults. A familial etiology is found in 30–50% showing autosomal dominant inheritance with incomplete penetrance and involves mutations in desmosomal proteins. There is diffuse or segmental progressive myocyte atrophy and fibrofatty infiltration of the right ventricular apex and outflow tract, and the left ventricle. There is progressive right ventricular or biventricular dysfunction and electrical instability leading to arrhythmias, heart failure, and increased risk of sudden cardiac death, especially in athletes. The estimated annual mortality is 2.3%.

**Presentation**   Diagnosis is often difficult early in the disease. Presentation is with palpitations, chest pain or syncope, or sudden cardiac death. Ventricular arrhythmias are precipitated with exercise. Ventricular tachycardia is usually of left bundle branch block morphology, and inferior QRS axis suggests a right ventricular outflow tract site of origin, while superior axis suggests the origin from the right ventricular apex. Many patients progress to right or biventricular cardiac failure, over a period of 4–8 years.

**Investigations**    The ARVC task force has outlined diagnostic criteria based on electrical and morphological features.

Electrocardiogram: May show right ventricular conduction delay as complete or incomplete right bundle branch block in the right precordial leads. Characteristic epsilon waves may be seen as terminal deflections in the right precordial QRS complexes in the presence of delayed activation of right ventricular myofibers.

Echocardiogram: Dilatation of the right ventricular outflow tract, right ventricular wall motion abnormalities/hypokinesia, and aneurysm formation.

Cardiac MRI: May show myocardial adipose infiltration and delayed hyperenhancement may identify areas of fibrosis. Definitive diagnosis is based on the finding of transmural fibrofatty replacement.

Endomyocardial biopsy: Rarely useful as the changes affect the free wall of the right ventricle.

## Management

- Antiarrhythmic therapy: Sotalol is more effective than other beta blockers or amiodarone in reducing malignant arrhythmias; however, pharmacotherapy does not prevent sudden cardiac death.
- An AICD is the most effective safeguard in high-risk individuals. Fibrofatty changes in the myocardium may interfere with proper sensing and pacing.
- Radiofrequency catheter ablation has also been studied. It may be useful but success often requires multiple ablation attempts and there is a high recurrence rate.
- Progression to ventricular failure requires usual anti-failure therapy and consideration for orthotopic heart transplant.

# Restrictive Cardiomyopathy (RCM)

Restrictive cardiomyopathy is rare in children, seen in 2–5% of all pediatric cardiomyopathies. Most are idiopathic, but may also be secondary to systemic disorders (pericardial disease, glycogen storage disease, amyloidosis, endomyocardial fibrosis) or associated with various skeletal myopathies. Mutations in sarcomeric proteins including troponin I, troponin T, and actin have been identified. Restrictive cardiomyopathy is characterized by diastolic dysfunction resulting in elevated ventricular filling pressures but preserved systolic function. In adults, it carries a relatively benign course with frequent survival beyond 10 years. Few children survive more than 2–5 years from diagnosis.

**Presentation**   Deterioration in diastolic function is insidious. Infants may present with failure to thrive. Older children present with decreased exercise tolerance, arrhythmias, syncope, congestive heart failure, or low cardiac output syndrome (LCOS). Thromboembolism is common (15–30%).

**Investigations**   Chest radiograph: May show a normal cardiothoracic ratio but almost half of patients display pulmonary venous congestion.

Electrocardiogram: Usually normal sinus rhythm, although atrial tachyarrhythmias and heart block occur. May suggest atrial enlargement but ventricular forces are usually normal.

Echocardiogram: Normal-sized ventricles, marked atrial dilatation, preserved systolic function but severe diastolic dysfunction in the form of a restrictive ventricular filling pattern.

Cardiac catheterization: Will differentiate restrictive cardiomyopathy from constrictive pericarditis.

Endomyocardial biopsy: Patchy endocardial and interstitial fibrosis.

## Management

- Mainstay of medical treatment is anticongestive therapy.
- Peripheral vasodilators have been used, but angiotensin converting enzyme inhibition shows no symptomatic or therapeutic benefit; sometimes detrimental effect on cardiac output with an abrupt drop in aortic pressure in the face of an inability to augment ventricular filling.
- Due to the increased risk of thromboembolism, antiplatelet or anticoagulant therapy should be started at diagnosis.
- It has been suggested that they should be listed for transplant at diagnosis. However, a subset of patients seems to have significantly better survival. Poor prognostic factors include age <5 years, high pulmonary vascular resistance, and syncope. In addition, sudden cardiac death due to malignant arrhythmia can

occur. Severe pulmonary hypertension (PVRI $>15$ U-m$^2$) may preclude heart transplant. PVRI should be closely monitored in these patients and any significant increase should prompt the consideration for transplant.

# Left Ventricular Non-compaction (LVNC)

Left ventricular non-compaction accounts for 9% of pediatric cardiomyopathies. It may be a primary lesion but it is also associated with congenital heart disease, especially ventricular septal defects and obstruction outflow lesions. Particularly in children, there is an association with neuromuscular disorders. Many affected children are described with minor facial dysmorphisms: micrognathia, lowset ears, and prominent forehead. The cardiomyopathy in Barth syndrome has mutations in tafazzin proteins. Some mutations in various cytoskeletal proteins such as dystrobrevin are identified in LVNC. Ventricular non-compaction is characterized by a thickened two-layered myocardium with a thinner compact outer layer and a thicker, spongy endocardial layer with prominent trabeculations and deep intertrabecular recesses. It may be due to an intrauterine arrest of normal development, whereby a spongy primitive myocardium condenses, producing the papillary muscles, trabeculae carnae, and chordae tendinae. Coronary artery distribution appears normal but abnormal intramural perfusion results in myocardial dysfunction. Prognosis in children suggest overall survival of 76–93%. Complications include heart failure, arrhythmias, and thromboembolic events, although these occur less frequently than with non-compaction.

**Presentation**    Most commonly congestive heart failure with poor systolic function. Many children are asymptomatic and identified because of an abnormal electrocardiogram or murmur. Some are diagnosed during investigation for neuromuscular disease. A subset shows rapid progression to death. A common pattern is one of transient recovery of function followed by later deterioration. An undulating phenotype has been described consisting of a changing pattern from dilated to hypertrophic cardiomyopathy over time.

**Investigations**    Chest x-ray: May be normal or show cardiomegaly.

Electrocardiogram: May show biventricular hypertrophy, intraventricular conduction delay, and abnormal repolarization.

There is an elevated incidence of Wolff-Parkinson-White syndrome associated with LVNC. Atrial and ventricular arrhythmias occur.

Echocardiogram: A thick myocardial wall is composed of a thicker non-compacted layer and an outer thin compact layer, with a ratio of 2:1 non-compacted to compacted, often considered necessary for diagnosis. Endocardial fibrosis may suggest myocardial ischemia.

## Management

- Children with depressed ventricular systolic function may benefit from beta blockade or calcium channel blockers.
- An antiplatelet agent should be started in all patients; those with poor ejection fraction are at higher risk of thromboembolism and may benefit from anticoagulation.
- Implantable cardioverter defibrillators are a primary prevention in patients with very poor ejection fraction or ventricular arrhythmias.
- Patients with heart failure not responding to medical therapy should be considered for orthotopic heart transplant.

## Myocarditis (Inflammatory Myocarditis)

Myocarditis is an acute or chronic inflammatory process of the myocardium with leukocytic infiltration and myocyte necrosis. Viral etiology is felt to be the most common etiology, especially cardiotropic viruses such as adenovirus and enteroviruses, although rarely proven. Bacterial, rickettsial, fungal, and parasitic infections, and various toxins and drugs may also cause myocarditis. Inflammation may trigger a secondary autoimmune response with myocyte damage and progression to a dilated cardiomyopathy phenotype. Mortality rates are reported as 10–25% in children. At least 50% of children with a well-defined preceding history of myocarditis may achieve normalization of cardiac function if they survive the acute phase.

**Presentation**   It is difficult to obtain a true estimate of the prevalence of myocarditis as its presentation may often be subclinical. There may be a mild flu-like illness with fever and gastrointestinal symptoms that resolves followed days to weeks later by the gradual onset of heart failure symptoms. Circulatory collapse or arrhythmia resulting in sudden cardiac death may be the initial presentation. Myocarditis should be included in the differential diagnosis of infants presenting with septic shock and negative blood cultures. Spontaneous recovery in weeks to months is frequent but progression to dilated cardiomyopathy occurs in 20% of cases.

**Investigations**    Diagnosis depends on a high index of suspicion.

Chest x-ray: May show pulmonary venous congestion; in the acute stages, the cardiac size may be normal.

Electrocardiography: Sinus tachycardia, low ($<$5 mm) QRS voltages, conduction abnormalities, diffuse ST flattening, and T wave inversion or ventricular ectopy. Arrhythmias include atrial tachyarrhythmias, ventricular tachycardia, and complete heart block.

Laboratory findings: May be lymphocytosis, elevated C-reactive protein or erythrocyte sedimentation rate, and elevated troponin levels. Creatine phosphokinase levels may be elevated. Viral cultures or viral serology titers may be obtained from blood, nasopharyngeal washings, cerebrospinal fluid, urine, or stool. Positive results do not imply etiology as most people have been exposed to these viruses.

Echocardiogram: Depressed ejection fraction, pericardial effusion, and wall motion abnormalities. If the course has been protracted, there may be an increased left ventricular end-diastolic dimension and mitral regurgitation due to the distended mitral valve annulus.

Cardiac MRI: Emerging as an important noninvasive imaging modality for diagnosis.

Endomyocardial biopsy (EMBx): The gold standard for diagnosis, demonstrating lymphocyte infiltration and myocardial necrosis (definitive diagnosis) or interstitial edema in association with lymphocyte infiltration (borderline diagnosis) (the Dallas criteria). EMBx carries the risk of inducing intractable arrhythmia or myocardial perforation. In addition, the disease process is often patchy and may be localized to the epicardium, yielding a high rate of false negative testing. A study in children found a better yield if biopsy was performed within the first 72 hours of presentation and within the first 6 weeks of the disease course when inflammatory changes were more likely to be present.

**Management**    The hemodynamic picture is often one of poor contractility and high systemic vascular resistance. Treatment is generally supportive.

- Oral captopril may be the only medication required in mild cases. ACEI may also help to limit myocyte hypertrophy and necrosis.
- Inotropic agents may augment contractility but both dopamine and dobutamine increase heart rate; milrinone has been useful in the acute setting but may increase mortality when used for longer periods.
- Metroprolol and carvedilol show some efficacy in more chronic heart failure, perhaps by relief of vasospasm.
- Immunosuppressive therapies including IVIG and corticosteroids may be useful only in the acute viremic phase of the illness. Unfortunately, presentation usually occurs well beyond this period. A recent meta-analysis has shown no supportive evidence for immunosuppressive therapy. The exception may be in children when the presentation may be more fulminant, and treatment may improve survival.
- Mechanical support with ECLS or ventricular assist devices as a bridge to recovery or heart transplantation has reported return to normal function after 9–10 days of support in up to 70% of cases requiring ECLS.

# Suggested Readings

Maron, BJ et al. Contemporary definitions and classification of the cardiomyopathies: An American Heart Association scientific statement from the Council on Clinical Cardiology, Heart Failure and Transplantation Committee; Quality of care and outcomes research and functional genomics and translational biology interdisciplinary working groups; and council on epidemiology and prevention. Circulation 2006;113:1807–16.

Maron BJ, McKenna WJ. ACC/ESC expert consensus document on hypertrophic cardiomyopathy. JACC 2003;42(9):1687–1713.

Maron BJ. Hypertrophic cardiomyopathy: a systematic review. JAMA 2002; 287:1308–20.

Yetman AT, McCrindle BW. Management of pediatric hypertrophic cardiomyopathy. Current Opinion in Cardiology 2005;20:80–3.

Towbin JA, et al. Incidence, causes, and outcomes of dilated cardiomyopathy in children. JAMA 2006;296:1867–76.

Elliott P. Cardiomyopathy: diagnosis and management of dilated cardiomyopathy. Heart 2000;84:106–112.

Kumar RK. A practical approach for the diagnosis and management of dilated cardiomyopathy. Indian J Pediatr 2002; 69(4):341–50.

Kies P. et al. Arrhythmogenic right ventricular dysplasia/cardiomyopathy: screening, diagnosis and treatment. Heart Rhythm 2006;3(2):225–34.

Gemayel C, Pelliccia A, Thompson PD. Arrhythmogenic right ventricular cardiomyopathy. JACC 2001;38:1773–81.

Piccini JP, et al. Predictors of appropriate implantable defibrillator therapies in patients with arrhythmogenic right ventricular dysplasia. Heart Rhythm 2005;2:1188–94.

Russo LM, Webber SA. Idiopathic restrictive cardiomyopathy in children. Heart 2005;91;1199–02.

Weller RJ, Weintraub R, Addonizio LJ, et al. Outcome of idiopathic restrictive cardiomyopathy in children. Am J Cardiol 2002;90:501–6.

Ammash NM, Seward JB, Bailey KR, et al. Clinical profile and outcome of idiopathic restrictive cardiomyopathy. Circulation 2000;101;2490–96.

Denfield SW, Rosenthal G, Gajarski RJ, et al. Restrictive cardiomyopathies in childhood: etiologies and natural history. Tex Heart Inst J 1997;24:38–44.

Freedom RM, et al. The morphological spectrum of ventricular noncompaction. Cardiol Young 2005;15:345–64.

Jenni R, Oechslin EN, van der Loo B. Isolated ventricular non-compaction of the myocardium in adults. Heart 2007;93:11–15.

Lilje C, et al. Complications of non-compaction of the left ventricular myocardium in a paediatric population: a prospective study. European Heart Journal 2006;27:1855–60.

Weiford BC, Subbarao VD, Mulhern KM. Noncompaction of the ventricular myocardium. Circulation 2004;109:2965–71.

Ellis CR, Di Salvo T. Myocarditis: basic and clinical aspects. Cardiology in Review 2007;15:170–7.

Bohn D, Benson L. Diagnosis and management of pediatric myocarditis. Pedatr Drugs 2002;4(3):171–81.

Feldman AM, McNamara D. Myocarditis. NEJM 2001;343(19):1388–1400.

Allen HD, Driscoll DJ, Shaddy RE, Feltes TF eds. Moss and Adams' heart disease in infants, children and adolescents: Including the fetus and young adults, 7th Ed. Lippincott Williams and Wilkins; 2008.

# E. Perioperative Care of the Child with CHD

Peter W Skippen

## Key Principles

- Accurate diagnosis of a specific cardiac lesion is not necessary before initiating basic emergency management in children.
- $PGE_1$ should be considered in any critically ill neonate with either cyanosis or poor pulses.
- Standard aspects of initial resuscitation include ABC, vascular access (IV/IO) with blood cultures, IV antibiotics, volume resuscitation, and checking of serum glucose.
- An understanding of the changes in vascular resistance and cardiorespiratory interactions is critical to successful management of the child with congenital heart disease.

This chapter is intended as a guideline to the management of infants and children with congenital heart disease, from initial presentation through definitive repair. It is not an exhaustive review of all lesions, nor a substitute for in-depth reading of specific aspects of care.

## Challenges

Successful management of infants and children with congenital heart disease (CHD) requires a multidisciplinary team approach. Management of these cases is challenging because of anatomic and physiological variations associated with age and maturation including:

- Issues relating to prematurity and low birth weight

  - Transitional circulation to adult maturational changes

- Secondary effects of congenital cardiac lesions on other organs
- Issues specific to neonates, including:

  - A less compliant myocardium (less tolerant and less responsive to afterload increases)
  - Greater vulnerability to the effects of cardiopulmonary bypass and circulatory arrest

- Immature renal and hepatic function
- Developing cerebral physiology
- Large total body water and altered capillary permeability (makes postoperative fluid management difficult)
- Vascular access challenges

The approach to management when faced with a newborn or older child will depend on the acuity of the presentation. Crises, such as infants in circulatory collapse or extreme hypoxemia, must be dealt with emergently. In all cases evaluation of a chest radiograph will provide clues to the underlying pathophysiology.

# Preoperative Resuscitation and Stabilization

Once it has been identified that the child is critically ill, standard aspects of urgent management include:

- ABC, including rapid assessment of the cardiorespiratory system including femoral pulses
- Vascular access: peripheral intravenous, intraosseous, central access, eg, UA/UV
- Blood cultures—antibiotics (if sepsis is a possibility)
- Volume resuscitation
- Prostaglandin $E_1$ ($PGE_1$) to open the duct (if hypoxemia is the predominant issue)
- Inotropes
- Calcium infusions in neonates improve cardiac function and may also be required for infants with 22q deletions (phenotype of Di George may be present)
- Monitor for hypoglycemia
- Cautious use of oxygen and bicarbonate with control of ventilation and $PaCO_2$ to balance the PVR and SVR to prevent pulmonary over-circulation

Although accurate diagnosis of the specific cardiac lesion is not necessary prior to initiating basic resuscitation, a physiologic approach to assessment and diagnosis should be taken. Based on this, a few key questions to be addressed following the initial management of these infants and children.

1. Is the baby blue or pink?
2. Is the circulation normal or inadequate?

3. Is pulmonary blood flow increased or decreased?
4. Is there obstruction to blood flow?
5. Is there mixing and shunting, and if so, at what level cardiac or extra-cardiac?
6. Is the circulation in series or in parallel?
7. How does systemic venous return reach the systemic arterial circulation to maintain cardiac output?
8. Is there a volume or pressure load on the ventricles?

PGE$_1$ infusions are used to open the duct or maintain ductal patency in any duct-dependent lesion in the newborn period. Any critically ill child deserves consideration of a trial of PGE$_1$ until cardiac disease is excluded.

Side effects are more common above doses 0.05 mcg/kg/min and include apnea, hypotension, and flushing, fever, and central nervous system (CNS) excitation. Recurrent apnea will require mechanical ventilatory support. PGE$_1$ usually improves arterial oxygenation by improving pulmonary blood flow from the aorta to the pulmonary vessels, and allows mixing of oxygenated blood with deoxygenated blood at either the atrial or ventricular shunt level.

Clinical deterioration after initiating PGE$_1$ in a baby with CHD may indicate:

- Obstructed pulmonary venous drainage such as HLHS with restrictive PFO
- TGA with IVS and restrictive PFO
- TAPVR with obstruction


## Specific Aspects of Management

*Cyanotic babies without significant respiratory distress:*

- Hyperoxia test for cyanotic babies
- PGE$_1$ infusion for stabilization prior to transfer to a pediatric center for definitive diagnosis and management

*Cyanotic babies with significant respiratory distress:*

- PGE$_1$ infusion, intubate and ventilate prior to transfer
  Reopening a duct may require higher doses of PGE$_1$ (0.05–0.1 mcg/kg/min) than maintenance of an open duct (0.01–0.05 mcg/kg/min)

*Transport of critically ill children with CHD:*
Consult with critical care physicians and pediatric cardiology. Most children require the following prior to and during transport:

- Intubation and ventilation, including advice regarding controlled oxygen administration and ventilation strategies
- Reliable vascular access
- $PGE_1$ infusion
- NG tube
- Antibiotics
- Treatment of shock and circulatory support

# Preoperative Evaluation

The advent of preoperative stabilization in a modern PICU and $PGE_1$ infusions means that surgery is very rarely needed emergently. During this stabilization period, ongoing evaluation includes identification of the cardiac lesion, other associated anomalies (including chromosomal), assessment of electrolyte and acid base status, and other organ function. Section 8A on assessment describes the more commonly used advanced investigations of children presenting with cardiac disease.

## Cardiorespiratory Interactions

An understanding and meticulous attention to cardiopulmonary interactions is the basis of pre- and postoperative care in the patients.

Changes in pulmonary vascular resistance (PVR) are an important determinant of cardiorespiratory function and impact systemic oxygen delivery. Factors affecting PVR include:

- Hypoxemia
- Hypercarbia
- Acidosis
- Lung over-distension with high tidal volumes or mean airway pressures
- High left atrial pressure
- Medications, humoral influence, eg, nitric oxide, catecholamines, alpha-blockers, vasopressin
- Sympathetic stimulation
- Mechanical obstruction
- Persistent L-R shunt
- Recurrent chest infections
- Pulmonary edema
- Cardiopulmonary bypass

The clinical impact of elevated PVR on the right side of the circulation includes:

- Increased RV afterload through PVR elevation
- Increased R-L shunt across ASD with RV hypertrophy/restrictive physiology
- Increased AV valve regurgitation across right-sided incompetent valve

The clinical impact of elevated PVR on the left side of the circulation includes reduced LV preload from the reduced PBF, unless there exists an atrial or ventricular shunt.

Left-sided afterload is reduced generally during positive pressure ventilation and increased during spontaneous ventilation, especially in situations associated with an increased work of breathing. On balance, systemic oxygen delivery generally improves when PPV is used to support a child with significant LV dysfunction. In addition, the reduced work of breathing for patients with stiff lungs allows cardiac output to be distributed to vital organs.

Positive end-respiratory pressure (PEEP) used appropriately will optimize functional residual capacity and minimize PVR. Zero PEEP for more than short periods of time will result in atelectasis causing an increase in PVR. However, it remains unclear what the optimal level of PEEP should be for different cardiac lesions, particularly those with passive pulmonary blood flow (Glen and Fontan).

## Cardiopulmonary Bypass (CPB)

The aim of CPB is to isolate the cardiopulmonary system to ensure optimal surgical exposure. At a minimum the circuit must remove carbon dioxide, oxygenate, adjust temperature, and provide adequate perfusion pressure. The extracorporeal circuit drains venous blood (usually passively, based upon cannulae diameter and the height of the right atrium above the venous reservoir) to a reservoir, pumps it through an oxygenator and filter, and then returns it to the arterial circulation, bypassing the heart and lungs.

During CPB, children are exposed to extremes of temperature, severe hemodilution, low perfusion pressures (20–30 mm Hg), wide variation in pump flows from normal cardiac output to circulatory arrest, and differing blood pH management strategies (alpha-stat or pH-stat). Cannulation techniques vary depending on the procedure and the cardiac lesion. Small changes in cannula position can significantly impact blood flow during bypass, particularly in the tiny babies. The presence of a patent duct requires either ligation prior to initiation of bypass, or cannulation to ensure body perfusion during bypass. In addition there are marked physiologic responses to CPB in the child.

- Cannulation

Bypass can be either total or partial. Most operative procedures in children require total bypass. Capturing most of the systemic venous return requires cannulation of the right atrium with either a single right-angle cannula or both an SVC and IVC cannula. Right atrial pressure approaches zero. Some cardiac lesions have other venous return that can create surgical exposure problems, such as persistent left SVC draining into the coronary sinus, interruption of the infra-hepatic IVC, or azygous continuation of the IVC. Snagging tapes around the vessels and cannulae prevents air entrainment.

Arterial return to the patient is generally achieved with a cannula placed in the lesser curve of the ascending aorta proximal to the innominate artery. With a hypoplastic arch, cannulating the ductus through the pulmonary artery achieves systemic perfusion. With an interrupted arch, proximal and distal arch cannulation is necessary.

Partial bypass via the femoral artery may be necessary in some patients presenting for repeat sternotomies if the heart or great vessels are adherent beneath the sternum as determined on chest radiograph or CT scan. As the cannula size and flows are limited by the small size of the femoral artery, this is a temporary measure until full bypass is achieved through the sternotomy.

- Circuit components

Two types of pump exist, double-headed roller and centrifugal. Each has its advantages and disadvantages. Most pediatric centers use roller pump technology as it allows fine control of flow rate and volume administration. Oxygenator technology has advanced and most pediatric centers use reverse hollow fiber microporous oxygenators. These are very efficient as the oxygen air mixture is inside the capillaries and the blood is in contact with the entire outer surface resulting in a large contact area interface with low prime volume. These newest oxygenators have incorporated heat exchangers. Most oxygenators are also coated to minimize the contact inflammatory response. Arterial microfilters prevent micro and macro air emboli.

In addition to the main venous cannulae, cardiotomy suction and ventricular vents are required. Blood collected through cardiotomy suction must first be filtered prior to pumping to the venous reservoir in order to remove procoagulant microparticles to reduce inflammatory mediator generation. Venting of the ventricles prevents ventricular over-distension and warming of the heart. Right heart filling during full CPB comes from either coronary or noncoronary blood flow. Left heart filling comes from thebesian veins, bronchial veins, and extra-cardiac left to right shunts (eg, unligated BT shunt, systemic aortopulmonary shunts) or aortic valve incompetence.

- Hypothermia

Hypothermic CPB is used to preserve organ function (especially cerebral function) during cardiac surgery. Systemic hypothermia reduces whole body and cerebral oxygen consumption by a factor of 2–4 for each 10 °C reduction in temperature in neonates and infants. The choice depends upon the required surgical condition, size of the patient, type of operation, and surgeon preference. Four methods are used:

1. Normothermic CPB
2. Moderate hypothermic CPB (25–32°C)
3. Deep hypothermia with low flow CPB (15–20°C)
4. Deep hypothermic circulatory arrest

Moderate hypothermic CPB is generally employed for older children. Deep hypothermic CPB allows complex repairs in neonates and infants by providing a near bloodless field. It may also sometimes be required for certain complex arch problems in older children. Flow is preferentially distributed to the brain when low pump flows are used. The contribution of CPB perfusion variables to the development of other organ dysfunction postoperatively is unclear (eg, renal function).

Hypothermic techniques require hemodilution to minimize viscosity effects. Limited hemodilution is more commonly used with Hct of 0.24 to 28.

- Circuit prime

Volume and composition of the prime have important physiologic consequences for the pediatric patient. The aim is to achieve a physiologically balanced prime while limiting the prime volume. Miniaturizing the exposure to the least amount of foreign circuit involves choosing the smallest oxygenator, the smallest tubing and cannulae capable of delivering the desirable blood flow with the least resistance. Despite best efforts, newborns still have 100% to 150% dilution of their blood volume (smallest circuit prime about 300 mL). The main constituents of the pediatric prime are Plasmalyte A® or equivalent, banked RBC reconstituted with FFP to achieve a desired Hct, and colloid. Other supplements such as mannitol, glucose, steroids, magnesium, and bicarbonate are surgeon and perfusionist specific. The larger child can have bloodless prime to limit donor blood product exposure.

• Anticoagulation

Newborns have different coagulation and fibrinolytic protein concentrations that impact CPB anticoagulation and postoperative bleeding complications. Systemic heparin anticoagulation is required to prevent circuit clotting and inflammatory responses to fibrin generation. Unfractionated heparin is the usual agent although thrombin generation is not completely inhibited even at massive doses. It also causes platelet activation. Heparin-induced thrombocytopenia, cold agglutinin vasculitis, and other rare conditions require hematology consultation prior to initiation of hypothermic CPB. The heparin dose is higher in neonates and infants due to greater blood volume dilution and greater clearance of heparin and binding of heparin to acute phase proteins. Protamine reversal can cause severe pulmonary hypertensive reactions, although these appear to be less common than in adults.

• Bypass

Venous cannula misplacement can cause problems such as obstructed venous return from either the IVC or SVC. IVC obstruction will manifest as ascites and hepatomegaly with reduced splanchnic and renal perfusion. SVC obstruction may result in cerebral edema or reduced cerebral blood flow. Neurologic monitoring using Doppler or near-infrared spectroscopy is a useful tool. Constant communication with the perfusionist regarding adequacy of venous return and temperature gradients is essential. Similarly, arterial cannula malposition in the small newborn arches or babies with complex anatomy or aortopulmonary communications (eg, PDA or large collaterals) may impair cerebral circulation. Once the surgeon has the cannulae placed, bypass is initiated by slowly starting the arterial pump. High arterial line pressure, reduced venous return, or inadequate flow rates would indicate a cannula problem. Once cannulae positions are verified, the venous line clamp is reduced and pump flow is increased rapidly to achieve the desired systemic flow, the adequacy of which is monitored using arterial blood gas analysis and blood lactate levels. Ventricular distension while on CPB indicates ineffective venous drainage.

Pump flow rates are based upon the patient's body mass and evidence of efficient organ perfusion as determined by blood gases, acid base, lactate, and whole body oxygen consumption. Hypothermia reduces metabolism, allowing flow rates to be reduced significantly while still providing sufficient flow to vital organs. Outcome data related to specific flows are lacking. Following the surgical repair and while on bypass, a transesophageal echocardiogram is often performed to assess adequacy of the repair and to evaluate for valvular regurgitation or stenosis.

- Myocardial Protection

   In addition to hypothermia and the prevention of myocardial distension during bypass, intracardiac repair requires cardiac arrest by one of two techniques:

   a. Cardioplegia (high potassium concentration causing the heart to arrest in diastole) is administered via a small cardioplegia cannula placed in the ascending aorta distal to the aortic valve, but isolated from the aortic inflow cannula by an aortic cross clamp. This gives rise to the term aortic cross clamp time.

   b. Deep hypothermia circulatory arrest (DHCA).

DHCA facilitates precise surgical repair of certain complex cardiac lesions under optimal conditions, free of blood and cannulae. DHCA should be maintained as short as possible to minimize the risks of cerebral ischemia. The duration of safe DHCA appears to be up to 45 minutes. The technique of cooling (eg, rapid cooling in less than 20 minutes is associated with more long-term neurologic deficits) and rewarming to ensure homogenous brain temperatures probably impacts ultimate neurologic recovery. Cerebral autoregulation is lost during extremes of temperature, and cerebral perfusion becomes highly dependent upon the conduct of extracorporeal perfusion and probably post CPB hemodynamics. Selective cerebral perfusion has been tried in an attempt to mitigate the adverse effects of prolonged DHCA although there are no long-term outcome studies.

- Weaning from bypass

During weaning from CPB, intravascular volume is monitored using right atrial or left atrial filling pressures. Once filling pressures are adequate, the patient is fully warmed, Hct is optimized, and acid base and electrolyte abnormalities are corrected. When heart rate and rhythm are adequate (paced or otherwise), the venous drainage is gradually occluded and weaning from bypass begins. The arterial cannula is left in place until the patient is fully weaned for slow infusion of pump blood to optimize filling pressures. Inotropes and afterload reduction are usually required to separate from bypass for a variable period of time. Direct heart visualization, acid base status, lactate levels, and central venous saturations are all used to assess adequacy of cardiac function prior to separation. Failure to separate successfully implies one of the following:

- Right or left ventricular dysfunction
- Pulmonary hypertension
- Residual anatomic abnormality

Diagnosis is made using selective chamber and vascular pressure measurements, catheter pullback measurements, cardiac echo, or cardiac catheterization. If there is no residual anatomic problem and the surgery deemed adequate, some children may be successfully weaned with some further myocardial rest and reperfusion on full CPB or require support in the PICU postoperatively using ECLS.

## Postoperative Care

Safe return from the operating room (OR) to the pediatric intensive care unit (PICU) is facilitated by adequate preparation and clear communication as to expected time of arrival and level of monitoring and support needed. The keys to successful transitioning from the operating room to the PICU are:

- Clear communication of the details of the surgery, CPB, and anesthesia
- Uninterrupted monitoring during conversion from transport to bedside monitoring equipment
- Uninterrupted delivery of vasoactive medications
- Maintenance of adequate gas exchange
- Calibration of vascular transducers, assessment of cardiac rhythm, assessment of atrial and arterial waveforms during the initial assessment in the PICU

Supporting cardiac output, treating low output and preventing cardiovascular collapse are the focus during the initial hours and days in the PICU. An assessment for residual anatomic lesions is also important because they may dictate further evaluation and treatment and may lead to adverse outcomes.

## Initial investigations in the PICU include:

- CXR to determine lung volumes and status and position of monitoring lines and endotracheal tube
- 12-lead ECG
- Hemoglobin and platelet count
- Arterial and mixed venous blood gas analysis
- Lactate
- Electrolytes
- Coagulation screen

## Routine monitoring includes:

- ECG
- Pulse oximetry
- Invasive arterial pressure
- Central venous pressure: Monitoring central venous pressure provides an assessment of filling pressures, allows waveform analysis that can assist in the analysis of cardiac rhythm, and allows sampling of central venous oxygen saturations. Elevated pressures indicate either poor RV function, pulmonary hypertension, a restrictive RV, right AV valve regurgitation, tamponade, volume overload or may reflect cannon waves and AV dyssynchrony.
- Pulmonary artery pressure, left atrial pressure, right atrial pressure. Left atrial catheters are useful in patients with left-sided AV valve disease and ventricular dysfunction. Pulmonary catheters are useful in patients at risk of developing postoperative pulmonary hypertension or for assessing the severity of residual shunts.
- Urine output
- Ventilation parameters, including end tidal carbon dioxide
- Other: niroscopy (near-infrared spectroscopy)

## Assessment of cardiac output includes:

- Clinical assessment of the patient
- Mixed venous oxygen saturations
- Arterial lactate
- Base deficit

An increasing metabolic acidosis with increasing serum lactate and falling mixed venous oxygen saturation indicates low cardiac output.

## Cardiorespiratory Care

Ensuring adequate ventilation is critical after transfer from the OR to optimize CO by minimizing PVR and prevention of postoperative pulmonary hypertensive crises. Patients at risk of elevated PVR postoperatively are those with:

1. Documented preoperative PH
2. Neonates in the first few days of life
3. Specific cardiac lesions such as pulmonary venous hypertension, mitral stenosis, long-term L-R shunts
4. Severely impaired systemic ventricular dysfunction with high LVEDP
5. Patients with parenchymal lung disease

Steps:

1. Determine targets of $SaO_2$ and $PaCO_2$ based upon preoperative data and the surgical repair.
2. Set ventilator in consultation with the cardiac anesthetist that cared for the child during the cardiac procedure. Initial ventilator settings and blood gas goals can be found in Table 1. The cause of unexpected blood gas abnormalities warrants

*Table 1*
**Ventilation Strategies**

General *Initial* Ventilation Guidelines for Different Lesions:

- Optimize FRC: minimum PEEP 5 cm $H_2O$
- Initial $F_iO_2$: based upon that required in the OR, weaned based upon the ABG and desired arterial saturations
- Initial TV: 8–10 mL/kg; if plateau pressures >30 cm $H_2O$, consult the PICU critical care physician
- RR/I time/I: E ratio: age/patient/condition dependent

Routine Neonate post CPB:

- Optimize FRC: initial PEEP 5–10 cm $H_2O$, depending on oxygenation and CXR
- Maintain pH between 7.4 and 7.45; $PaCO_2$ 35ish, depending on the metabolic component of the pH

Post Glen Procedure:

- Optimize FRC: initial PEEP 5 cm $H_2O$
- Maintain $PaCO_2$ 40–50 mm Hg
- Aim for spontaneous respirations once hemodynamically stable, followed by early extubation

Post Fontan Procedure:

- Optimize FRC: initial PEEP 5 cm $H_2O$
- Maintain $PaCO_2$ 35–40 mm Hg
- Aim for spontaneous respirations once hemodynamically stable, followed by early extubation

Pulmonary Hypertension:

- Maintain pH 7.45–7.5, with initial $PaCO_2$ ~35 mm Hg
- Consider PA pressure monitor
- Consider NO, preferably after ECHO or direct pressure confirmation of pulmonary hypertension

Single Ventricle Physiology:

- Optimize FRC
- Maintain pH 7.4, with initial $PaCO_2$ ~40 mm Hg
- Monitor central venous saturations hourly until hemodynamically stable
- Aim for arterial saturations 75–80%; however, arterial saturation is dependent upon both pulmonary blood flow, cardiac output and pulmonary ventilation/perfusion mismatch (see following examples)

$$Q_P/Q_S \sim (Saorta - Ssvc)/(Spv - Spa)$$

But, because of the BT shunt, $Spa = Saorta = SaO_2$
Substituting:

$$Q_P/Q_S \sim (SaO_2 - Ssvc)/(Spv - SaO_2)$$

Assuming normal lungs, Spv ~ 95–100%; if coexisting lung disease, Spv less, maybe ~90%.

Also assuming a normal cardiac output (and metabolic rate, eg, normothermia), and normal a-v sat difference ~20%, that is, $SaO_2 - Ssvc = 20\%$. With falling CO, a-v difference increases, up to 40–45%.

With normal lungs and normal CO, then $Q_P/Q_S \sim 20/(95 - SaO_2)$.

*(continued)*

If $SaO_2 = 90\%$, then $Q_P/Q_S \sim 4:1$
If $SaO_2 = 85\%$, then $Q_P/Q_S \sim 3:1$
If $SaO_2 = 75\%$, then $Q_P/Q_S \sim 1:1$

If associated lung disease and normal CO, then $Q_P/Q_S \sim 20/(90 - SaO_2)$
If $SaO_2 = 85\%$, and assoc. lung disease, then $Q_P/Q_S \sim 4:1$
If $SaO_2 = 70\%$, and assoc. lung disease, then $Q_P/Q_S \sim 1:1$

If low CO, then $Q_P/Q_S \sim 40/(95 - SaO_2)$
If $SaO_2 = 90\%$, then $Q_P/Q_S \sim 8:1$
If $SaO_2 = 85\%$, then $Q_P/Q_S \sim 4:1$
If $SaO_2 = 75\%$, then $Q_P/Q_S \sim 2:1$

If low CO and lung disease, then $Q_P/Q_S \sim 40/(90 - SaO_2)$
If $SaO_2 = 85\%$, then $Q_P/Q_S \sim 8:1$
If $SaO_2 = 70\%$, then $Q_P/Q_S \sim 2:1$

an immediate search for the cause and rapid intervention to correct the cause and the abnormality. Expect parameters to change over time and between patients. Frequent changes in the immediate postoperative period are likely. Unexpectedly low saturations or elevated $PaCO_2$ requires confirming patency and position of the ETT.

3. Interpret arterial and mixed venous blood gas in light of postoperative cardiac anatomy and physiology.
4. Review CXR early to ensure all catheters and tubes are appropriately located, to rule out unexpected air or fluid collections, and to assess airspace disease and lung volumes.

## Temporary Cardiac Pacing

In a child with an arrhythmia, early accurate diagnosis is important (Figure 1).

The following approach is recommended:

- Is the child stable or unstable?

  - If unstable, ABC and follow ALS algorithm

- Call pediatric cardiology
- Obtain accurate diagnosis

  - History of the lesion, procedure, anesthetic, CPB, etc.
  - Rhythm strip
  - 12-lead ECG

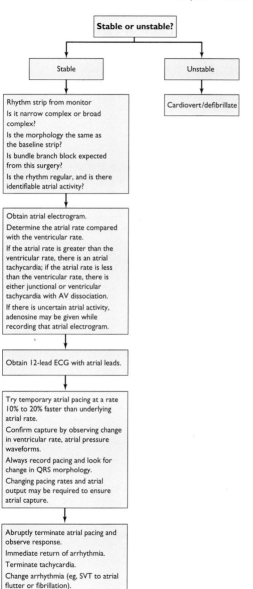

**Figure 1** Diagnostic approach to postoperative arrhythmia.

*Table 2*
## Setting up the Dual Chamber Pacemaker for the First Time (eg, Medtronic 5388)

In PICU, in patient already established on a pacemaker from the OR, reduce the pacing rate prior to testing pacing threshold to ensure there is an underlying rhythm.

Scenario A: patient not pacemaker dependent

*Step 1: Sensing Threshold*

Pacemaker must be ON:

Turn atrial and ventricular outputs to 0.1V or 0.1 mA

Set rate control less than patient's intrinsic rate

Turn atrial sensing threshold control anticlockwise to maximum threshold

Slowly reduce threshold (turn control clockwise) until sensing indicator flashes synchronously with patient's intrinsic rate

Set the sensing control to at least one half the original sensing threshold to allow a margin of safety

Typical atrial sensing thresholds <1 mA

Repeat procedure for ventricular threshold setting

Typical ventricular sensing thresholds ~2–5 mV

*Step 2: Capture Threshold*

Set rate control just above patient's intrinsic heart rate on ECG monitor

With output set below capture threshold, slowly increase atrial output, followed by ventricular output—with intact AV conduction, heart rate will increase with increasing atrial output; without AV conduction, there will be no increase in rate without increasing ventricular output

Once capture achieved, double the stimulation threshold to allow margin of safety

A-V interval is adjusted by observing P-R interval on a rhythm strip

AV sequential pacing with capture is indicated by:

    Increased regular heart rate
    Improved blood pressure
    Atrial spike immediately followed by P wave
    P-R interval
    Ventricular spike immediately followed by paced QRS complex
    Change in atrial waveform

> Scenario B: patient is pacemaker dependent
>
> Extreme caution is required during any manipulation of the pacemaker.
> If hemodynamic instability develops during rate reduction, or no intrinsic rate returns at low pacing rates, further manipulation should be abandoned and initial settings restored. Backup pacing equipment should be immediately available.

- Atrial electrogram
- Esophageal electrogram

- Observe waveform of atrial monitoring catheters

Table 2 outlines an approach to setting up the temporary pacemaker in the PICU following cardiac surgery. Management is determined by the specific rhythm disturbance. The most common indications for the use of temporary pacemakers in the postoperative period are as an aid in the diagnosis of postoperative arrhythmias; restoring an acceptable heart rate in cases of bradycardia and atrioventricular block; re-establishing atrioventricular synchrony; suppression of arrhythmias (junctional ectopic tachycardia, in particular); terminating certain re-entrant tachycardias; and improving coordination of ventricular contraction.

## Fluid and Electrolyte Management

Hemodilution and the stress response to the surgery and CPB result in aberrations in fluid and electrolyte balance. Patients are typically salt and water overloaded despite modified ultrafiltration. Neonates and young infants appear to develop greater volume overload than the older child. Most children produce adequate urine initially. Oliguria often follows 12–18 hours later as a result of elevated vasopressin levels and the nadir of decreased cardiac output that is typical following cardiac surgery. Renal function generally recovers spontaneously reflected by an increased urine output by 36–48 hours.

Intravenous fluid management consists of:

- Maintenance fluids are typically restricted to 50% while ensuring adequate glucose administration (10% glucose in normal saline for neonates).
- Intravascular volume support is determined by the surgical repair (eg, Fontan), degree of capillary leak and chest drain losses. The type of fluid used to replace chest drain losses or

support intravascular volume is determined by blood loss, the Hct, and possible need for coagulation factor replacement.

Maintaining normal ionized calcium levels is important in the neonatal group to ensure normal myocardial contractility. Hypocalcemia can arise as a result of hypoparathyroidism (22q chromosome deletion), or transfusion of large amounts of citrated blood products. A calcium infusion is the preferred approach to preventing hypocalcemia (initial dose: 1 mmol/kg/day via central line).

Diuretics are often required to excrete the excess water and sodium, usually furosemide, spironolactone and/or metolazone or other thiazide diuretic. Potassium and magnesium losses and replacement need to be anticipated to reduce the risk of arrhythmias. Metabolic alkalosis is common following diuretic therapy or massive transfusion. The combination of spironolactone and angiotensin-converting enzyme (ACE) inhibitors can cause hyperkalemia. Loop diuretics also increase calcium renal tubular excretion.

## Postoperative Complications

### Low Cardiac Output Syndrome (Figure 2)    The mean cardiac index in infants decreases by about 30%  6–12 hours after separation from CPB. Residual or undiagnosed structural lesions should always be excluded before attributing low output states to intrinsic depressed function. Numerous factors contribute to a low cardiac output:

- Surgical ventriculotomy
- Inflammatory response to CPB
- Myocardial ischemia time during aortic cross clamping
- Inadequate myocardial protection during CPB (eg, markedly hypertrophic ventricle)
- Hypothermia
- Reperfusion injury
- Persisting preoperative dysfunction
- Pulmonary hypertension
- Complication of surgery (eg, compromised coronary perfusion)
- Dysrhythmias

One or more of the following factors can be used to support the child with low cardiac output until recovery occurs, typically by day 2 or 3:

- An appreciation of the findings and course in the OR (good communication)
- Appropriate lesion specific and general monitoring

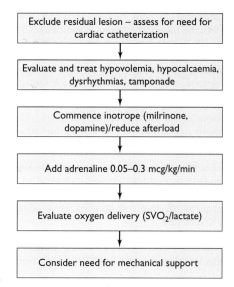

**Figure 2** Approach to low cardiac output syndrome.

- Optimize preload

  ○ Volume
  ○ Maybe lesion specific (eg, creating/preserving R-L shunt)

- Optimize afterload

  ○ Minimizing PVR
  ○ Reducing SVR

- Control heart rate and rhythm

  ○ Pacing/isoprenaline
  ○ AV sequential pacing
  ○ Antiarrhythmics

- Enhance contractility

  ○ Inotropes
  ○ Positive pressure ventilation

- Optimize heart lung interactions
- Mechanical support

Table 3 lists commonly used medications to treat low cardiac output syndrome. Low cardiac output is also caused by diastolic dysfunction. RV diastolic dysfunction results in a stiff noncompliant right ventricle, restricts filling, and manifests as high right-sided filling pressures (hepatomegaly, ascites, venous engorgement) with low systemic oxygen delivery and is seen following:

- Repair of tetralogy with ventriculotomy
- Myocardial edema with long bypass runs
- Inadequate myocardial protection in hypertrophied ventricles
- Residual right outflow tract obstruction

Management: Systemic oxygen delivery can be maintained by the creation of a surgical ASD (maintains left-sided preload and cardiac output) and a high hematocrit. Sedation and paralysis is often required, together with optimization of ventilation to minimize RV afterload.

LV diastolic dysfunction results in a stiff noncompliant left ventricle and manifests as high left atrial filling pressures, pulmonary edema, low cardiac output, and is seen in patients with:

- LV hypertrophy
- Myocardial edema

Management: Can be difficult but involves the usual attention to adequate preload, afterload reduction, minimizing inotropy to allow ventricular filling, and ensuring AV synchrony. Minimizing tachycardia allows increased time for diastolic filling. Mechanical cardiac support may be required.

## Bleeding

Postoperative bleeding results from suture lines or coagulopathy. Management: Correction of the coagulopathy begins in the OR with factor and platelet replacement. Persisting blood loss greater than 10 mL/kg for several hours after correction of the coagulopathy and normothermia requires re-exploration by the cardiac surgeon. Attention needs to be paid to the consequences of massive transfusion by the PICU team. Factor VIIa may then be considered for intractable bleeding in consultation with hematology.

## Tamponade

Usually results from mediastinal bleeding that is in excess of the drainage from the chest drains. Manifests with poor peripheral perfusion, rising right and left atrial pressures and occasionally

*Table 3*
## Common Cardioactive Agents

| Agent | low dose adrenaline | mod dose adrenaline | high dose adrenaline | noradrenaline | low dopamine | high dopamine | dobutamine |
|---|---|---|---|---|---|---|---|
| **Mechanism of action** | | | | | | | |
| Alpha | | ++ | ++++ | ++ | + | ++ | +++ |
| Beta 1 | + | ++ | ++++ | ++ | + | +++ | ++ |
| Beta 2 | ++ | ++ | +++ | | + | + | |
| Dopaminergic | | | | | ++++ | ++++ | |

| Agent | milrinone | nitroprusside | phenoxybenzamine | nitroglycerine | low dopamine / vasopressin | levosimendan |
|---|---|---|---|---|---|---|
| **Mechanism of action** | ↑cAMP | NO donor | alpha blocker | NO donor | V1 activation | Ca$^{++}$ sensitization |
| **Clinical effects** | inotropic vasodilator lusitropic | vasodilator Lusitropic Pulmonary vasodilator Systemic vasodilator | vasodilator | vasodilator | pulmonary vasodilator systemic vasoconstriction | inotrope vasodilator |

sudden cardiovascular collapse. High chest drain losses that suddenly decrease should raise an alert that the chest drains are blocked and that tamponade is imminent.

Opening the sternum and decompressing the mediastinum is the only definitive therapy. Emergent sternal opening places the patient at risk of sepsis through unsatisfactory aseptic technique.

Tamponade may occur in patients with preoperative cardiomegaly who develop myocardial edema, resulting in extrinsic compression of the cardiac chambers in the small mediastinum. This is usually anticipated by the cardiac surgeon dependent upon the surgical procedure and managed by leaving the sternum open for the first 24–48 hours until the myocardial edema resolves.

## Pulmonary Hypertension

Perioperative elevations in PVR complicate the postoperative course in many children following cardiac surgery. The increased PVR increases RV afterload and reduces LV preload. In children without an atrial communication, this can result in acute right heart failure and low systemic cardiac output. In children with an atrial communication, left atrial preload and systemic oxygen delivery may be maintained but systemic arterial desaturation results. Causes of an elevated PVR in the postoperative period include:

- Pulmonary disease
- Loss of FRC
- Endothelial injury resulting from CPB
- Elevated LAP
- Pulmonary venous obstruction
- Branch PA stenosis
- Residual L-R shunt

The best approach to managing pulmonary hypertension is to anticipate and treat the patient expectantly. General measures include adequate sedation and analgesia, optimizing ventilation and arterial pH, and minimizing stimuli known to accentuate elevations of PVR. Medications commonly used to reduce pulmonary artery pressures include milrinone, phenoxybenzamine, and nitroprusside. More specific agents include nitric oxide, sildenafil, and prostacyclin ($PGI_2$).

An acute pulmonary HT crisis, as defined by pulmonary artery pressures in excess of 50% of systemic mean pressures with an associated decreased systemic cardiac output, should prompt urgent interventions to prevent cardiac arrest.

Pulmonary compliance increases during acute elevations of pulmonary arterial pressures that may reduce ventilation at set ventilator settings, causing a viscous cycle of worsening pulmonary hypertension and reduced lung compliance.

- Hyperventilation with 100% oxygen using manual circuit
- Sodium bicarbonate given IV push
- Epinephrine given IV push may be required if bradycardiac and hypotensive
- Nitric oxide
- Milrinone infusion
- Prostacyclin (PGI$_2$) nebulized or infusion

**Chylothorax** Chylothoraces are not uncommon following pediatric cardiac surgery. Patients at risk include re-operations and aortic arch repairs. Depending upon the volume losses, large amounts of albumin, lymphocytes, and nutrients can be lost. Impaired immune function is a potential complication. Management includes (escalating therapy):

- Medical therapy

  ○ Pleural drainage
  ○ Special enteral formula (portogen or monogen)
  ○ Careful fluid and electrolyte management
  ○ TPN if special enteral formula fails to control losses

- Surgical therapy

  ○ Thoracic duct ligation
  ○ Pleuroperitoneal shunt

- Unproven medical therapy

  ○ Octreotide infusion
  ○ Low molecular weight heparin

## Diaphragmatic Paralysis

Diaphragmatic paralysis should be suspected in the child who experiences an increased work of breathing on low ventilator settings and/or an elevated hemidiaphragm on chest radiograph. It compromises infants in particular as it may impede weaning and successful extubation. It can be confirmed with chest ultrasound during spontaneous breathing or fluoroscopy. Although generally reversible over time, some smaller babies may require plication of the hemidiaphragm to achieve successful extubation.

## Neurologic Injury

There is a growing recognition of neurologic injury following congenital cardiac surgery and is related to:

- Pre-existing brain abnormalities
- Acquired events during bypass or the perioperative period

  - Children with shunts (paradoxical emboli)
  - Low-flow bypass or DHCA

Factors that are thought to contribute during CPB are:

- Duration of CPB
- Rate of core cooling and rewarming
- pH management during CPB
- Duration of circulatory arrest
- Depth of hypothermia
- Presence of arterial filtration
- Type of oxygenator
- Degree of inflammatory response

Seizures, delayed awakening, and choreoathetoid movements are the most common clinical signs. Intraventricular and subarachnoid bleeds are often asymptomatic, but basal ganglia lesions result in long-term developmental delay and learning disabilities. Deficits of varying degrees are being found in a significant proportion of these children.

**Infection**    Postoperative sepsis remains a serious cause of morbidity and mortality. Risk factors include central venous catheters, open chests, emergent opening of sternums for tamponade, and low cardiac output states. Lack of adherence to aseptic techniques by both surgeons and critical care team are important contributing factors.

**Necrotizing Enterocolitis (NEC)**    NEC presents with distended abdomen and feeding intolerance. It most commonly occurs in babies presenting in shock states, and in babies with HLHS and low cardiac output states. TPN, bowel rest, and broad-spectrum antibiotics are required.

**Inability to Extubate**    Failure to extubate in the absence of acute sepsis and excessive sedation requires a search for other causes:

- Tracheobronchomalacia
- Pulmonary disease
- Vocal cord paresis
- Diaphragm paresis
- Persisting left to right shunt (eg, patch leak, residual aorto-pulmonary collaterals)
- Residual anatomic lesion (eg, tracheal compression, arch obstruction, AV valve regurgitation, pulmonary vein stenosis)
- Marginal LV function
- Inadequate nutrition
- Persisting R-L shunt causing excessive hypoxemia (eg, hepatic vein connections to LA)

Cardiac catheterization, MR, and airway endoscopy may be required to exclude all possible causes. Once conditions that are amenable to surgical correction are excluded, many children can be supported with ventilatory support and adequate nutrition for weeks or months until successful extubation.

## Major Cardiac Pathology by Underlying Physiologic Derangement

### Left-Sided Obstruction

Figure 3 describes the basic physiology of a child with single ventricle. Hypoplastic left heart syndrome (HLHS) represents the most severe end of the spectrum of left-sided obstruction. The category also includes mitral and aortic valve stenosis, coarctation, and interrupted aortic arch. Initial management in patients presenting in the newborn period includes:

- Opening or maintaining ductal patency with $PGE_1$.
- Supporting systemic cardiac output.

Postoperative support following repair of a left-sided obstructive lesion depends upon many factors, including the specific lesion, the age of the patient at repair, perioperative complications, etc.

Postoperative systemic hypertension is not uncommon following a coarctation repair. These patients are often managed preoperatively with beta blockers and often require this continued postoperatively to treat postoperative hypertension. Resolution of LV hypertrophy occurs over time. Recurrent left

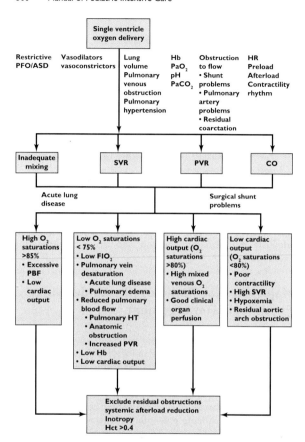

**Figure 3**   Single ventricle physiology.

sided laryngeal and phrenic nerve palsy are potential complications because of the location of the repair.

Interrupted aortic arch is often associated with a VSD. Postoperative problems to anticipate are low cardiac output, hypocalcemia, residual obstructions, nerve palsies, dysrhythmias, residual left to right shunts, and CNS injury.

Complications developing in children later in life include LV hypertrophy, systolic and diastolic dysfunction, pulmonary hypertension, and pulmonary edema.

## Right-Sided Obstruction

Tetralogy of Fallot covers a wide spectrum of disease that includes both cardiac anatomy and variations in pulmonary arterial anatomy. The need for a palliative BT shunt in the newborn period is determined by the degree of cyanosis and anatomy. The typical child with tetralogy of Fallot will be repaired by 6 months of age. Some centers are performing newborn tetralogy repairs in babies with favorable anatomy. Postoperative complications following definitive repair depend upon the presence of a ventriculotomy, the degree of RV hypertrophy, and the degree of pulmonary regurgitation through the reconstructed RV outflow tract. Restrictive physiology results in low cardiac output. Minimizing PVR reduces the RV afterload. High right-sided filling pressures may be required, but attempts to increase the CVP to more than 15 mm Hg will not improve cardiac output. Patients anticipated to develop low cardiac output in the postoperative period are often left with a residual ASD to ensure LV preload and systemic cardiac output at the expense of short-term cyanosis until the RV diastolic function improves over the following days. Arrhythmias and heart block are not uncommon and temporary AV sequential pacing is important to improve systemic cardiac output. A prolonged postoperative course results from significant residual VSDs, small pulmonary arteries, or compromised ventricular function.

Pulmonary atresia is likewise a spectrum of disease ranging from atretic PV but normal PAs and near normal-sized RV, to discontinued PAs and coronary fistulae with miniscule RV cavities. Pulmonary blood flow at birth is derived entirely through a ductus and requires $PGE_1$ to maintain patency. Patients with a small RV and intact septum have coronary perfusion dependent upon RV-coronary sinusoids. Decompression of the RV in these patients will cause myocardial infarction. Many of these children have aorto-pulmonary collaterals arising from the descending aorta supplying the lungs. Either an ASD or a VSD is required for systemic venous return to enter the systemic circulation. The bronchopulmonary collateral flow in some children may be enough to provide acceptable systemic saturations but an unacceptable volume load on the left ventricle. Surgical options are often staged and multiple and range from palliative BT or central shunt, unifocalization of larger collaterals and occlusive coiling of the smaller collaterals, to single-ventricle repair to two-ventricle repair with either outflow tract reconstruction of RV to PA conduit. Postoperative management and complications depend upon the surgical procedure.

## Transposition

Pulmonary and systemic circuits are in parallel with aorta arising from the RV and PA arising from the LV. The most common form is where the aorta is malposed anteriorly and rightward above the right ventricle, and the pulmonary artery is posterior and leftward above the aorta. Associated anomalies include:

- Coronary artery abnormalities (30%) are important to define prior to surgery
- Ventricular septal defect (40%)
- Coarctation or interrupted arch (10%)
- Left ventricular outflow tract obstruction (5–10%)

Systemic saturation depends on mixing at either ductal, atrial, or ventricular level, or bronchopulmonary collateral circulation. Babies born with TGA with intact ventricular septum can be extremely cyanotic and require urgent intervention to improve mixing. TGA with VSD are less cyanotic because of better mixing. Therapies to increase mixing preoperatively include $PGE_1$ to maintain ductal patency, and balloon atrial septostomy as the initial interventions. Persisting hypoxemia usually results from poor mixing, a restrictive ASD, or may be due to PPHN. Other interventions to consider include intubation and hyperoxic mechanical ventilation, hypothermia to reduce oxygen consumption, inotropes to increase systemic cardiac output, and ensuring a high hematocrit. Unresponsive hypoxemia may require early switch repair and postoperative ECLS.

## Bidirectional Cavopulmonary Connections

Indicated for children in whom two-ventricle repair cannot be achieved (eg, tricuspid atresia, HLHS). The SVC is transected and anastomosed end to side of the RPA allowing bidirectional flow from SVC to both pulmonary vascular beds. Pulmonary blood flow is passive. IVC flow returns to a common atrium. The procedure is not performed until several months of life to allow newborn high PVR to resolve. A large ASD or atrial septectomy is required for adequate mixing, and adequate-sized pulmonary arteries two-ventricle repair. The procedure is performed on bypass with a beating heart and minimizes complications of CPB and cross clamping the aorta. Postoperative recovery is usually uneventful and allows early extubation, which encourages better PBF. Usual saturations to expect in the postoperative period are greater than 80%. Persistent hypoxemia suggests:

- Anatomic problem with the anastomosis or pulmonary artery anatomy
- Low cardiac output
- Restrictive ASD

The Fontan procedure is the final stage repair to make complex single-ventricle lesions "physiologic," that is, systemic and pulmonary blood flow in series rather than parallel. The operation is the final stage of multiple operations, and involves adding an external conduit from the IVC to the pulmonary artery and completing the circuit of the bidirectional cavopulmonary connection. A fenestration is typically left to ensure adequate systemic cardiac output. Relative contraindications to this procedure include poor systemic ventricular function, small PAs and high PVR, and significant AV valvular regurgitation. Pulmonary blood flow is passive and determined by the transpulmonary gradient, that is, systemic venous pressure and left atrial pressure. An ideal transpulmonary gradient of 5–10 mm Hg with good systemic cardiac output indicates low PVR. Significant intravascular volume support is often required in the postoperative period. In those few children where early extubation is not possible, ventilatory techniques are important in order to minimize PVR. Some patients with an elevated transpulmonary gradient and confirmed good anatomic repair may require nitric oxide in the postoperative period until the elevated PVR resolves. Afterload reduction to improve cardiac output using milrinone is recommended to ameliorate the increase in wall stress that occurs following the procedure. Early resumption of spontaneous ventilation is recommended. Cyanosis may persist during the first few days postoperatively as a result of elevated PVR and flow across the fenestration. Over time, arterial saturations improve allowing device closure of the fenestration in the cardiac catheterization laboratory.

## Total Anomalous Pulmonary Venous Drainage

Children with total anomalous pulmonary venous drainage (TAPVD) are cyanotic. Obstructed veins cause greater degrees of cyanosis, right heart failure, poor systemic cardiac output and metabolic acidosis, and pulmonary edema in the newborn period. Pulmonary hypertension depends upon the degree of obstruction (most commonly occurs with infradiaphragmatic anomalous drainage). For survival, there must be a communication at the atrial level to allow blood from the right side to the left side of the heart; the size of the ASD determines the degree of mixing. The connections can be partial or total, supra-diaphragmatic, or infra-diaphragmatic. Resuscitation includes intubation, ventilation, PEEP, inotropic support, and urgent surgical intervention. $PGE_1$ may be initiated during initial resuscitation because of cyanosis but may make the pulmonary edema worse and should be discontinued once the diagnosis is made. Postoperative support is focused on managing pulmonary hypertension and supporting the RV and systemic cardiac output. Nitric oxide (NO) is effective in these patients until resolution of the reactive pulmonary vasculature. Postoperative mechanical support may occasionally be required.

**L-R Shunts**    These lesions can range from a persisting PDA, an ASD (with partial anomalous pulmonary venous return), to VSD, AVSD, and truncus arteriosus. In addition, some are associated with syndromes and their associated problems, of which trisomy 21 is the most common. The pathophysiology is similar in that the left to right shunt is determined by the size of the defect, and duration of the left to right shunt. PH is worse with volume and pressure overload (eg, large VSD/AVSD or truncus arteriosus). Postoperative problems include RV and LV dysfunction, and pulmonary hypertension. Truncal valve anomalies add to the complexity of the truncus repair.

## Other Issues

There is an increasing awareness of complex endocrine abnormalities occurring in some of these patients that contribute to low output states in the perioperative period. Of increasing interest is the use of steroids and thyroxine in postoperative low cardiac output states, but this remains experimental at this stage.

## Acknowledgments

Dr. John Mawson, Dept of Radiology, BC Children's Hospital

Doug Salt, Perfusion Services, BC Children's Hospital

Dr. Tex Kissoon, Division of Critical Care

Dr. Norbert Froese, Division of Critical Care

## Suggested Readings

Nichols DG, Ungerleider RM, Spevak PJ, et al. Critical Heart Disease in Infants and Children. 2nd ed. Philadelphia (PA): Mosby; c2006.

Nichols DG. Roger's Textbook of Pediatric Intensive Care. 4th ed. Philadelphia (PA): Lippincott Williams & Williams; c2008. Section IV, Cardiac Disease; pp. 997–1196.

# F. Extracorporeal Life Support in the PICU (ECMO)

Arthur Cogswell

## Key Principles

- Extracorporeal life support (ECLS) is a modified form of heart-lung bypass circuit used to provide temporary support of cardiovascular and respiratory function in patients with acute life-threatening disease.
- Extracorporeal membrane oxygenation (ECMO), the best known form of ECLS, provides an extracorporeal circuit containing an artificial gas exchange device (membrane) and a pump, and is capable of supporting patients with no native cardiac or respiratory function.
- Ventricular assist device (VAD) is another form of ECLS where the circuit provides pump support for a failing myocardium, but no gas exchange.
- Continuing improvements in technology and its medical application have led to the current expanding role of ECLS as the ultimate support for a wide variety of diseases manifesting with severe cardiac and/or respiratory failure.

## Introduction

Logistic and financial realities restrict the availability of ECLS to select referral intensive care units (ICUs), with a careful, QA controlled, program approach.

- With careful patient selection, specific staff training, and rigid quality control, ECLS support can provide survival figures exceeding those of conventional ICU support, and with minimal long-term morbidity. Conversely, when applied ad hoc by inexperienced or untrained staff, it can be a disaster.
- We suggest that for best results from ECLS, it should be considered early in the patient management strategy, and applied before disease progresses to multiple organ system failure and/or the conventional support itself becomes responsible for morbidity.

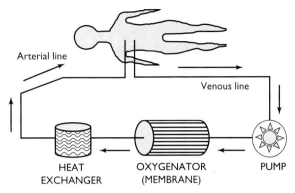

**Figure 1**    Diagram of basic ECMO circuit.

The Extracorporeal Life Support Organisation (ELSO) is a voluntary, international consortium of health care professionals dedicated to the development of ECLS techniques. Their website (http://www.elso.med.umich.edu) is an invaluable source of information and recommendations regarding the use of extracorporeal technology for organ support.

The basic ECMO circuit drains venous blood from the patient circulation to an extracorporeal plastic circuit, which runs the blood sequentially through a pump, a gas exchange device, and then a heat exchanger, and then returns the blood to the patient's circulation. Exposure of the blood to the plastic circuit components mandates the use of heparin for anticoagulation.

There are a number of different types of pump (roller, centrifugal, impeller), gas exchangers (silicone membrane, hollow fibre and polymethylpentylene) and heat exchangers (Figure 1), and each individual ECLS program has its own biases in terms of which is better. The physiology of the ECLS circuit is discussed below, and remains the same for all circuits and different components. However, troubleshooting a dysfunctional circuit is dependent on the specific components and requires detailed knowledge and training beyond the scope of this article.

Depending on the access and return points in the circulation, ECMO may be venovenous (VV) (Figure 2) or venoarterial (VA) (Figure 3), although the circuit for both is identical. VA ECMO runs in parallel with the native pulmonary circulation, and provides full respiratory and cardiac support, while VV ECMO runs

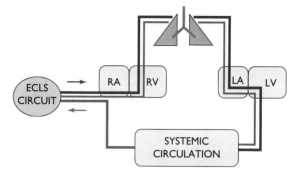

**Figure 2**  VV ECMO. Deoxygenated blood is drawn to the ECMO circuit from the large systemic veins and returned to the RV. Native pulmonary blood flow is normal, but gas exchange is done in the extracorporeal circuit pre-RV. VV ECLS provides full respiratory support, although the final patient systemic oxygen saturation will depend on the amount of recirculation in the circuit, and may be in low 80s. The patient's systemic cardiac output is dependent on the native left ventricle and is not supported by the extra-corporeal circuit, so systemic tissue oxygen delivery is very dependent on good ventricular function.

in series and does not provide any support for the systemic circulation. The use of each modality will be covered under Clinical Applications. $ECCO_2R$ is a low-flow form of VV ECMO

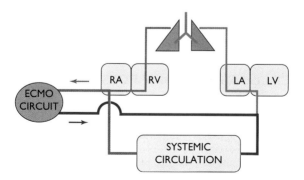

**Figure 3**  VA ECMO. Deoxygenated blood is drawn to the ECMO cir-cuit from the RA, and returned to a large artery. Native pulmonary blood flow is inversely proportional to the parallel circuit flow. Because the LV is "bypassed," this modality provides support for both heart and lungs.

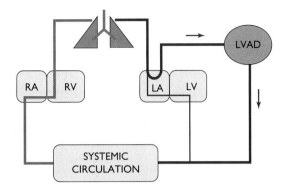

**Figure 4**    LVAD flow diagram. Cannulation for a VAD on either the right or left of the heart requires surgical access to the heart. The major advantage of removing the gas exchange device (membrane) is in reduction of platelet consumption by the circuit in the bleeding patient, and simplification of support.

that has found favor in Europe in the treatment of adults with respiratory failure. Ventricular assist device (VAD) is a generic term describing a pump which supports the circulation and may be left (LVAD) (Figure 4), right (RVAD), or both (BiVAD). The term infers surgical cannulation of the respective atrium and the circuit contains a pump only (no gas exchanger, no heat exchanger), with return to the respective circulation. The original VADs used the same pumps as for ECMO circuits, but modern technology has produced a variety of paracorporeal and intracorporeal devices for use as bridges to transplantation.

## Clinical Applications of ECLS Support

General indications for ECLS support include

- Acute, severe cardiac, and/or respiratory failure
- Underlying disease process treatable or reversible
- High predicted mortality with conventional management
- Patient otherwise has good prognosis with neurological and other organ function intact or recoverable
- Anticoagulation not contraindicated

Typical clinical applications for ECLS support in a pediatric setting include

- Neonatal respiratory failure: Many patients have persistent fetal circulation (PFC)—persistent pulmonary hypertension of newborn (PPHN)-associated disease, and respond rapidly (few days) to VV and/or VA ECMO support.
- Pediatric respiratory failure: Most patients have acute respiratory distress syndrome (ARDS)-type disease, which is well supported with VV ECMO but may require support duration measured in weeks rather than in days.
- Cardiac support: Most candidates are postoperative congenital heart disease (CHD) patients with low cardiac output. There are also a medical group of patients with cardiomyopathy/myocarditis who may require support. VA ECMO or VAD will be the likely mode of support in these patients and most patients likely to recover will declare themselves within a week. Patients who do not spontaneously recover may be bridged to transplant by either VA ECMO or VAD.

It must be remembered that ECLS is *not* a treatment per se, but rather a mechanical support system that keeps the patient alive while his native lungs or heart are recovering from injury, and removing the damaging effects of heroic ventilation or high-dose inotropic agents.

## Neonatal Respiratory Support

ECMO is accepted now by most as a "standard of care" for severe respiratory failure, and its use has been justified by three randomized controlled trials (see references). The ELSO database shows that worldwide use of ECMO for neonatal respiratory failure has progressively decreased since the early 1990s. This probably represents the combined effects of better conventional intensive care support in general, in addition to the use of exogenous surfactants, nitric oxide, and improved ventilation management.

Indications:

- The ELSO database details more than 20,000 neonates treated with ECMO for respiratory support—the most common diseases include meconium aspiration, congenital diaphragmatic hernia, pulmonary hypertension (PFC/PPHN), hyaline membrane disease, sepsis, and pneumonia. The average survival is around 70%.
- One of the difficulties in patient management is the ability to accurately quantify the severity of illness and link it to outcome. The oxygenation index (OI) has been accepted by most as a

reasonable selection tool for ECMO candidates, as it relates physiological parameters to level of ventilation support:

$$OI = \frac{MAP \ (cm \ H_2O) \times FiO_2 \ (\%)}{Post \ ductal \ PaO_2 \ (mm \ Hg)}$$

A sustained OI of 40 or more distinguishes neonates with a high mortality risk (59% in the UK ECMO trial). ECMO treatment in that group provided 68% survival with minimal morbidity. If a patient meets the OI criteria for severity of illness, then their eligibility for ECMO support should be based on the likelihood of a good outcome according to the following:

- birth weight greater than 2 kg
- gestational age greater than 34 weeks
- absence of specific contraindications

  - IVH no greater than grade I
  - no hypoxic ischemic cerebral injury
  - ventilation for less than 7–10 days

**Preferred Therapy**    The majority of neonatal respiratory cases are adequately supported by VV ECMO as the ECLS treatment option of choice as there is good evidence that the perfusion of the pulmonary vasculature with oxygenated blood may help resolution of the reactive component of any pulmonary vascular disease.

## Pediatric Respiratory Support

Unfortunately, there are no controlled trials to justify the use of ECMO support for respiratory failure in the postneonatal pediatric patient. However, a lot of anecdotal experience, case reports and small series suggest it has a place. Finding that place, and determining indications for abandoning conventional support in favor of the potentially complicated extracorporeal support, will ultimately be an individual ICU decision, and probably on an individual case basis. The absence of a controlled trial reflects the small numbers of patients seen in each center, the broad range of pathology leading to respiratory failure, and the shifting baseline of outcome with conventional therapy.

Indications:

- The ELSO database shows that over 3,000 patients have been ECMO supported for respiratory failure in the past 20 years, with an average survival approaching 60%.

- Conditions treated include viral and bacterial pneumonia, aspiration, ARDS, and significantly, a large "other" group with respiratory failure of obscure origin.
- Review of the case report literature shows a wide diversity of conditions in which ECMO has been successfully applied and our approach now is to consider ECMO support in any patient with severe respiratory failure, and decide on an individual case basis balancing contraindications and literature reported outcomes.
- General contraindications include ventilation for greater than 7–10 days, irreversible lung disease and immunosuppression.
- It is important to optimize the general patient condition, including temperature control, cardiac output and oxygen delivery, and avoiding fluid overload where possible. In some cases, early use of extracorporeal renal replacement to enhance free water clearance may avoid mechanical respiratory support.
- Because many patients remain without a specific diagnosis by the time they need a decision regarding ECMO, in that situation we would generally go ahead with ECLS support with a clear understanding among the team that with parental consent treatment would be withdrawn in the event that non-recovery of the underlying disease was inevitable. There are no specific data to help to decide when to intervene with ECMO support in the patient who is failing on more conventional respiratory support. We ensure that patients first have their ventilation optimized initially using protective strategies, including early use of high-frequency oscillation as needed.
- ECMO will be considered for:

  - Oxygenation failure as evidenced by OI $>35$, $P(A-a)O_2$ $>500$, or a PF ratio $<100$ (Figure 5)
  - Ventilation failure with severe acidosis, uncompensated
  - Air leak/barotrauma

## Type of ECLS:

- As for neonates, VV ECMO should adequately support uncomplicated respiratory failure and is the support mode of choice.
- Everyone involved should be clear that the patient's systemic oxygen saturations may be no better with VV ECMO than they were with conventional ventilation.
- This is not an issue provided that tissue oxygen delivery can be supported through improved cardiac output and optimized oxygen carrying capacity of the blood.
- The whole idea of starting ECMO is to rest the lungs by removing the lung damaging high pressure/high volume/high

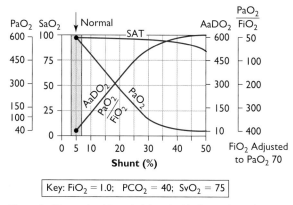

Key: FiO$_2$ = 1.0;   PCO$_2$ = 40;   SvO$_2$ = 75

**Figure 5**   Oxygenation failure physiology. As this diagram shows, the severity of oxygenation failure (shunt) may be expressed with a variety of physiological and interventional characteristics. Finding a clear "ECMO intervention point" has been difficult.

FiO$_2$ ventilation, and allowing the disease process to resolve with time allowing recovery of respiratory function.

## Cardiac Support

- As for pediatric respiratory failure, there are no controlled trials to guide the use of ECLS support in pediatric cardiac patients.
- Again this reflects limited individual ICU experience, a very diverse diagnostic group and difficulty in establishing a baseline control group or mortality rate.
- The ELSO database shows that ECLS support has been used progressively more frequently over the past 10 years in neonatal and pediatric patients for cardiac support, with now about 500 cases yearly worldwide.
- Survival currently averages 30–40% for neonates, 40–50% for infants, and 50–60% for older patients.
- The vast majority of reported patients require ECLS support following corrective congenital cardiac surgery (pre- or postoperatively),
- A smaller but significant group has either cardiomyopathy or myocarditis.
- In both groups, some patients with no recovery of native cardiac function have been supported for extended periods

whilst awaiting a donor transplant organ (so-called "bridge to transplant").

- In addition there are reports of cardiac support ECLS being performed for more unusual indications such as profound hypothermia, drug overdoses, malignant tachyarrhythmias, myocardial trauma, and transplant rejection.

Pediatric cardiac surgery is a rapidly evolving specialty and major invasive procedures are being done on younger and younger patients. The availability of ECLS support for pre- and postoperative management of neonatal patients would be regarded by some as mandatory.

Indications:

Short-term extracorporeal cardiac support such as VA ECMO or VAD should be considered in the following situations:

- Previously healthy patient, normal cardiac anatomy: any acute illness with severe acute heart failure, nonresponsive to optimized medical management (eg, myocarditis, drug intoxication, trauma).
- Known congenital heart disease, preoperative stabilization: acute pulmonary hypertensive crisis, TAPVR, hypercyanotic lesions.
- Known congenital heart disease, postoperative low cardiac output: either failure to separate from cardiopulmonary bypass or deterioration in the first few days postoperatively, despite optimized medical support. This is the most common scenario. A stunned myocardium is difficult to differentiate from an infarcted one, but the former will do well with temporary support of VA ECMO or VAD. If in doubt, support with ECLS and wait.
- Previous cardiac transplant, acute rejection.

Longer term mechanical support with paracorporeal or intracorporeal VAD is possible in pediatric patients but is offered by very few centers and is beyond the scope of this discussion. Some preliminary questions that have to be asked when considering a patient for cardiac support include:

- Is the patient's overall condition and prognosis good, or is the cardiac problem just the tip of the iceberg?
- Is there an accurate anatomical/physiological diagnosis? If there is time, detailed echocardiography and/or cardiac catheterization may be necessary. ALCAPA and TAPVR can be easily missed.

- Will the patient's anatomy support cannulation for support? The venous and aortic arch anatomy are important.
- Is there a residual surgical lesion that may be contributing to low cardiac output? If in doubt, cardiac catheter is the gold standard: No amount of ECMO will fix a residual surgical problem.
- Is there a reversible surgical lesion such as tamponade?

After these questions are addressed, then the decision has to be made when to intervene?

- Review in detail medical management to ensure that myocardial support is indeed optimized—this is well covered elsewhere.
- If no further optimization can be done, and the patient's hemodynamic profile is relentlessly deteriorating with signs of impending multiorgan system failure (rising lactate and worsening metabolic acidosis, oliguria/anuria, poor perfusion), or where the level of support could itself be damaging (eg, high-dose inotrope) then it is preferable to act in anticipation and start ECLS support rather than wait and have to resuscitate the patient, and then start ECLS as a rescue.

Once the decision has been made to proceed with ECLS support, the next question to address is the mode of support.

- The majority of patients end up on VA ECMO or LVAD as the primary problem is usually ventricular dysfunction and poor systemic cardiac output.
- However, VA ECMO is less than ideal for a hypoxic/ischemic/stunned LV, as the support itself imposes a significant afterload on the LV, and the coronaries are perfused by the native pulmonary blood flow which may well be hypoxic.
- In the event of proceeding with VA ECMO, it should be remembered that:

  - the lungs need some blood flow to survive, so avoid full bypass flow.
  - the coronaries will still be supplied by the native pulmonary circulation. Therefore, avoid the temptation to turn down the ventilation too far; pulmonary damage should not be an issue in most cardiac patients, so maintaining an $FiO_2$ of 0.40, physiologic PEEP, and low normal minute ventilation should not create any undue problems.

Complications:

- If there is no forward flow of blood through the aortic valve once on full flow, and no residual ASD or PFO, then the left atrium must be vented or there will be problems with pulmonary venous hypertension, pulmonary hemorrhage, and endocardial ischemia; the LA may be vented directly through a sternotomy and connected to the venous drainage side of the circuit, or via a balloon or blade septostomy in the cardiac catheter laboratory; addition of systemic afterload reduction may also be beneficial; the effect of the vent on circuit $SvO_2$ must be remembered, and the vent must also be restricted when the time comes to wean ECLS flow.

• If the patient being supported has either a single ventricle or shunt-dependent circulation, then allowances must be made for "double flow" when the ECLS circuit flow is prescribed. While postoperative cardiac patients may be cannulated transthoracically via the sternotomy incision, these cannulae are not as secure as cervical/femoral percutaneously inserted cannulae, especially if trips to the catheter laboratory or CT scan are envisaged. The latter also have the advantage of enabling better wound closure for avoidance of infection.

# The Physiology of ECLS Support

The technological advances that have permitted development of ECLS as an entity are extraordinary, but still have their limitations.

## Anticoagulation

• Exposure of the patient's blood to all the plastic components of the circuit results in activation of the coagulation system, and in the absence of heparinization the circuit will clot within minutes.

• Anticoagulation must be monitored at the point of care, and Activated Clotting Time (ACT) testing is the standard used by most centers in North America.

• A "normal" patient with no anticoagulation will have an ACT in the range 90–150, and the general target for running ECMO is 180–220. A bolus of 50–75 U/kg is given just prior to cannulation, and then an infusion is commenced and titrated to ACT: most neonates require 20–60 U/kg/hour, older children 15–30 U/kg/hour, depending on renal function.

• The necessary anticoagulation is responsible for the major complication of ECLS: Bleeding. In addition, even with the most modern devices, some blood cell damage occurs and hemolysis must be monitored by performing plasma-free Hb estimations.

## Cannulation

- The ECLS circuit, and the life-sustaining flow of blood that it provides, starts and ends with cannulae in major blood vessels, and these are the most likely source of limitation to the support that can be provided.
- The venous drainage cannula is the more important.
- As for any tube, resistance to blood flow through a cannula is directly proportional to cannula length and inversely proportional to the fourth power of the radius; therefore, we aim for the shortest and widest internal diameter cannula that will access the central circulation from the insertion point.
- Classical VA ECMO uses a venous drainage cannula inserted in the right internal jugular vein with the tip in the right atrium, and a right internal carotid return cannula placed so that the tip is just within the aortic arch.
- Most neonates will be supportable with this arrangement, but some babies and many larger patients will require augmentation of the venous drainage by using a second site: possible sites include a cephalad-directed right internal jugular vein cannula and a femoral vein cannulation.
- Venovenous ECMO can be achieved in neonates with a single, double lumen cannula placed in the right internal jugular vein, with the tip in the RA at the IVC.
- The lumens are designed to drain from the RA/IVC and the return flow is directed at the tricuspid valve so as to minimize recirculation.
- Again some babies and all larger patients require additional venous drainage sites, and the possibilities are the same as above.
- For patients over about 18 kg, no double lumen canulae are yet available, and so the standard approach is to drain from right internal jugular and right femoral, and return using a long left femoral cannula.

## Gas Exchange

**Parts of the Gas Exchange System**    The work of the ECLS circuit for respiratory support occurs in the gas exchange unit. Remember that the full circuit blood flow runs through the gas exchange unit, the equivalent of native pulmonary perfusion, and a countercurrent flow of gas (the "sweep gas") provides the equivalent of alveolar ventilation.

- There are three basic types of gas exchange unit in use, with different technology but similar physiology. All types use a membrane of some description to separate the blood and gas flow within the unit but to allow $CO_2$ and $O_2$ gas exchange between the two (alveolar capillary membrane equivalent).

- The traditional "membrane oxygenator" uses a huge surface area sheet of Silastic material as the separating membrane.
- Hollow fibre oxygenators use multiple small channels to separate blood and gas.
- The most recently developed polymethylpentylene units use a Silastic type material in a hollow fiber type design.
- Different sizes of unit are available to correlate with patient size and gas exchange requirements, and the blood and gas flow tolerances for the units are printed on the outside.
- The position of the gas exchange unit in the circuit is the same for both VV and VA ECMO: in series between the pump and the heat exchanger.
- The blood flow to the membrane ("pulmonary perfusion") is determined by the circuit pump flow, and this is manipulated to meet physiological requirements.
- The gas flow to the membrane ("alveolar ventilation") comes from a blender and flow meter so that $FiO_2$ and total flow can be manipulated, and $CO_2$ can also be added.
- The gas phase pressure is monitored and limited to ensure that it never exceeds blood phase pressure, or an air embolus could occur.
- Blood phase pressure is also monitored pre- and postmembrane and a small gradient will be present due to resistance to flow within the unit. This gradient will be seen to slowly increase over the life of the membrane as microthrombi accumulates with time.
- Membrane function as a gas exchange unit is monitored by checking blood gases taken pre- and postmembrane on a regular basis. Expected deviations with time are a slow decrease in oxygenation ability and ability to clear $CO_2$.

**Process of Exchange**   Gas exchange between blood and gas occurs by diffusion and therefore depends on the gas diffusion gradient between circuit blood and sweep gas, the surface area of the membrane interface between blood and gas, the diffusion characteristics of the membrane for the particular gas and the relative flow rates of blood and sweep gas.

- The membrane's diffusion characteristics are such that $CO_2$ transfers very much faster than $O_2$, with the effect that the rate-limiting step in net $CO_2$ transfer is the rate at which the transferred $CO_2$ is removed from the system, ie, the sweep gas flow rate.

- The rate-limiting step for net $O_2$ transfer is the rate at which the blood "takes away" the transferred $O_2$, ie, the circuit blood flow rate.
- This then explains how the blood and sweep gas flows can be manipulated in support of patient physiological demands:
  - If the patient ABG shows $PCO_2$ above desired limits, then the circuit sweep gas should be increased to improve $CO_2$ clearance.
  - If the patient ABG shows $PO_2$ below desired limits, then either increase the $FiO_2$ of the sweep gas or increase the circuit blood flow to improve $O_2$ transfer.
- Circuit $PO_2$ above 450 should be avoided because of the risk of $O_2$ bubbling out of solution.
- Be aware that for any given membrane, the physical characteristics are such that there is a point at which blood flow is so fast that there is insufficient time for $O_2$ to traverse the diffusion path: Turning blood flow up beyond this point will *not* further improve $O_2$ delivery: this is the "rated flow" of the particular membrane, and should be printed on the outside of the device.

The membrane lung is subject to problems which mimic pathophysiologic processes in the native lung such as pulmonary edema, ventilation-perfusion mismatch and pulmonary embolus. Most problems can be diagnosed by detecting changes in gas exchange and resistance to blood flow. Gas phase problems, such as fluid accumulation, will most likely manifest as problems with $CO_2$ clearance, while blood phase problems such as clot accumulation will manifest as $O_2$ problems.

**Pump**    There are a number of different types of technology available for use as pumps in ECLS circuits: roller pumps, centrifugal vortex pumps, and impellers. Each has its own pros and cons and requires specific training to manage properly. Roller pumps have traditionally been used for ECMO for neonatal respiratory failure, but a significant number of centers also use centrifugal vortex pump systems for patients of all ages.

**Flow**    After initial cannulation, circuit flow is slowly increased to a predetermined target with a view to assessing the adequacy of that flow to meet the patient's physiological needs, and then fine-tuned accordingly. For VA ECMO that initial target is around 100 mL/kg/min and for VV ECMO it will be of the order of 120–150 mL/kg/min. The final flow depends upon the patient arterial saturation and clinical assessment of adequacy of oxygen delivery.

## Physiologic Targets for Support

ECLS support in cardiorespiratory failure is targeted at replacing the crucial end point of the native circulation, tissue oxygen delivery:

$$\text{Oxygen delivery} = \text{Blood } O_2 \text{ Content} \times \text{Cardiac output}$$

$$= (Hb \times O_2 \text{ Sat}) \times CO$$

Hemoglobin should be monitored and maintained via transfusion for a hematocrit in the range 35–45. Most centers use monitors within the circuit that provide a continuous update of Hct.

Systemic oxygen saturation will be determined primarily by the ECLS circuit, in addition to patient oxygen consumption. As already noted, oxygenation is a blood flow determined variable: The more flow through the circuit, the better the oxygenation, within the rated flow limits. For VA ECMO, the more flow through the circuit, the less flow through the native pulmonary circulation, and this further enhances systemic saturation. For VV ECMO, recirculation becomes an increasing issue with increasing flow.

The $HbO_2$ dissociation curve should be remembered: A $PaO_2$ greater than 100 offers minimal additional $O_2$ content augmentation, and so targets need to remain realistic.

- Cardiac output manipulation for the patient on VV ECMO is no different to the non-ECLS patient: The physiologically directed targets of optimizing preload, myocardial contractility, and afterload reduction remain the basis of management.
- Cardiac output manipulation on VA ECMO is a little different, as the patient's cardiac output is determined directly by the circuit flow, and as that flow is progressively increased toward full cardiac index levels, the systemic arterial pulse contour (IA line trace) flattens. The adequacy of that flow to meet physiologic requirements will be determined by monitoring ABGs, serum lactate, $S_vO_2$, perfusion, urine output, and neurologic function:

    - Target $S_vO_2$ is 65–75, with lactate in normal range, good peripheral perfusion, and mean arterial pressure (MAP) and urine output 0.5–1 mL/kg/hour

- If $S_vO_2$ <65, try increasing ECMO flow: If unable to increase flow (roller pump) or unacceptably high negative access pressure on centrifugal pump, then assess for venous cannula obstruction or hypovolemia: Is BP low? Is urine output down? Is there tachycardia, or poor perfusion?

  Consider trial of volume support 10 mL/kg: What fluid is chosen is determined by latest hematocrit, CBC/platelet count, and coagulation profile. Target Hct 40–45 and transfuse packed red cells, FFP, platelets, albumin, or saline as appropriate.

- If $S_vO_2$ >80, then decrease circuit flow
- If patient hypertensive, consider:

  - fluid overload (low $PO_2$, large pulse pressure): give diuretic
  - anxiety/pain: give analgesic and/or sedation
  - idiopathic: give vasodilator

- If patient $PO_2$ low despite postmembrane $PO_2$ ≥100, consider fluid overload. Excess fluid traverses native pulmonary vasculature with ventilator on rest settings: essentially an R-L shunt.

# Medical Management of the Patient on ECMO

ECLS is a complex process with a high frequency of serious complications. Patients on ECMO require obsessive multisystem review on a daily basis and collaborative multidisciplinary support in order to achieve the best outcome with the shortest possible run and therefore the briefest exposure to the potential risks. Observe the following:

Cardiovascular system: for cardiac support ECLS,

- Wean all inotropes and rest the myocardium as soon as possible.
- Assess surgical repair if postoperative: Confirm no residual lesion/s using echocardiography or cardiac catheter as necessary.
- Assess recovery with serial echocardiography, if necessary with flow weaned.
- Hypertension is common and multifactorial and should be treated aggressively with vasodilators and diuretic if appropriate.

Pulmonary system for respiratory support ECMO, ventilation is weaned to "rest settings" as soon as good circuit flow is established: the purpose ECMO for respiratory support is to enable the lungs to be rested from injurious ventilation. Different centers use very different approaches to lung rest, ranging from zero PEEP/zero ventilation, to PEEP alone at various levels, to PEEP plus low rate, low tidal volume IMV, to HFOV. There are no definitive trials to guide therapy and therefore each case should be approached individually. We have had good experience with "lung rest" comprising pressure control ventilation 20/10, at a rate of 10 and $FiO_2$ $\leq$40%. As the lungs improve based on clearing CXR and improving compliance, recruitment maneuvers can commence, using either sustained positive pressure inflations or gentle HFOV.

- Avoid fluid overload/actively diurese as soon as hemodynamic stability permits.
- Surfactant use is controversial in this setting, even in the neonates.

Neurologic

- Most patients will be muscle relaxed initially, but this should be discontinued as soon as feasible in order to allow accurate neurological assessment.
- Analgesia and sedation are required to ensure comfort, amnesia and to avoid hypertension. Achieving adequate levels can be very challenging as most commonly used agents are adsorbed by the circuit, and patients frequently end up on "industrial" doses.
- Neurological imaging with serial cranial ultrasounds is standard for neonates. A visit to CT scan is quite feasible given an obsessive approach to patient safety and enough hands. EEG is entirely feasible and should be done as required or indicated. There has been a recent trend to use NIRS "cerebral oximetry" as an ongoing measure of cerebral perfusion/oxygenation: while the theory for this application is appealing, there is no gold standard to indicate just exactly what is being measured.

Renal system

- Renal dysfunction or failure is not uncommon in ECLS patients. Causes are multifactorial and include the pre-existing pathophysiologic abnormalities prior to ECLS (such as hypotension or asphyxia), or complications of ECLS such as hemolysis and hemoglobinemia with hemoglobinuria and sepsis. Most spontaneously recover with time and good ECLS support, but the majority requires a lot of diuretic to achieve a negative balance.

- Maintaining tight fluid balance is important although often challenging, requiring either aggressive diuresis or some form of renal replacement therapy. Continuous renal replacement therapy (CRRT) is a relatively easy addition to an already established ECLS circuit, and should be considered early in the ECLS run in order to promote adequate nutrition and good fluid balance.

### Nutrition

- Early initiation of nutrition and maintaining adequate caloric intake is important. Most occasions this can be achieved through the enteral route, preferably via nasojejunal tube placement.

### Infectious disease

- ECLS patients are at a high risk for sepsis due to invasive lines, relative immune compromise, frequent open surgical wounds, and often massive transfusion requirements. Despite this risk, prophylactic antibiotics should be avoided wherever possible. If antibiotics are prescribed, therapeutic monitoring should be used to optimize dosing: Behavior of drugs in the circuit, and with renal failure, may be difficult to predict.

## Complications of ECLS

It should come as no surprise that a support as invasive as ECLS can be extraordinarily complicated—one of the reasons that it is only undertaken when the patient has a high risk of mortality. Complications may be divided into those relating to the circuit and those that are patient related.

- Mechanical/circuit:
  - Cannula displacement/obstruction/kinking/perforation
  - Hemolysis
  - Clots or air in the circuit

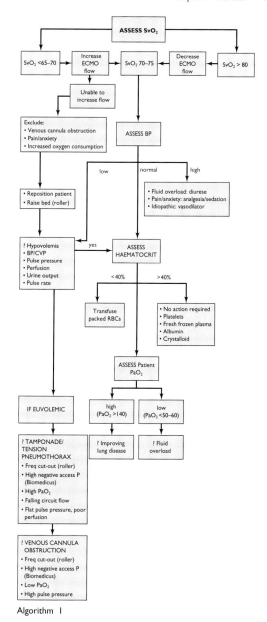

Algorithm 1

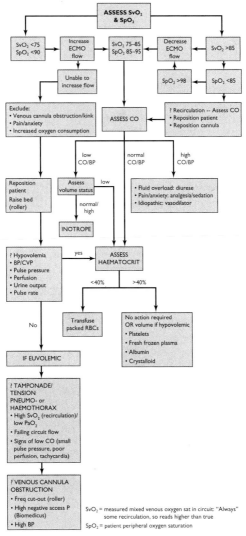

ASSESS SvO₂ & SpO₂

| SvO₂ <75 SpO₂ <90 | Increase ECMO flow | SvO₂ 75–85 SpO₂ 85–95 | Decrease ECMO flow | SvO₂ >85 |

Unable to increase flow

SpO₂ >98    SpO₂ <85

Exclude:
• Venous cannula obstruction/kink
• Pain/anxiety
• Increased oxygen consumption

ASSESS CO

? Recirculation -- Assess CO
• Reposition patient
• Reposition cannula

low CO/BP    normal CO/BP    high CO/BP

Reposition patient
Raise bed (roller)

Assess volume status    low

• Fluid overload: diurese
• Pain/anxiety: analgesia/sedation
• Idiopathic: vasodilator

normal/high

INOTROPE

? Hypovolemia
• BP/CVP
• Pulse pressure
• Perfusion
• Urine output
• Pulse rate

yes    ASSESS HAEMATOCRIT

<40%    >40%

Transfuse packed RBCs

No action required
OR volume if hypovolemic
• Platelets
• Fresh frozen plasma
• Albumin
• Crystalloid

No

IF EUVOLEMIC

? TAMPONADE/ TENSION PNEUMO- or HAEMOTHORAX
• High SvO₂ (recirculation)/ low PaO₂
• Failing circuit flow
• Signs of low CO (small pulse pressure, poor perfusion, tachycardia)

? VENOUS CANNULA OBSTRUCTION
• Freq cut-out (roller)
• High negative access P (Biomedicus)
• High BP

SvO₂ = measured mixed venous oxygen sat in circuit: "Always" some recirculation, so reads higher than true
SpO₂ = patient peripheral oxygen saturation

Algorithm 2

- Patient complications:
  - Bleeding
  - Thromboembolic events
  - Sepsis
  - Systemic inflammation
  - Renal dysfunction

## Outcome of ECLS Support

As described, mortality is very variable depending on age and disease being treated. Early patient identification and selection and careful timing of intervention, before multiorgan system damage, are critical to a good outcome. Provision of ECLS support by a multidisciplinary team, in a quality-controlled program setting, should provide the best outcome. All patients should be followed long term for assessment of morbidity. The majority of survivors are neurologically intact, developmentally normal, and free of ECLS-related complications.

## Resources

The Extracorporeal Life Support Organisation (ELSO) home page: http://www.elso.med.umich.edu: This site contains a wealth of information regarding extracorporeal life support in general and, in particular, practical information for centers considering involvement in ECLS. The site also contains an up-to-date bibliography on journal publications on ECLS.

ELSO also published the red "bible," *Extracorporeal Cardiopulmonary Support in Critical Care*, 3rd Ed (2005). Eds. Van Meurs, Lally, Peek and Zwischenberger.

Significant clinical trials using ECMO for neonatal respiratory failure:

- Bartlett RH, Roloff DW, Cornell RG, et al. Extracorporeal circulation in neonatal respiratory failure: a prospective randomized study. Pediatrics 1985;76:479–87.
- O'Rourke PP, Crone RK, Vacanti JP, et al. Extracorporeal membrane oxygenation and conventional medical therapy in neonates with persistent pulmonary hypertension of the newborn: a prospective randomized study. Pediatrics 1989;84:957–63.

- UK collaborative randomized trial of neonatal extracorporeal membrane oxygenation. UK Collaborative ECMO Trial Group. Lancet 1996;348:75–82.

The use of ECMO for pediatric respiratory failure:

- Green TP, Timmons OT, Fackler JC, et al. The impact of extracorporeal membrane oxygenation on survival in pediatric patients with acute respiratory failure. Crit Care Med 1996; 24:323–9.
- Bohn D. Acute hypoxic respiratory failure in children. Extracorporeal *Cardiopulmonary Support in Critical Care*, 3rd Ed. 2005, pp. 329–61.

The use of ECLS for pediatric cardiac support:

- Duncan BW. Pediatric cardiac failure: management and use of ECLS. *Extracorporeal Cardiopulmonary Support in Critical Care*, 3rd Ed. 2005, pp. 431–48.

# Chapter 9

# Neurology

## A. Monitoring the Central Nervous System

Paul M Shore

### Key Principles

- "Monitoring" requires real-time evaluation and assessment of the patient and of interventions
- Monitoring of the CNS is crude compared to other organ systems
- Many measures of brain physiology, such as blood flow or oxygenation, are local measurements that may fail to detect important regional variations
- All intracranial pressure monitoring is invasive, so the benefits must be weighed against the risks of bleeding or infection
- The best test of brain function is the clinical exam

### Definition of "Monitoring"

- "Monitoring" refers to continuous evaluation of the physiologic function of a patient in real time to guide management decisions and assessment of interventions
- Serial clinical exams are as much a form of monitoring as bedside electronic devices
- Not all bedside electronic devices are monitors; for example, continuous EEG or Holter recordings are generally

not evaluated in real time, and therefore do not qualify as monitors

# Monitoring Clinical Neurologic Status

- Serial neurologic exams in all patients should be recorded on a bedside flowsheet and, at the minimum, consist of

  - Mental status exam, quantified by the Glasgow Coma Scale score
  - Pupil size and reactivity
  - Presence of cough and gag

- Nonneurologic clinical findings may be relevant to neurologic status in particular disease states, for example:

| Disease | Clinical Finding | Concern |
|---|---|---|
| Head trauma, stroke, brain tumor, intracranial mass | Hypertension, bradycardia | Intracranial hypertension |
| Guillain-Barre syndrome | Weaker negative inspiratory force (NIF) | Progressive demyelination, leading to respiratory failure |
| Infantile botulism | Loss of facial expression, presence of drooling | Progressive neuromuscular junction dysfunction, leading to respiratory failure |

# Intracranial Pressure (ICP) and Cerebral Perfusion Pressure (CPP)

- Normal ICP is $<10$ mm Hg (may rise transiently to $>20$ mm Hg in normal subjects)

  - After brain injury, ICP $>20–25$ mm Hg is abnormal and concerning
  - ICP $>40$ mm Hg is considered critical

- CPP = Mean arterial pressure (MAP) − ICP

  - CPP corresponding to the normal adult autoregulatory range is 50−150 mm Hg (may be lower in infants and children)
  - CPP <50 mm Hg is associated with ischemia in adults, especially after brain injury
    - Regional ischemia may occur after brain injury, even with CPP ≥50 mm Hg
    - CPP >150 mm Hg may cause hypertensive encephalopathy
    - A CPP that is high, but within the autoregulatory range, may be generated spontaneously after brain injury, especially stroke

- An evidence-based treatment threshold for ICP or CPP after brain injury has not yet been determined

  - Current recommendations in children are
    - ICP monitoring is appropriate after head trauma if GCS score ≤8
    - Treat ICP >20–25 mm Hg
    - Maintain CPP 40–65 mm Hg
  - See Chapter 10, "Neurosurgery" for medical and surgical treatment of increased ICP

- All ICP monitors are invasive and require a craniotomy

  - The risk of inadequately treated intracranial hypertension must be weighed against the risk of hemorrhage, especially in coagulopathic patients
  - A ventriculostomy catheter is the "gold standard" for measuring ICP but carries a greater risk of hemorrhage than a fiberoptic monitor
  - ICP monitors carry a 1–10% risk of infection and 1–2% risk of intracranial bleeding

## Cerebral Blood Flow (CBF)

- Normal global CBF is 40–60 mL/100 g/minute

  - Low global CBF suggests ischemia, but may instead reflect lowered metabolic demands in a sedated or injured brain
  - CBF lower than 20 mL/100 g/minute is associated with ischemia
  - CBF may be measured by magnetic resonance imaging (MRI) techniques, computed tomography (CT) scan with inhaled xenon, or positron emission tomography (PET) scan

- Transcranial doppler ultrasound (TCD)

  - TCD assesses CBF indirectly, by measuring the cross-sectional area and velocity of blood flow of the middle cerebral artery
  - Velocity, area, and flow pulsatility can be used to estimate changes in CBF and to infer vasospasm, especially after subarachnoid hemorrhage

# Cerebral Oxygenation

- General principles

  - Cerebral oxygenation ($CMR_{O_2}$) reflects the balance between oxygen delivery and consumption
  - Oxygen extraction increases as delivery decreases (eg, ischemia, vasospasm, hypoxia) or metabolism increases (eg, hypermetabolism, seizure, agitation)
  - Monitoring cerebral oxygenation is not fully investigated in pediatrics and should be considered as an experimental therapy
  - Oxygen extraction decreases as delivery increases (eg, hyperemia) or metabolism decreases (eg, cell death, sedation/anesthesia)
    - The normal and injured brain are extremely heterogenous, thus measures of $CMR_{O_2}$, whether global or local, may fail to detect important regional differences

- Jugular venous oxygen saturation ($Sjv_{O_2}$)

  - $Sjv_{O_2}$, the oxygen saturation of blood in the jugular bulb, can be detected by intermittent sampling from an indwelling catheter or by continuous reflectometry
    - $Sjv_{O_2}$ is a global measure that may fail to detect regional ischemia

  - Important values
    - Normal $Sjv_{O_2}$ is 55–70%
    - $Sjv_{O_2}$ <50–55% is associated with worse outcome after TBI in adults and children

- Partial pressure of oxygen in brain tissue ($Pbt_{O_2}$)

  - $Pbt_{O_2}$ is the partial pressure of oxygen in the interstitial fluid of a small (~1 cm$^3$) region of brain tissue, detected by an invasive probe

- No consensus exists on whether to place the probe in normal brain or near regions of injury
  - Studies are underway to determine if normalizing the $PbtO_2$ improves outcome

- Important values
  - Normal $PbtO_2$ is 20–40 mm Hg
  - $PbtO_2$ <10–15 mm Hg is associated with worse outcome after TBI

- Near-infrared spectroscopy (NIRS)

  - NIRS uses reflectance absorptiometry to detect absorption of light emitted into the scalp and reflected from tissues under the scalp
    - The principle is similar to pulse oximetry, with the detection probe and software ignoring the pulsatile (arterial) signal and focusing on the steady-state (venous and capillary blood, tissue) signal

  - Precisely what the cranial NIRS signal measures is unclear
    - The NIRS signal has been used as a proxy for brain oxygenation, jugular and mixed-venous saturation, and brain mitochondrial redox state
    - Unpredictable thickness of scalp/skull, differences in blood flow between scalp and brain, regional differences in brain oxygenation, and variability in heme-containing moieties in all tissues make inter- and intra-individual variability great
    - Variability within a single individual may be clinically meaningful; the NIRS monitor has found use during and after cardiac surgery

## Electroencephalographic Monitoring

- Electroencephalography (EEG)

  - The surface EEG is the record of voltage potentials measured between multiple electrodes placed at standardized points on the scalp
    - Arrays (montages) of 4 to 22 leads can be used, with additional leads for specific purposes
    - EEGs require simultaneous electrocardiography (ECG) to identify cardiac artifacts

  - EEGs *can* detect several types of brain activity

- Normal background activity, typically visualized as rhythmic voltage variations from 4–20 Hz
- Normal sleep patterns
- Activation of cortical regions in response to stimuli
- Abnormal background activity, often visualized as disorganized patterns with slow frequencies
- Transient high-voltage waves ("spikes") that may be single or repetitive, focal or global
- Seizure involving the surface cortex at the time the EEG is being recorded, regardless of motoric component
- Lack of brain activity, whether intermittent ("burst-suppression") or total ("electrocortical silence")

- EEGs *cannot* detect
  - Brain activity obscured by medications or metabolic derangements
  - Completed seizures or seizures that will occur in the future
  - Seizures involving deep cortex or brain stem but not the surface cortex

- The EEG is not always an effective bedside monitor
  - The EEG may be a good burst suppression monitor, since this can easily be determined by most bedside caretakers
  - More involved interpretation of the EEG requires highly specialized physicians who generally do not read EEGs in real time, making the EEG a poor seizure monitor
  - Automatic seizure detection software is, at present, imperfect

- Bispectral index (BIS)

  - The BIS is a processed EEG signal that is reported as a number from 0 to 100
  - Lower BIS numbers correlate with depth of sedation in the operating room and ICU, even after brain injury
  - Important values
    - BIS of 100 correlates with full consciousness
    - BIS of 50 correlates with adequate surgical anesthesia in children

## Chemical Monitoring

- Chemical monitoring is still in the early investigational stages and should not be considered as standard care.

- Biochemical surrogates of organ function (eg, creatinine for renal function) or organ injury (eg, troponin I for myocardial injury) are frequently monitored in the ICU. At present, biochemical monitoring of the CNS is unavailable for clinical use.
- Potential biomarkers of CNS injury include neuron-specific enolase (NSE), the glial protein S100B, myelin basic protein (MBP). All can be detected in serum and cerebrospinal fluid.
- Potential biomarkers of CNS function include the excitatory amino acids glutamate and aspartate; the energy-state markers lactate, pyruvate and glucose; and the lipid breakdown product glycerol. These can be detected in brain interstitial fluid by invasive microdialysis, nearly in real time.

# References

Tobin MJ. Principles and practice of intensive care monitoring. New York: McGraw-Hill; 1998.

Carney NA, Chesnut R, Kochanek PM. Guidelines for the acute medical management of severe traumatic brain injury in infants, children, and adolescents. Pediatr Crit Care Med 2003;4(3 Suppl):S1.

Hlatky R, Robertson C. Advanced bedside neuromonitoring. In: Fink MP, Abraham E, Vincent JL, Kochanek PM, eds. Textbook of Critical Care. 5th ed. Philadelphia, PA: Elsevier Saunders; 2005:287–94.

Steiner LA, Andrews PJ. Monitoring the injured brain: ICP and CBF. Br J Anaesth 2006;97:26–38.

Hlatky R, Valadka AB, Robertson CS. Intracranial hypertension and cerebral ischemia after severe traumatic brain injury. Neurosurg Focus 2003;14:e2.

Perez A, Minces PG, Schnitzler EJ, Agosta GE, Medina SA, Ciraolo CA. Jugular venous oxygen saturation or arteriovenous difference of lactate content and outcome in children with severe traumatic brain injury. Pediatr Crit Care Med 2003;4:33–8.

Rosow C, Manberg PJ. Bispectral index monitoring. Anesthesiol Clin North America 2001;19:947–66, xi.

Deogaonkar A, Gupta R, DeGeorgia M, et al. Bispectral Index monitoring correlates with sedation scales in brain-injured patients. Crit Care Med 2004;32:2403–6.

Powers KS, Nazarian EB, Tapyrik SA, et al. Bispectral index as a guide for titration of propofol during procedural sedation among children. Pediatrics 2005;115:1666–74.

Berger RP. The use of serum biomarkers to predict outcome after traumatic brain injury in adults and children. J Head Trauma Rehabil 2006;21:315–33.

Bellander BM, Cantais E, Enblad P, et al. Consensus meeting on microdialysis in neurointensive care. Intensive Care Med 2004;30:2166–9.

# B.  Seizures and Status Epilepticus

Paul M Shore

## Outline

- Key Principles
- Definition of Seizure and Status Epilepticus
- Etiologies
- Incidence
- Potential Consequences of Untreated Status Epilepticus
- Treatment of Acute Seizures
- Status Epilepticus (Prolonged Seizures)

## Key Principles

- There is no consistent definition of status epilepticus, and insufficient research regarding its optimal treatment
- Conventionally, seizures should be treated aggressively to

  - Ensure that airway, breathing and circulation are secure
  - Administer antiepileptic medications of differing classes until seizures resolve
  - Treat the underlying cause of the seizure, if possible
  - Monitor for further seizure activity

## Definition of Seizure and Status Epilepticus

- Conceptually, "seizure" refers to abnormal, paroxysmal electrical activity of the brain with or without a motor correlate. Status Epilepticus (SE) refers to prolonged seizure without return to baseline activity or mental status.
- Operationally, there is no consistent definition of SE

  - Some authors consider any seizure lasting >5 min to be SE, while others argue for 30–60 min of seizure activity (whether consistent or intermittent) without return to baseline mental status.

- Seizures lasting 10–29 min may resolve without treatment (perhaps 40% rate of spontaneous resolution).
- Since spontaneous resolution cannot be predicted, all seizures lasting 5–10 min should be considered "impending SE" and treated. In animal models, seizures >30 min become self-sustaining, resistant to pharmacologic agents, and result in neuronal injury.
- Most authors consider seizure-like electrographic activity without motor activity to be seizure (known as subclinical seizure), but some feel motor activity is required.

## Etiologies

The list of etiologies of seizures and SE is extensive; a partial list of common causes is presented in Table 1.

*Table 1*
## Common Cause of Seizures

| Metabolic | Toxic | Brain injury |
|---|---|---|
| Electrolyte abnormalities | Drug ingestion | Traumatic brain injury |
|   Hypo- or hypernatremia | Medications | Stroke |
|   Hypocalcemia | | Intracranial Hemorrhage |
| Hypoglycemia | | Tumor |
| Temperature | | AVM |
|   Fever | | |
|   Hyperthermia | | |
|   Simple febrile seizure | | |
| Hypoxia | | |
| Hepatic encephalopathy | | |
| Infection | Malignant hypertension | Congenital/genetic |
|   Intracranial | HUS | Primary epilepsy |
|     Encephalitis | TTP | Inborn errors of metabolism |
|     Meningitis | Eclampsia | Leukodystrophies, etc. |
|   Extracranial | | Chromosomal abnormalities |
|     Shigella | | Mitochondrial disorders |

# Incidence of Seizure and Status Epilepticus

- Because of the inconsistent definition of SE, the true incidence is unknown.
- The lifetime risk of seizure for any individual is estimated at about 4%.
- The overall incidence of SE in adults has been estimated at 10–41 per 100,000 person-years.
- SE is likely under-recognized, even in the ICU.

  - A study of adults referred for continuous EEG (cEEG) studies found that 19% of patients monitored with cEEG had SE; 92% of these patients had exclusively subclinical SE and 88% were in the ICU at the time of diagnosis.
  - The incidence of SE in the ICU after traumatic brain injury rises from 9–14% to 14–33% in studies using clinical only vs electrographic criteria to diagnose SE.

# Potential Consequences of Untreated Status Epilepticus

*Denotes items that may be both a consequence and/or a cause of SE

**Taken from preclinical data

Airway disturbances
    Obstruction
    Aspiration
Breathing disturbances
    Apnea
    Hypopnea
Circulatory disturbances
    Hypertension (usually early)
    Hypotension (usually late)
Metabolic disturbances
    Hypermetabolism
        Hyperthermia/fever*
        Hypoglycemia*
        Lactic acidosis
    Tissue breakdown
        Rhabdomyolysis, possibly leading to renal insufficiency or failure
    Hyperkalemia, possibly leading to cardiac arrhythmias

CNS disturbances **

    Neuronal and glial necrosis

    Neuronal apoptosis

    Cerebral edema (vasogenic and cytotoxic)

    Disturbance of autoregulation, with compromised cerebral blood flow

    Lowering of threshold for subsequent seizures

    Synergistic compounding of damage with other forms of brain injury

# Treatment of Acute Seizures

- There is no single, universally recognized treatment algorithm for acute seizures.
- Conceptually, treatment consists of recognition of the seizure, stabilizing airway/breathing/circulation, administration of anti-epileptic drugs (AEDs), monitoring for further seizures, and investigation/treatment of the underlying cause of seizure.
- Recognition of seizure

  - Seizure nearly always presents with alteration of mental status or coma.
  - Motoric findings may be
    - Obvious, such as generalized tonic-clonic activity
    - Subtle, such as eye or head deviation, lip-smacking, or tonic-only activity
    - Absent

  - Tachycardia, hypertension, and pupillary dilation (or anisocoria) are often present.
    - These may be the only signs in a patient receiving neuromuscular blockade.
  - Electrographic findings

    - By definition, show seizure.
    - Subclinical seizure can be diagnosed only by EEG.
    - In a cohort of 500 adults referred for cEEG monitoring, seizures were detected in 88% on the first day of monitoring, but patients in coma were 4.5 times more likely to require $>$24 hrs of monitoring to detect seizure than patients who were not in coma (see Chapter 9C, "Coma").

- Stabilization of airway, breathing, and circulation (ABCs)

  - ABCs should be stabilized in standard fashion (see Chapter 5, "Resuscitation").

- Compromise of airway and breathing are common, especially after administration of AEDs, and should be anticipated.

    - Airway maneuvers, such as jaw thrust and/or chin lift, may be required.
    - Bedside suction should be on, and a Yankauer suction catheter attached to suction tubing.
    - An appropriate sized mask and a ventilation bag should be immediately available.
    - Oral and nasal airways should be immediately available.
    - Endotracheal intubation should be considered if airway and/or breathing compromise is expected to be ongoing or if the patient is to be transported to another facility.

- Intravenous or intraosseous access should be obtained rapidly if IV medication is to be administered.

- Administration of antiepileptic drugs

    - Well-designed comparative studies of AEDs are few in number; therefore, there is no single, universally recognized AED-of-choice.
    - Benzodiazepines, barbiturates, fosphenytoin, or phenytoin are generally the first-line AEDs.

        - In adults, lorazepam is a better single agent than diazepam or phenytoin. Phenobarbital is equally effective as lorazepam and diazepam/phenytoin.
        - A lack of data prevents firm conclusions from being drawn for children. Lorazepam, midazolam, and diazepam given IV, IO, IM, PR, or intranasally (IN) are all effective at resolving seizures, but none is consistently superior or has been compared to other classes of AEDs.
        - In a large adult trial comparing four seizure treatments, the first drug resolved 44–65% of seizures, the second resolved only an additional 7.3%, and the third an additional 2% of seizures.
        - Diazepam has been associated with a higher incidence of intubation in children than phenobarbital or phenytoin.

    - AEDs administration is generally recommended within 5–10 minutes of seizure onset—usually without EEG information.
    - The more refractory the seizure, the more urgent it is to get an EEG to accompany on-going treatment.

- In the ICU setting, IV administration is generally preferred.
- Midazolam IN and diazepam PR are acceptable alternatives prior to obtaining IV access.

- If the seizure does not resolve in 5–10 min,
  - Check to see that the IV is patent—if not, replace and re-administer the first AED
  - If the IV is patent, administer a different class of medication
  - If the second AED does not resolve the seizure, a third class of medication is unlikely to work but may be considered.
  - If seizure is refractory to an AED of >2 classes and/or 30 minutes have elapsed, treat as status epilepticus (see below).
  - Additional doses of phenobarbital (10 mg/kg) may be given and are likely to terminate the seizure eventually—although the risk of respiratory depression or hypotension increases with additional doses, these risks may be acceptable in order to terminate seizure.
  - Phenytoin and fosphenytoin can themselves be epileptogenic; therefore additional doses beyond a 20 mg/kg loading dose should not be given unless a serum phenytoin level is known to be sub-therapeutic.
  - Anti-epileptic medications may interact and affect serum levels, consider consultation with pharmacy to ensure optimal dosing.
  - Additional medications may be used in consultation with Neurology consultants and may include valproate, pyridoxine, or other chronic medications used by the patient.

- Monitoring for further seizures and when Refractory SE or SE present

  - Electroencephalography (EEG)
    - EEG is the "gold standard" of seizure diagnosis, but requires highly trained personnel to interpret the studies.
    - Serial or continuous EEGs should not be considered "monitoring," but rather "recording," since results are not available until the study is read (much like a Holter monitor).
    - Serial or continuous EEG should nevertheless be strongly considered in any patient in whom SE is not yet resolved, or who is at high risk of recurrence.

- Clinical monitoring

    - Currently, careful monitoring of vital signs and physical exam is the mainstay of SE monitoring.
    - Unexplained tachycardia, hypertension, and/or pupillary dilation or anisocoria may signal recurrence of seizure.

- Other modalities
    - See Chapter 9A on Neuromonitoring.

- Investigation/treatment of underlying cause of seizures/SE

    - Investigation and treatment of the cause of seizures and SE can be simultaneous with treatment of the seizure itself, and should begin as soon as seizure is recognized
    - Rapid, bedside tests for common causes of seizure should be used as it is being managed

        - Bedside glucometer
        - Bedside electrolytes (sodium and calcium)

    - Treatment of the underlying cause should begin when it is suspected or confirmed
        - Dextrose (10% or 50%) may be administered empirically if hypoglycemic seizure is suspected
        - Hyponatremic seizures
            - Do not generally resolve until the serum sodium is increased; typical AEDs are ineffective
            - Administer 2 mL/kg boluses of 3% NaCl (or 1 mL/kg of 7.5% NaCl) until seizure resolves
        - Hypocalcemic seizures
            - Do not generally resolve until the serum calcium is increased; typical AEDs are ineffective
            - Administer 100 mg/kg bolus of calcium gluconate (or 20 mg/kg calcium chloride if central or intraosseous access is present) until seizure resolves
            - Restoration of serum magnesium may be required to achieve normal serum calcium

    - Full workup of the causes of seizure should follow the etiologies listed in the Table 1. A partial list includes:

        - Thorough history and physical exam
        - Electrolytes, including calcium, magnesium and phosphate, and anion gap
        - Arterial blood gas
        - BUN and creatinine
        - Ammonia, transaminases

- Complete urine and/or serum toxicologic studies (not only for drugs of abuse)
- Serum osmolar gap
- Urine and/or serum pregnancy test
- Brain imaging, including CT scan and/or MRI
- Lumbar puncture with culture, Gram stain, cell count, protein, glucose
- PT and aPTT
- Genetic or metabolic workup if such a disorder is suspected
- Consultation with a neurologist and/or other required specialist(s)

# Status Epilepticus (Prolonged Seizures)

- Status epilepticus (SE) may be defined as clinical or electrographic seizures lasting ≥30 min without full recovery of consciousness

  - Failure of SE to resolve after administration of 2 AEDs is known as Refractory Status Epilepticus (RSE)

- As with acute seizure, there is no universally accepted treatment for SE

  - All on-going further treatment of SE or RSE should be guided by STAT cEEG monitoring
  - Anticipate the side effects of AED administration (particularly respiratory depression/apnea and hypotension) by intubating the trachea, placing arterial and central venous lines, and ordering inotropes to the bedside as treatment for SE is begun

- Treatment options include

  - Barbiturate infusion

    - Pentobarbital (load with 5 mg/kg IV, then 1–3 mg/kg/h IV infusion titrated to burst-suppression on cEEG)
    - Thiopental (load with 5 mg/kg IV, then 3–5 mg/kg/h IV infusion)
    - Drug infusion should be titrated to burst-suppression on cEEG
    - Patients very frequently become hypotensive on barbiturate infusions; patients should have an arterial line placed, and dopamine, epinephrine and/or norepinephrine infusions should be immediately available

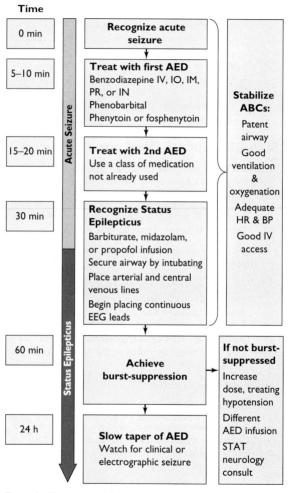

**Figure 1**  Management of status epilepticus.

- Midazolam infusion (0.1–0.2 mg/kg/h or 1–3 microgram/kg/min initially)
- Propofol infusion (load with 1–3 mg/kg IV, then 125–250 mcg/kg/min)

  - Use with caution in children, especially if used ≥24 hrs, due to small risk of metabolic acidosis that is occasionally fatal (propofol infusion syndrome)

- Ketamine (load with 1–2 mg/kg IV, then 1–4 mg/kg/h IV infusion)
- Pentobarbital may be more effective than midazolam or propofol for RSE, but produces more hypotension. Other agents have not been studied

- Once SE has resolved and/or burst-suppression achieved, the AED infusion should be weaned slowly, watching carefully for recurrence of clinical or electrographic seizures

The flow diagram for the management of status epilepticus is shown in Figure 1.

# References

DeLorenzo RJ, Garnett LK, Towne AR, et al. Comparison of status epilepticus with prolonged seizure episodes lasting from 10 to 29 minutes. Epilepsia 1999;40(2):164–9.

Chen JW, Wasterlain CG. Status epilepticus: pathophysiology and management in adults. Lancet Neurol 2006;5(3):246–56.

Hauser WA, Annegers JF, Kurland LT. Incidence of epilepsy and unprovoked seizures in Rochester, Minnesota: 1935–1984. Epilepsia 1993;34(3):453–68.

Claassen J, Mayer SA, Kowalski RG, Emerson RG, Hirsch LJ. Detection of electrographic seizures with continuous EEG monitoring in critically ill patients. Neurology 2004;62(10):1743–8.

Vespa P. Continuous EEG monitoring for the detection of seizures in traumatic brain injury, infarction, and intracerebral hemorrhage: "to detect and protect". J Clin Neurophysiol 2005;22(2):99–106.

Prasad K, Al-Roomi K, Krishnan PR, Sequeira R. Anticonvulsant therapy for status epilepticus. Cochrane Database Syst Rev 2005(4):CD003723.

Treiman DM, Meyers PD, Walton NY, et al. A comparison of four treatments for generalized convulsive status epilepticus. Veterans Affairs Status Epilepticus Cooperative Study Group. N Engl J Med 1998;339(12):792–8.

Appleton R, Martland T, Phillips B. Drug management for acute tonic-clonic convulsions including convulsive status epilepticus in children. Cochrane Database Syst Rev 2002(4):CD001905.

Orr RA, Dimand RJ, Venkataraman ST, Karr VA, Kennedy KJ. Diazepam and intubation in emergency treatment of seizures in children. Ann Emerg Med 1991;20(9):1009–13.

Claassen J, Hirsch LJ, Emerson RG, Mayer SA. Treatment of refractory status epilepticus with pentobarbital, propofol, or midazolam: a systematic review. Epilepsia 2002;43(2):146–53.

# C. Coma and Altered Mental Status

Lennox Huang

## Introduction

Altered mental status is a common presentation for a variety of pediatric disease processes. The differential diagnosis is lengthy and encompasses virtually all pediatric subspecialties. The priority for patients presenting with altered mental status to a pediatric intensive care unit (ICU) is to ensure cardiopulmonary stability, followed by interventions directed toward life-threatening and reversible causes of altered mental status. After initial stabilization, a thorough history and physical exam with focused investigations is essential to establish a working diagnosis.

## Key Principles

- Identify and manage life-threatening problems first.
- Perform a limited neurologic exam.
- Identify and treat easily reversible causes of altered mental status.
- Serial neurologic evaluations, including Glasgow Coma Scale (GCS) scores.

## Definitions

| | |
|---|---|
| Coma | A profound state of unconscious unresponsiveness; patient is not aware of self and surroundings. |
| Delirium | Fluctuating reduction in awareness, attention, orientation, and perception. Characterized by abnormal sleep wake patterns and psychomotor disturbances. |

(continued)

| Locked-in | Preservation of cerebral cognitive activity with an inability to move or speak secondary to motor pathway damage. |
| Obtunded/Lethargic | Decreased level of consciousness, interruptable by pain or direct examination followed by a return to depressed state. |
| Stupor | An increase above the patient's normal sleep/wake ratio. Responsive to pain and other stimuli. |

# Differential Diagnosis for Altered Mental Status

| Structural | Trauma<br>Tumor<br>Infectious abscess<br>Hydrocephalus<br>Intracranial hemorrhage or infarction<br>Venous thrombosis | |
| Nonstructural | Infectious | Meningitis<br>Encephalitis<br>Sepsis |
| | Metabolic | DKA<br>Uremia<br>Hepatic encephalopathy<br>Inborn errors of metabolism<br>(see Chapter 18, "Infection") |
| | Psychiatric | Conversion disorder<br>Psychosis |
| | Other | Shock state with compromised cerebral perfusion<br>Seizures, postictal state<br>Electrolyte abnormalities<br>Hypo- or hyperthermia<br>Hypercapnia<br>Toxins (see Chapter 23, "Pharmacology") |

# Initial Investigations/Management

Evaluate and initiate treatment as you go along

## Airway, Breathing, Circulation

- Altered mental status may lead to an inability to protect the airway, majority of patients with a GCS score less than 8 should be intubated
- Anticipatory management is essential, if a patient exhibits a rapid or fluctuating decline in mental status, it is essential to secure the airway even if there are no signs of respiratory distress or failure or if GCS is >8
- Unassisted respiratory pattern may provide clues to the underlying etiology:

  - Kussmaul—underlying acidosis, DKA, or metabolic cause
  - Cheyne-Stokes—bilateral cerebral dysfunction, increased intracranial pressure (ICP)
  - Tachypnea—midbrain lesions
  - Apneustic—medullary or pontine dysfunction

- Circulatory compromise especially in shock states may lead to altered mental status. Isotonic or hypertonic fluids and inotropic resuscitation may improve CNS perfusion
- Circulatory compromise may also occur secondary to primary brain pathology, especially in cases of brainstem injury
- Look for vital sign changes suggesting raised intracranial pressure: hypertension, bradycardia, abnormal respirations (Cushing response)

Focused neurologic exam—should take <3 minutes

- Ideally, exam should be performed in the absence of sedation, neuromuscular blockade, or narcotic analgesics
- Consider patient's developmental and chronologic age
- Pediatric Glasgow Coma Scale (GCS) or AVPU  (see Table 1)
- Cranial nerve exam
- Funduscopy to look for papilledema, retinal hemorrhages
- Examine for signs of meningismus
- Basic motor exam for tone, posturing, deep tendon reflexes
- Neurologic exam in a comatose patient may suggest a herniation syndrome requiring immediate measures to treat raised intracranial pressure (see Table 2)

*Table 1*
## Pediatric Glasgow Coma Scale

| | | |
|---|---|---|
| Eye Opening | Spontaneous | 4 |
| | To Voice | 3 |
| | To Pain | 2 |
| | None | 1 |
| Verbal Response | Oriented | 5 |
| (Over 5 yr) | Confused | 4 |
| | Inappropriate Words | 3 |
| | Nonspecific Sounds | 2 |
| | None | 1 |
| (2 to 5 yr) | Appropriate Words | 5 |
| | Inappropriate Words | 4 |
| | Cries and/or Screams | 3 |
| | Grunts | 2 |
| | None | 1 |
| (0 to 23 mo) | Smiles/Coos/Cries appropriately | 5 |
| | Cries/Inconsolable | 4 |
| | Inappropriate Cry | 3 |
| | Persistent Cry/Grunting | 2 |
| | None | 1 |
| Motor Response | Obeys Command | 6 |
| (Over 5 yr) | Localizes Pain | 5 |
| | Withdraw (Pain) | 4 |
| | Flexor Posturing (Pain) | 3 |
| | Extensor Posturing (Pain) | 2 |
| | None | 1 |
| (Up to 5 yr) | Obeys Command | 6 |
| | Localizes Pain | 5 |
| | Withdraw (Pain) | 4 |
| | Flexor Posturing (Pain) | 3 |
| | Extensor Posturing (Pain) | 2 |
| | None | 1 |
| Normal Scores by Age: | | |
| Birth to 6 mo | 9 | |
| 7–12 mo | 11 | |
| 1–2 yr | 12 | |
| 2–5 yr | 13 | |
| >5 yr | 14 | |

*Table 2*
## Herniation Syndromes

- Subfalcine (cingulate)
  - usually supratentorial etiology usually no specific clinical signs, detected on imaging precedes transtentorial herniation

- Lateral tentorial (uncal)
  - usually supratentorial etiology
  - uncus of temporal lobe through tentorial notch
  - unilateral dilated pupil, extraocular movement (EOM) paralysis from ipsilateral CN III compression

- Central tentorial (axial)
  - diencephalon and midbrain trough tentorial notch
  - supratentorial midline lesion
  - decreased level of consciousness, upward EOM impairment, brainstem hemorrhage, diabetes insipidus (late)

- Tonsillar (coning)
  - cerebellar tonsils through foramen magnum
  - infratentorial lesions, or after axial herniation, or after LP
  - rapidly fatal cardiorespiratory centers affected

---

- A more detailed neurologic exam should be performed once the patient has been stabilized and life-threatening etiologies have been treated or ruled out

Limited laboratory workup:

- Blood gas
- CBC
- Electrolytes/bedside metered glucose

Empirically treat acute life-threatening and easily reversible causes

IV dextrose if hypoglycemia proven or strongly suspected
Naloxone if narcotic overdose is suspected
Empiric reversal of benzodiazepines is not recommended
Empiric antibiotics with CSF penetration—eg, cefotaxime or ceftriaxone
Short acting antiepileptic medications if seizure is suspected (see Chapter 9, "Neurology")

Treat suspected raised intracranial pressure (see Chapter 10, "Neurosurgery")

> Head of bed raised 30 degrees
> Head midline
> Minimal stimulation
> Isotonic IVF
> Hypertonic saline or mannitol
> Normal $PaCO_2$

Imaging

- Early imaging is generally essential to obtain a diagnosis
- A non-contrast head CT is often the best initial imaging required to rule out hemorrhage, large space occupying lesions, herniation syndromes
- Contrasted CT or CT angiography may be required if vascular disease or infectious abscesses are suspected
- MRI should be performed for suspected stroke (emergently if within the therapeutic window for thrombolysis), tumors, encephalitis

Additional investigations

- Lumbar puncture

  - Opening and closing pressure should be obtained
  - Send CSF for cell count, protein, glucose, culture
  - Should be performed *after* imaging if there are focal neurologic findings or suspicion of raised intracranial pressure

- EEG if seizure activity or encephalopathy suspected
- Sensory evoked potentials (SEP)—bilateral absent SEPs in adults indicates a very poor prognosis with <1% likelihood of recovery; SEPs are less predictive of prognosis in children

ICU syndrome/delirium/psychosis

- Common complication of ICU admission
- Risk factors include prolonged intubation, sedation
- Often indistinguishable from medication withdrawal
- Patients may appear combative, agitated, disoriented with hallucinations

Management

- Presence of parents, pictures, familiar objects to orient patient

- Establish day-night cycle with lighting and activity; patient room with window is especially helpful
- Reduction of sedating medications or medications which alter sensorium including benzodiazepines, opioids. Weaning regimens may be helpful for some patients
- Symptoms generally resolve with time; haloperidol may be used for acute episodes where the patient becomes a danger to their self

Prognosis

- Prognosis of altered mental status is highly variable and dependent on the underlying etiology
- Prognosis of pediatric coma is also associated with the duration of the coma
- Persistent low serial GCS scores indicate a poor outcome

Things to note:

Minimum score is 3
Can be measured serially, deterioration in score by 2 or more should warrant reevaluation

# References

Altered States of Consciousness. In Clinical Pediatric Neurology. Feinchel G. 5th edition 2005, (pp. 47–76). Philadelphia, Pennsylvania: WB Saunders.

Avner JR. Altered states of consciousness. Pediatrics Rev 2006;27:331–7.

Holmes JF, Palchak MJ, Macfarlane T, Kuppermann N. Performance of the pediatric Glasgow Coma Scale in children with blunt head trauma. Acad Emerg Med 2005;12:814–9.

# D. Neuroprotection in the PICU

Haresh Kirpalani

## Key Principles

> - Moderate hypothermia may have a neuroprotective role in neonatal hypoxic encephalopathy and post-adult cardiac arrest.
> - Hypothermia for pediatric cardiac arrest and traumatic brain injury is not supported by current evidence.

## Introduction

This field is in a ferment with several new putative therapies. Sadly to date, there have been too few pivotal trials. Some promising therapies are either likely to be tested by RCTs shortly, or in the case of hypothermia have been already. The following references indicate the long list of agents being discussed for potential RCT testing over the next years. They cover a wide range of potential pathophysiology from erythropoietin to anesthetic agents to various gene-targeted therapies including hepatocyte growth factor. Mention should also be made that it appears corticosteroids are of no benefit.

## Moderate Hypothermia

Some human data does exist for this modality, and is discussed under three broad headings: neonatal hypoxic encephalopathy, hypothermia for pediatric head injury or traumatic brain injury (TBI), and hypothermia post cardiac arrest.

### Neonatal Hypoxic Encephalopathy

There have been some pivotal reported trials and two are awaiting completion prior to reporting. Although they have been amalgamated in the Cochrane library, various bodies are still recommending further study before declaring this a standard of care. This has created controversy, with some pointing to methodological deficits while others state these are outweighed by the evidence. Target ranges for therapy are 33.5°C for 72 hours, ideally within 6 hours of birth. Following the cooling period is a slow rewarming. Details of the two main therapeutic modalities (cooling blanket or head cooling) are in two main papers. Short-term safety is not in question at these ranges of temperature.

## Hypothermia for Pediatric Head Injury or Traumatic Brain Injury (TBI)

Hypothermia in adults in large trials showed short-term benefit was found. However, this was not present at long term, and these data are summarized in two meta-analyses. The neonatal and adult work impelled an RCT in children with TBI1. Cooling here was achieved with cooling blanket systems, to a target of 32.5°C for 24 hours, and was induced within a window of 8 hours of injury. There was no benefit in the primary outcome at 6 months age between normothermic and hypothermic groups. As well, there were an excess of deaths in the hypothermic group (21% versus 12%), more hypotension, and more vasoactive agents required in the hypothermia group during the rewarming period. Currently, it can be viewed only as experimental and advisable only in the context of informed consent within further randomized trials.

## Hypothermia Post-Cardiac Arrest

This area is also in a ferment. There have been three relevant adult trials composed of 381 patients, summarized in a meta-analysis. Patients in the hypothermia group were more likely to be discharged without neurological damage (risk ratio, 1.68; 1.29–2.07). This translates to a number-needed-to-treat of 6 (95% confidence interval, 4–13). Results have been followed in some of the patients up to 6 months. Target ranges for temperature are 32°C to 34°C with the use of an external cooling device. There have been some objections to the trials, including that of no allocation concealment in one trial, and that tight selection limits generalizability of this information, such that <10% of assessed patients were included in the European study. The European trialists agree that: "only a small proportion of patients with cardiac arrest may currently benefit from therapeutic hypothermia.... Nationwide implementation would prevent 3 percent of all unfavorable neurologic outcomes (the population attributable fraction) in patients with cardiac arrest."

The trials had marked differences from each other: Two trials; were multiple-center trials; and included only ventricular fibrillation patients. The other trial had patients with asystole and pulseless electrical activity. Three different methods were used to apply hypothermia. Active maintenance of hypothermia lasted either 4 hours, 12 hours, or 24 hours.

Nonetheless, on the basis of these data, the American Heart Association, together with ILCOR, has recommended that it be a standard of care as follows:

> Unconscious adult patients with spontaneous circulation after out-of-hospital cardiac arrest should be cooled to 32°C to 34°C for 12 to 24 hours when the initial rhythm was ventricular fibrillation (VF); such cooling may also be beneficial for other rhythms or in-hospital cardiac arrest.

This is not universally adopted, however, as shown by the statement of the National Association of EMS Physicians in 2007:

> Induced hypothermia in the post-resuscitative period has been shown to benefit select survivors of cardiac arrest. Whether the benefits of induced hypothermia extend to all cardiac arrest patients, and what the most effective means and best time of initiation of this modality are, remain unknown. A lack of evidence on induced hypothermia in the pre-hospital setting currently precludes recommending this treatment modality as standard of care for all emergency medical services (EMS) patients resuscitated from cardiac arrest. At present, it is more important to focus efforts on proper resuscitation techniques, including high-quality cardiopulmonary resuscitation and appropriate defibrillation, and attentive post-resuscitation monitoring and support.

No doubt, such confusion explains why the ILCOR recommendations have not been so widely adopted in practice currently.

For children, the situation is even less clear. The causes of cardiac arrest are quite different from adults, being largely driven by hypoxia and shock rather than by ventricular fibrillation or coronary artery disease. Although there are calls for further study before making such therapy "standard of care"—these authors propose that if it is to be used, it should be performed speedily and they give a protocol modified from a trial in head injury. This is given below, following the references. In addition, at the University of Pennsylvania website (http://www.med. upenn.edu.libaccess.lib.mcmaster.ca/resuscitation/hypothermia/ protocols.shtml), protocols of other sites using hypothermia are given.

## Neuroprotection While Undergoing Bypass and ECMO

Short- and long-term neurologic sequellae remain important components of morbidity related to cardiopulmonary bypass and ECMO. Cerebral injury during bypass surgery and ECMO is thought to mainly result from hypoperfusion and embolism. Optimal strategies to minimize neurologic damage during cardiopulmonary bypass surgery remain controversial but may include hypothermia, pH regulation, alternative perfusion methods, blood glucose regulation, and anti-inflammatory agents. To date, there is no evidence to support any specific neuroprotective measures for infants or children undergoing ECMO.

## Cooling Protocols for Children

Cooling should be started as soon as possible after the cardiac arrest because there is likely a therapeutic window:

- A cooling mattress is placed under the patient (5°C).
- Neuromuscular blocker (eg, pancuronium, 0.1 mg/kg) is administered intravenously as needed to prevent shivering.
- An esophageal temperature probe is placed, and the tip is confirmed to be in the lower third of the esophagus by chest radiograph.
- Crushed ice is placed in double plastic bags, air is removed, and the bags are sealed to prevent leakage. The bags are placed in cotton bags (pillow cases) to prevent injury to the skin. As much surface area as possible is covered with these bags of ice, and the skin is inspected frequently to prevent cold-induced injury.
- A cooling blanket (forced air) is placed over the ice and the patient.
- Once the patient's esophageal temperature reaches 34°C, the ice packs and upper cooling blanket are quickly removed, and the servo-controlled cooling mattress below the patient is on automatic at 33.5°C. Close temperature monitoring is done to prevent overcooling.
- We aim to keep the temperature between 33° and 34°C for 48 hours.

- We slowly rewarm the patient by increasing the set point on the servo-controlled cooling mattress by 0.5°C every 2 hours. Rewarming takes 14 to 18 hours.

# References

Thal SC, Engelhard K, Werner C. New cerebral protection strategies. Curr Opin Anaesthesiol 2005 Oct;18(5):490–5.

Mogi M, Iwai M, Horiuchi M. New paradigm for brain protection after stroke. Hypertension 2006 Apr;47(4):642–3.

Tasker RC. Pharmacological advance in the treatment of acute brain injury. Arch Dis Child 1999 Jul;81(1):90–5.

Christophe M, Nicolas S. Mitochondria: a target for neuroprotective interventions in cerebral ischemia-reperfusion. Curr Pharm Des 2006;12(6):739–57.

Fagan SC, Hess DC, Machado LS, et al. Tactics for vascular protection after acute ischemic stroke. Pharmacotherapy 2005 Mar;25(3):387–95.

Head BP, Patel P. Anesthetics and brain protection. Curr Opin Anaesthesiol 2007 Oct;20(5):39.

Alderson P, Roberts I. Corticosteroids for acute traumatic brain injury. Cochrane Database Syst Rev 2005 Jan 25;(1):CD000196.

Gluckman PD, Wyatt JS, Azzopardi D, et al. Selective head cooling with mild systemic hypothermia after neonatal encephalopathy: multicentre randomised trial. Lancet 2005;365:663–70.

Shankaran S, Laptook AR, Ehrenkranz RA, et al. National Institute of Child Health and Human Development Neonatal Research Network. Whole-body hypothermia for neonates with hypoxic-ischemic encephalopathy. N Engl J Med 2005;353:1574–84.

Jacobs S, Hunt R, Tarnow-Mordi W, et al. Cooling for newborns with hypoxic ischaemic encephalopathy. Cochrane Database Syst Rev 2007 Oct 17;(4):CD003311.

Blackmon LR, Stark AR, American Academy of Pediatrics, Committee on Fetus and Newborn. Hypothermia: a neuroprotective therapy for neonatal hypoxic-ischemic encephalopathy. Pediatrics 2006;117:942–8.

Higgins RD, Raju TN, Perlman J, et al. Hypothermia and perinatal asphyxia: executive summary of the National Institute of Child Health and Human Development workshop. J Pediatr 2006;148:170–5.

American Heart Association. 2005 American Heart Association (AHA) guidelines for cardiopulmonary resuscitation (CPR) and emergency cardiovascular care (ECC) of pediatric and neonatal patients: pediatric basic life support. Pediatrics. 2006 May;117(5):e989–1004.

International Liaison Committee on Resuscitation. The International Liaison Committee on Resuscitation (ILCOR) consensus on science with treatment recommendations for pediatric and neonatal patients: pediatric basic and advanced life support. Pediatrics. 2006. May;117(5):e955–77. Epub 2006 Apr 17.

Kirpalani H, Barks J, Thorlund K, Guyatt G. Cooling for neonatal hypoxic ischemic encephalopathy: do we have the answer? Pediatrics 2007;120:1126–30.

Hoehn T, Hansmann G, Bührer C, et al. Therapeutic hypothermia in neonates. Review of current clinical data, ILCOR recommendations and suggestions for implementation in neonatal intensive care units. Resuscitation 2008 Jul;78(1):7–12.

McIntyre LA, Fergusson DA, Hébert PC, et al. Prolonged therapeutic hypothermia after traumatic brain injury in adults: systematic review. JAMA 2003;289:2992–9.

Alderson P, Gadkary C, Signorini DF. Therapeutic hypothermia for head injury. Cochrane Database Syst Rev 2004 Oct 18;(4):CD001048.

Hutchison JS, Ward RE, et al; Hypothermia Pediatric Head Injury Trial Investigators and the Canadian Critical Care Trials Group. Hypothermia therapy after traumatic brain injury in children. N Engl J Med 2008 Jun 5;358(23):2447–56.

Hypothermia After Cardiac Arrest (HACA) study group. Mild therapeutic hypothermia to improve the neurologic outcome after cardiac arrest. N Engl J Med 2002;346:549–56.

Bernard SA, Gray TW, Buist MD, et al. Treatment of comatose survivors of out-of-hospital cardiac arrest with induced hypothermia. N Engl J Med 2002;346:557–63.

Hachimi-Idrissi S, Corne L, Ebinger G, et al. Mild hypothermia induced by a helmet device: A clinical feasibility study. Resuscitation 2001;51:275–81.

Holzer M, Bernard SA, Hachimi-Idrissi S. Collaborative group on induced hypothermia for neuroprotection after cardiac arrest hypothermia for neuroprotection after cardiac arrest: systematic review and individual patient data meta-analysis. Crit Care Med 2005 Jun;33(6):1449–52.

Ballew KA. Mild hypothermia improved neurologic outcome and reduced mortality after cardiac arrest because of ventricular arrhythmia. ACP J Club 2002 Sep–Oct;137(2):46.

Padosch SA, Kern KB, Böttiger BW. Therapeutic hypothermia after cardiac arrest. N Engl J Med 2002 Jul 4;347(1):63–5.

Moran JL, Peake SL. Editorial: hypothermia as therapy in cerebral injury. Critical Care and Resuscitation 2002;4:81–92.

Holzer M. Therapeutic hypothermia after cardiac arrest. N Engl J Med 2002 Jul 4;347(1):63–5.

International Liaison Committee on Resuscitation. International consensus on cardiopulmonary resuscitation and emergency cardiovascular care science with treatment recommendations. Circulation 2005;112:III-1–III136.

Nolan JP, Morley PT, Vanden Hoek TL, et al. Therapeutic hypothermia after cardiac arrest: an advisory statement by the advanced life support task force of the international liaison committee on resuscitation. Circulation 2003;108(1):118–21.

National Association of EMS Physicians. Induced therapeutic hypothermia in resuscitated cardiac arrest patients. Prehosp Emerg Care 2008 Jul–Sep;12(3):393–4.

Brooks SC, Morrison LJ. Implementation of therapeutic hypothermia guidelines for post-cardiac arrest syndrome at a glacial pace: seeking guidance from the knowledge translation literature. Resuscitation 2008 Jun;77(3):286–92.

Hutchison JS, Doherty DR, Orlowski JP, Kissoon N. Hypothermia therapy for cardiac arrest in pediatric patients. Pediatr Clin North Am 2008 Jun;55(3):529–44, ix.

# Chapter 10

# Neurosurgery

## A. Care of the Postoperative Neurosurgical Patient

Andrew Latchman
Robert Hollenberg

### Indications for PICU Admission

PICU admission should be considered in the following neurologic conditions:

1. Acutely and severely altered sensorium in which neurologic deterioration or depression is likely or unpredictable, or coma with the potential for airway compromise
2. After neurosurgical procedures requiring invasive monitoring or close observation
3. Acute inflammation or infections of the spinal cord, meninges, or brain with neurologic depression, metabolic and hormonal abnormalities, and respiratory or hemodynamic compromise or the possibility of increased intracranial pressure
4. Head trauma with increased intracranial pressure
5. Preoperative neurosurgical conditions with neurologic deterioration
6. Progressive neuromuscular dysfunction with or without altered sensorium requiring cardiovascular monitoring and/or respiratory support
7. Spinal cord compression or impending compression
8. Placement of external ventricular drainage device

# General Considerations for Postoperative Care

The most important component of caring for the neurosurgical patient is knowledge of their baseline neurologic status. Optimally, a joint examination of the patient by the PICU staff with the neurosurgeon and/or neurologist as well as discussion of areas involved with surgery should occur postoperatively.

## Changes in neurological status

A change in a patient's neurological status may be due to:

- Seizure/post-ictal state
- Increased ICP

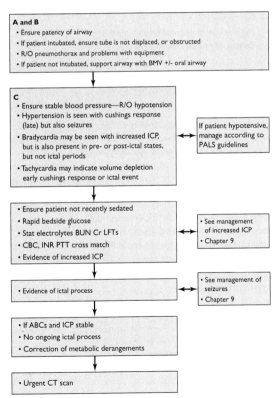

**Figure 1**   Approach to neurosurgical patient with altered LOC.

- Postoperative hemorrhage
- Medication
- Cortical injury secondary to surgery
- Electrolyte derangements
- Hypoglycemia
- Decompensation of cardio-respiratory status

Manifestations of increased ICP:

- Decreasing GCS score
- More subtle changes in mental status
- Headache
- Cranial nerve abnormalities (especially CN 6)
- Abnormality or changes in pupillary size and reaction to light
- Cushing's response—a late response (hypertension, bradycardia, tachycardia early on) and respiratory abnormalities
- Papilledema
- Focal seizures or focal neurological deficit
- Bulging of cranial defect if present

# Electrolyte Abnormalities in the Neurosurgical Patient

Regular monitoring of electrolytes, especially sodium, is essential in the postoperative care of the neurosurgical patient. Knowledge of the patient's electrolytes prior to surgery as well as fluids administered perioperatively and urine output is necessary to determine postoperative fluid management. Upon return from the operating room, serum electrolytes and urine electrolytes and osmolarity should be drawn and repeated every 6 hours for the first 24 hours and possibly more frequently if aberrations are present. The initial fluid should be NS at maintenance unless the patient is hypovolemic or there is a free water deficit.

## Hyponatremia

Hyponatremia is the result of a net gain of free water or a net loss of monovalent cations at a concentration greater than that of plasma. Clinical features of hyponatremia are rarely seen when serum sodium is greater than 125 mmol/L.

Features of hyponatremia include:

1. nausea
2. vomiting

3. headache
4. decreased level of consciousness
5. incontinence
6. seizures
7. respiratory arrest
8. features may be absent if patient is heavily sedated

Although there are many causes of hyponatremia, there are two etiologies specific to the neurosurgical patient:

1. cerebral salt wasting (CSW)
2. SIADH

- Differentiating between the two can be difficult, as hyponatremia, decreased serum osmolarity, inappropriately normal or high urine osmolarity, and high urine sodium (>20 mmol/L) exist in both SIADH and CSW.
- CSW often results in hypovolemia.
- SIADH generally results in euvolemia or volume overload.
- Management of CSW involves replacing the fluid deficit as well as maintaining and replacing sodium losses. This can be accomplished by measuring urine sodium and estimating fluid deficit, ie, using weight and fluid balance.
- SIADH should be managed with fluid restriction (urine output + insensible losses) if the hyponatremia remains refractory to restriction; then treatment with Lasix® (0.5–1 mg/kg) along with hypertonic saline to match urinary sodium losses is recommended.

## Hypernatremia

Hypernatremia is usually the result of net water loss relative to sodium loss.

- In the neurosurgical patient, special consideration must be given to osmotic diuresis, secondary to mannitol use and diabetes insipidus (DI).
- Diabetes insipidus is characterized by polyuria and polydipsia.
- In the conscious patient with access to free water and an intact thirst center, polyuria is compensated for by an increased water intake.
- However, postoperatively a patient's free water is determined by the medical team.
- Typically, the serum osmolarity is high and the urine is dilute 50–150 mmol/kg.
- Diabetes insipidus can be either neurogenic or nephrogenic. If it is neurogenic, it will respond to DDAVP®.

# Steroids

- Steroids re-enforce the blood brain barrier (BBB), making it less permeable to fluid moving from the blood into the tissue surrounding the brain.
- Steroids are effective in reducing edema caused by brain tumors.
- Suggested dosing is a 0.5–1 mg/kg IV loading dose followed by 0.25–0.5 mg/kg/d PO/IV divided q6h.
- For cerebral abscesses, steroids decrease the likelihood of fibrous encapsulation of the abscess, but may reduce the penetration of antibiotics into the abscess. In these cases, it is generally reserved for patients with radiographic and clinical evidence of mass effect and deterioration.
- Steroids are not recommended in head injuries, except when adrenal hormones are known to be depleted.

# Postoperative Infections

## CSF Infection

1. Presence of organism isolated from CSF
2. Presence of fever (>38°C) in the absence of other recognized causes with institution of appropriate antimicrobial treatment and any of the following: increased white cell count (>50% polymorph nuclear leucocytes), increased protein and/or decrease in glucose in CSF or organism visible on gram stain

   - Common organisms include *Staphylococcus epidermididis, Staphylococcus aureus*, enteric bacteria, diphtheroids, and *Streptococcus* species.
   - Antibiotic prophylaxis is controversial and varies between centers. The majority of neurosurgeons administer a dose of antibiotics prior to insertion of extraventricular drains (EVDs); however, positive cultures are still found in patients after such treatment.
   - It has been shown that drainage time of the catheter is not a significant risk factor for EVD infection, and that the most sensitive indicator of CSF infection is an increasing cell count.
   - Regular changes of the EVD catheter also have not resulted in decreased postoperative infections.

# The Aseptic Meningitis Syndrome

- Initially described after posterior fossa surgery in children but now recognized as a possible complication of other intracranial operations.

*Table 1*
## Aseptic vs Bacterial Meningitis

|  | Aseptic meningitis | Bacterial meningitis |
|---|---|---|
| Onset | May be febrile within hours of surgery |  |
| New focal deficit | 0% | 10% |
| Lactate level | <2 mmol/L | >3 mmol/L |
| Posterior fossa surgery | 50% | 25% |
| Associated features | CSF leak uncommon | CSF leaks |

- Diagnosis of exclusion.
- Characterized by spiking fever, neck stiffness, and headache, generally occurring during steroid tapering, 1–2 weeks after surgery.
- Spiking fevers may continue for days or weeks; however, meningismus rarely persists past second postoperative week.
- CSF generally shows pleocytosis (significant mononuclear component) hypoglycemia, and increased protein.
- Generally patients are not toxic-looking with the absence of persistent CSF leaks as well as new focal deficits.
- Symptoms of fever headache and malaise are usually controlled by reinstituting the steroid dosage.

## Posterior Fossa Syndrome

- Consists of mutism combined with ataxia cranial nerve palsies, bulbar palsies, hemiparesis, cognitive impairment, and emotional lability; however, the postoperative symptoms are often dominated by lack of speech.
- The onset is usually between 1 and 7 days postoperative and there is typically a period of normal speech before onset of symptoms.
- Mutism on its own may follow posterior fossa surgery, as well as head injury trauma to cerebellum, cerebellar hemorrhages, subarachnoid hemorrhage vertebral artery injury, and basilar artery occlusion.

- This syndrome is most often associated with medulloblastoma and sometimes with ependymomas or astrocytomas. The mutism is typically transient, lasting days to months; however, the other neurological manifestations are generally permanent.

Differential diagnosis includes:

- Post-ictal aphasia
- Manifestation of basilar migraine, possibly without headache
- Sudden onset of deafness (ie, after bacterial meningitis)
- Vascular lesions
- Landau-Kleffner syndrome (acquired epileptic aphasia)
- Visual impairment has also been associated with the posterior fossa syndrome

## Considerations for Specific Operations

### Craniosynostosis Repair

- Common elective operation with low risk of mortality
- May be admitted to PICU overnight postoperatively for pain control and neurological monitoring
- Facial swelling
- Blood loss

  - Historically, patients required significant postoperative blood transfusions.
  - Blood salvage and changes in surgical technique have reduced this need.
  - Assessing overall fluid status can be difficult.
  - Patients are at risk for developing respiratory insufficiency from volume overload.

- Cerebral edema, dural tears
- Use of newer endoscopic minimally invasive techniques may result in fewer complications and reduce need for PICU care

## Posterior Fossa Surgery

- Mortality 1%
- Increased neurological deficits 25%
- Pseudobulbar syndrome 5%
- Aseptic meningitis 8%
- Bacterial meningitis 2–8% vs 0.64–1.9%

# Pituitary Surgery

- Pituitary surgery carries high risk for disturbances of water balance. Both SIADH and DI may present in alternating fashion over the first 24–48 hours if there has been hypothalamic damage.
- Overriding principle of management is to achieve a normovolemic, normosmolar state and then "lock in" by replacing only **U/O + Insensible losses.** The choice of fluid replacement in this setting depends on urine composition.
- High urine losses do not necessarily represent DI. It may simply be an appropriate response to hypervolemia.
- DDAVP is an adjunct-only treatment for therapy of DI. It is not mandatory. Use of DDAVP in effect creates a state of SIADH, with all of its attendant risks.

## Diagnostic and Management Principles

DIABETES INSIPIDUS (DI)

- Serum Na+ (Osmo) abnormally elevated
- Dilute urine (Urine osmol < Serum osmol)
- U/O >4 cc/kg/h

Rx: Fluid replacement (U/O + Insens)
　　Choice of replacement fluid reflects urine composition
　　　+/− DDAVP®

SYNDROME OF INAPPROPRIATE ADH (SIADH)

- Serum Na+ (Osmo) low or decreasing
- Concentrated urine (Ur osmol > Serum osmol)
- U/O decreasing
- Euvolemia or hypervolemia

Rx: Fluid restriction

1. **Immediately post-op (in recovery room):**

    a) Send serum electrolytes, creatinine, and blood sugar
    b) Send urine electrolytes, osmolarity, and specific gravity

2. **The following should be monitored in the recovery room and throughout the PICU admission:**

    a) Accurate I&O: fluid intake and urine output hourly (q1h) with complete tally q12 hours (q12h); Foley catheter must be in place

b) Serum electrolytes and osmolarity q4h

c) Urine electrolytes and osmolarity, specific gravity q4h

d) If on steroids: blood glucose b.i.d.

3. **If urine output >4cc/kg/hour:** (may be due to either DI or hypervolemia)

a) Serum electrolytes and osmolarity now and q4h

b) Urine electrolytes and osmolarity now and q4h

4. **If serum Na+ <135:**

a) Urine electrolytes and osmolarity now and q4h

b) Page PICU resident and staff

# References

Gordon N. Mutism: elective selective and acquired. Brain and Development 2001;23:83–7.

Pfisterer W, Muhlbauer M, Czech T, Reinprecht A. Early diagnosisi of external ventricular drainage infection: results of a prospective study. J Neurol Neurosurg Psychiatry 2003;74:929–32.

Wong GKC, Poon WS, Wai S, Yu LM, Lyon D, Lam JMK. Failure of regular external ventricular drain exchange to reduce cerebrospinal fluid infection: result of a randomized control trial. J Neurol Neurosurg Psychiatry 2002;73:759–61.

Mainprize TG, Taylor MD, Rutka JT. Perspectives in pediatric neurosurgery. Child's Nerv Syst 2000;16:809–20.

Venes JL. Infections of CSF Shunt and Intracranial Pressure Monitoring Devices. Infections Diseases of North America 1989;3:289–99.

Bookallil T, Ruggier R. Sodium abnormalities in the neurosurgical patient. Current Anaesthesia and Critical Care 2002;13:153–8.

Bohn D. Salt water and cerebral edema. Critical Care Rounds 2002;3:2.

Harrigan MR. Cerebral salt wasting syndrome: a review. Neurosurgery 1996;38:152–8.

Doxy D, Cruce D, Sklar, F, Swift D, Shapiro K. Posterior fossa syndrome: identifiable risk factors and irreversible complication. Pediatr Neurosurg 1999;31:131–6.

Kestle JRW. Pediatric hydrocephalus: current management. Neurologic Clinics 2003;21:1–9.

Chumas P, Tyagi A, Livingston J. Hydrocephalus what's new? Arch Dis Child Fetal Neonatal Ed 2001;85:F149.

Frawley CP, Dargaville PA, Mitchelle PJ, Tress BM. Clinical course and medical management of neonates with severe cardiac failure related to vein of Galen Malformation. Arch Dis Child Fetal Neonatal Ed 2002;87:F144.

Drake JM, Kestle JR, Milner R, Cinalli G. Randomized trial of cerebrospinal fluid shunt valve design in pediatric hydrocephalus. Neurosuregery 1998;43:294.

Shapiro S, Boaz J, Kleiman M, Kalsbeck J. Origin of organisms infecting ventricular shunts. Neurosurgery 1988;22:868.

Siomin V, Cinalli G, Grotenhuis A, Golash A. Endoscopic third ventriculostomy in patients with cerebrospinal fluid infection and/or hemorrhage. J Neurosurg 2002;97:519.

International PHVD Drug Trial Group. International randomized controlled trial of acetazolamide and furosemide in posthemmorrhagic ventricular dilatation in infancy. Lancet 1998;352:433.

Haines SJ, Lapointe M. Fibrinolytic agents in the management of posthemmorrhagic hydrocephalus in preterm infants: the evidence. Childs Nerv Syst 1999;15:226.

Whitelaw A. Repeated lumbar or ventricular punctures in newborns with intraventricular hemorrhage. Cochrane Database Syst Rev 2001;CD00216.

Kang JK, Lee SW, Baik MW, et al. Perioperative specific management of blood volume loss in craniosynostosis surgery. Childs Nerv Syst 1998 Jul;14:(7):297–301.

Ross D, Rosegay H, Pons V. Differentiation of aseptic and bacterial meningitis in postoperative neurosurgical patients. J Neurosurg 1988;69:669–74.

# B. External Cerebral Ventricular Drainage and Intracranial Pressure Monitoring

Lennox Huang

## Key Principles

- Intracranial pressure (ICP) is affected by changes in pressure or volume of intracranial blood, brain, or cerebrospinal fluid (CSF).
- CSF affects ICP in the following ways:
    - Changes in rate of production of CSF
    - Changes in the rate of absorption of CSF
    - Obstruction to CSF flow
- ICP monitoring with or without external ventricular drainage is a useful therapeutic tool.

## Indications

- Monitor ICP
- Drain free fluid from ventricles and relieve increased ICP
- Treatment of infected internal CSF drain

## Insertion

- Generally performed by a pediatric neurosurgeon
- Should be done in a sterile environment
- May be performed in the operating room or at the bedside in the pediatric intensive care unit (PICU)

## Types of Monitors and Drains

See Figure 1.
- Intraventricular
    - Tip is usually located in the anterior horn of lateral ventricle

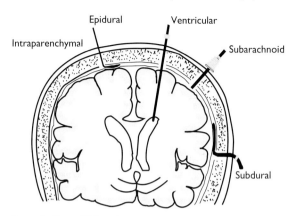

**Figure 1** Types of ICP monitors.

- Can drain CSF and monitor ICP
- Can be calibrated against CSF fluid column
- Gold standard of ICP monitoring

- Intraparenchymal catheter

  - Relatively easy to insert
  - Only monitors ICP, does not drain CSF
  - May have measurement drift

- Subarachnoid bolt

  - Does not drain CSF
  - May be occluded by clots, brain tissue

- Subdural

  - May lose accuracy over time and with cerebral edema

- Epidural

  - Dura not penetrated
  - Less reliable
  - Infrequently used

- Lumbar drain

  - L4–L5 or L5–S1 interspace
  - Not used for ICP monitoring

Catheters may be attached to a variety of transducers. The simplest is an external fluid filled transducer that allows for manual measurement of ICP in the event of electronic equipment failure. Pressure may also be transduced by internal microchip, fiberoptic-diaphragm, or air-filled balloon pouch.

## Monitoring

- Zero point is foramen of Munro—generally at the level of earlobe using a laser level
- ICP waveform has three peaks that correlate with arterial pulsations
- ICP is normally between 0–15 mm Hg
- Cerebral perfusion pressure (CPP) = mean blood pressure-ICP

## Therapeutic Use

- Randomized controlled trial data specifically evaluating outcome of ICP monitoring and therapy is not available and is not likely to be studied in isolation.
- Outcomes from traumatic head injury have improved with the implementation of multiple therapies including better emergency response systems, changes in general ICU care, more sophisticated imaging technologies, and ICP-directed management.
- Despite the paucity of data, ICP monitoring and therapy is considered standard practice in the management of severe traumatic brain injury. Invasive ICP monitoring is more controversial in the setting of coma, encephalopathy, and infectious brain pathology.
- Dose response curve has been demonstrated between CSF drainage and ICP in trauma patients.
- For persistent raised ICP, sterile drainage of a small amount of CSF (3 mL) may decrease ICP.
- CSF drainage may be used to relieve signs or symptoms resulting from pseudotumor cerebri.
- External CSF drainage may be used to relieve pressure and promote healing of persistent CSF leaks—generally lumbar drains are used for this purpose.
- May be used for intrathecal administration of medications.

- Structured therapy including ICP monitor directed interventions can decrease morbidity and mortality for traumatic brain injury (see Chapter 20, "Trauma").

# Complications

- Improper calibration/measurements leading to improper ICP interventions
- Drain blockage leading to increased ICP/herniation
- Excessive drainage may lead to
    - ventricular collapse, cerebral hemorrhage (see below for definitions)
    - inadvertent infusions into external ventricular drain
    - infection

# Infection

- Infection rate about 4–10%
- Diagnosis established by combination of the following: increasing CSF cell counts, positive cultures, clinical symptoms—fever, headache
- Associated with drain blockage, site leakage, duration of external ventricular drain
- Tends to be skin flora; coagulase negative staph and *Staphylococcus aureus*
- Prophylaxis with first-generation cephalosporin, nafcillin, or vancomycin may or may not decrease infection rates—prophylaxis practices vary between centers
- Antibiotic impregnated drains may have lower infection rates

# Troubleshooting

- Ensure proper patient and system position
- Ensure proper calibration/zeroing if applicable
- Inspect drainage system for debris, air
- Temporarily lower drain to increase drainage
- Drainage system may be gently flushed with small amount of sterile saline to clear debris—generally performed by experienced physician
- Excessive drainage—varies depending on patient size and underlying pathology >50 mL/hour is generally considered excessive, drainage may be decreased by raising drain

# References

Drake JM, Crawford MW. Near miss injection of an anesthetic agent into a cerebrospinal fluid external ventricular drain: special report. Neurosurgery 2005;56:E1161.

Guide to the care of the patient with intracranial pressure monitoring. AANN Reference series for clinical practice, American Association of Neuroscience Nurses. 2005.

Kerr ME, Weber BB, Sereika SM, Wilberger J, Marion DW. Dose response to cerebrospinal fluid drainage on cerebral perfusion in traumatic brain-injured adults. Neurosurg Focus 2001;11:1–7.

Schade RP, Schinkel J, Visser LG, et al. Bacterial meningitis caused by the use of ventricular or lumbar cerebrospinal fluid catheters. Neurosurg 2005;102:229–34.

Korinek A-M, Reina M, Boch AL, et al. Prevention of external ventricular drain-related ventriculitis. Acta Neurochirurgica 2005;147:39–46.

# Chapter 11

# Anesthesia/Sedation

Design Reddy

## Pain Assessment

The International Association for the Study of Pain (IASP) defines pain as "an unpleasant sensory and emotional experience associated with actual or potential tissue damage, or described in terms of such damage." Pain can be classified as acute, chronic, and malignant. Untreated or inadequately treated pain produces negative physiological, psychological, behavioral, and psychological problems.

Short-term adverse effects:
  Respiratory
      Tachypnea/respiratory distress
      Splinting leading to atelectasis, V/Q mismatch
  Cardiovascular
      Tachycardia
      Hypertension
  Endocrine
      Stress response: increased cortisol, catecholamines
      (more prolonged in infants vs older children)

Long-term effects manifest as emotional disorders, alteration in subsequent response to stimuli, developmental delays, and alterations in cerebral neuroanatomy.

Pain assessment is a fundamental and essential part of pain treatment; however, it remains one of the most difficult challenges. Many scales are available, but a useful one has to be appropriate for the age of the child, practical, reliable, valid, and reproducible. Scales can be classified into one of three categories. Effective assessment of pain often requires the use of multiple scales, placing the scores in a physiologic context and involving the child's parent or caregiver.

## Self-Report Scales

**Visual Analog Scale (VAS)**    10 cm ruler, markings between "No pain" and "Worst possible pain." Applicable to age 8 years and older.

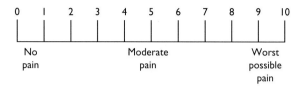

## Faces Scale (eg, Bieri, Wong-Baker, Oucher)

One of the most common pain scales in use: Faces representing different levels of pain intensity. Applicable to children 4 years and older.

### Wong-Baker FACES Pain Rating Scale

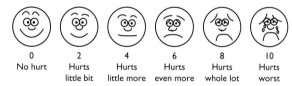

From Wong D.L., Hockenberry-Eaton M., Wilson D., Winkelstein M.L., Schwartz P.: Wong's Essentials of Pediatric Nursing, ed. 6, St. Louis, 2001, p. 1301. Copyrighted by Mosby, Inc. Reprinted by permission.

## Behavioral Scales

**Children's Hospital of Eastern Ontario Pain Scale (CHEOPS)**    Widely validated behavior scale that is applicable to patients from 1 to 7 years of age. Observational scale involving six areas. Scores greater than 4 indicate pain.

Cry      None, Moaning, Crying, Screaming
Facial   Composed, Grimace, Smiling
Verbal   None, Other, Pain, Both, Positive
Torso    Neutral, Shifting, Tense, Shivering, Upright, Restrained
Touch    None, Reach, Touch, Grab, Restrained
Legs     Neutral, Squirming, Drawn-up, Standing, Restrained

**Neonatal Infant Pain Scale (NIPS)**    Developed to measure neonatal response to needle puncture. Recommended for infants less than 1 year old. Scores greater than 3 suggest pain.

| Score | Pain Assessment |
|---|---|
| **Facial Expression** | |
| 0 – Relaxed muscles | Restful face, neutral expression |
| 1 – Grimace | Tight facial muscles; furrowed brow, chin, jaw, (negative facial expression – nose, mouth and brow) |
| **Cry** | |
| 0 – No Cry | Quiet, not crying |
| 1 – Whimper | Mild moaning, intermittent |
| 2 – Vigorous Cry | Loud scream; rising, shrill, continuous (Note: Silent cry may be scored if baby is intubated as evidenced by obvious mouth and facial movement.) |
| **Breathing Patterns** | |
| 0 – Relaxed | Usual pattern for this infant |
| 1 – Change in Breathing | Indrawing, irregular, faster than usual; gagging; breath holding |
| **Arms** | |
| 0 – Relaxed/Restrained | No muscular rigidity; occasional random movements of arms |
| 1 – Flexed/Extended | Tense, straight legs; rigid and/or rapid extension, flexion |
| **Legs** | |
| 0 – Relaxed/Restrained | No muscular rigidity; occasional random leg movement |
| 1 – Flexed/Extended | Tense, straight legs; rigid and/or rapid extension, flexion |
| **State of Arousal** | |
| 0 – Sleeping/Awake | Quiet, peaceful sleeping or alert random leg movement |
| 1 – Fussy | Alert, restless, and thrashing |

## Physiologic Scales

**Premature Infant Pain Profile (PIPP)**    Measures changes in heart rate, oxygen saturation, and facial action. Pain assessment is best accomplished by correlating self-report, behavioral, and physiologic parameters with the child's overall clinical practice.

**Sedation Assessment** Assessment of sedation varies depending on whether short-term procedural sedation is being performed vs long-term sedation in an ICU setting. Sedation is often assessed in a qualitative fashion as outlined in Table 1 and the Ramsay scale. Numeric sedation scales such as the COMFORT score add an objective element to therapy, allowing multiple observers to achieve similar goals with sedation.

"Conscious sedation" is a term that is discouraged, as it is impossible to achieve this level of sedation.

Table 1
**Levels of Sedation**

| Levels of sedation | Verbal response | Pain response | Airway response | Breathing | Circulation |
|---|---|---|---|---|---|
| No sedation | +++++ | +++++ | ++++++ | +++++ | +++++ |
| Minimal sedation | +++ | ++++ | ++++ | +++++ | +++++ |
| Moderate sedation | + | ++ | +++ | +++++ | +++++ |
| Deep sedation | 0 | + | + | ++ | +++ |
| General anesthesia | 0 | 0 | 0 | 0/+ | ++ |

**Ramsay Scale** The Ramsay scale is a six-point scale initially designed to test rousability in adults. While the scale has not been validated for use in PICUs, it does provide a rough qualitative guide to assessment of sedated patients.

1. Patient is anxious and agitated or restless, or both.
2. Patient is co-operative, oriented, and tranquil.
3. Patient responds to commands only.
4. Patient exhibits brisk response to light glabellar tap or loud auditory stimulus.
5. Patient exhibits a sluggish response to light glabellar tap or loud auditory stimulus.
6. Patient exhibits no response.

**COMFORT Scale/Modified Comfort Score** The most commonly utilized tool in pediatric intensive care units. A score designed for and validated in PICUs. It is applicable to all ages for children on a ventilator or unconscious and observes six behavioral and two physiologic indicators:

> Alertness
> Calmness/agitation
> Respiratory response
> Physical movement
> Blood pressure
> Heart rate
> Muscle tone
> Facial tension

Scores range from 8 to 40 with an optimal target range of 17–26. Note that children on neuromuscular blockade cannot be accurately assessed using the COMFORT scale.

**Neuromuscular Function Assessment** Patients with neuromuscular blockade require regular monitoring to assess depth of blockade. For patients on continuous infusions, one approach is to have intermittent windowing of the infusion to assess time until spontaneous movement is regained. For patients in whom full reversal of blockade is necessary (eg, post operative patients), there are four common measures of adequacy.

1. Response to peripheral nerve stimulator
2. Sustained head lift for >5 seconds

3. Sustained hand grip for >5 seconds
4. Maximum negative inspiratory pressure >25 cm $H_2O$

**Peripheral Nerve Stimulation**    A number of patterns can be obtained with a peripheral nerve stimulator. The most common pattern is the Train-of-Four (TOF) ratio (Figure 1). It consists of four supramaximal stimuli causing a muscle to contract. The two patterns involving the TOF are:

1. TOF count: Number of contractions present when muscle is stimulated four times.
2. TOF ratio: Division of the amplitudes of the fourth twitch by the first twitch.

When only one response is present, the degree of neuromuscular blockade is 90–95%. When the fourth twitch reappears, blockade is 60–80%.

The TOF ratio must exceed 0.9 to exclude clinically important residual blockade. The ulnar nerve is stimulated and the adductor pollicis is monitored commonly.

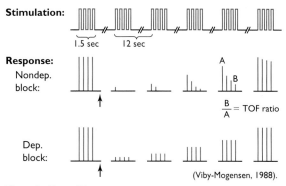

**Figure 1**    Train-of-Four testing.

**Pain Management**    Effective pain management in children starts with behavioral and non-pharmacologic techniques such as psychologic preparation, distraction, imagery, relaxation, anxiolysis, and reduction of parental perception of pain.

Involving the child's parent or caregiver as well as child-life specialists can reduce the need for pharmacologic intervention.

## Simple Measures

1. Sucrose analgesia:
   Safe and effective for procedural pain, such as heel prick blood sampling in neonates.

2. Topical anesthesia:
   EMLA (Eutectic Mixture of Local Anesthetics: prilocaine and lidocaine) Effective when applied 60–90 minutes prior to procedures such as a lumbar puncture, bone marrow sampling, or skin graft donor sites.

3. Wound infiltration (Table 2):
   Useful for surface wounds and tunneling procedures such as placing central venous catheters, arterial lines, and large bore peripheral intravenous lines.
   Useful tips: Use 27–32-gauge needle to infiltrate.
   Bupivicaine will last three times longer than lidocaine.

4. Systemic medications (Table 3):

*Table 2*
### Medications for Wound Infiltration

| Drugs | Maximum doses |
| --- | --- |
| Lidocaine 1% or 2% | 3 mg/kg |
| Lidocaine 1% or 2% with | |
|   epinephrine 1:100 000 | 7 mg/kg |
| Bupivicaine 0.25% or 0.5% | 2 mg/kg |

*Table 3*
### Systemic Analgesic Medications

| Drugs | Route | Dose |
| --- | --- | --- |
| Diclofenac | Oral, rectal | 1 mg/kg/8h |
| Ibuprofen | Oral | 10 mg/kg/8h |
| Ketorolac | Intravenous | 0.5 mg/kg/8h |
| Acetaminophen | Rectal | 40 mg/kg; followed by 30 mg/kg/8h |
| | Oral | 20 mg/kg followed by 30 mg/kg/8h |
| | Newborn, rectal | 20 mg/kg and 30 mg/kg/12h |
| Ketamine | IV | 0.5–2 mg/kg |
| | IM | 3–5 mg/kg |

A multimodal approach with different medications acts synergistically to enhance the analgesic effects with a reduction in the side effects of individual drugs.

## Opioids

- Opiods may be used to provide analgesia and/or sedation
- Opiods commonly used in the PICU are listed in Table 4

*Table 4*
## Opoid Medications

| Drugs | Situation | Dose |
|-------|-----------|------|
| Morphine | Newborn – intermittent dose | 0.02 mg/kg/8h |
| | Newborn (infusion) | 5–15 mcg/kg/h |
| | Children – intermittent dose | 0.05–0.1 mg/kg/6h |
| | Children (infusion) | 0–30 mcg/kg/h |
| Fentanyl | Intermittent dose | 2–10 mcg/kg |
| | Infusion | 2–5 mcg/kg/h |
| Remifentanil | Infusion | 0.1–1 mcg/kg/min |
| Codeine | In combination with acetaminophen | 0.5–1 mg/kg/4h |

## Sedation

### Sedation Goals
- Anxiolysis
- Analgesia
- Amnesia
- Safety
- Behavior control
- Baseline return

## Common Sedative Medications (Table 5)    Note that all of the systemic analgesic medications previously discussed may also be used for sedation. Combining two different medication classes (eg, benzodiazepine + opioid) often results in a synergistic effect. Many sedative medications (especially benzodiazepines) may result in paradoxical reactions with increased agitation and disinhibition.

*Table 5*
## Common Sedative Medications

| Drug | Route | Dose | Comments |
|---|---|---|---|
| **Chloral hydrate** | PO/PR | 25–100 mg/kg/ dose (max 2 g) | Slow onset, variable absorption, and prolonged duration |
| **Pentobarbital** | IV | 2 mg/kg, then 1–2 mg/kg q5–10 min as needed | |
| **Midazolam** | Oral | 0.5–0.75 mg/kg (max 20 mg) | Reversible with flumazenil |
| | IV | 0.05–0.1 mg/kg/ dose | Tolerance develops quickly in young children |
| | | 1–5 mcg/kg/min continuous infusion | Reversible with flumazenil |
| **Lorazepam** | IV | 0.05–0.1 mg/kg/ dose | Reversible with flumazenil |
| | | 1–4 mcg/kg/min | Caution should be used with continuous infusions secondary to accumulation of propylene glycol leading to lactic acidosis |
| **Ketamine** | IV | 0.5–2 mg/kg | Secretagogue, contraindicated with increased ICP |
| **Propofol** | IV | 1–3 mg/kg/dose and/or 50–200 mcg/kg/min | Long-term (>24 hr) use in the PICU is associated with increased mortality in pediatric patients & propofol infusion syndrome |

## Neuromuscular Blockade

Paralysis results when the acetylcholine receptors at the neuromuscular junction are blocked by neuromuscular blocking drugs. There are two types of agents: depolarizing and nondepolarizing drugs (differentiated by mechanism of blockade, reversal of effects, and monitoring response to a nerve stimulator). Neuromuscular blockade should never be administered without accompanying sedation. ICU indications include but are not limited to the following:

Rapid-sequence intubation
Invasive or operative procedures in ICU

*Table 6*
## Neuromuscular Blockade

| Classification | Drugs | Doses | Duration (min) | Infusions |
|---|---|---|---|---|
| **Depolarizing** | Succinylcholine | 1–2 mg/kg | 10 | |
| **Nondepo-larizing** | Mivacurium | 0.2 mg/kg | 15–20 | 10–14 mcg/kg/min |
| | Cisatracurium | 0.1 mg/kg | 35–45 | 1–2 mcg/kg/min |
| | Vecuronium | 0.1 mg/kg | 35–45 | 1–2 mcg/kg/min |
| | Rocuronium | 0.6–1.0 mg/kg | 30–40 | 5–12 mcg/kg/min |
| | Pancuronium | 0.1 mg/kg | 60–120 | |

Ventilator dysynchrony
Reduction of metabolic demand
Assisting in the control of ICP spikes

Notes:

1. Succinylcholine is metabolized by endogenous pseudocholin-esterase in the plasma and liver.
2. Beware of succinylcholine-induced hyperkalemia, particularly in burn patients, spinal cord injury patients, and patients with myopathies (eg, Duchenne's dystrophy).
3. Nondepolarizing drugs are reversed by acetylcholinesterase inhibitors such as neostigmine (0.05 mg/kg).
4. Cisatracurium undergoes degradation by Hoffman elimination (self-destructs at a certain pH and temperature, independent of hepatic and renal function). Therefore, it is useful in patients with hepatic or renal dysfunction.
5. Other nondepolarizing drugs prolonged in the presence of renal or hepatic failure.
6. Succinylcholine is contra indicated in patients susceptible to malignant hyperthermia.

## Withdrawal

Withdrawal may occur in children who have a sudden discontinuation or reduction of prolonged sedative/analgesic medications. Assessment of withdrawal may be difficult as symptoms are often nonspecific and can be confused with age-appropriate responses to illness/hospitalization. Likelihood of withdrawal is associated with duration and dose of the medication administered. Synthetic opioids such as fentanyl may be associated with a higher likelihood of withdrawal. Risk of withdrawal should not limit the use of sedative or analgesic medications in the PICU.

The Neonatal Abstinence Score (NAS) was developed to assess symptoms in infants following in utero exposure to opiates, but has been adopted/modified to be used in PICU environments. Elements of the NAS reflect the behavioral manifestations of a hyper-adrenergic drive in infants and are outlined in Table 7.

Withdrawal may be treated with a variety of modalities:
Behavioral

    In infants, tight swaddling, rocking, holding
    Presence of parent/family members
    Establishing day-night cycle

Pharmacologic

The principles of pharmacologic treatment of withdrawal are as follows:

    1) Short-term control of CNS and adrenergic symptoms
    2) Gradual tapering of medication dose

These principles can be achieved by a number of medications, including:

    1) Slow wean of continuous infusions including:
      a. Opioids
      b. Benzodiazepines
      c. Dexmetetomidine

*Table 7*
**NAS Scoring Elements**

| | |
|---|---|
| Cry | Seizures |
| Sleep | Sweating |
| Moro reflex | Fever |
| Tremors | Respiratory rate/pattern |
| Tone | Feeding |
| Yawning | Stooling |
| Excoriation | |

2) Wean with intermittent dosing of long-acting medications, including:
   a. Opioids (methadone)
   b. Benzodiazepines (lorazepam/diazepam)
   c. Clonidine
   d. Phenobarbital

# Suggested Readings

Marx CM, Smith PG, Lowrie LH, et al. Optimal sedation of mechanically ventilated pediatric critical care patients. Crit Care Med 1994 Jan;22(1):163–70.

Polaner DM. Sedation-analgesia in the pediatric intensive care unit. Pediatr Clin North Am 2001 Jun;48(3):695–714.

Reed MD, Yamashita TS, Marx CM, et al. A pharmacokinetically based propofol dosing strategy for sedation of the critically ill, mechanically ventilated pediatric patient. Crit Care Med 1996 Sep;24(9):1473–81.

Tobias JD. Sedation and analgesia in the pediatric intensive care unit. Pediatr Ann 2005 Aug;34(8):636–45.

Twite MD, Rashid A, Zuk J, Friesen RH. Sedation, analgesia, and neuromuscular blockade in the pediatric intensive care unit: survey of fellowship training programs. Pediatr Crit Care Med 2004 Nov;5(6):521–32.

# Chapter 12

# Intravenous Fluid and Electrolyte Management

Karen Choong

## Overview

This chapter will provide the principles for the acute management of common fluid and electrolyte disorders encountered in the critically ill pediatric patient. There is some overlap with the shock, endocrine, and nephrology chapters. Hence, for elaborated discussions on the pathophysiology of individual disorders, please refer to Chapter 16, "Endocrine," Chapter 5, "Resuscitation," and Chapter 13, "Nephrology."

## Key Principles

- Fluid requirements and management in the critically ill child differ from that of a well or mildly ill patient.
- Safe fluid administration in the PICU is a therapy that requires close assessment and monitoring.
- Electrolyte abnormalities occur frequently in the PICU and may be life-threatening.
- Electrolyte abnormalities should be anticipated based on the patient's clinical condition and managed in a timely manner.

## Maintenance Fluid Requirements

Intravenous (IV) maintenance fluids are designed to provide free water and electrolyte requirements in a fasting patient. Traditional recommendations in children are derived from energy expenditure calculations of three convenient weight-based categories (<10 kg, 10–20 kg, >20 kg) (Table 1). These guidelines also call for sodium and potassium requirements of 3 and 2 mmol/100 kcal/24 hours, respectively, and thus suggest that the ideal maintenance solution in all children and adolescents should be hypotonic (0.2% saline). Advances in our understanding of water and electrolyte handling in health and disease have called into question these recommendations. There is emerging data that there is impaired free-water excretion during illness, and that the most important role of sodium in acute illness is the maintenance of plasma tonicity. Hence isotonic/near isotonic maintenance solutions may be more appropriate in the critically ill patient. Our recommendations for maintenance fluid therapy in the critically ill child are targeted at maintaining tonicity balance, rather than nutritional $Na^+$ calculations. It needs to be emphasized that *no single* solution or formula can be appropriate for *all* patients, and the administration of IV fluids should be individualized and considered an invasive procedure, and therefore should be treated with the same vigilance as medication prescription. Please note that these guidelines do not extend to term and preterm infants, who have unique physiology.

## Baseline Assessment

Hospitalized children receiving parenteral fluid therapy should be considered at risk for developing hyponatremia and monitored closely. Always assess the following prior to ordering and during the administration of IV maintenance fluids.

*Table 1*
**Traditional Recommendations for Determining the Maintenance Calories (and Water) Requirements in Hospitalized Patients**

| Weight | Daily requirements: Kcal/d or mL/d | Hourly requirements: Kcal/h or mL/h |
| --- | --- | --- |
| <10 kg | 100/kg/d | 4/kg/hour |
| 11–20 kg | 1000 + (50/kg/d)* | 40 + (2 mL/kg/h)* |
| >20 kg | 1500 + (20/kg/d)ψ | 60 + (1 mL/kg/h)ψ |

* For each kg >10 kg
ψ For each kg >20 kg

- Extracellular fluid (ECF) volume status
- Accurate weight in kg
- Electrolytes: take plasma sodium into consideration
- Patient risk factors: eg, surgery, central nervous sytem (CNS) disorder, burns, diabetic ketoacidosis (DKA), ECF volume overload, preexisting electrolyte disorder

## Maintenance Fluid Volume

Intravascular volume depletion should be resuscitated first (Chapter 5, "Resuscitation"). Fluid resuscitation and replacement of ongoing losses should be considered and prescribed separately. The traditional recommendations for maintenance fluid volume are shown in Table 1.

## Deviations from this formula

Consider decreasing maintenance fluid volume in the following:

- Decreasing maintenance fluid requirements by 30–50% in *euvolemic, nonfebrile*, ventilated patients. Energy expenditure in physically immobile critically ill children may be less than 40 kcal/kg/day. Insensible water losses may be reduced as much as 30% in patients on a warm humidified air through a ventilator circuit.
- Patients with clinical evidence of ECF volume overload (eg, nephrosis, cirrhosis, congestive heart failure, glomerulonephritis).
- Patients with ALI/ARDS.
- Catabolic patients, acute renal failure (production of endogenous water from tissue catabolism may be increased in acute disease).

Consider increasing maintenance fluid volume in:

- Patients with increased insensible losses—eg, fever, burns, tachypnea in nonventilated patients.
- Volume and rapidity of fluid replacement in patients who are intravascularly depleted is dependent on the severity of their hemodynamic status (see Chapter 5, "Resuscitation"). There are generic tables for estimating degree of volume depletion in hemodynamically stable patients (see Table 2). It is important to bear in mind that the clinical estimation of extracellular volume status in a critically ill child is often difficult and may require adjunctive measurements to these clinical signs (eg, acid-base balance, central venous pressure, serum lactate, central venous oxygen saturation).

*Table 2*
**Estimating Fluid Deficits**

| Severity | Age <1 yr | Age >1 yr | Clinical signs |
|---|---|---|---|
| Mild | 5% (50 mL/kg) | 3% (30 mL/kg) | Few, mild oliguria, thirst, essentially normal exam |
| Modeate | 10% (100 mL/kg) | 6% (60 mL/kg) | Tenting skin turgor, severe thirst, dry mucous membranes, irritability, oliguria |
| Severe | 15% (150 mL/kg) | 9% (90 mL/kg) | Cardiovascular compromise, tachycardia, hypotension, lethargy, sunken fontanelle, anuria |

## Choice of Fluid

Fluid for intravascular volume expansion: should be isotonic (crystalloid or colloid).

Replacement Fluid:

Should reflect volume and composition of fluid loss (eg, GI, renal losses) (Table 3).

Maintenance IV Solutions:

Think of maintenance fluids as containing not just electrolytes, but % electrolyte-free water (EFW) (Table 4).

*Table 3*
**Electrolyte Composition of GI Fluids (mmol/L or mEq/L)**

| Fluid | $Na^+$ | $K^+$ | $Cl^-$ | $H^+$ | $HCO_3$ |
|---|---|---|---|---|---|
| Gastric | 20–80 | 5–30 | 100–120 | 80 | 0 |
| Bile | 120–140 | 2–10 | 90–120 | 0 | 50 |
| Ileostomy | 100–140 | 5–15 | 80–120 | 0 | 30 |
| Diarrheal | 10–90 | 10–80 | 10–110 | 0 | 40 |

*Table 4*
**Electrolyte Free Water (EFW) Content of Parenteral Fluids**

| IV solution | Na (mmol/L) | K⁺ | Cl⁻ | In vitro osmolality$^\Phi$ (mOsm/L) | In vivo tonicity$^\Psi$ (mOsm/L) | % Electrolyte free water* |
|---|---|---|---|---|---|---|
| 5% dextrose in water | 0 | 0 | 0 | 252 | 0 | 100 |
| 0.2% NaCl in 5% dextrose in water | 34 | 0 | 34 | 321 | 68 | 78 |
| 0.45% NaCl | 77 | 0 | 77 | 154 | 154 | 50 |
| 0.45% NaCl in 5% dextrose in water | 77 | 0 | 77 | 406 | 154 | 50 |
| Lactated Ringer's | 130 | 4 | 109 | 273 | 160 | 16 |
| 5% dextrose lactated Ringer's | 130 | 4 | 109 | 525 | 160 | 16 |
| 0.9% NaCl | 154 | 0 | 154 | 308 | 308 | 0 |
| 0.9% NaCl in 5% dextrose in water | 154 | 0 | 154 | 560 | 308 | 0 |

* Based on a sodium plus potassium concentration in the aqueous phase of plasma of 154 mmol/L, assuming that plasma is 93% water with a plasma sodium of 140 mmol/L and a potassium concentration of 4 mmol/L.
$^\Phi$ In vitro osmolarity refers to the number of osmoles of solute per liter of solution.
$^\Psi$ In vivo tonicity refers to the total concentration of solutes that exert an osmotic force across a cell membrane. This excludes the effect of dextrose as it is rapidly metabolized in blood.

When to consider isotonic maintenance solutions.

- Isotonic (eg, 0.9% saline) or near isotonic (lactated Ringer's) solutions may minimize changes in Plasma Na⁺ (PNa)
- Isotonic fluids are indicated when the objective is to maintain high effective osmolality (ie, a patient with or has potential for cerebral edema, eg, CNS disorder, DKA).

- Isotonic fluids should be considered in patients who are at increased risk of developing hyponatremia, eg, in conditions where there are non-osmotic stimuli for antidiuretic hormone secretion (acute infection, hypoxia, acute postoperative period, particularly orthopaedic and craniofacial surgery).
- Add dextrose (eg, 5% concentration) with the goal of maintaining normoglycemia.
- Add $K^+$ to provide 1–2 mEq/kg/day.

When to consider EFW/hypotonic maintenance solutions:

- Hypotonic solutions should be administered if the goal is to create a positive balance for EFW, eg,

    1. To match daily loss of EFW in sweat in a patient with PNa >138 mmol/L
    2. PNa significantly >145 mmol/L and patient is symptomatic
    3. Ongoing free water losses (renal, GI, skin) or a free-water deficit

- To avoid solute loading in patients with established third space overload, eg, congestive heart failure, nephritic syndrome, cirrhosis.
- Neonatal population.
- Do NOT give hypotonic solutions when PNa <138 mmol/L in the absence of hypoglycemia, unless patient is expected to have a rapid water diuresis, and the goal is to limit the rise in PNa.
- Caution in patients at greater risk of developing a more severe decline in PNa with EFW administration:

    - Young age (brains have larger ICF volume/total skull volume)
    - Small skeletal muscle mass

## Daily Monitoring

Maintenance IV fluid therapy should be monitored and individualized daily and dictated by patient's clinical status and response. EFW prescription should be adjusted in response to changes in PNa. High PNa implies free-water deficit; low/falling PNa indicates EFW excess. The frequency of monitoring will be dependent on the individual patient's condition, expected fluid shifts or losses, and their clinical course. Fluid volume and composition should be adjusted depending on the following minimal parameters:

- Intravascular volume status
- Fluid balance—should be assessed at least every 12 hours
- Daily weights
- Biochemistry: maintain electrolyte balance
- Glucose: maintain normoglycemia

# Salt and Water Balance

## Total Body Water (TBW)

- Proportion of body weight that is body water varies with age, sex, fat content. There is a nonlinear change in TBW with age:

  - 85% in premature infant
  - 78% in full-term infant
  - 55–60% in an adult

- TBW is distributed between the intracellular and extracellular space. The ECF:ICF ratio also changes with age, being the highest in the fetus, and progressively decreases during childhood, to reach lowest point in early adulthood (at which time 60% of TBW is intracellular, 40% extracellular). Three-fourths of ECF is distributed in the interstitial space, and ¼ in plasma.
- Integrated role of thirst, vasopressin and renin-angiotensin-aldosterone system, and renal handling of filtered $Na^+$ are responsible for maintaining the tight balance between $Na^+$ and water. $Na^+$ is the major osmotically active extracellular cation, and hence is the main determinant of ECF volume. Abnormalities in ECF volume are, therefore, primarily related to abnormalities in $Na^+$.
- Normal range for plasma Na: 136–145 mmol/L.

# Hyponatremia

Definition: PNa <136 mmol/L

Manifestations: Severity of symptoms is proportional to the rate of drop in PNa and degree of hyponatremia. A rapid decline in PNa (over several hours) results in intracellular edema, which is well tolerated by most tissues, but not well tolerated within the boney calvarium. Hence clinical manifestations of hyponatremia are primarily related to cerebral edema. Gradual decline (days–weeks) in PNa allows compensatory mechanisms to occur, and hence symptoms are milder. Children with hyponatremia are at higher risk of neurologic morbidity than adults.

Nonspecific symptoms: nausea, vomiting, headache, lethargy.
Severe hyponatremia (typically PNa <125 mmol/L or higher in patients at risk) may progress to seizures, coma, and brainstem herniation.

Etiology: Almost always due to a defect in water balance

- See diagnostic approach—Figure 1

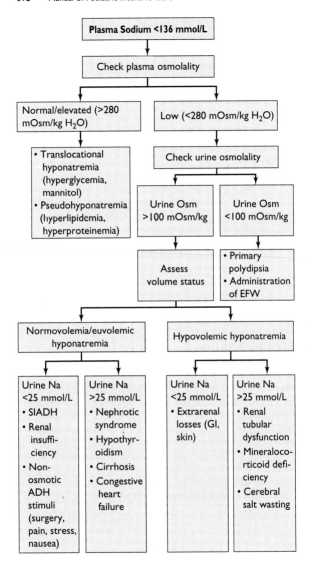

**Figure 1**   Diagnostic approach to hyponatremia.

- Extent of investigation depends on history and degree of clinical suspicion
- Plasma and urine osmolarity and electrolytes are useful in assessing etiology

Management: Management strategy depends on the underlying cause and severity of symptoms.

## Severe Acute Hyponatremia

- Defined arbitrarily as PNa ≤125 mmol/L or any PNa associated with symptoms.
- Symptomatic hyponatremia is a medical emergency.
- Principles of treatment: Rapidly raise PNa to a "safe" level, eg, to a PNa of 130 mmol/L, or when neurological symptoms improve and patient stops seizing, whichever occurs first. Then gradually correct remaining sodium deficit

  - For immediate correction:
    3–5 mL/kg of hypertonic saline (3% NaCl) over 30 minutes (1.2 mL/kg of 3% NaCl raises the PNa about 1 mmol/L).
  - Gradual correction—replace estimated sodium deficit:

    $Na^+$ deficit = %TBW × lean body weight in kg × (target plasma sodium − present plasma sodium).

    Target a maximum rate of serum sodium increase of 0.5 mmol/L–1.0 mmol/L per hour to decrease the risk of central demyelinating lesions.

- Furosemide may be added to enhance water excretion if urine osmolality is high (>300 mOsm/kg), and patient is not hypovolemic.

Management of hyponatremia otherwise depends on (a) the assessment of the volume status of the patient and (b) the underlying cause (Figure 1a).

# Hypernatremia

Definition: PNa >145 mmol/L

Manifestations: Nonspecific—irritability, progressive lethargy, listlessness, may progress to seizures and coma. Signs: doughy or velvety skin, signs of volume loss is less pronounced due to

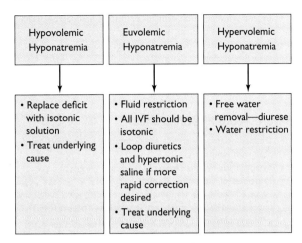

**Figure 1a**  Management of underlying cause of hyponatremia.

preservation of ECF volume. Risks/sequelae: transient cellular dehydration, central demyelenating lesions, venous sinus thrombosis, intracranial hemorrhage, rhabdomyolisis with severe hypernatremia.

Etiology: often multifactorial. See diagnostic approach Figure 2.

- Check urine volume, fluid balance, urine specific gravity, osmolality, and electrolytes
- Urine <800 mOsm/L (less than maximally concentrated)— implies renal concentrating defect
- Urine specific gravity: low (often <1.005) in diabetes insipidus

Management principles:

- Restore circulating volume depletion first—volume expansion with isotonic crystalloid or colloid.
- Estimate and correct EFW deficit—rate of correction depends on a) underlying cause and b) severity of hypernatremia.

Rule of thumb: EFW deficit (mL) = 4 mL × lean body weight (kg) × desired change in PNa mmol/L

- Volume of fluid will depend on EFW composition of solution used (Table 3).

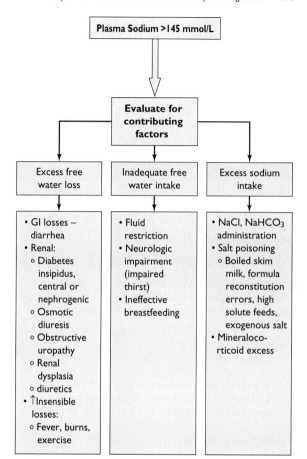

**Figure 2**   Diagnostic approach to hypernatremia.

- Rapid correction may lead to cerebral edema.
- Ideal rate of correction is unknown, but in general, unless encephalopathic, lower PNa by no more than 0.5 mmol/L per hour or maximum of 15 mmol/L/day. Hence start with isotonic fluid (depending on severity of hypernatremia), and progress to fluid with more EFW composition to achieve target rate of drop in PNa.

- Monitor neurologic status and electrolytes hourly in acute phase of therapy to ensure target correction rate.

# Potassium

Plasma $K^+$ concentration is determined by the relationship between $K^+$ intake, distribution of $K^+$ between cells and ECF, and urinary $K^+$ excretion. $K^+$ is tightly regulated because cellular and urinary adaptations prevent significant $K^+$ accumulation in the ECF. Plasma $K^+$ doesn't reflect total $K^+$ body stores, as nearly 98% of $K^+$ is intracellular. Small changes in the extracellular potassium level can have profound effects on the function of the cardiovascular and neuromuscular systems. The reference range for plasma $K^+$ is 3.5–5 mmol/L.

# Hyperkalemia

Definition: Plasma $K^+$ greater than 5.5 mmol/L.

Manifestations: symptoms generally don't manifest until $K^+$ exceeds 7.0 mmol/L, unless that rate or rise is very rapid. Symptoms are otherwise related to the underlying cause.

- Neuromuscular: paresthesia, weakness, may progress to flaccid paralysis.
- Cardiac conduction abnormalities—sequence of electrocardiographic (ECG) changes is illustrated in Figure 3. Large interpatient variability exists with respect to actual $K^+$ and progression of ECG changes, partly related to concomitant associated abnormalities in acid-base balance, $Ca^+$, or $Na^+$.

Etiology:

Increased $K^+$ release from cells

- Pseudohyperkalemia (leakage of $K^+$ out of cells which occurs after specimen collected, eg, hemolyzed specimen)
- Transmembrane shifts
  - Metabolic acidosis
  - Medications: acute digitalis toxicity, beta-blockers

$K^+$ supplements

Reduced urinary $K^+$ excretion
- Renal failure
- Hypoaldosteronism
- Hyperkalemic type I RTA
- Uterojejunostomy
- Drugs: $K^+$-sparing diuretics, cyclosporine, NSAIDS
- Sickle cell disease
- Urinary obstruction

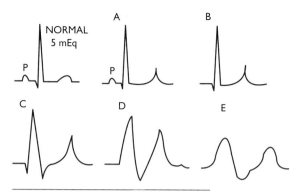

| K⁺ (mmol/L or mEq/L) | ECG Changes |
|---|---|
| 5.5–6.5 | Peaking of T waves |
| >6.5 | Lengthening of QRS interval |
| >7 | P wave amplitude diminished and P-R interval increases |
| >8 | P wave disappears |
| 12–14 | VF or asystole |

**Figure 3**   Classical ECG changes of hyperkalemia.

- Cell breakdown (eg, tumor lysis syndrome, burns, rhabdomyolysis, blood transfusions)
- Succinylcholine in patients with burns, extensive trauma, neuromuscular disease

Management:

- Ensure specimen was not factitious or hemolyzed
- Individualize treatment based upon the patient's presentation, K⁺ level, and ECG changes
- Assess ABCs and promptly evaluate the patient's cardiac status with an ECG
- Ensure continuous ECG monitoring with frequent vital sign checks
- Treat underlying cause

Specific treatment: If the hyperkalemia is severe (potassium >7.0 mmol/L) or the patient is symptomatic or has ECG changes, begin treatment before identifying underlying cause (Table 5).

# Hypokalemia

Definition: Plasma K less than 3.5 mmol/L

Manifestations:

- Nonspecific and may involve the GI, renal, musculoskeletal, cardiac, and nervous systems. Severe hypokalemia may result in hypotension, brady- or tachyarrhythmias, ventricular arrhythmias, and respiratory depression.
- ECG changes

    - T-wave flattening or inverted T waves
    - Prominent U wave that appears as QT prolongation
    - ST segment depression
    - Ventricular or arrhythmias

Etiology: Hypokalemia may result from the movement of potassium into cells without loss of potassium from the body.

### Renal losses

- Renal tubular dysfunction
- Mineralocorticoid excess
- Salt wasting nephropathies
- Hypomagnesemia
- Leukemia (mechanism uncertain)
- Drugs: diuretics, amphotericin B, aminoglycosides
- Metabolic acidosis (degree of $K^+$ depletion masked by transcellular shift of K to ECF)

### Malnutrition or decreased dietary intake

### Excess removal/dilution

- Dialysis, plasmapheresis

### GI losses

- Vomiting or nasogastric drainage
- Diarrhea
- Enemas or laxative use
- Ileal loop

### Transcellular shift (increased $K^+$ entry into cells, resulting in transient hypokalemia)

- Insulin
- Alkalosis
- Beta$_2$-adrenergic agents
- Hypothermia

*Table 5*
## Emergency Management of Acute Hyperkalemia

| Effect | Agent | Dose | Comment |
|---|---|---|---|
| Antagonize cell membrane effects of ↑K$^+$ | Calcium chloride | 10–20 mg/kg/dose, max 1 g (0.1–0.2 mL/kg/dose of 10% calcium chloride, max 10 mL) | Infuse over 2–5 min |
| | Calcium gluconate | 50–100 mg/kg/dose, max 3 g (0.5–1 mL/kg/dose, max 30 mL) | Infuse over 2–5 min |
| Shift K from ECF into ICF space | NaHCO$_3$ | 1–2 mEq IV max 50 mEq (1–2 mL/kg of 8.4% solution, max 50 mL) | Infuse over 5–10 min |
| | Insulin and dextrose | 0.1 unit/kg regular insulin with dextrose infusion (0.5 g/kg or 2 mL/kg D25) IV over 30 min | Monitor glucose to avoid hypoglycemia |
| Increase cellular reuptake of K$^+$ | Beta$_2$-adrenergic agonists | Salbutamol: Inhaled: 2.5–5 mg (0.5–1 mL of 5 mg/mL solution) IV: 4 microgram/kg over 20 min | |
| Remove K$^+$ from body | Binding resins | Sodium polystyrene sulfonate: PO/PR: 0.5–1 g/kg (usual maximum 30–60 g/dose) | |
| | Diuretics | Furosemide 1 mg/kg/dose IV | |
| | Dialysis | | |

Management:

- Therapy depends on severity of symptoms, $K^+$ levels, and underlying cause. If the patient is severely bradycardic or manifesting cardiac arrhythmias, appropriate pharmacologic therapy and/or cardiac pacing should be considered.
- Patients with mild or moderate hypokalemia (potassium of 2.5–3.5 mmol/L), and are asymptomatic, or have only minor symptoms need only oral potassium replacement therapy—1–4 mmol/kg/24 h of KCl PO divided bid/qid. If patient is nothing by mouth (NPO), ensure adequate $K^+$ in maintenance IV.
- Patients in whom severe hypokalemia (less than 2.5 mmol/L) is suspected should be placed on a continuous ECG monitor; establish intravenous (IV) access and assess respiratory status. IV potassium should be given 0.5–1 mmol/kg/dose *slowly*. Maximum rate of administration 0.5 mmol/kg/h or 20 mmol/h, whichever is less.
- Plasma $K^+$ is difficult to replenish if magnesium is also low. Look to replace both.

# Calcium

Calcium regulation is critical for normal cell function, neural transmission, membrane stability, bone structure, blood coagulation, and intracellular signalling. Calcium regulation is maintained by parathyroid hormone (PTH), vitamin D, and calcitonin through complex feedback loops. These compounds act primarily at bone, renal, and GI sites. Calcium also is affected by magnesium and phosphorus. Calcium is measured either bound to protein, or as unbound (ionized) cation $Ca^{2+}$. The ionized $Ca^{2+}$ should be measured whenever low serum protein or pH is abnormal. Adjusted $Ca^{2+}$ mmol/L

*Table 6*
**Normal Reference Ranges for $Ca^{2+}$**

|  | Total Ca mmol/L | Ionized Ca mmol/L |
| --- | --- | --- |
| <2 weeks | 1.80–2.65 | 0.9–1.30 |
| >2 weeks | 2.10–2.65 | 1.10–1.35 |

for hypoalbuminemia: corrected $Ca^{2+}$ = total $Ca^{2+}$ + 0.02 (40—albumin).

Note: none of the various correction factors for determining the effects of hypoalbuminemia on the plasma calcium concentration has proven reliable.

# Hypocalcemia

Manifestations:

- Neuromuscular: irritability, confusion, hallucinations, dementia, extrapyramidal manifestations, and seizures (Chvostek sign and Trousseau sign)
- Cardiovascular: depressed myocardial contractility, hypotension, bradyarrhythmias, decreased response to exogenous catecholamines
- Respiratory: laryngospasm, bronchospasm

Causes:

- PTH deficiency/resistance

  - Congenital hypoplasia/aplasia—eg, DiGeorge syndrome
  - Autoimmune hypoparathyroidism
  - Hypo- or hypermagnesemia
  - Pseudohypoparathyroidism—eg, Albright disease

- Vitamin D deficiency/resistance

  - Inadequate intake, lack of sunlight
  - Renal and hepatic dysfunction
  - Malabsorption
  - Medications: eg, phenobarbital and phenytoin

- Acute loss of $Ca^{2+}$ from circulation

  - Rhabdomyolysis, tumor lysis syndrome

- Chelation or precipitation

  - Hyperphosphatemia, EDTA, citrate (transfused blood), lactate, bicarbonate, medications: eg, calcitonin, bisphosphonates, forcarnet, ethylene glycol

- Acute pancreatitis
- Malignancy: Osteoblastic skeletal metastases

Management:

- Mild hypocalcemia: The majority of hypocalcemic emergencies are mild and require only supportive treatment and further laboratory evaluation.

  - Confirm ionized hypocalcemia and check other pertinent laboratory tests.
  - If the cause is not obvious, send for a PTH level.
  - Depending on the PTH level, the endocrinologist may do further laboratory workup, particularly an evaluation of vitamin D levels.
  - Oral repletion may be indicated for outpatient treatment; patients requiring intravenous (IV) repletion should be admitted.

- Severe hypocalcemia (potential life-threatening symptoms—ie, CNS irritability or hemodynamic instability)

  - Supportive treatment often is required prior to directed treatment of hypocalcemia (ie, IV, oxygen, monitoring). Be aware that severe hypocalcemia often is associated with other life-threatening conditions.
  - Check ionized calcium and other pertinent screening laboratory tests.
  - IV replacement:

    - Calcium gluconate: 50–100 mg of calcium gluconate/kg/dose IV (usual maximum 3 g/dose) or add 1 g of calcium gluconate to a total of 50 mL NS (0.046 mmol/mL) and give 0.05–0.1 mmol/kg/h (1–2 mL/kg/h), adjust rate q4h.
    - Calcium chloride: 10–20 mg of calcium chloride/kg/dose IV (usual maximum 1 g/dose).

  - $Ca^{2+}$ should be infused *slowly*, under continuous cardiorespiratory monitoring.

# Hypercalcemia

Manifestations: nonspecific—weakness, lethargy, depression, anorexia, nausea, vomiting, abdominal pain, constipation, polyuria.

Causes:

- Hyperparathyroidism
- Pharmacologic agents—thiazide, calcium carbonate (antacid), hypervitaminosis D, hypervitaminosis A, lithium, milk-alkali syndrome, and theophylline toxicity

*Table 7*

**Normal Ranges for Mg: Approximately a Third of Mg is Protein-Bound Analogous to Plasma Calcium, the Free (ie, Unbound) Fraction of Magnesium Is the Active Component**

|  | mmol/L | mEq/L |
|---|---|---|
| Newborn | 0.75–1.15 | 1.5–2.3 |
| Child | 0.7–0.95 | 1.4–1.9 |
| Adult | 0.65–1.0 | 1.3–2.0 |
| Ionized | 0.54–0.67 | |

- Endocrinopathies (nonparathyroid)—hyperthyroidism, adrenal insufficiency, and pheochromocytoma
- Immobility
- Chronic renal failure with aplastic bone disease
- Acute renal failure
- Tertiary hyperparathyroidism—postrenal transplant and initiation of chronic hemodialysis
- Familial hypocalciuric hypercalcemia
- Neoplasm related: ↑ osteoclastic bone activity
- Granulomatous disease

Management: therapy should be tailored depending on degree of hypercalcemia, severity of dehydration, and underlying cause

Goals of acute management:

- Stabilization and reduction of the calcium level
- Adequate hydration: volume expansion with IV crystalloid/colloid
- Increased urinary calcium excretion: loop diuretics (furosemide)
- Inhibition of osteoclast activity in the bone
- Discontinuation of pharmacologic agents associated with hypercalcemia
- Treatment of the underlying cause
- Dialysis is necessary to correct hypercalcemia in patients with renal failure

# Magnesium

Magnesium (Mg) is the second-most abundant intracellular cation. Mg is involved in nearly every aspect of biochemical metabolism (eg, deoxyribonucleic acid [DNA] and protein synthesis, glycolysis, oxidative phosphorylation). Almost all enzymes involved in phosphorus reactions (eg, adenosine triphosphatase [ATPase]) require magnesium for activation. Magnesium serves as a molecular stabilizer of ribonucleic acid (RNA), DNA, and ribosomes. Because magnesium is bound to ATP inside the cell, shifts in intracellular magnesium concentration may help regulate cellular bioenergetics such as mitochondrial respiration. Approximately 60% of total body magnesium is located in bone, and the remainder is in the soft tissues. Because less than 2% is present in the ECF compartment, serum levels do not necessarily reflect the status of total body stores.

# Hypomagnesemia

Manifestations:

- Neuromuscular irritability: hyperreflexia, muscle cramps, Trousseau and Chvostek signs, esophageal dysmotility
- CNS hyperexcitability, disorientation, psychosis, ataxia
- Cardiac arrhythmias
- Neonates: apnea, weakness, jitteriness, seizures

Etiology: The causes of hypomagnesemia are numerous. Most causes are related to renal and GI losses.

- GI losses: malabsorption, chronic diarrhea, laxative abuse, inflammatory bowel disease, or neoplasm
- Decreased dietary intake
- Renal losses: primary renal disorders or secondary causes (eg, drugs, hormones, osmotic load)
- Drugs: diuretics, cisplatin, pentamidine, fluoride poisoning
- Endocrine disorders: primary aldosteronism, hypoparathyroidism
- Osmotic diuresis: eg, diabetic ketoacidosis

Management: Treatment of hypomagnesemia depends on the degree of deficiency and the clinical effects. Oral replacement is appropriate for mild symptoms, while IV replacement is indicated for severe clinical effects.

- Routine replacement: 25–100 mg/kg of magnesium sulfate (maximum 5 g) IV. Usual maximum rate is 20 mg/kg of magnesium sulfate/h.
- Treat life-threatening dysrhythmias: 25–50 mg/kg of magnesium sulfate (maximum 2 g) rapid infusion.
- Usual dilution for infusion is 10 mg of magnesium sulphate/mL.

- Risks involved with IV magnesium therapy include hypermagnesemia, hypocalcemia, and sudden hypotension. Continuously monitor electrolytes and hemodynamic parameters during replacement under high infusion rates.
- Treat seizures with benzodiazepines.
- Perform history, physical examination, and appropriate laboratory tests.
- Treat underlying cause.

# Hypermagnesemia

The most common cause of hypermagnesemia is renal failure. Other causes include the following:

- Excessive intake
- Lithium therapy
- Hypothyroidism
- Addison disease
- Familial hypocalciuric hypercalcemia
- Milk alkali syndrome
- Depression

Manifestations: Symptoms of hypomagnesemia usually are not apparent unless the serum magnesium level is greater than 2 mmol/L. Concomitant hypocalcemia, hyperkalemia, or uremia exaggerates the symptoms of hypermagnesemia at any given level.

- Neuromuscular: hyporeflexia, weakness, flaccid paralysis, apnea
- CVS: conduction abnormalities, bradyarrhythmias, vasodilation and hypotension, cardiac arrest
- Hypocalcemia
- Platelet clumping and delayed thrombin formation
- Nonspecific: nausea, vomiting

Management:

- In patients with symptomatic hypermagnesemia that is causing cardiac effects or respiratory distress, antagonize the effects by infusing calcium. Calcium directly antagonizes neuromuscular and cardiovascular effects of magnesium. Use for patients with symptomatic hypermagnesemia that is causing cardiac effects or respiratory distress.

  (See hyperkalemia section for dosing and administration of calcium.)

- Glucose and insulin—May help promote magnesium entry into cells (see hyperkalemia section for dosing and administration).
- Furosemide may promote excretion of magnesium.

# References

Holliday MA, Segar ME. The maintenance need for water in parenteral fluid therapy. Pediatrics 1957;19:823–32.

Wallace WM. Quantitative requirements of infant and child for water and electrolytes under varying conditions. American Journal of Clinical Pathology 1953;23:1133–41.

Darrow DC, Pratt EL. Fluid therapy, relation to tissue composition and expenditure of water and electrolytes. JAMA 1950;143:432–9.

Duke T, Molyneux EM. Intravenous fluids for seriously ill children: time to reconsider.[see comment]. Lancet 2003;362:1320–3.

Taylor D, Durward A. Pouring salt on troubled waters. Arch Dis Child 2004; 89:411–4.

Gerigk M, Gnehm H, Rascher W. Arginine vasopressin and renin in acutely ill children: implication for fluid therapy. Acta Paediatr 1996;85:550–3.

Hoorn EJ, Geary D, Robb M, et al. Acute hyponatremia related to intravenous fluid administration in hospitalized children: an observational study. [see comment]. Pediatrics 2004;113:1279–4.

Judd BA, Haycock GB, Dalton RN, et al. Antidiuretic hormone following surgery in children. Acta Paediatrica Scandinavica 1990;79:461–6.

Moritz ML, Ayus JC. Prevention of hospital-acquired hyponatremia: a case for using isotonic saline. [see comment]. Pediatrics 2003;111:227–30.

Neville K, Verge C, Rosenberg A, et al. Isotonic is better than hypotonic saline for intravenous rehydration of children with gastroenteritis: a prospective randomised study. Arch Dis Child 2006;91:226–32.

Choong K, Kho M, Menon K, et al. Hypotonic versus isotonic saline in hospitalised children: a systematic review. Arch Dis Child 2006;91: 828–35.

Shafiee MAS, Bohn D, Hoorn EJ, et al. How to select optimal maintenance intravenous fluid therapy. [see comment]. Q J Med 2003;96:601–10.

Sosulski R, Polin RA, Baumgart S. Respiratory water loss and heat balance in intubated infants receiving humidified air. J Pediatr 1983;103:307–10.

Lewis CA, Martin GS. Understanding and managing fluid balance in patients with acute lungs injury. Curr Opin Crit Care 2004;10:13–7.

Choong K, Bohn D. Maintenance parenteral fluids in the critically ill child. Jornal de Pediatria 2007;83:S3–10.

# Chapter 13

# Nephrology

## A. Hypertensive Emergencies
Emad Zaki

### Key Principles

- Hypertensive emergencies may result in multi-system organ damage and should be managed initially in the PICU.
- Initiation of treatment should not be delayed for diagnosis.
- Continuous close monitoring is needed to prevent precipitous blood pressure drops.
- Ideal PICU management includes a short-acting titratable parenteral agent.

### Hypertensive Emergencies

Hypertension is common in the pediatric intensive care unit (PICU). It may be the primary reason for hospitalization or it may develop as a complication during the course of a hospital admission.

### Definition

Hypertension: Average systolic or average diastolic greater than the 95th percentile for age, gender, and height. Note that normal blood pressures also have variation according to race and nation. (See Table 1.)

"Hypertensive emergency" replaces the previously used term "hypertensive crisis." Hypertensive emergencies occur when elevated blood pressure results in target organ damage

*Table 1*

**95th Percentile for Blood Pressure Assuming 50th Percentile for Height**

| Age | Boys | Girls |
|---|---|---|
| 1 year | 103/56 | 104/58 |
| 5 years | 112/72 | 110/72 |
| 10 years | 117/80 | 119/78 |
| 15 years | 131/83 | 127/83 |

Adopted from NHLBI 2004 tables.

this is distinguished from hypertensive urgencies where no target organ damage has occurred. Hypertensive emergencies should also be distinguished from increased blood pressure from a known underlying primary pathology such as head injury with increased ICP.

Examples of target organ damage include hypertensive encephalopathy, heart failure, intracranial and/or retinal hemorrhage and papilledema, and renal failure. The term malignant hypertension refers to a hypertensive emergency with neuroretinopathy complications.

## Pathophysiology

Hypertension may have numerous pathophysiologic implications for a variety of organ systems. Hypertensive encephalopathy is the most common critical complication of severe hypertension in pediatrics. It is the cerebral dysfunction that results from an acute rise in blood pressure that overcomes the autoregulatory mechanism of the central nervous system.

Normally, cerebral blood flow is maintained at a constant level despite fluctuations in blood pressure. This is due to the protective autoregulatory mechanism that involves dynamic alterations of intracerebral vascular resistance. If there is a chronic hypertension, the range of tolerance increases to higher ranges of blood pressure. However, even then, an acute rise in the hypertension may overwhelm autoregulation. This results in an increased cerebral perfusion due to impaired blood-brain barrier integrity, with a hydrostatic capillary leak. Unless the systemic blood pressure is dropped, arteriolar damage and necrosis occur—with cerebral edema, and papilledema. This leads to decreased blood flow that may result in ischemic changes, micro-infarcts, and necrosis.

# Etiologies of Hypertension

## Renal

- **Parenchymal renal disease**
  - Post-infectious glomerulonephritis
  - Nephrotic syndrome
  - Membranoproliferative glomerulonephritis

- **Vasculitis/Renovascular**

  - Systemic lupus nephritis
  - Henoch-Schönlein purpura (HSP)
  - Hemolytic uremic syndrome (HUS)
  - Thrombotic thrombocytopenic purpura (TTP)
  - Scleroderma
  - Polyarteritis nodosa (PAN)
  - Kawasaki disease
  - Takayasu's arteritis
  - Renal artery stenosis or thrombosis
  - Sickle cell nephropathy

- **Congenital malformation**
  - Cystic kidney disease (autosomal dominant or recessive)
  - Renal dysplasia
  - Tuberous sclerosis
  - Obstructive uropathy
  - Reflux nephropathy

- **Renal tumors**

  - Wilms' tumor
  - Renal cell carcinoma
  - Hemangiopericytoma

- **Acute and chronic renal insufficiency**

## Cardiovascular

- Aortic coarctation
- Arteriovenous fistula
- Polycythemia

## Endocrine

- Cushing's syndrome
- Hyperaldosteronism
- Hyperthyroidism

- Catecholamine excreting tumor (pheochromocytoma and neuroblastoma)

## Central nervous system

- Intracranial tumor
- Increased intracranial pressure
- Meningoencephalitis
- Dysautonomia (Riley-Day syndrome)

## Drugs

- Corticosteroids
- Amphetamines
- Clonidine withdrawal
- Cyclosporine
- Drugs of abuse (cocaine)

## Miscellaneous

- Insect bites (scorpion venom)
- Posttransplant hypertension
- Intravascular volume overload
- Pain
- Severe anxiety
- Severe burn

## Clinical Features

Clinical features are related to the underlying cause. Characteristic clinical features of hypertensive encephalopathy include severe headache, vomiting, blurred vision, papilledema, altered sensorium, localized neurological signs, and/or convulsion. In the PICU, this constellation of symptoms may be confused with other disease processes such as delirium or withdrawal.

## Evaluation

A focused history should be obtained and directed toward renal, endocrine, cardiac, and neurological disorders. Be sure to inquire about current medications and substance abuse. Physical examination should be performed with emphasis on the cardiovascular, abdominal, neurological, and fundus evaluation. A four-limb blood pressure should be obtained to rule out coarctation of the aorta or other vascular anomalies.

Initial investigations should be guided by patient presentation and may include:

- Complete blood count (CBC)
- Serum electrolytes
- Serum calcium and phosphorus
- BUN, creatinine
- Glucose
- Plasma catecholamine
- Aldosterone level
- Plasma renin activity
- Thyroid stimulating hormone/T4
- Urine analysis and culture
- Toxicology screen
- Chest x-ray—screening
- Renal ultrasound with Doppler
- Echocardiogram—for ventricular hypertrophy or cardiac lesions
- CT head—for acute bleeds/mass lesions
- MRI for posterior reversible encephalopathy syndrome or other changes associated with chronic hypertension

## Acute and Continuing Management

Initiation of immediate and effective control of hypertension is a key factor in determining the eventual outcome in hypertensive emergencies. Rapid normalization or overcorrection of blood pressure may increase the risk of cerebral and cardiac ischemia, especially when target organ damage is not present. Therefore, a reasonably safe approach is to decrease blood pressure by one-third of the desired reduction over the first 6 hours and the remainder over the following 12 to 36 hours.

- Adequate intravenous access and placement of an intra-arterial blood catheter for continuous blood pressure monitoring are essential in management.
- Knowledge of the underlying cause is helpful. This may aid in the proper selection of a first line antihypertensive treatment.
- Selection of first line antihypertensive agents is, to some degree, a matter of preference. If not contraindicated, oral nifedipine is the treatment of choice in emergency departments before the initiation of parenteral therapy.

- Common antihypertensive agents used in the treatment of hypertensive crisis are included in Table 2. Guidelines for choosing the appropriate medication are included in Table 3.
- In general, a continuous infusion of a short-acting titratable vasodilator is appropriate parenteral therapy. It is better to start with one antihypertensive medication and increase the dosage until a maximum dose is attained, or side effects start to develop before adding a second antihypertensive agent.

Table 2
## Antihypertensive Therapy

| Agent | Route | Onset of action | Duration | Side effect |
|-------|-------|-----------------|----------|-------------|
| Labetalol | Continuous IV infusion | 5 minutes | 2–4 hours | Bronchospasm, premature ventricular contractions |
| Nitroprusside | Continuous IV infusion | Immediate | During infusion only | Cyanide and thiocyanate toxicity |
| Hydralazine | IV | 5–20 minutes | 2–6 hours | Tachycardia, headache, flushing, palpitation, myocardial ischemia |
| Esmolol | Continuous IV infusion | 5 minutes | 10–30 minutes | Bronchospasm, bradycardia, heart failure |
| Nicardipine | Continuous IV infusion | 10–20 minutes | Up to 8 hours | Tachycardia, flushing |
| Enalapril | IV | 15 minutes | 4–6 hours | Contraindicated in acute renal insufficiency |
| Nifedipine | PO | 30 minutes (1–5 minutes if capsule is bitten and swallowed) | 4–8 hours | Syncope, tachycardia, flushing<br><br>Contraindicated in ICH |

*Table 3*
## Selection of Antihypertensive Agent

| Clinical condition | Drug of choice |
| --- | --- |
| Hypertensive encephalopathy | Labetalol, nitroprusside, nicardipine |
| Head trauma/intracranial hemorrhage | Labetalol, nitroprusside |
| Acute glomerulonephritis | Loop diuretics, nifedipine, hydralazine |
| Catecholamine production | Phentolamine |
| Renovascular disease | ACE inhibitor |
| Obstructive uropathy or reflux nephropathy | ACE inhibitor |
| Post surgery | Pain management, labetalol, nifedipine, hydralazine |

## Contraindications in Selection of Antihypertensive Therapy

| Medication | Contraindication |
| --- | --- |
| ACE inhibitor | Pregnancy, bilateral renal artery stenosis, renal artery stenosis in solitary kidney, renal transplant graft, acute renal failure |
| Nifedipine | Intracranial hemorrhage |
| Beta blocker | Asthma, congestive heart failure, atrioventricular conduction disturbance other than 1st degree heart block |
| Hydralazine | Cerebrovascular disease, coronary vascular disease, rheumatic valve disease, dissecting aortic aneurysm |

Once therapy is initiated, continuous reassessment and modification of management based on clinical findings, laboratory results, and response to initial therapy are necessary for successful and appropriate management.

# Suggested Readings

Blaszak RT, Savage JA, Ellis EN. The use of short acting nifedipine in pediatric patients with hypertension. J Pediatr 2001;139:34–7.

Flynn JT, Mottes TA, Brophy PD, et al. Intravenous nicardipine for treatment of severe hypertension in children. J Pediatr 2001;139:7–9.

Flynn JT: Neonatal hypertension: diagnosis and management. Pediatric Nephrology 2000;14:332–41.

Fossali E, Signorini E, Intermite RC, et al. Renovascular disease and hypertension in children with neurofibromatosis. Pediatr Nephrol 2000;14:806–10.

Kay JD, Sinaiko AR, Daniels SR. Pediatric hypertension. American Heart Journal 2001;142:422–32.

Lopes HF, Bortolotto LA, Szlejf C, et al. Hemodynamic and metabolic profile in offspring of malignant hypertensive patients. Hypertension 2001;38(pt2):616–20.

National Heart Lung and Blood Institute. Fourth report on the diagnosis, evaluation and treatment of high blood pressure in children and adolescents. 2004.

Neutel JM, Smith DH, Wallin D, et al. A comparison of intravenous nicardipine and sodium nitroprusside in immediate treatment of severe hypertension. Am J Hypertens 1994;7:623.

# B. Hemolytic Uremic Syndrome
## Emad Zaki

## Hemolytic Uremic Syndrome (HUS)

HUS is characterized by microangiopathic hemolytic anemia, thrombocytopenia, and impaired renal function. It is a leading cause of acute renal failure (ARF) in infants and children. HUS is a clinical syndrome resulting from a heterogeneous group of disorders that is traditionally classified into typical (classic) and atypical HUS.

### Typical HUS (D + HUS)

- Results most commonly from infection with verotoxin-producing strain of *Escherichia coli* (0157:H7)
- Other associated infections

  1. *Shigella dysenteriae*
  2. *Salmonella typhimurium*
  3. *Compylobacter jejuni*
  4. *Yersinia enterocolitica*

- Commonly occurs as an epidemic—mode of transmission usually ingestion of contaminated common foods. Bacterial contamination of hamburger has been incriminated in the largest reported outbreak; other vehicles have included contaminated water, soft drinks including cider.
- Occurs in children from ages 6 months to 10 years with peak incidence in children 1 to 4 years old
- Peak incidence is between April and September
- Clinical course varies from subclinical illness to life-threatening disease
- Clinical presentation includes a prodrome of watery diarrhea (enteropathic) with or without abdominal cramps in a previously healthy child
- Hemorrhagic colitis (bloody diarrhea) then develops after a few days
- Decreased urine output might develop and progress to ARF
- GI symptoms such as vomiting, severe abdominal pain, pancreatitis, and intussusception could also be associated
- CNS involvement presents in the form of seizure, lethargy, disorientation, and coma

## Atypical HUS (D − HUS)

- May be associated with following infections: *S. pneumoniae*, coxsackie virus, influenza, epstein-barr virus
- Also referred to as nondiarrhea-associated HUS
- Drug associated such as tacrolimus, cyclosporine A, OKT3, ATG, OCP
- Thrombotic microangiopathy (TTP)
- BMT-associated HUS
- Cancer-associated HUS
- Lupus-associated HUS
- Pregnancy-associated HUS
- Associated with higher incidence of serious complications

## Diagnosis and workup

- Primarily a clinical diagnosis
- History
- Anemia, hyperbilirubinemia, increased Retic counts, increased LDH
- Thrombocytopenia
- Fragmented RBCs, schistocytes, burr, or helmet cells on blood smear
- Negative Coombs test (+ in Lupus-associated HUS)
- Decreased C3, C4 (Familial HUS, SLE, PSGN)
- Increased blood urea nitrogen (BUN), creatinine, P, and uric acid
- Hyperkalemia
- Identification of *E. coli* 0157:H7 or other bacteria from stool

## PICU management

- Patients with oligo-anuria, dehydration, WBC >20 × 10(9)/L, and hematocrit >23% are at risk for fatal HUS and should be cared for in a tertiary care center.
- Empiric antibiotics are not recommended as they may increase toxin release.
- Pediatric intensive care unit (PICU) monitoring during active phase of hemolysis.

## ARF management (please refer to Chapter 12, "Intravenous Fluid and Electrolyte Management")

- Hyperkalemia should be closely monitored and aggressively treated as it can reach fetal levels with ongoing hemolysis.
- Hypertension.

- Up to 50% of patients require hemodialysis or continuous renal replacement therapy (CRRT).
- Consider PRBC transfusion if patient hematocrit <20% or if symptomatic.
- Platelet transfusion if platelet count <10, or if active bleeding is resent.
- Anticonvulsants if seizure.
- Aggressive fluid management with isotonic fluids may be nephroprotective.

**Prognosis**

HUS is a self-limited disease with greater than 90% survival rate, 3–5% mortality rate, and 3–5% chronic changes such as chronic renal failure (CRF) or hypertension.

# Suggested Readings

Ake JA, Jelacic S, Ciol MA. Relative nephroprotection during *Escherichia coli* O157:H7 infections: association with intravenous volume expansion. Pediatrics 2005;115:e673–80.

Corrigan JJ Jr, Boineau FG. Hemolytic-uremic syndrome. Pediatr Rev 2001;22:365–9.

Oakes RS, Siegler RL, McReynolds MA, et al. Predictors of fatality in postdiarrheal hemolytic uremic syndrome. Pediatrics 2006;117:1656–62.

# C. Acute Renal Failure

Emad Zaki

## Acute Renal Failure

## Definition

The sudden deterioration or cessation of the kidney function, with an inability to appropriately regulate fluid and electrolyte homeostasis and the retention of nitrogenous waste products.

- Acute renal failure (ARF) may occur with or without oliguria.
- The nonoliguric form of ARF is often associated with a nephrotoxic insult or interstitial nephritis rather than an ischemic insult.
- Severity of the insult is thought to be less than that of oliguric renal failure.

## Key Principles

- ARF occurs in approximately 4.5% of PICU admissions.
- ARF is associated with an increased risk of mortality.
- There are many risk factors and etiologies for ARF.
- Treatment consists of careful fluid, lectrolyte, and acid-base management, which must be tailored to the specific clinical picture and the underlying condition.

## Physiology

- Urine formation begins with glomerular filtration and is completed by tubular reabsorption and secretion.
- More than 98% of the enormous amount of glomerular filtrate is reabsorbed.
- Approximately 85% of filtered sodium and fluids are reabsorbed by the renal proximal tubule.
- The harmony between glomerular filtration and the tubular reabsorption is regulated mostly by the feedback mechanism between the macula densa and the juxtaglomerular cells of the afferent arteriole involving the renin-aldosterone system.

- When blood flow to the kidney increases, the glomerular filtration rate (GFR) increases. This, in turn, leads to the increase of sodium chloride delivered to the macula densa. The increase in the sodium chloride at the macula densa stimulates a negative feedback loop which results in increased vascular tone and decreased blood flow and GFR.
- When renal blood flow decreases, positive feedback results in the vasodilation of the afferent arteriole in an attempt to increase renal blood flow.
- In ARF, the proximal tubule is injured (due to an ischemic/toxic insult) and is unable to efficiently reabsorb the filtered solute. This results in an inappropriate increase of the sodium chloride delivered to the macula densa. This ultimately results in decreased GFR, secondary to the stimulation of the negative feedback loop. The continued failure of the proximal tubule to reabsorb sodium will result in progressive and sustained reduction of renal blood flow and GFR. In this setting, the feedback mechanism is highly protective as it prevents circulatory collapse, from salt and fluid loss if GFR was maintained in spite of the inefficient reabsorption of sodium and fluid.
- Several other factors contribute to the decrease in GFR such as the blockage of the tubular lumina by casts formed from the necrotic tubular cells. Partial or complete blockage of the tubule decreases tubular fluid flow and increases intra-tubular pressure which leads to a decrease in GFR.

## Etiology

A wide range of etiologies can produce ARF via different mechanisms. ARF is usually a multifactorial process. It is unlikely that a single mechanism can explain all of the dimensions of ARF.

Traditionally, the causes of ARF are classified as prerenal (renal hypoperfusion), intrinsic renal, and postrenal (obstructive uropathy).

### Prerenal Failure

Decreased true intravascular volume

- Dehydration
- Hemorrhage
- Third space losses (nephrotic syndrome, acute pancreatitis, sepsis, peritonitis)

Decreased effective intravascular volume

- Congestive heart failure
- Pericarditis and cardiac tamponade
- Septic shock
- Anaphylaxis

Renal vascular obstruction

- Renal artery embolus
- Aortic thrombosis
- Renal vein thrombosis

# Intrinsic Renal Failure

- Nephrotoxicity

  - Drug-induced (eg, aminoglycosides, IV contrast dye, cisplatin, nonsteroidal anti-inflammatory drugs (NSAIDs), ifosfamide, amphotericin B, cyclosporine, angiotensin-converting enzyme (ACE) inhibitors in patients with pre-existing renal insufficiency)
  - Toxin-mediated

    - Exogenous (ethylene glycol, methanol, mushroom poisoning, mercury, gold, lead, cadmium, platinum)
    - Endogenous (myoglobinuria in rhabdomyolysis, uric acid in tumor lysis syndrome)

- Glomerulonephritis

  - Post-infectious glomerulonephritis
  - Membranoproliferative glomerulonephritis
  - Systemic lupus glomerulonephritis
  - Henoch-Schönlein purpura nephritis
  - Idiopathic rapidly progressive glomerulonephritis
  - Acute interstitial nephritis due to hypersensitivity

- Vascular injury

  - Hemolytic uremic syndrome (HUS)
  - Drug-induced HUS (mitomycin, quinine, tacrolimus)
  - Thrombotic thrombocytopenic purpura (TTP)
  - Disseminated intravascular coagulopathy (DIC)

- Congenital disorders

  - Polycystic kidney disease
  - Renal hypoplasia/dysplasia
  - Congenital nephrotic syndrome

- Renal agenesis (Potter syndrome)

- Infections

  - Severe acute pyelonephritis
  - Sepsis

- Tumor

  - Tumor cell infiltrate (ALL and AML)
  - Tumor lysis syndrome
  - Wilms' tumor with associated glomerular nephropathy

## Postrenal (Obstructive Uropathy)

- Ureteral obstruction

  - Congenital urethral valves
  - Obstructed Foley catheter
  - Foreign body/calculus
  - Ectopic ureterocele

- Bladder outlet obstruction

  - Neoplasm
  - Functional (neurogenic bladder)

- Ureteral obstruction (mostly in solitary kidney as bilateral obstruction is rare)

  - Congenital ureteropelvic junction obstruction
  - Congenital ureterovesical junction obstruction
  - Ureterocele
  - Stricture secondary to infection or instrumentation

Common causes of ARF in the PICU include the following:

- Hemolytic uremic syndrome
- Oncologic emergencies
- Multifactorial acute tubular necrosis
- Cardiac surgery
- Septic shock

Risk factors for ARF in the PICU include:

- Age greater than 12 years
- Hypotension
- Hypoxemia
- Thrombocytopenia
- Coagulopathy

## Clinical Features

The clinical manifestations of ARF vary according to the severity, underlying cause, and the presence or absence of other systemic complications. The most common findings include increased blood urea nitrogen (BUN) and creatinine, oliguria (urine volume less than 1 mL/kg/hour), anuria (less than 0.5 mL/kg/hour), volume overload, hypertension, hyperkalemia, metabolic acidosis, hyperphosphatemia, and anemia in HUS.

## Investigations

Initial workup should be directed toward identifying the cause of the ARF and other life-threatening abnormalities that require immediate intervention such as hyperkalemia. The laboratory workup of ARF should include:

1. Urine culture and analysis with urine electrolytes and creatinine to differentiate between prerenal and renal causes of ARF (Table 1)
2. Urine microscopic examination to elucidate the presence or absence of specific casts and red blood cells
3. Complete blood count (CBC) with differential analysis
4. Electrolytes including sodium, potassium, chloride, bicarbonate, total and ionized calcium, phosphate, magnesium, and uric acid
5. BUN and creatinine
6. Total protein and albumin
7. Blood smear for red cell morphology if vasculitis is suspected such as in HUS
8. Blood culture in septic patients or infants with pyelonephritis
9. Creatinine phosphokinase (CPK) level if rhabdomyolysis is suspected
10. LDH if HUS is suspected
11. PT, PTT, INR if a coagulation disorder is suspected

Imaging studies are also useful in the workup of ARF. These include:

1. Renal/bladder ultrasound
2. Renal ultrasound with duplex if hypertension is present or renal artery or vein thrombosis is suspected

Other imaging studies may be indicated for further evaluation in specific situations, and are beyond the scope of this chapter.

*Table 1*

**Differentiating Prerenal ARF from Intrinsic ARF**

| Diag-nostic Index | Prerenal Azotemia | | Intrinsic ARF | |
|---|---|---|---|---|
| | Adults/children | Neo-nates | Adults/children | Neo-nates |
| U Na (mEq/L) | <20 | <30 | >50 | >50 |
| U Osm (mOsm/kg $H_2O$) | >500 | >350 | <300 | <300 |
| FENa | <1 | <2.5 | >1 | >2.5 |
| RFI | <1 | <2.5 | >1 | >2.5 |

FENa (fractional excretion of sodium) = [urine sodium/serum sodium]/[urine Cr/serum Cr] × 100

RFI (renal failure index) = Urine sodium/[urine Cr/serum Cr]

**Note:** none of the above indices should be used in patients on diuretics

## Management

- First, target life-threatening complications such as hyperkalemia and pulmonary edema regardless of the cause. Thorough investigation for the underlying cause of ARF should be conducted after controlling these potentially fatal complications.
- Treament of ARF consists of conservative management under close monitoring and renal replacement therapy. Consider:

  1. Fluid balance
  2. Electrolyte balance
  3. Acid Base balance
  4. Hypertension
  5. Medication dose adjustment
  6. Nutritional support

### Monitoring During Management

- Strict intake and output records and frequent weights are critical.
- Frequent laboratory evaluation is essential. This includes electrolyte and total carbon dioxide evaluation up to every 4 to

8 hours. BUN and creatinine, ionized calcium, phosphate, magnesium, uric acid, blood gas, and CBC should be monitored every 12 to 24 hours. The frequency of testing varies according to the underlying cause and associated medical complications. For example, more frequent blood gas evaluation is required for a patient with respiratory dysfunction.

## Fluid Management

- Fluid management is key and appropriate fluid management is the hallmark of successful treatment.
- The ARF patient may be hypovolemic, euvolemic, or fluid overloaded according to the cause of the ARF.
- The goal of management is to maintain or reach the fluid balance state dictated by the overall status of the patient's organ systems.
- Converting oliguric to nonoliguric ARF facilitates fluid management, helps to maintain electrolyte homeostasis, and to provide appropriate nutritional requirements.
- Fluid status assessment is guided by history (emesis, diarrhea, etc.) and physical examination which includes weight, blood pressure, heart rate, skin turgor, and capillary refill.

**Fluid intake = insensible water loss + measured fluid losses.**

- Insensible water loss is roughly estimated to be 400 mL/m2/day.
- Other factors may affect insensible water loss. Increased loss may result with fever and an increased metabolic state while a decreased loss may be seen with assisted ventilation.
- Examples of measured fluid losses include urine, stool, vomiting, or fluids lost from any surgical indwelling catheters.

## Hypovolemia

- In the intravascular volume depleted (dehydrated) patient, who is oliguric, restores intravascular volume with 10 to 20 mL/kg of 0.9% normal saline.
- If the oliguria improves, continue with fluid replacement and monitor urine output.
- If the oliguria persists after restoring intravascular volume, an attempt to induce diuresis is reasonable.
- If attempted diuresis fails and oliguria persists, CVP-guided fluid management may be implemented with the target pressure of 4–6 cm $H_2O$.

## Fluid Overload

- Management is driven according to the presence or absence of complications such as hypertension, congestive heart failure (CHF), and pulmonary edema.
- In the presence of CHF, rapid fluid removal may be mandatory with dialysis or hemofiltration if adequate diuresis cannot be achieved.
- Severe fluid restriction is not recommended for more than 24 to 48 hours as it adversely affects nutritional status, and in turn, worsens the hypercatabolic state of ARF.

## Euvolemic State

- When euvolemic status is established, appropriate fluid management should be aimed toward replacing ongoing losses and removing indwelling surgical drains or chest tube, etc.

## Conversion of Oliguric to Nonoliguric ARF

- In a nondehydrated patient, a trial of IV furosemide is recommended starting with 1 mg/kg per dose.
- If diuresis is not achieved after 1 hour, a second trial with a higher dose of up to 5 mg/kg may be administered. Continuous loop-diuretic infusions may also be efficacious.
- If diuresis is still not achieved, further attempts are unlikely to be successful and carry the risk of ototoxicity.
- Osmotic diuresis using mannitol is not recommended for pediatric patients as there is a high risk for circulatory overload if unsuccessful.

## Electrolyte Management

### Sodium Abnormalities

- Conservative fluid management is usually successful in correction of serum sodium abnormalities in nonoliguric patients.
- Nonoliguric hyponatremic ARF patients may have large urinary sodium losses and appropriate management should be guided by urinary losses of sodium with 4 to 6 hours of pooled urine samples.
- Hyponatremia is often dilutional in oliguric patients. In this setting, serum sodium concentration reflects fluid status and there is no actual sodium deficit. Oliguric ARF patients lose

minute amounts of sodium and the management requires sodium restriction as overload can lead to circulatory congestion, edema, and hypertension. Appropriate free-water restriction will usually slowly correct serum sodium.

- Hemodialysis must be considered in oliguric hypervolemic patients with severe (sodium <125 mEq/L) or symptomatic hyponatremia.
- If serum sodium level is less than 120 mEq/L, 3% hypertonic saline should be considered to avoid risk of seizure with a target of serum sodium level of 125 mEq/L. Slow IV infusion over several hours is important to avoid central pontine myelinolysis.

The replacement formula is as follows:

---

**Replacement amount = {Desired Sodium Level − Current Sodium Level} × Weight in kg × 0.6 {Volume of Sodium Distribution}**

---

- In the oliguric hypernatremic patient, hemodialysis/hemofiltration should be considered if conservative fluid management fails or if it is unlikely to correct the electrolyte imbalance within an appropriate time period of 24–48 hours.

## Hyperkalemia

- Hyperkalemia is one of the most serious life-threatening complications of ARF as it can cause fatal arrhythmias through its depolarizing effect on the cardiac conduction pathway.
- Other factors may also influence the effects of hyperkalemia on cardiac muscle such as serum calcium level and acid base balance. Hypocalcemia, which is a common feature of renal failure, exacerbates the adverse effect of hyperkalemia on the cardiac muscle. Therefore, arrhythmias may occur with lower than expected potassium levels in the context of hypocalcemia.
- EKG changes are a sensitive indicator and useful method to monitor the effect of hyperkalemia on cardiac muscle. This usually manifests with a peaked T wave which may progress to a prolonged PR interval and ultimately to ventricular fibrillation if the hyperkalemia persists.
- The first step in the treatment of the hyperkalemia with EKG changes is directed toward stabilizing the myocardium with supplemental calcium therapy.

- Hyperkalemia is also aggravated by acidosis as acute acidemia shifts potassium from the intracellular to the extracellular fluid space. Acidosis also inhibits distal tubule potassium secretion.

Please refer to Table 2 for the treatment of hyperkalemia.

# Hyperphosphatemia

- This is a common electrolyte abnormality associated with acute and chronic renal failure.
- Hyperphosphatemia is usually tolerated in pediatric patients; however, resulting hypocalcemia may cause seizures.
- Severe hyperphosphatemia is more common in tumor lysis syndrome.

Treatment of hyperphosphatemia includes:

1. Diet restriction
2. Oral calcium binders
3. Frequent or continuous dialysis as phosphorus is mainly stored in non-extracellular fluid space and postdialysis rebound is common

# Hypocalcemia

- Hypocalcemia usually results from hyperphosphatemia, but exacerbating this is: inadequate production of active vitamin D by the kidney, and the skeletal resistance to the action of parathyroid hormone (PTH).
- Acid-base balance directly affects the level of ionized calcium and the severity of the acidosis dictates the choice of therapy.
- Calcium gluconate is administered in severe hypocalcemia or in borderline hypocalcemia if bicarbonate therapy is instituted.
- Bicarbonate therapy is often used for the treatment of acidosis and hyperkalemia. Ten percent calcium gluconate 100 mg/kg with a maximum dose of 3 g should be slowly infused over 30 to 60 minutes with EKG monitoring.
- Profound hypocalcemia may develop early in the course of ARF secondary to crush injury, electric injury, and severe muscle damage. However, later in the course of the injury, hypercalcemia can be a serious complication as calcium mobilizes from muscle tissue.
- Aggressive dialysis is often indicated with a calcium-free bath to adequately treat these special conditions.

*Table 2*
## Treatment for Hyperkalemia

| Drug | Dosage/route | Onset | Comments |
|------|--------------|-------|----------|
| Calcium gluconate | 50–100 mg/kg (maximum 3 g) IV over 5 min | Immediate | Protects cardiac muscle from hyperkalemic effect. This should be used for patients with EKG changes until potassium lowering therapy is instituted. |
| Dextrose/ insulin | Regular insulin 0.1 unit/kg AND dextrose 0.5 g/kg (D50W: 0.5 mL/ kg or D10W: 5 mL/kg) | 15 min | Shifts serum potassium to intracellular space. Watch for hypoglycemia. |
| Sodium polystyrene sulfonate | 1 g/kg PO or PR | 30 min | Potassium binder decreases total body potassium in exchange for sodium. |
| Dialysis | Hemodialysis | Immediate | Peritoneal dialysis and CRRT can be used in nonemergent situations. |
| Sodium bicarbonate | 1–2 mEq/kg IV | 20 min | Adequate ventilation is necessary. This should not be given simultaneously with calcium. |

## Acid-Base Balance

- Metabolic acidosis is a common feature of ARF due to the impaired ability of the kidney to excrete acid.
- Severe acidemia may adversely affect the myocardial contractility and vascular tone resulting in hypotension and fibrillation.
- Correction of metabolic acidosis with a pH greater than 7.15 is controversial and may not benefit the patient.
- IV sodium bicarbonate is used to correct severe acidemia. The correction should be slow except in the setting of hyperkalemia or hemodynamic instability.
- When correcting acidosis, a target total $CO_2$ level of 15 mEq/L is acceptable for the initial goal.
- To calculate the proper bicarbonate dose use the following formula:

---

**Bicarbonate Dose = [15 − {patient T $CO_2$}] × weight in kg × 0.3**

---

- Therapy should be monitored with hourly blood gas and pH levels.
- Check ionized calcium level before starting the base correction as correction of acidemia will decrease the ionized calcium level and may result in tetany or seizure.
- A supplemental dose of 1 to 3 mEq/kg/day of IV or oral sodium bicarbonate or oral sodium citrate can be used for maintenance in stable patients.
- Dialysis or hemofiltration should be considered if the patient is oliguric or hypervolemic and is unlikely to tolerate the intravascular expansion associated with the IV bicarbonate infusion.
- Dialysis/hemofiltration is the treatment of choice in mixed respiratory and metabolic acidosis as the bicarbonate therapy ultimately generates $CO_2$.
- An intact respiratory system is essential to remove excessive $CO_2$, otherwise the therapy will be ineffective. In intubated patients, hyperventilation is an effective emergency treatment for acidemia (but see respiratory system for possible complications from this).

## Hypertension

- In ARF, hypertension is usually the result of volume overload and/or altered vascular tone.

- Volume overload should be managed by fluid removal with diuretic therapy or renal replacement therapy if diuresis fails.
- The choice of antihypertensive therapy depends on the severity, cause of ARF, and the presence or absence of symptoms or complications. For a more comprehensive discussion, please refer to elsewhere in this chapter.

## Nutritional Support

- Due to the marked catabolic state in ARF patients, proper nutritional support is necessary to enhance recovery and reduce complications.
- For all ARF patients, a diet with a minimal potassium and phosphate content should be implemented. For conservatively managed patients, the dietary protein content restriction varies according to the creatinine clearance. It should be restricted to 0.5 to 1 g/kg/day to avoid an increase in BUN, phosphate, and acidosis.
- Total parental nutrition (TPN) through a central line should be considered if elemental feeding is not possible. An appropriate TPN solution should include high dextrose concentration (25%), lipid (10% to 20%), and larger protein intake of 1 to 2 g/kg/day using an essential amino acid preparation.
- In oliguric patients, if appropriate nutrition cannot be achieved because of fluid restriction, renal replacement therapy should be considered.

## Indications for Renal Replacement Therapy

The choice of renal replacement modality between hemodialysis, peritoneal dialysis, and continuous renal replacement therapy is determined for each individual according to multiple factors beyond the scope of this chapter. The most common indications for renal replacement therapy include:

1. Volume overload unresponsive to conservative management
2. Volume overload associated with complications such as congestive heart failure (CHF) and pulmonary edema
3. Severe hyperkalemia
4. Acidosis unresponsive to conservative therapy
5. Severe azotemia or uremic complications such as encephalopathy or bleeding
6. Severe resistant hypo- or hypernatremia
7. Fluid removal in an oliguric patient for supplemental nutritional needs, IV medications, or blood products

The two indices FENa and RFI are used interchangeably as the end numeric value is similar. Both indices are designed based on the premise that a healthy nephron will respond to hypoperfusion by increasing reabsorption of filtered sodium resulting in decreased urinary sodium and urine volume. Alternately, urine creatinine concentration increases as tubular secretion of creatinine is maintained despite the decrease in renal blood flow.

## Suggested Readings

Chan JC, Williams DM, Roth KS. Kidney failure in infants and children. Pediatr Rev 2002;23:47.

Andreoli SP. Acute renal failure. Curr Opin Pediatr 2002;14:183–8.

Feld LG, Springate JE, Fildes RD. Acute renal failure I. Pathophysiology and diagnosis. J Pediatr 1986;109:401–8.

Fildes RD, Springate JE, Feld LG. Acute renal failure II. Management. J Pediatr 1986;109:567–71.

Bailey D, Phan V, Litalien C, et al. Risk factors of acute renal failure in critically ill children: a prospective descriptive epidemiological study. Ped Crit Care Med 2007;8:29–35.

# D. Renal Replacement Therapy

Lia Lowrie

Beth A Vogt

## Introduction

Renal replacement therapy (RRT) is initiated when acute renal failure (ARF) occurs. An acute decline in glomerular filtration results in fluid overload and metabolic derangements. Historically, pediatric ARF occurred most commonly during hemolytic uremic syndrome (HUS); but more recent data show that pediatric ARF etiology mirrors that of adult patients occurring as a result of heart surgery, sepsis, and acute tubular necrosis as a part of multi-organ failure. Timing of RRT initiation depends on the degree of fluid overload and electrolyte derangement and signs and symptoms of uremia such as pericarditis and encephalopathy. Early initiation of RRT may be associated with improved mortality and morbidity, but studies are hampered by poorly standardized definitions of ARF in small numbers of patients. Due to the complex nature of ARF and multiple treatment options available for RRT children with ARF are best managed in close consultation with a pediatric nephrologist.

## Indications for RRT

Electrolyte abnormality: hyperkalemia, hyperphosphatemia, acidosis

Catabolic patients with increased nutritional needs

Sepsis—removal of inflammatory cytokines

Diuretic–unresponsive volume overload

Poisoning

Hyperammonemia or control of other products of in-born errors of metabolism

Hepatic or drug-induced coma

## Contraindications

There are few contraindications to renal replacement therapies, especially continuous renal replacement therapy.

- Hemodynamic instability limits the use of intermittent hemodialysis in the ICU.
- Active bleeding is a relative contraindication; however, there are protocols that do not require heparinization.
- Peritoneal dialysis may not achieve necessary clearance and fluid removal needed in critically ill patients.
- Surgical abdominal conditions may contraindicate peritoneal dialysis.

# RRT Modalities

## Peritoneal Dialysis (PD)

- Historically this was the earliest form of RRT available for children.
- PD uses the peritoneal membrane as the site for diffusion of solute and removal of fluid from the vascular compartment by the instillation of hypertonic dialysate solution into the peritoneum.
- It is inexpensive, easy to perform, requires little specialized equipment, is effective in hemodynamically stable children without respiratory embarrassment, and can be easily extended into a chronic supportive mode in the outpatient arena.
- Complications include a high risk of peritonitis, failure of the peritoneum as a semipermeable membrane, respiratory distress from abdominal distension, hyperglycemia, and slow and poorly controlled fluid removal rates.

## Intermittent Hemodialysis

- The process of hemodialysis employs blood passage over an artificial semipermeable membrane (the dialyzer) through which solute diffuses into the dialysate solution flowing over the other side of the membrane. Anticoagulant is generally necessary to prevent clotting within vascular access or the extracorporeal circuit.
- The blood flow and dialysate flows achievable with modern technology provide for very efficient and rapid small molecule and fluid clearance and removal. Chronic renal failure patients have stable catabolic and fluid management needs and a schedule of three to four 3-hour treatments per week is often a sufficient "dose" of hemodialysis.
- Complications of hemodialysis include hemodynamic instability and solute disequilibrium states resulting from the rapid

removal of fluid and solute from the extracellular compartment. The "dose" of dialysis needed for effective fluid and solute clearance in the often catabolic and hemodynamically unstable ICU patient is often higher, producing more potential for treatment intolerance and inadequate dialytic support.

# Continuous Renal Replacement Therapies (CRRT)

- Similar to hemodialysis, CRRT circulates blood through an extracorporeal circuit over an artificial, semipermeable membrane. Solute and fluid are removed by convection diffusion, or both. Blood flow, fluid removal, and solute clearance are slower than with intermittent hemodialysis but therapy is continuous allowing potentially equivalent therapy over a 24-hour period.
- Hemodynamically unstable patients, patients with ongoing metabolic derangement, and children with relatively small vascular volumes may tolerate the less intense fluid and solute shifts of CRRT better and derive benefit from fewer periods of toxin and fluid buildup between intermittent treatments.
- In adults, a meta-analysis of 1400 patients in 13 studies (3 randomized and 10 observational) found lower mortality in patients treated with CRRT after adjustment for severity of illness and study quality.

# Modes of CRRT

- Slow continuous ultrafiltration (SCUF)

  Provides fluid removal by ultrafiltration only. No dialysate or replacement fluids are used.

- Continuous venovenous hemofiltration (CVVH) with replacement fluid

  Provides solute removal primarily by convection. Plasma water is removed from the blood while a sterile replacement solution is simultaneously infused into the blood prefilter to maintain intravascular volume. Because unwanted solutes are removed by taking off plasma water. Increased clearances are achieved by using higher ultrafiltration rates to remove more plasma water. Compared to CVVHD, CVVH provides less efficient removal of solutes of small molecular weight (<350 Dalton), but more efficient removal of solutes of larger molecular weight.

- CVVHD with dialysate (continuous venovenous hemodialysis)

  Provides solute removal primarily by diffusion. Dialysate is continuously pumped through the fluid side of the filter, and the concentration gradient between the filter's blood and fluid side causes unwanted blood solutes to diffuse into the dialysate where they can be removed. Replacement fluid is not used.

- CVVHDF with replacement fluid and dialysate (continuous venovenous hemodiafiltration)

  Provides solute removal by convection and diffusion. Plasma water is removed from the blood while a sterile replacement solution is simultaneously infused into the blood prefilter to maintain intravascular volume. At the same time, dialysate is continuously pumped through the fluid side of the filter, and the concentration gradient between the filter's blood and fluid side causes unwanted blood solutes to diffuse into the dialysate where they can be removed.

| Modality | Mechanism of Fluid Removal | Mechanism of Solute Removal |
|----------|----------------------------|------------------------------|
| SCUF | Ultrafiltration | Some with small molecular weight only |
| CVVH | Ultrafiltration | Convection Efficient for large molecular weight |
| CVVHD | Ultrafiltration | Diffusion Efficient for small molecular weight |
| CVVDHF | Ultrafiltration | Convection and diffusion |

## Management Issues in Pediatric CRRT

**Vascular access** may be the limiting factor in establishment of successful CRRT in pediatric patients. Blood flow is enhanced and clotting risk diminished with the shortest, largest catheters available. In general, blood flow from the patient should be obtained through a lumen no smaller than 5 French gauge size, although blood return from the extracorporeal circuit to the patient can sometimes be successful through smaller, longer catheters. Subclavian or internal jugular sites are usually the better choices when compared to the femoral veins because of size of the vessels, less kinking with patient movement, and potentially less infection risk. CRRT has been successfully established in neonates using an umbilical arterial catheter for blood access and an umbilical venous catheter for blood return. Double lumen catheters with appropriate resistance characteristics to attain 3 to 5 mL/kg/minute blood flows are available in a range of sizes appropriate for infants and children. Flow is most successfully attained with the subclavian or internal jugular approach as opposed to the femoral approach because:

- Less effect on blood flow when the child moves
- Larger size of blood vessels in the cardiac region
- Lower infectious risk
- Ability to ambulate as the child recovers

| Suggested catheter sizes | Child's weight |
|---|---|
| 5 Fr single lumen (2 separate catheters needed) | Neonate <3 kg |
| 7 Fr double lumen | <25 kg |
| 8 Fr double lumen | <30 kg |
| 9 Fr double lumen | <35 kg |
| 11.5 Fr double lumen | >35 kg |
| 12 Fr double or triple lumen | >40 kg |

**Blood flow** is usually initiated at 3 to 5 mL/kg/minute. Filter and circuit clotting is generally lessened with higher flow rates, but pressure alarms may be more frequent. Commercially available CRRT machines usually control flow by pressure sensors.

**Access pressure** is a negative pressure and represents the pulling power needed to pull blood from the catheter. The more negative the number, the more effort is needed to pull the blood out of the catheter indicating high resistance that may be caused by inadequate vascular access size, clotting, or vessel wall collapse across catheter holes.

**Filter pressure** is the positive pressure measured as the blood is pushed through the filter. If the pressure becomes too positive, it indicates that the filter is clotting.

**Effluent pressure** may be positive or negative, and is the pressure required to control the fluid removal programmed into the machine. The more fluid to be removed, the more negative the number.

**Return pressure** is the positive pressure encountered when the blood is pumped back into the patient's catheter. The more positive the pressure, the greater the resistance, suggesting obstruction/kinking of the return port of the catheter.

**Dialysate solutions** are now commercially available; prior to 2000 most pediatric programs mixed customized solutions in their pharmacies at great expense and risk of contamination and compounding error. Standard dialysis solutions were often lactate based which, with continuous use during CRRT, led to high serum lactate concentrations in patients. *Normocarb* (Dialysis Solutions, Richmond Hill, Ontario, Canada) was approved by the FDA for CVVHD and has the added advantage of being calcium free allowing citrate anticoagulation schema. The total dialysate (and replacement fluid) flow rate may be initiated at 2000 mL/1.73 m$^2$/hour.

**Replacement fluid** for CRRT is often prepared by in-house pharmacies, although *Normocarb* was recently FDA approved for use as a replacement fluid.

The total replacement fluid (and dialysate) flow rate may be initiated at 2000 mL/1.73 m$^2$/hour.

| Normocarb composition: | |
| --- | --- |
| Na (meq/L) | 140 |
| K (meq/L) | 0 |
| Cl (meq/L) | 105 |
| HCO$_3$ (meq/L) | 35 |
| Ca (meq/L) | 0 |
| PO$_4$ (meq/L) | 0 |
| Mg (meq/L) | 0.75 |
| Dextrose (g/L) | 0 |

**Potential additives to Normocarb:**

| | |
|---|---|
| KCl (meq/L) | 0–2 |
| KPO$_4$ (meq/L) | 0–2 |
| Dextrose (g/L) | 1 |

**Pharmacy-prepared CRRT replacement fluid composition:**

| | |
|---|---|
| Na (meq/L) | 140 |
| K (meq/L) | 0 |
| Cl (meq/L) | 105 |
| HCO$_3$ (meq/L) | 35 |
| Ca (meq/L) | 2.4 |
| PO$_4$ (meq/L) | 0 |
| Mg (meq/L) | 1.4 |
| Dextrose (g/L) | 1 |

**Additives to pharmacy-prepared replacement solution:**

| | |
|---|---|
| KCl (meq/L) | 0–2 |
| KPO$_4$ (meq/L) | 0–2 |

**Anticoagulation** may be achieved with heparin or citrate protocols. In patients with severe coagulopathy, CRRT can be attempted without anticoagulation at the risk of more frequent circuit clotting.

**Heparin protocol:** A heparin bolus of 50 units/kg (maximum 2000 units) should be administered at the onset of CRRT. A continuous infusion of heparin at 5 to 10 units/kg/hour may be administered for ongoing anticoagulation. Activated clotting time (seconds) should be monitored from the venous side of the filter as ordered and heparin administration modified as follows, to maintain ACT within goal range of 180 to 220 seconds:

| ACT (seconds) | Action |
|---|---|
| <160 | Heparin bolus 10 units/kg<br>Increase herparin drip by 20% |
| 160–180 | Heparin bolus 5 units/kg<br>Increase heparin drip by 10% |
| 180–220 | No action |
| 220–260 | Decrease heparin drip by 10% |
| >260 | Decrease heparin drip by 20% |

Risks: Hemorrhage, heparin-induced thrombocytopenia

**Citrate protocol:** Infuse Citrate ACD(A) Solution (Baxter Health Care, Deerfield, IL) prefilter at 1.5 times the blood flow rate of the CRRT machine. Run 0.8% calcium chloride solution through central venous line into patient to run at 40% of the citrate flow rate. Titrate citrate and calcium infusions as suggested below:

| Circuit ionized Ca++(mmol/L) | Citrate infusion adjustment |
|---|---|
| <0.25 | Decrease rate by 10 mL/hour |
| 0.25–0.39 | No adjustment |
| 0.4–0.5 | Increase rate by 10 mL/hour |
| >0.6 | Increase rate by 20 mL/hour (Up to 200 mL/hour) |

| Patient ionized Ca++(mmol/L) | Calcium infusion adjustment |
|---|---|
| >1.3 | Decrease rate by 10 mL/hour |
| 1.1–1.3 | No adjustment |
| 0.9–1.1 | Increase rate by 10 mL/hour |
| <0.9 | Increase rate by 20 mL/hour (Up to 150 mL/hour) |

Risks: Citrate toxicity, metabolic alkalosis, hypocalcemia

# Special Cautions

**Bradykinin release syndrome (BRS)** appears to occur when acidotic blood comes in contact with certain synthetic membranes used in dialyzers for RRT resulting in arrhythmia, severe hypotension, vasodilation, and anaphylaxis. This is specifically a problem in infants under 10 kg in whom the CRRT machine may be primed with acidotic, banked blood. BRS has also been reported to occur when initiating therapy in adults with acidosis. The reaction can be avoided by buffering the blood prime appropriately with tris-hydroxy-methyl aminomethane, calcium and sodium bicarbonate or by carefully diverting the initial volume of membrane exposed blood prime from reaching the patient and infusing an equivalent amount of blood into the patient through the patient side of the filter.

**Drug dosing** during RRT particularly in pediatric patients is difficult. A nice approach is outlined by Veltri et al. including many medications commonly used in the pediatric intensive care unit (PICU).

# References

Williams DM, Sreedhar SS, Mickell JJ, Chan JC. Acute kidney failure: a pediatric experience over 20 years. Arch Pediatr Adolesc Med 2002;156:893–900.

Abramson S, Singh AK. Continuous renal replacement therapy compared with intermittent hemodialysis in intensive care: which is better? Curr Opin Nephrol Hypertens 1999;8:537–41.

Guerin C, Girard R, Selli JM, Ayzac L. Intermittent versus continuous renal replacement therapy for acute renal failure in intensive care units: results from a mulicenter propective epidemiological survey. Intensive Care Med 2002;28:1411–8.

Kellum JA, Angus DC, Johnson JP, et al. Continuous versus intermittent renal replacement therapy: a meta-analysis. Intensive Care Med 2002;28:29–37.

http://www.ltpro.com/pcrrt.com/index.html

Brophy PD, Mottes TA, Kudelka TL, et al. AN-69 membrane reactions are pH-dependent and preventable. Am J Kidney Dis. 2001 Jul;38(1):173–8.

Veltri MA, Neu AM, Fivush BA, et al. Drug dosing during intermittent hemodialysis and continuous renal replacement therapy. Special considerations in pediatric patients 2004;6:45–65.

Bunchman TE, Maxvold NJ, Barnett J, et al. Pediatric hemofiltration: Normocarb dialysis solution with citrate anticoagulation. Ped Nephrology 2002;17:150–4.

# E. Renal Transplantation
Emad Zaki

## Key Principles

- Renal transplantation is the definitive treatment for irreversible renal failure.
- Postoperative management in the PICU requires meticulous care to ensure preservation of graft function.
- Close monitoring of cardiac output, intravascular volume, and urine output are essential.
- Complications are rare but may include vascular/urologic complications, rejection, infection.

## Renal Transplantation

- Renal transplantation is the definitive treatment for children with irreversible renal failure.
- Successful transplantation provides a significantly better quality of life compared to dialysis.
- It also enhances skeletal growth, sexual maturation, cognitive performance, and psychosocial function.
- Seven-year patient survival exceeds 90% in all recipients older than 1 year of age of living related or deceased donors. Five-year patient survival ranged from 97% to 99% in children older than 1 year of age who received living donor grafts, 90% to 97% among children who received deceased donor grafts.

## Indication and Timing of Renal Transplantation

- Indicated in irreversible end-stage renal disease.
- Consider when renal replacement therapy is indicated and a suitable donor is available.
- Dialysis may be required until the patient reaches an optimal minimum weight of 8–10 kg and a suitable donor is available.

- Successfully organ transplantation requires a coordinated multidisciplinary team which may include the following disciplines: pediatric transplant surgeons, nephrologists, intensivists, nurses, social workers, ethicists, child life, nutritionists, and pharmacists.
- Extensive evaluation workup is done for both recipient and donor prior to transplantation in order to increase success rate.

Recipient evaluation includes:

- Serology testing: CMV, EBV, HIV, varicella virus, herpes virus, hepatitis A, B, and C, and syphilis serology
- PPD
- Echocardiography and CXR
- VCUG to detect and surgically manage anatomical abnormalities that might adversely affect the transplanted graft
- HLA typing

Donor exclusion criteria:

- Hypertension
- Impaired renal function
- Hematuria
- Proteinuria
- Nephrocalcinosis, or recurrent renal stones
- Significant urologic abnormality
- Chronic illness as diabetes, cardiac, hematologic, neurologic, pulmonary, or liver disease
- History of malignance
- Chronic viral infection as HIV, hepatitis B or C
- Family history of renal cell carcinoma
- Substance abuse
- Active psychosis

# Underlying Diagnoses in the Pediatric Renal Transplant Recipients

- Dysplastic/hypoplastic kidneys
- Obstructive uropathy
- Focal segmental glomerulosclerosis
- Reflux nephropathy
- Systemic immunologic disease
- Chronic glomerulonephritis
- Congenital nephrotic syndrome
- Prune-belly syndrome

- Polycystic kidney disease
- Hemolytic uremic syndrome (HUS)
- Medullary cystic disease
- Cystinosis
- Familial nephritis (Alport syndrome)
- Pyelonephritis
- Interstitial nephritis
- Membranoproliferative glomerulonephritis
- Renal corticomedullary necrosis (infarction)
- Idiopathic crescentic glomerulonephritis
- Membranous nephropathy
- Wilm's tumor

# Postoperative Management of Renal Transplant Patients

- Admission to the PICU
- Preservation of graft function requires adequate intravascular volume, good cardiac output, and continuous urine output to prevent urinary tract blockage
- Electrolyte abnormalities and acute renal failure are the most common PICU complications postop
- Obtain baseline ultrasound with doppler
- Renal isotopic scanning within the first 24 hours
- Chest and abdominal plain films
- Monitor

  - Vital signs every hour for 24 hours, then every 4 hours when the patient is stable
  - Intake and output every hour for the first 48 to 72 hours
  - Daily weight
  - Urine output; notify physician if <2.0 mL/kg/hour × 3 hours
  - CVP; notify physician if <8
  - Systolic blood pressure; notify physician if <100 or >140 (varies according to age and size)
  - Temperature; notify physician if >38°C
  - Patients with severe preoperative uremia may be at risk for cerebral edema secondary to osmol shifts postop—mental status should be closely monitored
  - Daily physical exam should look for signs and symptoms of blood loss including hypotension and tachycardia or for fluid overload resulting in hypertension, pulmonary edema, and/or heart failure

- Labs

  - CBC with differential every 6 to 8 hours × 3, then every 12 hours if stable levels

    1. Hemoglobin and hematocrit levels to ensure there is no evidence of internal hemorrhage
    2. WBCs for signs of infection
    3. Platelet count for HUS secondary to immunosuppressive therapy (Tacrolimus)

  - Blood gas analysis every 6 to 8 hours × 3, then every 12 hours if stable levels while patient is intubated; also watch for evidence of persistent metabolic acidosis (this is indication of graft malfunction)
  - Serum sodium, potassium, chloride, $CO_2$, BUN, creatinine, ionized calcium, and phosphorus levels
  - Urine electrolytes—to help adjust replacement fluids. Urine creatine is expected to increase after transplantation indicating a well-functioning graft

- Fluids

  - Careful monitoring of fluid balance is essential especially in the initial diuretic phase postoperatively
  - Urine output replacement mL for mL with 0.45% normal saline for the first 48 hours
  - Insensible water losses replacement with dextrose containing crystalloid
  - Potassium replacement if required

# Immunosuppressant Protocol

- Immunosuppressive protocols vary from one center to another. An outline is given below.
- Several factors such as living related versus cadaveric donor and first transplantation versus repeat transplantation will determine the exact protocol.
- Most pediatric centers use monoclonal antibodies such as basiliximab or daclizumab for induction.
- Combination drug therapy, calcineurin inhibitor (cyclosporine or tacrolimus), and corticosteroids with an adjunctive agent usually MMF (mycophenolate mofetil).
- Other immunosuppressive agents may be used in different protocols or for various medical or financial reasons. These include azathioprine, sirolimus, and thymoglobulin.

- Special attention should be directed toward the adverse reactions associated with immunosuppressants and drug interactions. Please refer to the pharmacology section.

# Complications Associated with Transplantation

- Vascular and urological technical complications

  - Vascular thrombosis (incidence increases with pediatric cadaver donors younger than 6 years old and prolonged cold ischemic time >24 hours)
  - Transplant artery stenosis
  - Urinary leak
  - Urethral obstruction
  - Vesicoureteric reflux

- Rejection

  - Rates are approximately 15% to 20% over the first year, but center variations may be large.
  - Usually not encountered in the immediate postoperative period.
  - Signs and symptoms include fever, graft tenderness, hematuria, proteinuria, decreased urine output, increased BUN, or creatinine.
  - Hyperacute form of rejection occurs as soon as the graft is revascularized and may be evident in the first 48 hours post-transplant.

    - Due to presensitization and is mediated by antibodies to donor HLA, which usually causes irreversible vascular rejection.
    - Doppler ultrasound and isotopic scanning will show evidence of diminished renal perfusion.
    - Prompt surgical exploration is mandatory.
    - Treatment is usually graft removal.

  - Acute rejection occurs 2 to 7 days post-transplantation.

    - Is mainly cell mediated and requires more immune suppression.
    - Imaging studies will illustrate good renal perfusion.

  - Chronic allograft nephropathy is the most common cause of late graft failure.

- Due to immune causes such as recurrent acute graft rejection, histocompatibility mismatch, prior sensitization, or insufficient immune suppression.
- Due to nonimmune causes such as ischemic injuries, calcineurin-inhibitor nephrotoxicity, and infections as CMV.

- Opportunistic infection

Renal transplant recipients are at increased risk for infection by many organisms with viruses as the most problematic.

- CMV
- EBV
- Other herpes viruses (HSV, VZV, HHV)
- Hepatitis B and C
- HIV
- Human T-lymphocytic viruses
- Polyoma virus
- Coccidioidomycosis
- Histoplasmosis

- Post-transplant hypertension

- Due to volume overload, steroid use, calcineurin-inhibitor use
- May resolve or sustain
- Short-acting antihypertensive is favored in the postop period

# Renal Transplantation Success and Long-Term Outcome Depend on Numerous Factors

- Donor source (living/cadaveric)
- Recipient age (younger than 2 years of age has a lower graft survival rate)
- Donor age (lower survival rate for age less than 5 or older than 60 years)
- Human leukocyte antigen (HLA) matching
- Presensitization (previous transplantation or blood transfusion)
- Technical factors and delayed graft function

Renal transplantation remains a challenge for clinicians in many settings including the PICU. It is essential that the treating physician is aware of the many intricate aspects of caring for these patients and is able to recognize possible complications early in their presentation. It has been reported that more favorable outcomes are present in high-volume centers.

## Suggested Readings

Jungraithmayr TC, Wiesmayr S, Staskewitz A, et al. German Pediatric Renal Transplantation Study Group. Five-year outcome in pediatric patients with mycophenolate mofetil-based renal transplantation. Transplantation 2007;15;83:900–5.

Pape L, Offner G, Ehrich JH, Sasse M. A single center clinical experience in intensive care management of 104 pediatric renal transplantations between 1998 and 2002. Pediatr Transplant 2004;8:39–43.

Smith JM, Stablein DM, Munoz R, et al. Contributions of the Transplant Registry: The 2006 Annual Report of the North American Pediatric Renal Trials and Collaborative Studies (NAPRTCS). Pediatr Transplant 2007;11:366–73.

# Chapter 14

# Gastroenterology

## A. Gastrointestinal Bleeding

Lara Bauman

Samra Sarigol Blanchard

### Introduction

- Gastrointestinal (GI) bleeding is a common problem in the pediatric intensive care unit (PICU) setting, but unlikely to be an emergency. One prospective study found 10.2% of pediatric patients developed upper GI bleeding while in the PICU, but only 1.6% of them were considered significant bleeds. Of the initial cohort, 37% were excluded because they came to the PICU already with an upper GI bleed.
- Lower GI bleeding is also common, with only a low percentage of a serious nature. In 104 children presenting to the emergency department (ED) with rectal bleeding, allergic colitis, infectious gastroenteritis, and anal fissure were the most common causes of rectal bleeding. Only four children had potentially life-threatening diagnoses (one Meckel's diverticulum and three ileocolic intussusception).

### Definitions and Descriptions of Bleeds

- An upper GI bleed (UGIB) is located proximal to the ligament of Treitz.
- A lower GI bleed (LGIB) is defined as distal to the ligament of Treitz.
- Determining the level of bleeding can usually be done with nasogastric lavage and clinical findings.
- Hematemesis is indicative of UGIB.

- Malena may result from UGIB or bleeding from the proximal small intestine.
- Hematochezia is generally indicative of bleeding lower in the GI tract; however, blood can have a cathartic action and rapid bleeding higher in the intestines may result in rapid GI transit and subsequent hematochezia.
- Currant jelly stools are usually a result of vascular congestion and hyperemia such as with intussusception. Large volume bleeds proximal to the rectosigmoid region may produce maroon-colored stools.

## Differential Diagnosis

- Based on age and symptoms (see Tables 1 and 2). While many GI diagnoses can occur at any age, typically there are specific age presentations.
- Determine whether a patient is experiencing a true GI bleed? Hematemesis: Is there an expulsion of swallowed blood from another source? These include ear, nose, and throat (ENT) surgery, recent epistaxis, pharyngitis, or oropharyngeal trauma. Red food coloring, fruit juices, red cabbage, and beets can resemble blood when vomited. Consider hemoptysis.
- Melena: Consider ingestion of iron supplements, bismuth, spinach, cranberries, blueberries, grapes, and licorice.
- Rectal bleedings: Ensure there is no hematuria or menstrual bleeding.

*Table 1*
**Upper GI Bleeding by Age Group**

| Neonatal | Infants | Younger children | Older/ adolescents |
| --- | --- | --- | --- |
| Swallowed maternal blood | Gastritis | Gastritis | Gastritis |
| Gastritis | Esophagitis | Mallory-Weiss tear | Peptic/duodenal ulcer |
| Duodenitis | Mallory-Weiss tear | Esophagitis | Mallory-Weiss tear |
| Stress ulcer | Stress ulcer | Varices | Esophagitis |
| Esophagitis | Esophageal varices | Vascular malformation | Varices |

*(continued)*

| Neonatal | Infants | Younger children | Older/ adolescents |
|---|---|---|---|
| Coagulopathy | Aortoesoph-ageal fistula | Toxic ingestion | Toxic ingestion |
| Vascular malformation | G/E duplication | Stress ulcer | Stress ulcer |
| Gastric/ esophageal duplication | Vascular malformation | Foreign body | Thrombocy-topenia |
| | Vascular lesions | Vascular lesions | Vascular lesions |

*Table 2*
## Lower GI Bleeding (GIB) by Age Group

| Neonatal | Infants | Younger children | Older/ adolescents |
|---|---|---|---|
| Swallowed maternal blood | Anal fissure | Juvenile polyps | Infectious colitis |
| Anal fissure | Allergic colitis | Anal fissure | Polyps |
| Allergic colitis | Infectious colitis | Infectious colitis | Inflammatory bowel disease |
| Infectious colitis | Volvulus | HSP | Hemorrhoids |
| NEC | Intussusception | Lymphono-dular hyperplasia | Anal fissure |
| Coagulopathy | Meckel's diverticulum | Intussuscep-tion | Meckel's diverticulum |
| Meckel's diverticulum | Vascular malformation | Meckel's diverticulum | HUS |
| Volvulus | Intestinal duplication | Inflammatory bowel disease | HSP |
| Intussusception | Pseudomem-branous colitis | HUS | Pseudomem-branous colitis |

| Neonatal | Infants | Younger children | Older/ adolescents |
|---|---|---|---|
| Hirschsprung's colitis | Ischemic colitis | Pseudomembranous colitis | Ischemic colitis |
| Intestinal duplication | Vascular lesions | Ischemic colitis | AV malformation |
| | | Vasculitis | Vasculitis |
| | | Vascular lesions | Vascular lesions |

# Assessment

## History

- Description of current bleeding episode
- Estimation of blood loss
- Medications, including recent antibiotic use
- Ingestions
- Trauma
- History of other bleeding episodes, peptic ulcer disease
- Stool history
- Family history of peptic ulcer disease
- Tendency to bruise or bleed easily

## Physical Examination/Findings

- Blood pressure and pulse (tachycardia is an early sign, postural hypotension is a late but emergent sign heralding cardiovascular collapse)
- Pallor, capillary refill time
- Signs of recent epistaxis
- Indications of liver disease such as jaundice, ascites, abdominal distension, hepatosplenomegaly, prominent abdominal veins, spider nevi, bruits
- Perianal disease, rectal masses, stool inspection
- Ecchymoses, petechiae
- Oral mucosal and lip freckling (polyposis syndrome)
- Palpable purpura (Henoch-Schönlein purpura—HSP)
- External hemangiomas and telangiectasia may indicate similar lesions in the GI tract

## Investigations

- Hemoccult (stool)
- Gastroccult (vomitus)
- Nasogastric lavage. Bloody aspirate can confirm an active bleed, but an active duodenal bleed may still result in clear aspirate

Use caution in placing the nasogastric (NG) tube if there is evidence of portal hypertension. The risk of variceal bleeding warrants the use of caution but does not contraindicate the placement of the NG tube.

- Complete blood count (CBC)

  - Low mean corpuscular volume (MCV) suggests microcytic anemia and a more chronic blood loss.
  - Low white blood count (WBC) and platelets: may be related to hypersplenism and portal hypertension, therefore suspect esophageal varices. May be due to sepsis, with a stress ulcer as the source of bleeding.

- Prothrombin (PT)/partial prothrombin (PTT)
- Hepatic function—elevated bilirubin, transaminases, PT, and low albumin may all suggest hepatic dysfunction with esophageal varices
- Elevated blood urea nitrogen (BUN) or BUN: creatinine ratio may indicate blood resorption from an upper GI bleed
- Blood type and cross
- Electrolytes
- Apt test (denaturation of fetal hemoglobin) to differentiate swallowed maternal blood versus fetal blood
- Meckel's scan for large volume lower GIB
- Stool cultures—as indicated for hematochezia

## Management/Treatment

### Resuscitation

- After addressing airway and breathing, hemodynamic stabilization is the first priority in all GIB cases. Volume replacement should be cautiously aggressive. Use of isotonic crystalloid solutions and packed red blood cells (RBCs) is essential.
- Assess degree of intravascular blood volume loss.

- Tachycardia: >10% loss
- Positive orthostatic maneuvers (ie, symptoms of dizziness, faintness, or lightheadedness on standing, with low blood pressure): 20% loss
- Prolonged capillary refill: 25% loss
- Mental status changes: 30–40% loss

- Place NG tube and assess aspirate.
- Monitor BP, heart rate, and urine output.
- Correct any coagulopathies or electrolyte imbalances
  - In patients with active bleeding, fresh frozen plasma FFP should be given if the PT is at least 1.5 times the control value.
  - Platelet transfusion is indicated if the platelet count is <50,000 mm$^3$.

- Airway protection with endotracheal intubation is necessary in certain cases. There is a high risk of aspiration in patients with massive GI bleeding or in those who have an altered mental status.
- In patients with a history or clinical signs of liver disease, an octreotide infusion should be started.
- Once the patient is hemodynamically stable, endoscopic evaluation should be done to fully assess the bleed and guide further treatment.
- If the patient cannot be stabilized, emergency surgical assessment is needed.
- Five mL/kg/hour of ongoing blood loss is generally considered a surgical threshold.
- See hematology section for considerations relating to massive blood transfusion.

# Management of Upper GI Bleeding

Early endoscopy after stabilization is the cornerstone of management of upper GI bleeding and provides the most accurate method available for identifying the source of bleeding.

# Variceal Bleeding

- Volume resuscitation with colloids, avoid overexpansion of the blood volume. In children with esophageal varices exceeding the portal venous pressures may lead to worsening of the variceal bleeding.
- Correct clotting factors.

- Careful NG placement to monitor bleeding.
- Octreotide 1 microgram/kg bolus followed by 1 microgram/kg/hour continuous infusion.

    - Octreotide is an analog of somatostatin and is widely used for reduction of collateral blood flow in patients with esophageal varices. Octreotide also tempers increases in portal pressure, which can lead to rebleeding, often seen with postprandial hyperemia from enteral feeding or entrance of blood into the stomach.

- Start intravenous H2 blocker or PPI therapy.
- Start prophylactic antibiotic therapy.

    - Cirrhotic patients warrant the use of antibiotics with an upper GIB.
    - There is an increased incidence of bacterial infections in cirrhotic patients after gastrointestinal bleeding.
    - The most common agents are enteric bacteria. Though there are no standard protocols for pediatrics, seven days of antibiotic prophylaxis is standard treatment for adult patients. Options include norfloxacin, ciprofloxacin, and cefotaxime or ceftriaxone.

- Endoscopic banding in combination with an octreotide infusion is more effective.
- Endoscopic sclerotherapy is an alternative option in infants and young children when band ligation is technically not possible.
- If there is a persistent bleeding despite banding or sclerotherapy, consider transjugular intrahepatic protosystemic shunt (TIPS) or emergency surgical shunt depending on technical availability and patency of portal vein. If there is a decompensated hepatic function, patient should be listed for liver transplantation.
- If bleeding is controlled, recurrence of bleeding can be prevented with propranolol prophylaxis or regular endoscopic band ligation sessions.

# Nonvariceal Upper GI Bleeding

## Endoscopy

Endoscopic evaluation is essential to fully assess the source and cause of bleeding. Hemostasis of nonvariceal bleeds may be achievable with injection, thermocoagulation, or laser therapy.

## Acid Suppression

Ulcers, gastritis, and duodenitis are commonly associated with upper GI bleeding. This justifies the empiric use of acid suppressing agents in the initial treatment of an UGIB. Either proton pump inhibitors (PPIs) or H2-receptor antagonists (H2RAs) can be used. Ranitidine and famotidine need to be dose-adjusted for renal insufficiency. There is a concern for the possible development of tolerance to H2RAs. PPIs are increasing in popularity. PPIs generally provide more effective suppression of acid production.

Sucralfate is cytoprotective and is used to reduce the risk of rebleeding or in some cases to treat or prevent ulcers. Sucralfate works by coating the esophageal or gastric mucosa and can be especially helpful in protecting ulcerated tissue, Mallory-Weiss tears, and banded or treated varices. It also stimulates the release of prostaglandin E2, promoting the mucosal defense system. The primary disadvantage of this agent is that it can interfere with the absorption of other medications. This can sometimes be avoided by prudent dosage scheduling. Be aware that sucralfate may cause constipation.

## Surgery

Surgical management of UGIB from peptic ulcer disease is uncommon. Medical management with H2RAs and PPIs, as well as antibiotic therapy for *Heliobacter pylori*, has advanced significantly and reduced the need for surgical intervention. Esophageal varices that fail banding and sclerotherapy will need surgical management. See Table 1 for vascular lesions and malformations, which are suitable for surgical assessment.

## **Management of Lower GI Bleeding**

### Endoscopy

Early endoscopic evaluation after stabilization allows for full assessment of the colon and also the terminal portion of the ileum. Visual inspection and biopsy can confirm and differentiate types of colitis and the presence of vascular lesions (see Table 2). Polypectomy is done endoscopically for colon polyps.

## Surgery

Surgical intervention is required in some cases. Surgical emergencies include volvulus and nonreducible intussusception. Surgical treatment will also be required for Meckel's diverticulum, vascular lesions, and malformations.

## Capsule Endoscopy

If the source of the GI bleed cannot be located, and the patient continues to bleed, capsule endoscopy is warranted in patients large enough to tolerate placement of the capsule and safely pass it through the intestines. An upper GI series with small bowel follow-through imaging should be done prior to use of capsule endoscopy. Capsule endoscopy may not be available in all settings.

## Stress Ulcer Prophylaxis

- Stress ulcers result from severe physiologic stress as can be found in the intensive care unit. These ulcers develop rapidly and are primarily a result of mucosal ischemia. They can be seen in any serious illness and measures should be taken to prevent them. Stress ulcer prophylaxis has not been well studied in children.
- The goal of pharmacologic therapy is to prevent stress ulcer formation and the related complications. Medications must be chosen based on available routes of administration and individualized needs of a patient. Prevention of damage may be achieved by keeping the gastric pH above 4 and by maintaining mucosal defense mechanisms. A caution in the prophylaxis of stress-related mucosal damage: increasing the gastric pH above 4 allows gram-negative organisms to live in the stomach. Aspiration of these can lead to nosocomial pneumonia, which is the most frequent infection in patients on mechanical ventilators.
- H2RAs are more effective than sulcrafate in adults, but sucralfate may be considered in some instances. It coats and protects the mucosa without raising the gastric pH. It also stimulates the release of prostaglandin E2, promoting the mucosal defense system. The use of sucralfate instead of H2RAs may decrease the risk of pneumonia in ventilator

patients. Sucralfate may be administered by NG tube, but it is not an option for patients requiring intravenous medications. Be aware of drug interactions with sucralfate. PPIs offer more effective acid suppression but have not been systematically studied as stress ulcer prophylaxis.

Refer to Table 3 for medication dosing.

*Table 3*

**Acid Suppression and Cytoprotective Therapy with Pediatric Dosages**

| Medication | Pediatric dose | How supplied** |
|---|---|---|
| **H2 RECEPTOR ANTAGONISTS** | | |
| Ranitidine | Oral: 4–10 mg/kg/d Divided twice or 3 times per day Maximum: 300 mg/d IV: 2–6 mg/kg/d. May be given as a continuous infusion or divided q6–12 h (usual maximum 50 mg q6–8h or 200 mg/d) | Syrup: 15 mg/mL Tablets: 75, 150, 300 mg Injectable: 50 mg |
| Famotidine | PO/IV: 1–2 mg/kg/d Divided twice a d Max PO: 80 mg/d Max IV: 40 mg/d | Syrup: 8 mg/mL Tablets: 10, 20, 40 mg Injectable: 20 mg |
| Cimetidine | PO/IV: 10–40 mg/kg/d Divided 2–4 times/d Adult max: 1200 mg/d | Syrup: 10, 60 mg/mL Tablets: 200, 300, 400, 800 mg |

*(continued)*

| Medication | Pediatric dose | How supplied** |
|---|---|---|
| **PROTON-PUMP INHIBITORS*** | | |
| Esomeprazole | Adult dose: 20–40 mg once daily 0.5–1 mg/kg/d has been used in children | Capsules: 20, 40 mg Injectable: 20 mg, 40 mg |
| Omeprazole | 1–2 mg/kg/d, up to 3.3 mg/kg/d has been used, or: <20 kg: 10 mg/d >20 kg: 20 mg/d Adult dose: 20–40 mg/d | Capsules: 10, 20, 40 mg Powder packet: 20, 40 mg |
| Lansoprazole | 0.8–1.6 mg/kg/d, up to 4 mg/kg/day has been used, or: <15 kg: 7.5 mg/d <30 kg: 15 mg/d >30 kg: 30mg/d Adult dose: 30 mg/d Approved for use over the age of 1 year | Capsules: 15, 30 mg Powder packet: 15, 30 mg Solu-tab: 15, 30 mg Injectable: 30 mg |
| Rabeprazole | Adult dose: 10–20 mg/d | Tablets: 10, 20 mg |
| Pantoprazole | Adult dose: 40–80 mg/d 0.5–1 mg/kg/d has been used in children | Tablet: 20, 40 mg Injectable: 40 mg |
| **CYTOPROTECTIVE AGENT** | | |
| Sucralfate | 40–80 mg/kg/d Divided into 3–4 doses maximum 1 g/dose | Suspension: 100 mg/mL Tablet: 1 g |

PPI use in pediatrics is widespread though not all PPIs have pediatric data. These are dosing guidelines based on common practice. Some pharmacies may prepare oral liquids formulations.
*For neonatal dosing refer to appropriate pharmacologic resources.
**Not all dosage forms may be available in all settings.

# References

Chaibou M, Tucci M, Dugas MA, et al. Clinically significant upper gastrointestinal bleeding acquired in a pediatric intensive care unit: a prospective study. Pediatrics 1998;102:933–8.

Teach SJ, Fleisher GR. Rectal bleeding in the pediatric emergency department. Ann Emerg Med 1994;23:1252–4.

Olson AD, Hillemeier AC. Gastrointestinal hemorrhage. In: Wyllie R, Hyams JS, eds. Pediatric Gastrointestinal Disease: Pathophysiology, Diagnosis, Management. Philadelphia: WB Saunders Co.; 1993:251–70.

Chameides L, Hazinski MF, eds. Textbook of Pediatric Advanced Life Support. Dallas: American Heart Association; 1994:2-1–10.

Garcia-Tsao G. Current management of the complications of cirrhosis and portal hypertension: variceal hemorrhage, ascites, and spontaneous bacterial peritonitis. Gastroenterology 2001;120:726–48.

Heikenen JB, Pohl JF, Werlin SJ, Bucavalas JC. Octreotide in pediatric patients. J Pediatric Gastroenterol Nutr 2002;35:600–9.

Peters JM. Management of gastrointestinal bleeding in children. Curr Treat Options in Gastroenterol 2002;5:399–413.

Spirt MJ. Stress-related mucosal disease. Curr Treat Options in Gastroenterol 2003;6:135–45.

# B. Short Bowel Syndrome

## Samra Sarigol Blanchard
## Lara Bauman

## Key Principles

- Short bowel syndrome (SBS) is caused by significant intestinal resection.
- Prognosis is related to degree of bowel loss and subsequent adaptation.
- Management is based on advancing enteral nutrition and preventing complications.
- Early recognition of intestinal failure for timely intestinal transplantation is essential.

## Pathophysiology

Short bowel syndrome (SBS) is characterized by a state of malabsorption after extensive resection of the small bowel. Absorption is related to the amount of residual length and the functional integrity of the remaining small intestine.

SBS can be due to either congenital or acquired conditions. The main causes are summarized in Table 1 depending on age groups. Functional SBS may also occur in cases of severe malabsorption in which the bowel length is often intact or near normal. Such conditions may include microvillus inclusion disease, chronic intestinal pseudo-obstruction, radiation enteritis, and tufting enteropathy.

The anatomic site of pathology (eg, following a bowel resection) affects the presentation of SBS.

- The jejunum is the site for the greatest nutrient absorption due to its long villi, large absorptive surface, and highly concentrated digestive enzymes. Jejunum is also relatively leaky, allowing the rapid flux of water and electrolytes throughout the mucosa to the intraluminal space. As a result, marked fluid secretion occurs in response to feeding, which is subsequently reabsorbed primarily in the ileum. After ileal resection, there is substantial fluid and electrolyte loss. Since the ileum is also the primary site of absorption of vitamin B12 and bile salts

*Table 1*
**Etiology of Short Bowel Syndrome**

| Infants | Older children |
|---|---|
| Necrotizing enterocolitis | Midgut volvulus |
| Total colonic aganglionosis (Hirschsprung's disease) | Crohn's disease |
| Intestinal atresia | Arterial/venous thrombosis |
| Gastroschisis | Post-trauma resection |
| Congenital short bowel syndrome | Tumor |
| Midgut volvulus | Radiation enteritis |

through site-specific receptors, these could be permanently malabsorbed. Bile salt malabsorption impairs fat and fat-soluble vitamin absorption. The delivery of unabsorbed bile acids to the colon can cause choleretic diarrhea. The ileum is also the site of synthesis for many gastrointestinal hormones such as enteroglucagon, epidermal growth factor, and peptide YY. Ileal resection impairs the ileal break phenomenon (which normally slows gut motility) due to lack of peptide YY and fat malabsorption. Also, the normal negative feedback mechanism for gastrin is lost, and hypergastrinemia causing acid-peptic disease is common in patients with SBS.

- Resection of the ileocecal valve compounds effects of ileal resection. It serves as a major barrier for reflux of colonic bacteria into the small intestine, preventing bacterial overgrowth. It also slows the intestinal transit time allowing nutrient absorption.

## Intestinal Adaptation

Residual small intestine undergoes an adaptive process characterized by mucosal hyperplasia. In humans, intestinal adaptation begins within 24 to 48 hours of resection and includes both structural adaptation and functional adaptation. Structural adaptation includes increase of the bowel diameter and lengthening of the villi, resulting in increased absorptive surface area. Functional adaptation entails increased nutrient absorption by up-regulation of carrier-mediated transport mechanisms.

Intestinal adaptation is highly dependent on the use of enteral nutrition. The intraluminal nutrients stimulate the mucosa directly or stimulate secretion of trophic gastrointestinal hormones (enteroglucagon, gastrin, secretin, cholecystokinin, insulin, neurotensin, growth hormone, glucagons peptide II, and epidermal growth factor are involved in intestinal adaptation).

Citrulline is a nonprotein amino acid produced by the intestinal mucosa. Serum measurements of citrulline correlate linearly with intestinal adaptation.

## Prognosis

At birth, the estimated small bowel length is 250 ± 40 cm. Infants left with only a duodenum or at most 10 cm of jejunum, and no ileocecal valve, will remain permanently dependent on parenteral nutrition (PN). Small bowel length of less than 30 to 40 cm, absence of an ileocecal valve, resection of some colon, minimal tolerance of enteral feeding within the first months after intestinal resection, and multiple surgical procedures are risk factors for intestinal failure. Older children and adolescents have less potential for structural adaptation and therefore generally a worse prognosis than in neonatal cases. The presence of a functioning colon is also important after extensive small bowel resection because it not only gives added bowel length but also slows intestinal transit. The colon is capable of increasing its absorptive capacity threefold to fivefold. Sodium, water, and some amino acids are absorbed in the colon as well as energy from absorbed short-chain fatty acids (SCFAs).

## Clinical Findings

- The severity of symptoms and the occurrence of short- and long-term complications relate to the site and the extent of the bowel excised, the residual surface area, and gut motility (see above).
- Diarrhea is the dominant finding and is caused by one or more of the following: decreased surface area, carbohydrate (CHO) and fat malabsorption, bile salt malabsorption, bacterial overgrowth ($>10^5$/mL), and intestinal inflammation.
- Other symptoms are abdominal pain/distention/bloating, and increased flatus. Perianal rash can be seen due to excessive diarrhea or zinc deficiency. Appropriate growth and development will depend on the management of nutritional needs.

# Medical Management

## Early Management

- Early postoperative management is done in the PICU.
- In the immediate postoperative period, maintain fasting and support with total parenteral nutrition (TPN).
- Closely monitor volume status including fecal/stomal losses of water and electrolytes to ensure optimal electrolyte and water balance.
- Patients with high jejunostomies are at high risk for large volume diarrhea, hyponatremia, hypokalemia, and hypomagnesemia. In addition to TPN, these patients require additional sodium-containing fluid replacement to match the losses.
- Patients should be started on acid blockers to prevent gastric hypersecretion.

## Enteral Feeding

- Start continuous enteral nutrition with pumped breast milk or an elemental diet when patients are hemodynamically stable with stable ostomy output.
- Protein hydrolysate infant formulas with higher medium-chain triglycerides (MCT) such as Pregestimil (Mead Johnson) or Alimentum (Ross) are well tolerated. MCTs are important because they are readily absorbed in the stomach and proximal small bowel, thereby improving fat and total energy absorption. MCTs should be the main source of fat and energy needs.
- Long-chain fatty acids are required to prevent essential fatty acid deficiency and should make up approximately 10% of the patient's energy needs. Long-chain fatty acids may have a trophic effect on the intestinal mucosa.
- An amino acid–based formula such as Neocate (SHS) can be used when breast milk or protein hydrolysate formulas are not tolerated.
- In older children (>12 months) Peptamen Jr (protein hydrolysate, Nestle), Neocate Jr (elemental, SHS), or Vivonex (elemental, Novartis) are recommended formulas to start enteral feedings.
- Continuous nasogastric feedings are recommended in early stages to improve absorption. Small bolus feeding should be introduced gradually to prevent dumping syndrome.
- It is often necessary to place a gastrostomy button for long-term administration of enteral feeds. Minimal amount of oral feeding can be carefully offered to prevent oral aversion.

- The success of enteral feeding can be assessed by measuring enteral fluid output, which reflects the degree of carbohydrate malabsorption. CHO malabsorption can be easily screened with stool/ostomy pH and reducing substances.
- Soluble fibers (pectin, guar gum, or psyllium) increase viscosity, decrease gastric emptying, and slow gut transit. They pass undigested into the colon where colonic bacteria ferment them to SCFAs. SCFAs (primarily acetate, propionate, and butyrate) stimulate sodium and water absorption and also induce a trophic effect on the colon. Butyrate is the major energy source for colonocytes. The fiber intake should be titrated based on response. Exceedingly high fiber intake (>0.5 gm/kg) in children can induce malabsorption.

## Long-Term Management

Long-term management includes advancing of enteral feeding while tapering parenteral nutrition and preventing or treating complications of SBS

## Complications of SBS

**Diarrhea:** This is the most common complication due to osmotic load and it may occur any time that enteral nutrition is advanced—often forcing a retreat to slower regimens. Consider:

- Switching from bolus to continuous feedings and changing to a low osmolar, low CHO, high fat formula.
- Use of somatostatin analogs (octreotide) especially in patients with jejunostomy who have high stoma output. It may cause biliary sludge.
- Add soluble fiber (eg, pectin, guar gum, psyllium)
- Cholestyramine (250–500 mg/kg per day, bid/tid) can be used to bind malabsorbed bile acids after ileal resection to decrease secretory diarrhea.
- Antisecretory agents, Immodium (loperamide) and Lomotil (diphenoxylate HCl + atropine) can be used to slow gastrointestinal motility in children.

**Catheter-related complications:** Central line sepsis, catheter breakage and occlusion, and catheter exit site infections eventually occur in most patients. Bacterial translocation from the gut epithelium can be a factor in recurrent line infection. Broad-spectrum antibiotic coverage should be started immediately in patients with suspected line infection.

**Acid-peptic disease** occurs due to gastric hypersecretion. Increased acidity also inactivates pancreatic enzymes and causes further fat malabsorption. H2 blockers can be added to TPN or proton pump inhibitors can be given IV or with enteral feedings (see GI Bleeding section for dosage of acid blockers).

**Bacterial overgrowth:** The absence of the ileocecal valve allows colonic bacteria to enter and populate the small intestine. Small bowel bacterial overgrowth (SBO) causes mucosal inflammation, which further may exacerbate nutrient malabsorption, deconjugate bile salts, and deplete bile salt pool with subsequent steatorrhea and fat-soluble vitamins malabsorption. It is usually associated with anorexia, diarrhea, abdominal pain and distention, metabolic acidosis from D-lactic acidosis, and failure to thrive. The diagnosis is made by hydrogen breath test. Antibiotic treatment with metronidazole or rifaximin is effective and in many patients empiric cyclical dosing can prevent bacterial overgrowth. Recalcitrant bacterial overgrowth has been successfully treated with periodic small bowel irrigation with a balanced hypertonic electrolyte solution, colonic flushes, encouraging frequent stooling, intestinal lengthening procedure, or probiotic therapy with Lactobacillus plantarium 299V and Lactobacillus GG.

**D-lactic acidosis** is a rare complication seen in patients with a preserved colon and bacterial overgrowth. Gram-positive anaerobes in the colon produce D-lactate from unabsorbed carbohydrates. An increased carbohydrate load in the diet can induce metabolic acidosis, headache, encephalopathy, ataxia, and dysarthria. The diagnosis is confirmed by an elevated measurement of D-lactate in the blood. Treatment consists of correction of acidosis, reduction of carbohydrate intake, and treatment of SBO with metronidazole or vancomycin for 7 to 10 days.

**Nutritional deficiencies:** Children with SBS are at risk for vitamin and trace element deficiencies when they are weaned from parenteral nutrition. Fat-soluble vitamin, iron, and zinc deficiencies can occur; these levels should be followed on regularly. Patients with ileal resection will need regular B12 replacement through either intranasal (Nascobal nasal spray 500 ug/week) or parenteral (cyanocobalamin 100 mcg/month IM for maintenance) administration. In the presence of significant steatorrhea, water-soluble forms of vitamins *ADEK* are available commercially. Other micronutrients, including manganese and selenium, can be provided in pharmacologic doses as required.

Selenium deficiency has been associated with cardiomyopathy, peripheral neuropathy, and proximal muscle weakness. Periodic measurements of zinc and selenium are merited for individuals on long-term parenteral nutrition.

**Osteoporosis** occurs due to calcium, magnesium, and vitamin D deficiencies as well as altered acid-base status. Patients can be screened with serum calcium, phosphorus, magnesium, and 1, 25 hydroxy vitamin D levels.

**Hyperoxaluria:** Normally oxalate in the diet binds to calcium and is excreted in the stool. Because of fat malabsorption, dietary calcium binds to free fatty acids and the oxalate is absorbed in the colon and filtered through the kidneys. This results in hyperoxaluria and kidney stones. Patients with intact colons should be regularly assessed for urinary oxalate excretion. Treatment of hyperoxaluria is to decrease oxalate intake in the diet and uses oral calcium supplementation.

**Hepatobiliary disease:** The following factors can contribute to chronic liver disease: impaired intestinal function and bacterial overgrowth (endotoxinemia), excessive glucose intake leading to hyperinsulinism and subsequent steatosis, prematurity, recurrent catheter infection, protracted bowel rest, continuous instead of cyclic TPN infusion, and direct toxicity of TPN.

Prevention of liver disease may be possible with the following: early introduction of enteral feeding, suppressing intraluminal bacterial overgrowth by giving empiric antibiotics in cyclical dosing, avoiding catheter-related sepsis by appropriate daily care of the line, optimizing and cycling TPN, and use of ursodeoxycholic acid, which can help decrease liver injury.

Patients with SBS are also at risk of developing gallstones. Diminished enteral stimulation and interruption of enterohepatic circulation of bile acid after ileal resection can cause biliary stasis and supersaturation of bile, which will lead to formation of biliary sludge and gallstones. Ursodeoxycholic acid at dose of 15 to 30 mg/kg/day may be helpful in prevention.

## Surgical Management

Additional surgical procedures are often indicated in SBS. There are two major categories of surgery:

- Increase the intestinal mucosal surface area. Intestinal lengthening and tapering have been performed in selected patients with dilated bowel segments. The intestinal lengthening procedure involves transection of the bowel longitudinally, preserving the blood supply and creating a bowel segment twice the length. The second type of surgery is the creation of artificial ileocecal valves and the reversal of anti-peristaltic intestinal segments to slow the motility.

- Intestinal transplantation is considered when there is reasonable certainty that intestinal dysfunction is permanent, impending loss of catheter site access for TPN, and development of TPN-related liver disease. Patients should be referred to small bowel transplant centers for the complexity of management.

# References

DiBaise JK, Young RJ, Vanderhoof JA. Intestinal rehabilitation and the short bowel syndrome: part 1. Am J Gastroenterol 2004;99:1386–95.

Goulet O, Ruemmele F. Causes and management of intestinal failure in children. Gastroenterology 2006;130(2 Suppl 1):S16–28.

Nightingale JM, Kamm MA, van der Sijp JR, et al. Gastrointestinal hormones in short bowel syndrome. Peptide YY may be the 'colonic brake' to gastric emptying. Gut 1996;39:267–72.

Buchman AL. Etiology and initial management of short bowel syndrome. Gastroenterology 2006;130(2 Suppl 1):S5–15.

Jeejeebhoy KN. Management of short bowel syndrome: avoidance of total parenteral nutrition. Gastroenterology 2006;130(2 Suppl 1):S60–6.

Cisler JJ, Buchman AL. Intestinal adaptation in short bowel syndrome. J Investig Med 2005;53:402–13.

Rhoads JM, Plunkett E, Galanko J, Lichtman S, et al. Serum citrulline levels correlate with enteral tolerance and bowel length in infants with short bowel syndrome. J Pediatr 2005;146:542–7.

Vanderhoof JA. Short bowel syndrome and intestinal adaptation. In: Walker WA, Sherman PM, Goulet O, et al., eds. Pediatric gastrointestinal disease. 4th ed. Hamilton: BC Decker; 2004:742–61.

Kollman KA, Lien EL, Vanderhoof JA. Dietary lipids influence intestinal adaptation after massive bowel resection. J Pediatr Gastroenterol Nutr 1999;28:41–5.

Kles KA, Chang EB. Short-chain fatty acids impact on intestinal adaptation, inflammation, carcinoma, and failure. Gastroenterology 2006;130(2 Suppl 1):S100–5.

Westergaard H. Short-bowel syndrome. Curr Treat Options Gastroenterol 2000;3:45–50.

DiBaise JK, Young RJ, Vanderhoof JA. Enteric microbial flora, bacterial overgrowth, and short-bowel syndrome. Clin Gastroenterol Hepatol 2006;4:11–20.

Scarpignato C, Pelosini I. Experimental and clinical pharmacology of rifaximin, a gastrointestinal selective antibiotic. Digestion 2006;73(Suppl 1):13–27.

Vanderhoof JA, Young RJ, Murray N, Kaufman SS. Treatment strategies for small bowel bacterial overgrowth in short bowel syndrome. J Pediatr Gastroenterol Nutr 1998;27:155–60.

Petersen C. D-lactic acidosis. Nutr Clin Pract 2005;20:634–45.

AGA Technical review on short bowel syndrome and intestinal transplantation. Gastroenterology 2003;124:1111–34.

Nightingale JM, Lennard-Jones JE, Gertner DJ, et al. Colonic preservation reduces need for parenteral therapy, increases incidence of renal stones, but does not change high prevalence of gall stones in patients with a short bowel. Gut 1992;33:1493–7.

Kelly DA. Intestinal failure-associated liver disease: what do we know today? Gastroenterology 2006;130(2 Suppl 1):S70–7.

Al-Hathlol K, Al-Madani A, Al-Saif S, et al. Ursodeoxycholic acid therapy for intractable total parenteral nutrition-associated cholestasis in surgical very low birth weight infants. Singapore Med J 2006;47:147–51.

Jain R. Biliary sludge: when should it not be ignored? Curr Treat Options Gastroenterol 2004;7:105–9.

Vanderhoof JA, Young RJ, Thompson JS. New and emerging therapies for short bowel syndrome in children. Paediatr Drugs 2003;5:525–31.

Bianchi A. From the cradle to enteral autonomy: the role of autologous gastrointestinal reconstruction. Gastroenterology 2006;130(2 Suppl 1):S138–46.

# C. Pancreatitis

Lara Bauman
Samra Sarigol Blanchard

## Key Principles

- Pancreatitis has been considered as rare in childhood, but incidence is rising. One center reports 25 cases per year instead of the 5 to 10 previously estimated.
- The most common clinical symptoms of acute pancreatitis are abdominal pain, vomiting, abdominal tenderness, and abdominal distension. Less common clinical findings include fever, tachycardia, hypotension, jaundice, abdominal guarding, rebound tenderness, and decreased bowel sounds. Pancreatitis in children is usually a single acute self-limited episode, unlike the adult population.
- Main etiology remains idiopathic, but a large variety of causes must be investigated.
- Always consider in a critically ill patient with abdominal symptoms, or with significant abdominal trauma.
- Management is primarily supportive and expectant, and aimed at the underlying cause.

## Pathophysiology

- The pancreas performs two major functions. The **endocrine** pancreas consists of islet cells and excretes hormones.
- The exocrine pancreas produces and secretes over 20 digestive enzymes including lipase, amylase, trypsin, elastase, and phospholipase. These enzymes are stored as inactive precursors (zymogens) that are normally activated on in the duodenum. If these zymogens are activated early, auto-digestion of the pancreas can occur resulting in pancreatitis. Triggers of early activation are the underlying causes of pancreatitis: trauma, obstruction, medications, systemic disease, or infection.
- There are local and systemic effects of pancreatitis. The initial auto-digestion of the gland triggers systemic cytokines and a systemic inflammatory response.

- Prognosis and treatment of pancreatitis depend on the cause and the degree of injury. If there is a treatable underlying condition, such as inflammatory bowel disease or obstruction, once this is addressed the pancreatitis should improve. Severe disease is characterized by organ failure or local complications such as necrosis or pseudocyst. Scoring systems to predict prognosis (Ranson criteria and the APACHE II scoring system) are mostly used in adults.

# Acute Pancreatitis

Most pancreatitis in children is a single self-limited episode, contrary to adults. More serious pancreatitis (necrotizing pancreatitis) worsens the prognosis and recovery time (see Table 1 for causes of pancreatitis).

# Chronic Pancreatitis

Irreversible structural changes in the pancreas can lead to chronic pancreatitis and pancreatic insufficiency. Pancreatic insufficiency is usually a late finding because of the large reserve capacity of the pancreas. There are two major classifications of chronic pancreatitis: calcific and obstructive. Calcific forms involve strictures, replacement of cells with fat, epithelial atrophy, and fibrosis. Obstructive disease of the pancreatic duct involves congenital anomalies, mass lesions, or sclerosis. Trauma is primarily associated with acute pancreatitis, but can also cause permanent change by destruction or obstruction of ducts, strictures, or compression.

*Table 1*

**Conditions Associated with Acute and Chronic Pancreatitis in Children**

| Systemic Conditions/ Disease | Obstructive |
|---|---|
| • Hypertriglyceridemia | • **Cholelithiasis** |
| • Cystic fibrosis | • **Pancreas divisum** |
| • Hypercalcemia | • **Pancreatic duct abnormalities** |
| • Alpha-1 antitrypsin deficiency | |
| • Crohn's disease | • **Biliary tract malformations** |
| • Hereditary pancreatitis | |
| • Diabetes | • **Tumor/mass** |

## Systemic Conditions/Disease

- Kawasaki's disease
- Malnutrition (including anorexia nervosa and bulimia) and refeeding
- Hemolytic Uremic Syndrome (HUS)
- Henoch-Schönlein Purpura (HSP)
- Metabolic disease (eg, organic acidemias, propionic academia, lactic acidosis, glycogen storage disease type 1, homocystinuria)
- Hemochromatosis
- Hyperparathyroidism
- Renal failure
- Transplantation (pancreas, kidney, heart, bone marrow, liver)
- Peptic ulcer disease
- Brain tumor

## Drugs/Toxins

- **Azathioprine**, 6-MP
- **L-asparaginase**
- **Valproic acid**
- **Estrogen**
- **Salicylates,** sulindac
- **Vincristine, vinblastine**
- **Tetracyclines, sulfonamides**, metronidazole, erythromycin
- Sulfasalazine, 5-ASA
- Furosemide, thiazide diuretics
- Didanosine, pentamidine
- Tamoxifen
- Alcohol
- Steroids

## Obstructive

- **Strictures**
- **Surgical complications**
- **ERCP complications**
- **Sphincter of Oddi dysfunction**
- **Duplication cyst**
- **Ampullary disease**

## Autoimmune

## Trauma

- **Blunt abdominal injury**
- **accidental and nonaccidental**
- **Surgical trauma**
- **Head trauma**

## Infectious

- **Coxsackie virus**
- **Mumps**
- **CMV**
- **EBV**
- **Hepatitis A and B**
- **Varicella-zoster**
- **HSV**
- **Measles**
- **Rubella**
- **Influenza A and B**
- **Mycoplasma**
- **Legionella**
- **Salmonella**
- **Malaria**
- **Leptospirosis**
- **Rubeola**
- **Aspergillus**
- **Toxoplasma**
- **Cryptosporidium**
- **Ascariasis (obstructive)**

Medications in bold are considered to have a stronger association in the etiology of acute pancreatitis.

# Clinical Features

- Diagnosis of acute pancreatitis may be difficult. There are no gold standard protocols for its diagnosis. Diagnosis depends on a clinical suspicion and test results.
- Diagnosis of chronic pancreatitis is difficult, and requires a recurring pattern.
- Common signs and symptoms may include:

  - Abdominal pain, often aggravated by eating
  - Nausea/vomiting, often worse with eating
  - Abdominal tenderness
  - Abdominal distension
  - Low-grade fever
  - Tachycardia
  - Decreased or absent bowel sounds

- Other possible findings:

  - Palpable epigastric mass (pseudocyst)
  - Hypotension
  - Mild jaundice
  - Severe cases may include ascites, renal failure, pleural effusion, bluish discoloration of the abdomen

# Differential Diagnosis

- Once pancreatitis is diagnosed based on clinical features including elevated pancreatic enzymes, the key is to determine whether there is a removable or treatable cause of the pancreatitis.
- Hyper-amylasemia may have non-pancreatic causes. The amylase level can be fractionated to determine whether it is predominantly pancreatic or salivary. Salivary amylase levels may increase from causes such as mumps, salivary duct obstruction, trauma, ovarian disease, diabetic ketoacidosis, eating disorders, or malignancies.
- Distinguishing causes of acute versus chronic pancreatitis is not easy in practice. The causes of chronic pancreatitis may also cause acute disease (see Table 1).
- Medications: Many conditions cause pancreatitis, and the medications to treat these conditions may also cause pancreatitis. Look for the temporal causality with the use of the medication and resolution with the withdrawal of the medication (see Table 1).

# Investigations

- Serum amylase is usually elevated within the first few hours of the initial pancreatic insult and remains elevated for 4 to 5 days. There are many cautions with the use of serum amylase level. Hyper-amylasemia may arise for many other reasons than pancreatitis. There are also rare cases (mostly adult) in which the serum amylase remains normal in pancreatitis.
- Serum lipase is more accurate for acute pancreatitis than amylase, though there are still false-positives and false-negatives. Specificity for both tests improves with a threefold increase in levels. Lipase generally rises within hours after onset of pancreatitis, but because it is reabsorbed in the glomerular tubules, it remains elevated for 8 to 14 days. After the first 24 hours of illness, the lipase is considered more accurate than amylase for the diagnosis of pancreatitis.
- Radiology (ultrasound and computed tomography [CT]) may be normal in up to 30% of cases at the time of presentation. However, radiologic evaluation should be performed to look for a definitive cause of the pancreatitis.

    - Ultrasound allows direct evaluation of the pancreas without exposure to radiation. One may find typical findings of pancreatitis such as enlargement, poorly defined border, decreased echogenicity, dilated ducts, or pseudocysts, or cholelithiasis and bile duct obstruction.
    - Abdominal CT may be useful if the ultrasound is inconclusive.

- MRCP (magnetic resonance cholangiopancreatography) can be useful to visualize the pancreatobiliary ductal system if needed in more difficult cases.
- Other tests include infectious disease evaluation, triglyceride levels, cystic fibrosis screening, serum calcium, screening for diabetes, malnutrition, vasculitis, metabolic disease, renal failure, and many other conditions. The clinical picture will guide these other evaluations.
- ERCP (endoscopic retrograde cholangiopancreatography) is used both in diagnosis and in treatment of pancreatitis. In diagnosis it is useful in the diagnosis of ductal abnormalities. Consultation with your institution's gastroenterologist will help to determine when ERCP or MRCP is indicated for this evaluation. ERCP carries complication risks such as exacerbation of pancreatitis, pain, perforation, and cholangitis.

# Complications

Complications of pancreatitis are reviewed in Table 2. Systemic complications are managed according to intensive care unit protocols. Common abdominal complications in children are pancreatic pseudocyst and infection.

Pancreatic pseudocsyt: A collection of pancreatic fluid encased by granulation tissue and collagen occurring in or around the pancreas as a result of auto-digestive fat necrosis or ductal leakage.

Development of an acute pseudocyst requires at least 4 weeks and is usually preceded by the presence of an acute peri-pancreatic fluid collection.

Pseudocyst presents with persistent pain, vomiting, persistently high serum amylase levels, or failure of an episode of pancreatitis to resolve.

Consider in patients with stable chronic pancreatitis who describe worsening of their abdominal pain.

Pseudocysts complicate acute pancreatitis in less than 5% of cases and chronic pancreatitis in 20% to 40% of cases—mainly in the most severe cases.

Pseudocyst development in chronic pancreatitis results from large duct occlusion causing smaller duct obstruction and dilatation. Occasionally, pseudocysts develop after trauma-related ductal disruption or after surgical injury.

Complications of pseudocyst: Infection occurs in approximately 10% of pseudocysts, usually with enteric flora, and systemic sepsis may occur. Pseudocysts can rupture into a neighboring viscus (stomach, duodenum, or colon) or directly into the peritoneal cavity, presenting with an acute abdominal

*Table 2*
## Complications of Pancreatitis

| *Abdominal* | *Systemic* |
|---|---|
| Pancreatic pseudocyst | Disseminated intravascular coagulation |
| Pancreatic abscess | Pleural effusion/pneumonia |
| Pancreatic necrosis | Hypoglycemia |
| Splenic vein thrombosis | Hypocalcemia |
| Hemorrhage | UGI bleeding due to stress |
| | Acute respiratory distress syndrome |
| | Multi-organ failure |

emergency or with pancreatic ascites (rich in amylase and protein) or a pleural effusion. Portal or splenic vein thrombosis may complicate pancreatitis and pseudocysts.

Treatment of pseudocyst: If pseudocysts are uncomplicated, asymptomatic, and not increasing in size, they can be managed expectantly. If intervention is indicated, endoscopic or surgical drainage is the treatment of choice.

## Infection

Risk of infection is high in patients with necrotizing pancreatitis. Broad-spectrum antibiotic therapy is generally recommended. Imipenem, cefuroxime, and the combination of ofloxacin and metronidazole have shown a benefit in the prevention of infectious complications but the spectrum of activity is probably more relevant than the individual agents used.

## Management

Treatment for mild to moderate pancreatitis is primarily supportive and expectant. There are no medications to suppress the secretion of the damaging pancreatic enzymes. Octreotide is not generally recommended but may have a role when used postoperatively. If there is a treatable cause, therapy involves addressing the trigger (such as removal of obstruction, control of Crohn's disease).

Fluid and electrolyte support is the basis of treatment for all patients with acute pancreatitis. Use intravenous fluids for resuscitation of the shock state as needed and to maintain hydration (see Chapter 18, "Infection"). Monitor electrolytes closely.

Nutrition is important to prevent further decompensation of the patient. Nasogastric or nasojejunal feeding may be tolerated sooner than oral feedings. Total parenteral nutrition can be used in patients who do not tolerate these feeding methods. TPN carries a higher rate of sepsis complications; therefore, it is recommended that if a patient with severe acute pancreatitis can tolerate jejunal feedings, that is the preferred route. A low fat enteral formula should be used. Lipids may be used with parenteral nutrition at less than or equal to 30%. Monitor triglyceride levels.

Analgesia is another important consideration in the pancreatitis patient. Opiates are commonly used in standard pediatric doses to control pain related to acute pancreatitis. Meperidine is not recommended. There is no evidence to suggest that sphincter of Oddi spasm secondary to morphine administration is clinically significant.

All medications should be reviewed. Considering possible pancreatotoxic drugs.

Acid suppression does not have a defined role in mild to moderate pancreatitis. Consider its use in more severe cases for the prevention of stress ulcers and GI bleeding.

ERCP with a sphincterotomy or stone extraction may be indicated. ERCP is also useful in some cases for presurgical evaluation.

Surgery may be indicated in a variety of situations. It is needed for the repair or resection of damaged or strictured pancreatic ducts. Necrotic or abscessed tissue will need surgical intervention for removal and debridement. Cholecystectomy is done after the acute phase has resolved unless there is an obstructive stone that cannot be removed endoscopically.

Chronic pancreatitis presents different management issues such as chronic pain control and nutritional support. These are usually managed on an ongoing basis by the child's gastroenterologist.

# References

Werlin SL. Acute pancreatitis in children. Curr Treat Options Gastroenterol 2001;4:403–8.

Benifla M, Weizman Zvi. Acute pancreatitis in childhood: analysis of literature data. J Clin Gastroenterol 2003;37:169–72.

Weizman, Z. Acute pancreatitis. In: Wyllie R, Hyams JS, eds. Pediatric Gastrointestinal Disease: Pathophysiology, Diagnosis, Management. Philadelphia: WB Saunders Co.; 1993:873–9.

Werlin, SL. Pancreatitis. In: Wyllie R, Hyams JS, eds. Textbook of Pediatric Gastroenterology. Philadelphia: WB Saunders Co.; 1999:681–93.

Byrne M, Mitchell RM, MB, Baillie J. Pancreatic pseudocysts. Curr Treat Options Gastroenterol 2002;5:331–8.

Martin SP, Ulrich CD. Complicated acute pancreatitis. Curr Treat Options Gastroenterol 1999;2:215–26.

Sainio V, et al. Early antibiotic treatment in acute necrotizing pancreatitis [see comments]. Lancet 1995;346:663–7.

Nompleggi, DJ. Nutrition in acute pancreatitis. Curr Gastroenterol Rep 1999;1:319–23.

Runzi M, Layer P. Drug associated pancreatitis: fact and fiction. Pancreas 1996;13:100–9.

Chari ST, Vege SS. Etiology of acute pancreatitis. In: Rose BD, ed. UpToDate. Wellesley, MA: UpToDate, 2005.

Lowe ME. Pancreatic function and dysfunction. In: Walker WA, et al., eds. Pediatric Gastrointestinal Disease. Ontario: BC Decker Inc.; 2004:98–111.

Stefan H, Schäfer M, Rousson V, Clavien P. Evidence-based treatment of acute pancreatitis: a look at established paradigms. Ann Surg 2006;243:154–68.

# D. Fulminant Hepatic Failure

Samra Sarigol Blanchard
Lara Bauman

## Key Principles

- Fulminant hepatic failure (FHF) is a syndrome of rapidly evolving hepatic synthetic dysfunction complicated by coagulopathy and encephalopathy.
- The etiology of FHF is age-dependent. Acute viral hepatitis is the most common in all series followed by metabolic diseases in neonates and infants.
- The major complications of FHF that require preventive measures or specific therapy include cerebral edema, coagulopathy, renal failure, hypoglycemia, and infection.
- Application of prognostic criteria associated with mortality from FHF can be to determine which patients are likely to recover and which are likely to die without liver transplantation.
- Care of children with FHF may include anticipatory transfer to a liver transplant center.

## Definition of Fulminant Hepatic Failure

(1)  Traditional (Adult) Definition

- Acute hepatic dysfunction (coagulopathy, poor synthetic function)
- Development of encephalopathy within 8 weeks

This is difficult to operationalize; however, since children are different because:

- Encephalopathy is difficult to assess
- Encephalopathy may not develop until terminal stages

Therefore, the accepted definition within pediatric age groups is as follows:

(2) Pediatric Acute Liver Failure Study Group (PALFSG) Definition

- No evidence of chronic liver disease
- Evidence of acute liver injury (increased liver enzymes, hyperbilirubinemia)
- Coagulopathy unresponsive to vitamin K

  - Prothrombin time (PT) >15 seconds or international normalized ratio (INR) >1.5 with encephalopathy
  - PT >20 seconds or INR >2.0 with or without encephalopathy

# Pathophysiology

- Normal liver functions include the following:

  - Protein/Enzyme synthesis
  - Glucose regulation
  - Cholesterol synthesis
  - Oxidative phosphorylation
  - Excretion of metabolic waste products

- Injury to the liver may be direct, ischemic, infectious, immune, or unknown
- Physiology in the initial stages of FHF may include the following:

  - Increased cardiac output, decreased systemic vascular resistance
  - Increase portal pressure
  - Renal vasoconstriction
  - Pulmonary shunting, V/Q mismatch
  - Total body fluid overload

# Etiology of Acute Liver Failure— (see Table 1)

*Table 1*
**Etiology of Acute Liver Failure**

| Infectious | Metabolic |
|---|---|
| • Viral hepatitis A, B, B&D, E | • Neonatal hemachromatosis |
| • Epstein-Barr virus | • Galactosemia |
| • Cytomegalovirus | • Tyrosinemia |

- Herpes 1, 2, and 6
- Varicella
- Adenovirus
- Leptospirosis

Drug-induced

- Acetaminophen
- Halothane
- Isoniazid
- Rifampicin
- Phenytoin
- Valproic acid
- Penicillin
- Ketoconazole
- Isoflurane
- Herbal supplements

Toxins

- Amanita phalloides
- Carbon tetrachloride

Recreational drugs

- Cocaine
- Ecstasy
- Amphetamines

- Hereditary fructose intolerance
- Niemann-Pick disease type C
- Wilson's disease
- Mitochondrial cytopathies
- Zellweger syndrome
- Urea cycle defects
- Crigler-Najjar type I

Autoimmune

- Type I or II autoimmune hepatitis

Vascular/Ischemic

- Budd-Chiari syndrome
- Veno-occlusive disease
- Acute circulatory failure

Infiltrative

- Histiocytosis
- Leukemia
- Lymphoma

HELLP syndrome
(Hemolysis, Elevated Liver enzymes, Low Platelet)

# Hepatic Failure in Chronic Liver Disease

- This is the development of advanced signs of liver disease or acute decompensation with pre-existing liver disease.
- The most common cause of chronic liver failure in infants is biliary atresia.
- Cirrhosis with portal hypertension eventually develops in all forms of progressive chronic liver disease.
- Malnutrition, ascites, variceal bleeding, encephalopathy, spontaneous bacterial peritonitis, pruritus, hepatorenal syndrome, and hepatopulmonary syndrome are common presentations.
- The goal of management is to prevent disease progression, provide adequate nutritional support, and prevent or treat complications.

- It is essential that children with chronic liver disease receive timely referral to a transplantation center. Persistently elevated bilirubin level, a prolongation of prothrombin time, failure to thrive despite nutritional intervention, a fall in albumin level, a delay in psychosocial development, refractory ascites, recurrent variceal bleeding, intractable pruritus are all indications for considering liver transplantation.

# Etiology of Chronic Liver Failure in Children

## Cholestatic Liver Disease

- Biliary atresia
- Alagille's syndrome
- Progressive familial intrahepatic cholestasis (PFIC)

## Metabolic Liver Disease

- Alpha-1-antitrypsin deficiency
- Tyrosinemia
- Cystic fibrosis
- Wilson's disease
- Neonatal hepatitis
- Viral hepatitis
- Autoimmune hepatitis
- Congenital hepatic fibrosis

# Initial Assessment and Diagnosis

- The clinical presentation varies with etiology

# History

- Risk factors

  - IV drug use or other illicit drugs
  - Transfusion history
  - Foreign travel
  - Contact with jaundiced person
  - Sexual contact

- Medication list

  - Over-the-counter and prescription medications
  - Herbal supplements or alternative medicines

# Physical Examination

- Look for evidence of any chronic liver disease.
- Look for signs of coagulopathy, hypoglycemia.
- Jaundice may be a late feature, especially in metabolic diseases.
- Acute decompensation may be secondary to an undiagnosed chronic condition.

  - Spider angioma, petechia
  - Ascites, splenomegaly
  - Eye exam for cataracts or Kayser-Fleischer ring
  - CNS evaluation to assess baseline level of consciousness and degree of coma (Tables 2 and 3)

# Investigations

## General Laboratory Evaluation

- Liver function tests
- Serum electrolytes including glucose, calcium, phosphorus, magnesium
- Lipid profile
- Blood gas analysis
- Complete blood count
- Prothrombin time (PT) and INR
- Blood type
- Urine toxicology screen
- Blood acetaminophen level

*Table 2*
### Clinical Stages of Hepatic Encephalopathy in Infants

| Stage | Clinical | Reflexes | Neurological |
|-------|----------|----------|--------------|
| Early (I and II) | Inconsolable crying Poor sleep | Unreliable: Normal or hyperreflexic | Unstable |
| Mid (III) | Somnolence, stupor combativeness | Unreliable: Normal or hyperreflexic | Unstable |
| Late (IV) | Comatose or no response | Absent | Decerebrate or decorticate |

Adapted from Bucuvalas J, Yazigi N, Squires RH.

*Table 3*
**Clinical Stages of Hepatic Encephalopathy: Older Children and Adolescents**

| Stage | Mental state | Reflexes | EEG |
|---|---|---|---|
| I | Mild confusion | Slight asterixis Normal tone and reflexes | Normal/minimal changes |
| II | Drowsiness Inappropriate behavior | Asterixis Increased muscle tone Brisk reflexes | Abnormal Generalized slowing |
| III | Marked confusion Sleeps most of the time Incoherent speech | Hyperreflexic (+) Babinski sign | Grossly abnormal slowing |
| IV | Unconscious Decerebrate or decorticate response | Absent | Abnormal with appearance of delta waves |

## Radiologic Evaluation

- Ultrasound of abdomen with Doppler studies to evaluate portal and hepatic veins

# Disease-Specific Evaluation

- Viral hepatitis: anti-HAV IgM, HBsAg, HBeAg, hepatitis D antigen and antibody, anti-hepatitis C antibody, anti-hepatitis E antibody, serology for CMV, EBV, HIV, HSV, adenovirus
- Autoimmune hepatitis: antinuclear antibodies (ANA), smooth muscle antibody (SMA), antibodies to liver/kidney microsome 1 (anti-LKM1), serum immunoglobulin levels to confirm IgG elevation
- Wilson's disease (WD): serum ceruloplasmin, 24-hour urine copper collection before and after penicillamine. Direct Coombs test for Coombs-negative hemolytic anemia. Very low serum alkaline phosphatase or uric acid levels are indirect indicator of WD

- Galactosemia: blood galactose-1-phosphate uridyl transferase level
- Neonatal hemochromatosis: ferritin and iron studies to look for high transferrin saturation
- Tyrosinemia: fasting serum amino acid levels and urinary succinyl acetone
- Budd-Chiari/veno-occlusive disease: Doppler ultrasound
- Mitochondrial hepatopathies: urine organic acids, lactate/pyruvate, plasma acyl-carnitines, liver or muscle tissue for direct measurement of respiratory chain enzyme

## Diagnosis

- The diagnosis is established by the combination of clinical and biochemical findings and specific diagnostic tests.
- Liver biopsy to establish histology is rarely helpful and is usually contraindicated due to coagulopathy.
- The risk of biopsy can only be justified when there are atypical features.
- Transjugular approach to biopsy should be considered in the presence of coagulopathy.

## Management

### General Measures

- To prevent cerebral edema

  - All patients should be in a quiet environment with little stimulation to minimize acute increases in ICP
  - Raise head of bed
  - Avoid hypotension, hypoxia, hypercarbia

- Careful monitoring of intake/output and hemodynamics

  - Heart rate, respiratory rate, blood pressure
  - Central venous pressure

- Frequent neurologic exam

  - Sedation should be avoided if possible
  - If necessary, administer sedation as intermittent doses to minimize accumulation
  - If neuromuscular blockade is required drugs such as cis-atracurium, which do not require hepatic metabolism, should be considered

- Close follow up of electrolytes, glucose level, and coagulation (PT/INR)
- Lactulose titrated to produce 2 to 4 stools a day
- Maintenance of nutrition

  - Intravenous glucose infusion or adequate enteral intake
  - Parenteral nutrition if ventilated

- Prevention of gastrointestinal hemorrhage

  - Keep gastric pH >5

- Remember cytochrome p450 drug interactions may be further exaggerated

# Disease-Specific Therapies

- Infection

  - Herpes/CMV: acyclovir or ganciclovir
  - Enterovirus: pleconaril/Immunoglobulin

- Acetaminophen toxicity: N-acetylcysteine infusion
- Neonatal Hemochromatosis: antioxidant cocktail as follows:

  - N-Acetylcysteine (100 mg/kg/day IV/NG)
  - Selenium (3 mcg/kg/day)
  - Alprostadil (prostaglandin E1) (0.4–0.6 mcg/kg/hour IV)
  - Vitamin E (25 units/kg/day)

- Hereditary tyrosinemia: NTBC (2-Nitro-4-trifluoromethylbenzoyl-1,3-cyclohexanedione)
- Galactosemia: remove lactose from diet
- Mushroom (Amanita species) poisoning:

  - Consider, in consultation with Poison Information Center:

    - Silibinin (silymarin or milk thistle) (30–40 mg/kg/day IV/PO for 3–4 days)
    - Penicillin G (300,000–1,000,000 units/kg/day)
    - Hemodialysis or hemofiltration

- Autoimmune disease: high-dose steroids
- Hemophagocytic syndrome: steroid and etoposide
- Acute circulatory failure: also referred to as "shock liver," cardiovascular support is the treatment of choice (see Chapter 18, "Shock")

- HELLP syndrome: early recognition in third trimester to expedite prompt delivery and supportive care

# Complications—Prevention and Management

## Neurologic Complications

Hepatic encephalopathy (HE) is defined as any brain dysfunction that occurs as a result of acute hepatic dysfunction. The pathophysiology of HE is still unknown but is likely multifactorial.

- HE can be exacerbated by sepsis, hypoglycemia, electrolyte imbalances, gastrointestinal bleeding, and sedation.
- Grading for HE in infants and older children are reviewed in Tables 2 and 3.
- Baseline electroencephalogram (EEG) is helpful to stage coma.
- Increased serum ammonia is linked to increased gamma-aminobutyric acid (GABA) transmission and may correlate to the level of HE. Frequent evaluation of neurological status and blood ammonia levels are essential. HE may still persist in the face of normalizing ammonia levels.
- Use of lactulose and control of the precipitating factors are important preventive tools.
- The use of intracranial pressure (ICP) monitoring devices in children with FHF is controversial due to coagulopathy and high complication rates.
- The aim of ICP monitoring is to maintain the ICP below 20–25 mm Hg and the cerebral perfusion pressure (mean arterial blood pressure—ICP) at over 50 mm Hg.
- Vasopressor agents may be needed to increase blood pressure in order to maintain adequate cerebral perfusion pressure (see Chapter 20, "Trauma" for more details).

Cerebral edema and increased ICP are usually seen in grade III and IV HE.

- Brain death associated with cerebral edema is the most common cause of both death in FHF and also poor outcome after liver transplantation.
- Fluid restriction to 75% maintenance while maintaining circulating volume with colloids is the key measure.

- Mannitol and hypertonic saline are used to treat acutely increased ICP. With concomitant careful monitoring of serum osmolarity (it should not exceed 320 mosmol/L).
- Intubation should be performed if cerebral edema is suspected. Gentle hyperventilation can reduce ICP temporarily, but excessive hyperventilation should be avoided due to paradoxical effect on cerebral perfusion pressure.
- Barbiturate coma may be used to treat persistent raised intracranial pressure that is refractory to other therapies.
- Seizures should be treated with phenytoin or phenobarbital, but persistent seizures are a poor prognostic sign.
- Hypothermia (decreasing core body temperature to 32°C) has been shown to be effective in lowering ICP in adults.
- Corticosteroids have been shown to be ineffective in preventing or reducing cerebral edema.

## Pulmonary Complications

- Hepato-pulmonary syndrome (HPS)

  - HPS is defined by a widened age-corrected alveolar-arterial oxygen gradient on room air with or without hypoxemia, resulting from intrapulmonary vasodilatation, with increased intrapulmonary shunting, seen in the presence of hepatic dysfunction or portal hypertension. This can be clinically measured with a narrowed difference between the arterial and the mixed-venous oxygen content.
  - The hallmark of HPS is microvascular dilatation occurring within the pulmonary arterial circulation that appears to result from decreased tone in precapillary arterioles.
  - HPS is characterized by hypoxia, dyspnea, digital clubbing, and platypnea (dyspnea induced by the upright position and relieved by recumbency) and orthodeoxia (arterial deoxygenation accentuated in the upright position and relieved by recumbency).
  - If HPS is suspected, contrast echocardiography (bubble ECHO) is the preferred screening test for intrapulmonary vasodilatation.
  - Treatment consists of supplemental oxygen and consideration of orthotopic liver transplantation if significant hypoxemia is present.

- Pulmonary hypertension
- CXR shows a range of abnormalities including pleural effusions, pneumonia, and sometimes "mottled" shadows—or "spidery" lesions.

## Metabolic Abnormalities

- Hypoglycemia

  - Present in 40% of patients.
  - It can worsen hepatic encephalopathy and cause rapid neurologic deterioration.
  - Frequent bed side monitoring every 2 to 4 hours.
  - Maintain blood glucose level >40 mg/dL.

- Electrolyte and acid-base disturbances

  - Metabolic acidosis is commonly seen with acetaminophen overdose.
  - Metabolic alkalosis is the most common acid-base abnormality in FHF and is often accompanied by hypokalemia and central hyperventilation.

# Infection

- Sixty percent of deaths in FHF have been attributed to sepsis.
- The presence of encephalopathy has been shown to be associated with bacterial infection in about 80% of cases and fungal infections in about 32% of cases.
- Surveillance cultures can be used to guide antibiotic therapy in the event of suspected infection.
- *Staphylococcus aureus, streptococci,* and Gram-negative organisms are the most common bacterial infections. *Candida* spp. are the most common fungal isolates and fluconazole is the preferred agent.
- Prophylactic antibiotics and antifungal agents may be considered but have not been shown to improve overall outcomes.

# Renal Failure

- Renal insufficiency (RI) can be caused by acute tubular necrosis, hepato-renal syndrome, or the direct effect of toxin (acetaminophen).
- Hepato-renal syndrome is the commonest cause of RI. The etiology is due to electrolyte imbalance, sepsis, and hypovolemia. Features include reduced urine output, normal urinary sediment, and urine sodium concentration <10 mmol/L.
- The aim of management is to maintain circulating volume to provide adequate renal perfusion.

- Patients may require continuous renal replacement therapy to achieve treatment goals (see Chapter 13, "Renal Replacement Therapy").

# Coagulopathy and Hemorrhage

- The prothrombin time (PT/INR) is elevated in patients with FHF and is used as an indicator of the severity of liver damage.
- The coagulation factors synthesized by hepatocytes include fibrinogen, factors II, V, VII, IX, and X.
- Factor V, which is independent of vitamin K, is one of the important indicators of prognosis in FHF. Factor V levels are significantly decreased in nonsurvivors as compared with survivors.
- Administration of vitamin K intravenously should be done to assure there are adequate stores, but it rarely improves the coagulation in FHF.
- Significant disseminated intravascular coagulation (DIC) is unusual in FHF. The presence of DIC usually indicates sepsis. The level of factor VIII may help to differentiate between DIC and FHF as it is normal or increased in FHF.
- The risk of hemorrhage correlates with thrombocytopenia.
- Common sites of internal hemorrhage include the gastrointestinal tract, lungs, nasopharynx, retroperitoneum, and needle puncture sites.
- Prophylactic acid suppressive therapy has been shown to decrease the incidence of gastrointestinal bleeding.
- It is not necessary to correct mild coagulopathy (PT <25 seconds). Marked coagulopathy (PT >40 seconds) should be corrected to prevent the risk of bleeding. Use fresh frozen plasma (FFP) 10 mL/kg every 6 to 12 hours. Factor VIIa (rFVIIa, Novo-Seven®, Novo Nordisk) can be used as an adjunctive (40–80 mcg/kg) to correct coagulopathy. Factor VIIa has been effective to correct coaguoplathy in FFP-resistant patients.
- The use of rFVIIa to rapidly improve coagulopathy before invasive procedures is an important innovation in management of patients with FHF.

# Hemodynamic Complications

- Cardiac output is increased secondary to reduced vascular resistance and arteriovenous shunting. These changes are similar to those seen in the systemic inflammatory response syndrome where endotoxins reduce vascular resistance.

- Hypotension can occur due to hemorrhage, sepsis, or increased capillary permeability. Volume replacement and vasopressor agents are needed to treat hypotension.

# Predicting Outcomes in Fulminant Hepatic Failure

- The prognosis of FHF depends on the underlying etiology. The prognosis is better for children with FHF resulting from acetaminophen overdose or hepatitis A.
- Factor V has been used as a prognostic marker. In children, a factor V level less than 25% of normal suggests a poor outcome.
- Studies from the liver unit at Kings College in London have established prognostic criteria for determining the increased probability of need for liver transplantation. Refer these patients to a liver transplant center urgently.

  I. Acetaminophen toxicity patients
     A. pH >7.3
     B. PT >100 (INR >6.5) and serum creatinine >3.4 mg/dL
  II. Other patients
     A. PT >100 (INR >6.5)
     B. Any three of the following variables
       1. Age
       2. Etiology: non-A, non-B Hepatitis, Halothane idiosyncratic drug reaction
       3. Duration of jaundice before encephalopathy >7 d
       4. PT >50 (INR 3.5)
       5. Serum bilirubin level >17.5 mg/dL

# Supportive Management—Liver Support Systems

These *experimental* therapeutic options may provide support during liver regeneration or serve as a bridge to transplantation while awaiting a donor organ and they should only be used in the context of clinical trials.

- Plasmapheresis/double-volume exchange
- Liver assist device—noncell-based

  - Hemoperfusion
  - Molecular absorbent regenerating system (MARS)
    - Removes protein-bound toxins by perfusion over resins

- Liver-assist device—cell-based

  - HepatAssist—porcine cells
  - ELAD—human hepatoblastoma cells
  - Bioartificial liver (BAL)—cryopreserved human hepatocytes

A recent meta-analysis including all forms of liver-assist devices demonstrated reduction in mortality in acute-on-chronic liver failure compared with standard medical therapy. Artificial and bioartificial support systems did not appear to affect mortality in FHF.

- Auxiliary liver transplant

  - The rationale behind this technique is that the allograft provides liver function while native liver regenerates.
  - Once the native liver has returned to normal function, immunosuppression is gradually weaned off.
  - There has been no universally accepted indication for auxiliary liver transplant in the setting of FHF.

- Hepatocyte transplant

  - Hepatocyte transplantation is an emerging procedure, consisting of infusing mature adult hepatocytes in the portal system of the recipient.
  - It aims to correct inborn errors of liver metabolism, bridge unstable patients to transplantation, or even allow bridge to recovery in fulminant liver failure. The technique addresses ideally patients with inborn errors of metabolism, unstable but not sick enough for orthotopic transplantation.
  - Best results have so far been obtained in metabolic diseases, such as urea cycle disorders, glycogenosis type I, Crigler Najjar, Refsum disease, and factor VII deficiency.

## Liver Transplantation

- Care of children with FHF may include anticipatory transfer to a liver transplant center.
- Liver transplantation (LT) should be considered in any patient with severe progressive liver injury from FHF who meets the fatal prognostic criteria.
- Etiology of FHF and patient age may be important prognostic factors.

- Children with FHF with severe coagulopathy, lower transaminase on admission, and prolonged duration of illness before the onset of hepatic encephalopathy are more likely to require liver transplantation.
- See this chapter for more details.

# References

Bucuvalas J, Yazigi N, Squires RH. Acute liver failure in children. Clin Liver Dis 2006;10:149–68.

Kelly DA, Wilson DC. Chronic liver failure. Curr Paediatr 2006;16:51–8.

Bansal S, Dhawan A. Acute liver failure. Curr Paediatr 2006;16:36–42.

Polson J, Lee WM. AASLD Position paper: the management of acute liver failure. Hepatology 2005;41:1179–97.

Nowak-Wegrzyn A, Phipatanakul W, Winkelstein JA, et al. Successful treatment of enterovirus infection with the use of pleconaril in 2 infants with severe combined immunodeficiency. Clin Infect Dis 2001;32:E13–4.

Broussard CN, Aggarwal A, Lacey SR, et al. Mushroom poisoning—from diarrhea to liver transplantation. Am J Gastroenterol 2001;96:3195–8.

Jalan R, Damink SW, Deutz NE, et al. Moderate hypothermia for uncontrolled intracranial hypertension in acute liver failure. Lancet 1999;354:1164–8.

Arguedas MR, Fallon MB. Hepatopulmonary syndrome. Clin Liver Dis 2005; 9:733–46.

Rolando N, Harvey F, Brahm J, et al. Prospective study of bacterial infection in acute liver failure: an analysis of fifty patients. Hepatology 1990;11:49–53.

Rolando N, Philpott-Howard J, Williams R. Bacterial and fungal infection in acute liver failure. Semin Liver Dis 1996;16:389–402.

Macdougall BR, Bailey RJ, Williams R. H2-receptor antagonists and antacids in the prevention of acute gastrointestinal hemorrhage in fulminant liver failure. Two controlled trials. Lancet 1977;1:617–9.

Shami VM, Caldwell SH, Hespenheide EE, et al. Recombinant activated factor VII for coagulopathy in fulminant hepatic failure compared with conventional therapy. Liver Transpl 2003;9:138–43.

Brown JB, Emerick KM, Brown DL, et al. Recombinant factor VIIa improves coagulopathy caused by liver failure. J Pediatr Gastroenterol Nutr 2003;37:268–72.

O'Grady JG, Alexander GJM, Hayllar KM, et al. Early indicators of prognosis in fulminant hepatic failure. Gastroenterology 1989;97:439–55.

Singer AL, Olthoff KM, Kim H, et al. Role of plasmapheresis in the management of acute hepatic failure in children. Ann Surg 2001;234:418–24.

Kjaergard LL, Liu J, Als–Nielsen B, et al. Artificial and bioartificial support systems for acute and acute-on-chronic liver failure: a systematic review. JAMA 2003;8:217–22.

Horslen SP, Fox IJ. Hepatocyte transplantation. Transplantation 2004;77:1481–6.

Fox IJ, Chowdhury JR, Kaufman SS, et al. Treatment of the Crigler-Najjar syndrome type I with hepatocyte transplantation. N Engl J Med 1998; 338:1422–6.

# E. Liver Transplantation

## Samra Sarigol Blanchard
## Lara Bauman

## Introduction

- Advances in immunosuppressive therapy and improvements in surgical techniques have brought liver transplantation (LT) from an experimental procedure to an effective therapeutic option for children with fulminant liver failure and end-stage liver disease.
- Use of cyclosporine and improved surgical expertise allowed 1-year survival rates to improve dramatically, from less than 40% in the 1970s to 70% to 80% in the 1980s. Now additional refinements of technique and immunosuppression have further improved outcomes with a 1-year survival rate between 85% and 90%.
- The posttransplant care of patients involves monitoring and stabilizing major organ systems, evaluation of graft function, and achieving adequate immunosuppression.
- Early recognition in the pediatric intensive care unit (PICU) of technical complications is essential to reduce the risk for both patient and graft loss.
- Long-term care focuses on maintaining graft function, screening for drug-related toxicity, and assessing for complications of chronic immunosuppression.

## Key Principles

- Liver transplantation (LT) management is a natural continuation of management of fulminant hepatic failure.
- Approach is multidisciplinary and requires collaboration between gastroenterologists, intensivists, and transplant surgeons.
- Knowledge if perioperative and postoperative complications is essential to anticipatory care of liver transplant patients.

# Indications for Liver Transplantation

## Cholestatic Liver Disease

- Extra-hepatic biliary atresia
- Progressive familial intrahepatic cholestasis (PFIC, Byler syndrome)
- Syndromic bile duct paucity (Alagille syndrome)
- Non-syndromic bile duct paucity
- Other biliary tract disease (sclerosing cholangitis)

## Metabolic Diseases

- Alpha-1-antitrypsin deficiency
- Tyrosinemia
- Galactosemia
- Urea cycle defects
- Organic acidemia
- Wilson's disease
- Glycogen storage disease (types I, III, and IV)
- Neonatal hemochromatosis
- Crigler-Najjar syndrome type I
- Hyperoxaluria type I

## Fulminant Hepatic Failure (reviewed in previous chapter in detail)

- Viruses
- Toxins
- Drugs
- Metabolic

## Chronic Hepatitis/Cirrhosis

- Viral
- Neonatal
- Autoimmune
- Idiopathic

## Tumors

- Hepatoblastoma
- Hepatocellular carcinoma
- Hemangioendothelioma

## Miscellaneous

- Cystic fibrosis
- Congenital hepatic fibrosis
- Cirrhosis from prolonged total parenteral nutrition
- Budd-Chiari syndrome

Biliary atresia is the most common indication for liver transplantation in children in the United States. Even after (under 60 days post birth) Kasai portoenterostomy, successful bile flow is achieved in 30% to 40% of patients. Two-thirds of the patients will require LT eventually.

Alagille syndrome typically presents with facial dysmorphism, pruritus, xanthomas, ocular abnormalities, cardiac defects, growth retardation, and skeletal abnormalities. These patients usually do not develop early cirrhosis and can be treated with nutritional support, ursodeoxycholic acid for cholestasis, and cholestyramine or rifampin for pruritus. For the few patients who have progressive biliary cirrhosis or poor quality of life, LT should be considered. A full cardiovascular evaluation should be performed before transplantation because cardiac and vascular defects are common.

Metabolic diseases are the second most common group of diseases for which children have received an LT. The most straight-forward indications for LT occur when the metabolic disease is associated with the development of end-stage or fulminant liver disease, and transplantation not only replaces the defective enzyme but also restores the liver function (eg, tyrosinemia and bile acid synthesis defects). In many circumstances the metabolic defect leads to potentially fatal complications even though liver synthetic function is generally normal (primary hyperoxaluria and Crigler-Najjar type I).

Alpha-1-antitrypsin deficiency is the most common metabolic disease leading to transplantation. Approximately 5% of phenotype PiZZ patients develop end-stage liver disease.

Wilson's disease is an autosomal recessive disorder linked to a mutation on chromosome 13 resulting in defective copper transport. The accumulation of copper can cause liver disease, cirrhosis, and neurologic complications. Chelation therapy stabilizes copper accumulation, but LT may be necessary if fulminant liver failure occurs before the initiation of therapy.

Neonatal hemochromatosis is a rare disorder in which the severe accumulation of iron in the liver and other organs leads to liver failure and death in infancy. It mimics sepsis with disseminated intravascular coagulation.

## Cystic Fibrosis.

Approximately 5% of patients develop cirrhosis requiring orthotic liver transplant (OLT). Survival rates are lower than for other disorders and approach 62%.

## Contraindications to LT

- Fulminant hepatic failure secondary to a nonreversible condition (eg, mitochondrial disease)
- HIV infection
- Uncontrollable systemic sepsis of nonhepatic origin
- Multi-organ irreversible system failure
- Malignancy not confined to liver
- Irreversible neurologic injury

## Pediatric Pretransplantation Evaluation

### History and Physical

- Previous surgery
- Congenital anomaly
- Immunizations
- Dietary history
- Medications

### Nutritional Assessment

- Anthropometrics
- Albumin, transferrin, pre-albumin
- Serum vitamin A, D, E levels
- Lipid profile
- Wrist X-ray for rickets

### Laboratory and Imaging

- CBC
- Renal panel
- Liver function tests
- PT, PTT, factor V
- Doppler US
- CT/MRI/MRA

## Infectious Disease Evaluation

- Viral hepatitis screen
- Serology for CMV, EBV, HSV, VZV, HIV
- Travel history
- Tuberculosis exposure (CXR and PPD)

## Other Studies

- Liver biopsy
- Cardiac assessment: ECHO/EKG
- Dental assessment
- Upper endoscopy

## Timing for the Transplant

- Diminished hepatic synthetic function
- Cerebral edema
- Symptomatic portal hypertension
- Intractable ascites
- Spontaneous bacterial peritonitis
- Recurrent variceal hemorrhage
- Failure to thrive or malnutrition
- Intractable pruritus
- Hepato-renal syndrome
- Hepato-pulmonary syndrome

## Donor Procurement

- Liver allocation is based on matching donor and recipient blood groups and body weight.
- In the United States, the United Network for Organ Sharing (UNOS) performs the matching process first on a local then a regional basis, and then nationally.
- In 2002, a new system for donor liver allocation was introduced by UNOS to determine medical urgency for children. The Pediatric End-Stage Liver Disease (PELD) scoring system is based on total bilirubin, international normalized ratio (INR), albumin, evidence of growth failure, and age younger than 1 year. Centers may request addition of exception PELD points from their regional review board if the providers judge that the calculated PELD score does not reflect the severity of the patient's disease.
- Donor shortage is the single most important challenge of the transplantation field. Seven percent of children died while

awaiting OLT in 1997. Children <1 year of age have a fivefold higher death rate on the waiting list than any other age group.

## Donor Organ Options

- Whole organ cadaveric grafts
- Reduced size liver transplantation

  - Surgically reducing an adult-sized or large organ to fit in the abdominal cavity. The most commonly used parts in children are left lateral segment (segments 2 and 3) or left lobe (segments 2, 3, 4) (Figure 1). The obvious disadvantage of reduction hepatectomy is that only one child benefits while suitable liver tissue is discarded. This shortcoming led to the development of split liver transplantation, whereby two recipients benefit from one donor graft.

- Split liver transplantation

  - Splitting a liver allows one donor graft to be transplanted into two recipients, generally an adult and a child. It is performed either ex vivo after harvest of a whole liver or in situ prior to cross clamping and perfusion in a hemodynamically stable donor. Overall patient and graft survival compare favorably with results obtained from whole organ transplantation.

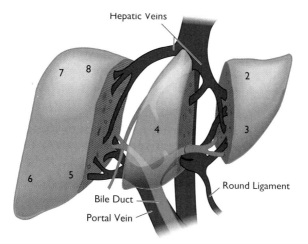

**Figure 1**  Segmental anatomy of liver. Segments 2 and 3 (left lateral segment) and segments 2, 3, and 4 (left lobe) are used in children.

- Living-related transplantation

  - The left lateral segment may also be removed from a living donor. The hepatic venous anastomosis is performed in an end-to-end fashion with an extension made onto the vena cava from the recipient left and middle hepatic vein orifice. This allows proper orientation without kinking that might predispose to outflow obstruction. Alternatively, the hepatic vein may be anastomosed directly "en-face" to the cava. Biliary reconstruction is by Roux-en-Y hepaticojejunostomy.
  - Liver donors face significant surgical risk and the decision to donate should be undertaken only after rigorous preoperative consultation and evaluation.

## Immediate Postoperative Management

Transplant centers each have their own postoperative and immunosuppressive protocols. Complete blood count, PT, PTT, electrolytes, and arterial blood gas levels should be monitored every few hours for the first 2 days after LT. Liver function tests and tacrolimus/cyclosporine levels are followed on a daily basis.

- Analgesia/sedation/neuromuscular blockade

  - Sedation should be titrated as needed for the specific clinical situation, with a goal of early extubation.
  - Pain control can be achieved with patient-controlled devices in older children.
  - If possible avoid neuromuscular blockade; cis-atracurium is preferred over other agents.

- Ventilatory support

  - Timing of extubation varies between transplant centers.
  - Extubate next day if patient has improving synthetic function and Doppler ultrasound shows normal vasculature.
  - Early extubation has been shown to prevent nosocomial pneumonia.
  - Some centers advocate immediate extubation following surgery for stable patients.

- Fluid management

  - Avoid hypovolemia as it is a risk for clotting the hepatic artery.

- Maintain a high-normal central venous pressure (7 to 10 mm Hg), urine output of 1 to 2 mL/kg/hour and normal mean arterial pressure.
- Follow electrolytes closely. Calcineurin inhibitors such as cyclosporine and tacrolimus may cause hypomagnesemia.
- Watch for glucose intolerance.
- Consider colloid replacement in the setting of hypoproteinemia.

- Nutritional management

  - Start slow continuous nasogastric (NG) tube feedings when postoperative ileus resolves within 3 to 4 days.

- Prophylaxis for infection

  - Broad-spectrum antibiotic coverage for 48 hours:

    - Piperacillin/tazobactam
    - Or, ampicillin/sulbactam
    If penicillin allergy
    - Third-generation cephalosporin, addition of vancomycin may be warranted if gram-positive infection is suspected

  - CMV prophylaxis: ganciclovir/acyclovir
  - Antifungal:
    - Nystatin swish and swallow
    - Prophylactic use of systemic antifungal therapy (flucanazole) in high-risk patients

  - PCP prophylaxis
    - Trimethoprim-sulfamethoxazole (TMP/SMX) 3 times a week
    - Alternative regimens if TMP/SMX is not tolerated:
      - Aerosolized pentamidine once a month
      - Dapsone

- Anticoagulant and antiplatelet therapy (per transplant center protocol)

  - Heparin
  - Aspirin
  - Dipyridamole

- Ulcer prophylaxis

  - An antacid can be given via NG-tubeo
  - H2 receptor blocker
  - Proton pump inhibitor

- Immunosuppression

While there is significant variability in immunosuppression protocols, all centers initially use steroids and calcineurin inhibitors (cyclosporine and tacrolimus).

The phases of immunosuppression are induction, maintenance, and treatment of rejection. During induction very high levels of immunosuppression with steroids (prednisolone) and calcineurin inhibitors are maintained.

Acute postoperative period:

- Tacrolimus (0.1–0.15 mg/dose PO bid) target levels of 10–15 ng/L
- Cyclosporine (5–10 mg/dose PO bid) target levels of (200–250 ng/L)

(See Table 1 for immunosuppressive drugs and Table 2 for drug interactions.)

*Table 1*
## List of Immunosuppressive Drugs

| Medication | Mechanism | Clinical use | Side effects |
|---|---|---|---|
| Corticosteroids | Inhibits T-cell and antigen presenting cells | Used in induction and acute cellular rejection | Truncal obesity Growth failure Fluid retention Osteoporosis Cataracts Glucose intolerance |
| Cyclosporin | Calcineurin inhibitor Inhibits IL-2 | Maintenance therapy | Gingival hyperplasia Hypertrichosis Hypertension Neurotoxicity Nephrotoxicity |
| Tacrolimus | Calcineurin inhibitor Inhibits IL-2 | Maintenance therapy More potent than cyclosporin | Nephrotoxicity Hyperglycemia Neurotoxicity |
| Azathioprine | Nucleoside synthesis Inhibitor Inhibits purine synthesis | Maintenance therapy Not commonly used | Bone marrow suppression Hepatotoxicity Pancreatitis |

| Medication | Mechanism | Clinical use | Side effects |
|---|---|---|---|
| Mycophenolate mofetil | Nucleoside synthesis inhibitor Inhibits guanine formation | Maintenance therapy Calcineurin toxicity Chronic rejection | Diarrhea Nausea Abdominal pain Leukopenia |
| Rapamycin | Inhibits both T & B cell activation and thymocyte proliferation | Calcineurin toxicity | Hyperlipidemia Delayed wound healing HAT in early postop use |
| OKT-3 | Anti-CD3 monoclonal antibody | Steroid resistant rejection | Infusion reaction Pulmonary edema |
| Antithymocyte globulin | Binds both B & T cells | Not used routinely in induction anymore | Anaphylaxis Serum sickness |
| Basiliximab | Monoclonal IL-2 antibody | Induction | Infusion reaction |
| Daclizumab | Monoclonal IL-2 antibody | Induction | Infusion reaction |

*Table 2*
## Cyclosporin and Tacrolimus Drug Interactions

| Increase levels | Decrease levels | Potentiate nephrotoxicity |
|---|---|---|
| Ketoconazole/ Fluconazole | Phenytoin | Aminoglycosides |
| Omeprazole | Carbamazepine | Amphotericin B |
| Erythromycin | Barbiturates | Acyclovir |
| Oral contraceptives | Rifampin | |
| Verapamil Imipenem | Cimetidine | |

# Complications in First Postoperative Week in PICU

## Technical

- Primary graft nonfunction
- Hepatic artery thrombosis
- Hemorrhage
- Bile leak

## Infectious

- Sepsis

## Complications Due to Immunosuppression

- Neurologic (tacrolimus)
- Renal insufficiency (cyclosporine/tacrolimus)
- Diabetes (steroids/tacrolimus)

## Primary Graft Nonfunction

- It is rare in children but has very poor outcome
- Patients have severe coagulopathy, encephalopathy, and transaminases over 10,000 U/L and acidosis
- Patients unlikely to survive without retransplantation
- Risk factors

  - Donor factors: Injury to donor organ prior to harvest, hypoxia, hypotension, donor organ steatosis
  - Transplant factors: Prolonged cold ischemic storage, complex vascular anastomosis requiring revision, significant size discrepancy
  - Recipient factors: Postreperfusion hypotension, vascular thrombosis, ABO incompatible cross-match

## Hepatic Artery Thrombosis (HAT)

### Early

- It occurs most often within the first 30 days of OLT.
- It is three to four times more frequent in children than in adults due to the smaller diameter of arterial vessels.
- Patients have elevated transaminases, acidosis, and coagulopathy.
- Ultrasound of liver with Doppler is usually diagnostic.

- It presents with a variable clinical picture, composed of
- Fulminant allograft failure with necrosis
- Biliary disruption or obstruction
- Systemic sepsis
- Urgent thrombectomy is a therapeutic option if HAT is detected early in the course. Otherwise urgent retransplantation is required.

## Late

- HAT can be asymptomatic or present slowly progressive biliary complications causing cholangitis, strictures, intrahepatic abscesses, and sepsis.
- Treatment includes management of biliary complications while planning for elective retransplantation.

# Portal Vein Thrombosis (PVT)

- PVT occurs less frequently than HAT and may present as ascites or variceal bleeding.
- Doppler ultrasound (US) is helpful to make the diagnosis. Early intervention with thrombectomy and reanastomosis can be curative.

# Postoperative Hemorrhage

- Coagulopathy, thrombocytopenia, and disseminated intravascular coagulation are risk factors for early postoperative hemorrhage.
- Recipients of lobar or segmental grafts are at particular risk for bleeding from the multiple small arteries transected on the cut surface of the liver.
- Persistent bleeding despite multiple transfusions would be an indication for re-exploration.

# Bile Leak

- Bile duct leaks may occur with either duct to duct or Roux-en-Y anastomoses.
- Early leaks can be noted by the appearance of bile in the drains, and are confirmed with T-tube cholangiogram or HIDA scan.
- Children with segmental grafts may leak from the cut edge of the graft while patients with a whole graft are more likely to have an anastomotic leak.

- In case of biliary complications, Doppler liver US should be done to evaluate patency of the hepatic artery since the artery is the only supply of oxygenated blood to the bile ducts.
- Leaks are either treated with decompression with additional drains or repaired surgically.

## Acute Cellular Rejection

- Clinical symptoms: fever, jaundice, abdominal pain, lethargy
- Elevated liver enzymes
- Histologic features

  - Mixed portal mononuclear inflammation
  - Portal and central vein endothelialitis
  - Bile duct damage

- Primary treatment: Short course of high dose steroids is successful in 75% to 80%
- Steroid-resistant cases are treated with a monoclonal antibody, OKT3 (muromonab-CD3)

# Infection

Infections represent the most common source of morbidity and mortality following OLT.
Infections affect up to 70% of liver transplant recipients.

Infections within the first month of OLT:

- Early postoperative infections are related to surgical complications and nosocomial infections.
- The majority of infections are due to bacterial, followed by fungal, pathogens.
- Risk factors:

  - Prolonged duration of surgery
  - Graft failure requiring retransplantation
  - Prolonged ICU stay
  - Prolonged intubation or need of renal dialysis
  - Biliary anastomosis with the Roux-en-Y choledochojejunostomy predisposes the patient to cholangitis

Infections in the period 1 to 6 months post-OLT:

- The greatest risk is for the development of opportunistic infections.

- CMV, EBV, RSV, HHV6, adenovirus, hepatitis
- *Pneumocystis jiroveci* pneumonia (PCP), Aspergillus, Nocardia

- Posttransplant lymphoproliferative disease associated with EBV is also occasionally seen during this period.

More than 6 months post-OLT:

Common community infections
Opportunistic infections

# Bacterial

- Bacteria are the most common causes of infection affecting 35% to 70% of patients.
- Gram-negative organisms, Enterococcus and Staphylococcus are the common pathogens.
- All intraoperative lines should be removed as early as possible.
- Antibacterial prophylactic therapy should be discontinued within 48 hours to minimize the development of resistant infections.

# Fungal

- Candida is the most common fungal infection.
- Aspergillosis and Cryptococcus can cause more severe infections.
- Risk factors for fungal infections:

  - Multiple courses of antibiotics
  - Multiple operative procedures

Pneumocystis jiroveci (formerly carinii) pneumonia

- PCP can occur at anytime and presents as dyspnea and cough.
- When index of suspicion is high, urgent bronchoscopy for bronchioalveolar lavage should be done.
- Treatment:

  - Trimethoprim-sulfamethoxazole
  - Pentamidine
  - Steroids

# Viral

## CMV

- CMV infection occurs between 4 and 12 weeks post-OLT in 30% to 70% of recipients.

- Symptoms:

    - Flu-like symptoms: fever, malaise, and myalgias
    - Gastrointestinal ulcers with bleeding
    - Pulmonary involvement with progression to acute respiratory distress syndrome

- The prophylactic use of ganciclovir and acyclovir has markedly decreased morbidity and mortality.
- High-risk patients:

    - Seronegative recipient/seropositive allograft
    - Intensified immunosuppression

## Herpes Virus 6

- It can be a primary infection or reactivation of the virus.
- It presents with fever, rash, hepatitis, and/or encephalopathy.

## EBV

- It can present as a primary or as a reactivated past infection.
- Clinical manifestations:

    - Mono-like syndrome
    - Hepatitis simulating rejection
    - Lymphadenopathy
    - Tonsillar hypertrophy
    - Extranodal lymphoproliferative infiltration of gastrointestinal tract

        - Diarrhea, heme-positive stools, protein-losing enteropathy

    - Encephalopathy
    - Posttransplant lymphoproliferative disease (PTLD)

## Posttransplant Lymphoproliferative Disease (PTLD)

- PTLD is more common in children compared to adults
- Potentially fatal abnormal proliferation of B-lymphocytes
- Clinical presentations:

    - Benign polyclonal lymphoproliferation-like syndrome
    - Early malignant transformation
    - Malignant monoclonal lymphoma

## Risk Factors:

- Young age
- Seronegative patients receive a seropositive graft
- More potent immunosuppression (OKT3 > tacrolimus > cyclosporine)

Patients are now monitored routinely with quantitative polymerase chain reaction (PCR) for EBV DNA. Immunosuppressive drugs should be reduced when EBV DNA PCR counts reache 200 copies per $10^5$ peripheral blood leukocytes. Antiviral therapy with ganciclovir and CMV-IgG is also used in some cases. PTLD can also develop without an increase in EBV-PCR viral load.

## Management

- Withdrawal of immunosuppression
- High-dose ganciclovir
- Anti-CD 20 monoclonal antibody (rituximab)

In malignant form:

- Stop immunosuppression
- Chemotherapy
- Surgical resection/radiation

# Long-Term Outcome

The ultimate goal of liver transplantation is to allow the child long-term survival with good quality of life. Survival rate after liver transplantation depends on primary illness, age, and status of the patient before surgery. Overall 1 year patient and graft survival reached 88% and 82% respectively and long-term survival beyond 1 year is 83% and 74% respectively in the SPLIT (Studies of Pediatric Liver Transplantation) registry.

Long-term outcome depends on allograft function, medical compliance, and the complications of long-term exposure to immunosuppressive drugs.

The most common late complication is graft dysfunction due to infection, chronic rejection, lymphoproliferative disease, and recurrent disease.

# Late Complications and Issues

Infections, late hepatic artery thrombosis, and PTLD can present as late complications and are reviewed in previous section.

Chronic rejection is seen in 8% to 20% of patients. It presents with a progressive rise in alkaline phosphatase, gamma glutamyl transpeptidase, and progressive cholestasis. The patients can be asymptomatic or have a prior history of acute rejection. Diagnosis is confirmed on liver biopsy. Histologic features include ductopenia, foam cell arteriopathy, and fibrointimal hyperplasia and fibrosis.

## Biliary Complications

There is an increased risk of recurrent cholangitis or anastomotic stricture in patients who received reduced size grafts.

## Renal Insufficiency

- Nephrotoxicity is a complication of calcineurin inhibitor treatment.
- Glomerular filtration rate drops close to 40% within the first year after OLT.
- After 5 years, 20% have normal renal function, 4% develop renal insufficiency, and 1% to 2% develop end-stage renal disease.

## Cardiovascular Disease

- Hyperlipidemia and hypertension are prevalent among organ transplant recipients occurring in 25% to 75% of patients.

## Cancer

The chronic use of immunosuppressive drugs increases the long-term risk of development of malignancy. Skin cancer, non-Hodgkin's lymphoma, PTLD, and sarcoma occur with increased frequency in solid organ transplant recipients.

## Growth and Development

- Despite OLT, persistent growth failure occurs in 20% to 25% of children.
- Important factors: Pretransplant malnutrition, steroid therapy, graft dysfunction, behavioral feeding problems, genetic disorders.
- Malnutrition and prolonged hospital stay after OLT predicted poor neurodevelopmental outcome in children with biliary atresia during the first year after liver transplant.
- Learning problems can be seen in 25% of LT recipients.

# References

Abramson O, Rosenthal P. Current status of pediatric liver transplantation. Clin Liver Dis 2000;4:533–52.

Ghobrial RM, Amersi F, McDiarmid SV, et al. In: Maddrey WC, ed. Transplantation of the liver. Philadelphia, PA: Lippincott Williams & Wilkins; 2001, pp. 79–100.

Kelly DA, Mayer D. In: Kelly DA, ed. Diseases of the liver and biliary system in children. Malden, MA: Blackwell Publishing Ltd; 2004, pp. 378–401.

Rykman FC, Alonso MH, Bucuvalas JC, et al. Liver transplantation in children. In: Suchy F, et al. eds. Philadelphia, PA: Lippincott Williams & Wilkins; 2001, pp. 949–70.

Kinkhabwala M, Emond JC. The transplant operation. In: O'Grady JG, Lake JR, Howdle PD, eds. Comprehensive clinical hepatology. London: Mosby; 2000. pp. 35.1–4.

Krasko A, Desphande K, Bonvino S. Liver failure, transplantation, and critical care. Crit Care Clin 2003;19:155–83.

Brady L. Liver Transplantation: indication, modalities, and medical follow-up. In: Guandalini S, ed. Essential pediatric gastroenterology, hepatology, and nutrition. McGraw-Hill; 2005, pp. 319–33.

Rand EB, Olthoff KM. Overview of pediatric liver transplantation. Gastroenterol Clin North Am 2003;32:913–29.

McDiarmid SV. Current Status of liver transplantation in children. Pediatr Clin N Am 2003;50:1335–74.

Paya CV, Sia IG. Infective Complications. In: O'Grady JG, Lake JR, Howdle PD, eds. Comprehensive clinical hepatology. London: Mosby; 2000, pp. 37.1–18.

Green M. Viral infections and pediatric liver transplantation. Pediatr Transplantation 2002;6:20–4.

Faye A, Vilmer E. Post-transplant lymphoproliferative disorder in children. Incidence, prognosis, and treatment options. Pediatr Drugs 2005;7:55–65.

Tiao G, Ryckman FC. Pediatric liver transplantation. Clin Liver Dis 2006;169–97.

Porayko MK, Textor SC, Krom RA, et al. Nephrotoxic effects of primary immunosuppression with FK-506 and cyclosporine regimens after liver transplantation. Mayo Clin Proc 1994;69:105–11.

Bucuvalas, JC, Ryckman FC. Long-term outcome after liver transplantation in children. Pediatr Transplant 2002:6:30–6.

# Chapter 15

# Nutrition

## A. Nutrition in Critical Illness
Diana Calligan
Lennox Huang

### Introduction

A key component in the reduction of morbidity and mortality in critically ill children is the provision of proper nutrition. Unfortunately, many variables alter our ability to provide optimal nutrition. Underfeeding is frequently present and mainly due to prescription and administration of energy amounts inferior to measured energy expenditure values in enterally fed patients.

### Key Principles

- Optimize nutrition early in patient's course
- Caloric needs must be individualized to each clinical scenario
- Enteral is the preferred mode of delivery
- Underfeeding or overfeeding can adversely affect ICU course and outcome

# Goals of Nutrition Support

- Provide substrates required to minimize catabolism
- Support the immune system
- Reduction of morbidity and mortality
- Promote gastrointestinal (GI) integrity
- Facilitation of wound healing
- The pediatric intensive care unit (PICU) is *not* a feeding and growing center

## Nutritional Physiology in the Critically Ill

Injury, sepsis, and severe inflammation all result in a surge of neuroendocrine mediators such as catecholamines. This causes a hemodynamic state that augments oxygen delivery and demand and the availability of energy substrates to meet the increased demands of the body. This response of the body results in a combined hypermetabolic and hypercatabolic state leading to rapid malnutrition in the already vulnerable pediatric patient. Cumulative negative nutrition deficits are associated with poorer outcomes. During this phase, hepatic protein synthesis is redirected away from synthetic proteins (ie, albumin) and to acute phase reactant proteins (ie, CRP). Rapid proteolysis supplies amino acids for cellular substrate.

Technology, type of injury, and pharmacologic supports alter requirements (see Table 1).

*Table 1*
**Factors Affecting Nutrition in the PICU**

| Factors increasing caloric needs | Factors decreasing caloric needs | Limits on ability to provide nutrition |
|---|---|---|
| Major surgery | Sedation | Severe shock state with impaired organ perfusion |
| Multiple trauma | Mechanical ventilation | Gut integrity and motility |
| Burns | Non-ambulatory | Vascular access |
| Sepsis | No activity | Fluid limitations |
| Fever | | Use of IV lipids in septic states/ARDS (omit ARDS) |
| Pain | | Airway management |
| Anxiety | | Procedures |
| Growth (long term) | | Vomiting |
| | | Abdominal distention |
| | | Diarrhea |

Nutrition should be started as soon as possible if the patient is hemodynamically stable. Ideally, start feeds within 24 to 48 hours of PICU admission.

# Consequences of Inadequate Nutrition in the ICU

- Accelerated weight loss and muscle atrophy
- Prolonged post-ICU recovery
- Increased ICU stay
- Increased risk of nosocomial infections
- Increased risk of sepsis
- Increased mortality and morbidity

# Complications with Overfeeding

Overfeeding can have severe consequences on the liver, lungs, and kidney. Overfeeding may also result in volume overload with subsequent cardiopulmonary implications.

Excess carbohydrate

Increased $CO_2$ production

Increased minute ventilation

Hepatic steatosis

Hyperglycemia

Elevated triglycerides

Increased risk for sepsis

Excess protein

Increased ureagenesis

Can impair renal function or worsen pre-existing dysfunction

Hypertonic dehydration

Contribute to metabolic acidosis

Excess fat

Increased triglycerides

Increased transaminases

Hepatomegaly

Cholestasis

# Assessment of Nutritional Needs

- **History**: medical history, diagnosis and anticipated PICU course, diet history, premorbid nutritional status
- **Anthropometrics**: weight (include estimate of dry weight), length/height, head circumference ($<$3 years)

*Table 2*
**Serum Markers of Nutrition**

| | |
|---|---|
| Ferritin | Half-life 2–3 days, also acute phase reactant |
| Albumin | Half-life 18–21 days. Poor indicator of nutrition, better reflects acuity of illness and synthetic liver function |
| Prealbumin | Half-life 2 days, preferred marker in ICU if used in conjunction with CRP, will reflect shift to anabolic state (recovery) allowing for more aggressive feeding |
| Glucose | Can indicate excessive carbohydrate infusion |
| Triglycerides | Can indicate overfeeding of carbohydrate or fat |

- **Physical assessment**: edema, muscle wasting, fat stores
- **Medications**: prior to admission and current. Include vitamin/mineral supplements
- Biochemistry and the impact of nutrition on lab values and lab values' impact on nutrition (see Table 2)

In some cases management of fluid balance supersedes nutrition; for example, if goal is to reach a certain dry weight to tolerate specific/definitive surgery, nutrition may be limited.

# Determining Energy Requirements

There is no consensus on how to best estimate energy requirements of the critically ill child. Energy requirements vary between individual patients and over the course of their ICU stay. Indirect calorimetry is the best indicator of energy expenditure, assuming a steady state, no air leaks, or high $FiO_2$. However, most facilities do not have a metabolic cart, so equations must be used to estimate energy requirements.

- Admission weights or last dry weight should be used for estimating requirements.
- Increased serum glucose, urea, or bicarbonate can be due to overfeeding.

Initial caloric goals should be basal metabolic rate (BMR)

| Age (years) | BMR (kcal/kg) |
|:---:|:---:|
| 0–3 | 55 |
| 4–6 | 47 |
| 7–10 | 40 |
| 11–14 | 30 |
| 15+ | 25 |

Source: World Health Organization

Stress factors can then be used to calculate additional energy required

ICU on vent 1.0

Major surgery 1.2–1.3

Multiple fractures 1.2–1.35

Peritonitis 1.25–1.5

Pneumonia 1.3–1.4

Head injury 1.3–1.4

Liver failure 1.4–1.5

Sepsis 1.4–1.5

Burns 1.5–2.0

- Energy requirements will increase as child improves as demonstrated by weaning ventilation and sedation, extubation, and the resumption of growth.
- Clinical judgment and individual patient characteristics must be used when estimating energy requirements.

## Protein Requirements

- Can be as high as 2 to 2.5 times the recommended daily allowance (RDA).
- Post-severe injury, proteolysis occurs with a concurrent inhibition of the protein-sparing mechanisms of ketogenesis from fat.
- Protein depletion is associated with respiratory failure, sepsis, muscle weakness, and death.
- Extra protein losses need to be accounted for losses from CRRT, chest tubes, peritoneal drains, and fistulas.
- See Table 3 for list of normal protein requirements by age.

*Table 3*
**Protein Requirements by Age**

| Age (years) | Protein (g/kg/d) |
| --- | --- |
| 0–1 | 2–3.5 |
| 1–6 | 2–2.5* |
| >6 | 1.5–2* |

*higher for burns

## Monitoring Response to Nutrition Therapy

- Weight will reflect fluid shifts during acute and prolonged critical illness. Weight is useful in the recovery stage of illness.
- Growth curves are useful for chronic patients. Include weight, length, and head circumference.
- Serum markers in ICU are unlikely to reflect nutritional status. They are useful for electrolyte and mineral modifications and monitoring response to nutrition support.

## References

Briassoulis G Zavaras N, Hatzis T. Malnutrition, nutritional indices and early enteral feeding in critically ill children. Nutrition 2001;17:548–57.

Cresci G (ed). Nutrition support for the critically ill patient: A guide to practice. Boca Raton, FL: Taylor & Francis, 2005.

Gurgueira GL, Leite HP, Taddei JA, de Carvalho WB. Outcomes in a pediatric intensive care unit before and after the implementation of a nutrition support team. JPEN J Parenter Enteral Nutr 2005;29:176–85.

King W, Petrillo T, Pettignano R. Enteral nutrition and cardiovascular medications in the pediatric intensive care unit. JPEN J Parenter Enteral Nutr 2004;28:334–8.

Taylor RM, Preedy VR, Baker AJ, Grimble G. Nutritional support in critically ill children. Clin Nutr 2003;22:365–9.

Turi RA, Petros AJ, Eaton S, et al. Energy metabolism of infants and children with systemic inflammatory response syndrome and sepsis. Ann Surg 2001;233:581–7.

Oosterveld MJ, Van Der Kuip M, De Meer K, et al. Energy expenditure and balance following pediatric intensive care unit admission: a longitudinal study of critically ill children. Pediatr Crit Care Med 2006;7:147–53.

# B. Enteral Nutrition

Kevan Jacobson

Diana Calligan

## Introduction

Enteral nutrition (EN) is the most natural way in which humans meet their caloric needs. EN includes normal oral, as well as tube feeds. In the pediatric intensive care unit (PICU) setting, oral intake is often not possible or sufficient to meet metabolic demands.

EN rather than parenteral nutrition support is generally considered the preferred modality for a number of reasons:

- More physiologic
- Easier to administer
- More economical
- Safer
- Fewer metabolic and infectious complications
- Decreased risk of bacterial translocation
- More complete supply of nutrients
- Provides a trophic effect on the gut
- Facilitates transition to home care more rapidly

Conditions where inadequate oral intake may warrant tube feeding:

Preterm infants
Gastrointestinal disease

- Anorexia
- Inflammatory bowel disease (Crohn's disease)
- Protracted diarrhea
- Short bowel syndrome
- Gastroesophageal reflux disease
- Failure to thrive (FTT)
- Chronic liver disease

Cardiorespiratory illness

- Chronic lung disease
- Cystic fibrosis
- Severe trauma/closed head injury
- Congenital heart disease
- Mechanical ventilation

Renal disease
Hypermetabolic states

- Burn injury
- Severe trauma/closed head injury
- Cancer

Presurgery/postsurgery
Neurologic disease/cerebral palsy

## Routes of Delivery

Routes of delivery are classified by orifice of entry and location of the tube tip. There are various ways in which patients can be enterally fed including:

Nasogastric/orogastric (NG/OG)
Nasojejunal (NJ)
Gastrostomy (G)
Gastrojejunostomy (GJ)
Jejunostomy (J)

- Gastric feeding is usually the first choice with NG being the preferred route to the stomach. Jejunal feeding should be considered for infants and children with impaired gastric emptying, severe gastroesophageal reflux, with severe respiratory compromise and at risk for formula aspiration or if the child has failed gastric feeding. Jejunal feedings are typically safer patients without a secure airway (eg, noninvasive ventilation).

  - NG and NJ tubes are common procedures in the PICU. Insertion is contraindicated in the presence of severe facial

trauma. Correct positioning prior to commencement of feeds is necessary. Placement should be verified by x-ray.
- Occasionally, an NG may migrate across the midline to become a nasoduodenal tube. ND tube may be pulled back into the stomach or can be used to deliver continuous infusions.
- Jejunal placement may be achieved with the help of positioning, prokinetic agents, and/or fluoroscopy.

- Ostomy tubes (G, GJ, and J) inserted percutaneously via endoscopy, radiology, or surgery and are intended for more long-term use (>3 months).

## Methods of Delivery

Enteral feeds can be administered by either bolus feeds, intermittent infusion, or continuous infusion (Table 1). Indications for continuous feeds include:

- Failed bolus feeds
- Delayed gastric emptying
- Impaired absorption (chronic diarrhea, short gut)
- Ventilated patients
- Treatment of active small bowel Crohn's disease
- Nighttime augmentation in malnourished states

*Table 1*
**Modes of Delivery**

| Bolus feeds | Intermittent infusion | Continuous infusion |
|---|---|---|
| Delivered over short periods (15–60 min) every 3–6 hr Administered by pump or gravity More physiologic May not be used with jejunal or duodenal tubes | Delivered via pump Infused over more prolonged periods (eg, overnight) Can be used with all routes of delivery | Delivered via pump Infused continuously Preferred method of delivery in critically ill patients Can be used with all routes of delivery |

# Complications

Complications that may arise from tube feeding include:

- Persistent regurgitation
- Nausea and vomiting
- Pulmonary aspiration
- Formula intolerance
- Abdominal distention
- Diarrhea
- Skin infection (G, GJ, J tubes)
- Granulation tissue formation at skin site (G, GJ, J tubes)

## Signs and Symptoms of Feeding Intolerance

- Increased abdominal girth
- Abdominal distention
- Absence of bowel movements
- Increased frequency/volume of bowel movements
- Vomiting
- Persistent, consecutive large residuals

The utility of gastric residuals in determining feeding intolerance is controversial. Consecutive measurements may provide some indication of gastric emptying. Gastric residuals should be used in conjunction with other signs and symptoms of feeding tolerance.

## Management of Feeding Intolerance

If the child is having difficulty with enteral feeds, consider the following:

- Rate of infusion (too rapid)
- Method of infusion
- Enteral product
- Osmolality of formula
- Caloric density
- Bacterial contamination of feed (ie, hang time)
- Temperature of feed
- Consider adding promotility medications
- Consider adding bowel motility medications

# Guidelines for Initiation of Enteral Tube Feeding

Suggested guidelines for initiation and advancement of intermittent bolus feeds in children:

| Weight (kg) | Initial bolus q4h | Daily increases | Goal |
|---|---|---|---|
| 2–15 | 2 mL/kg/feed | 2 mL/kg/feed | Varies depending on illness and fluid restrictions |
| 16–30 | 1–2 mL/kg/feed | 1–2 mL/kg/feed | |
| 30–50 | 1–2 mL/kg/feed | 1–2 mL/kg/feed | |
| >50 | 2 mL/kg/feed | 1–2 mL/kg/feed | |

Suggested guidelines for initiation and advancement of continuous feeds in children:

| Weight (kg) | Initial infusion | Daily increases | Goal |
|---|---|---|---|
| 2–15 | 0.5–1 mL/kg/h | 1–2 mL/kg/h q4–8 hr | Varies depending on illness and fluid restrictions |
| 16–30 | 0.5–1 mL/kg/h | 0.5–1 mL/kg/h q4–8 hr | |
| 30–50 | 0.5 mL/kg/h | 0.5 mL/kg/h | |
| >50 | 25 mL/h | 25 mL/h | |

# Formula Selection

Formula selection varies between institutions. Formula selections should be based on age of the child, disease state, or clinical condition and formula composition.

## Classification of Infant Formulas

Breast milk if available
Standard cow's milk formulas: iron-fortified versions recommended
Soy-based formulas
Cow's milk-based formulas lactose free
Specialty formulas include: preterm formulas, thickened formula, protein hydrolysawtes, semi-elemental, and amino acid-based formula

Infant formulas can be concentrated stepwise from 20 kcal/oz to 24 kcal/oz, 27 kcal/oz, and 30 kcal/oz. Dietitian involvement advised.

Nutrient analysis per 100 mL

| FEED | Kcal | Protein grams | Fat source | mOsm/ kg $H_2O$ | Indications for use |
|---|---|---|---|---|---|
| **INFANT (0–1 YR)** | | | | | |
| HUMAN MILK (mature) | 70 | 1.1 | Human milk fat | 290 | Preferred feeding for term and preterm infants. |
| SIMILAC ADVANCE + IRON Ross | 68 | 1.4 | Safflower, coconut sunflower, soy | 300 | Iron fortified term infant formula with added DHA and ARA. |
| ENFAMIL A+ Mead Johnson | 67 | 1.4 | Palm olein, soy, coconut, sunflower | 300 | Iron fortified term infant formula with added DHA and ARA. |
| GOODSTART Nestle | 67 | 1.5 | Palm olein, soy, coconut, safflower | 265 | Iron fortified hydrolyzed whey- for infants *at risk* for milk protein allergy, poor gastric emptying or mild reflux. DHA & ARA added. |
| ENFAMIL A+ THICKENED Mead Johnson | 68 | 1.7 | Palm olein, soy, coconut, sunflower | | For babies with reflux. Formula thickens when combines with stomach acids. Cannot be concentrated beyond 24 kcal/ oz. ARA & DHA added. |

*(continued)*

| FEED | Kcal | Protein grams | Fat source | mOsm/ kg H$_2$O | Indications for use |
|---|---|---|---|---|---|
| **INFANT (0–1 YR)** | | | | | |
| ENFAMIL LACTOSE FREE Mead Johnson | 67 | 1.4 | Coconut, sunflower soy, palm olein | 180 | Milk-based, lactose-free formula. |
| ENFAMIL SOY Mead Johnson | 68 | 1.7 | Coconut, sunflower soy, palm olein | 182 | Soy-based formula. Milk, lactose and sucrose free. Use powdered form for galactosemia, vegan diet. |
| ALIMENTUM Ross | 68 | 1.9 | MCT 33% safflower, soy | 370 | Hydrolyzed casein for milk protein allergy (33% MCT). Lactose free. |
| NUTRAMIGEN Mead Johnson | 67 | 1.9 | Palm olein, soy, coconut, sunflower | 320 | Hydrolyzed casein for milk protein allergy. Lactose and sucrose free. |
| PREGESTIMIL Mead Johnson | 68 | 1.9 | MCT, corn, soy, high oleic sunflower | 273 | Hydrolyzed casein for milk protein allergy, fat malabsorption. (55% MCT). Lactose and sucrose free. |
| NEOCATE Nutricia | 67 | 2.1 | Safflower, coconut, soy | 375 | Amino acid-based for milk protein allergy, malabsorption. Contains long chain fats. |
| PORTAGEN Mead Johnson | 67 | 2.4 | MCT, corn, coconut | 230 | Fat malabsorption, chylothorax, defective lymphatic transport. Recipe on can = 1 cal/mL; consult RD. |
| SIMILAC ADVANCE NEOSURE 22 Ross | 74 | 2.1 | Soy, coconut, MCT (25%) | 224 | Preterm discharge formula with increased energy, vitamin D and minerals. Added DHA & ARA. √ ODB. |
| SIMILAC SPECIAL CARE 24 Ross | 81 | 2.4 | MCT (50%), soy, coconut | 270 | For preterm Infants <2 kg birthweight when human milk not available. |

| FEED | Kcal | Protein grams | Fat source | mOsm/ kg H$_2$O | Indications for use |
|---|---|---|---|---|---|
| **INFANT (0–1 YR)** | | | | | |
| SIMILAC HMF (Ross) (100 mL EBM + 4pkg HMF ) | 79 | 2.3 | MCT oil | 385 | To fortify human milk fed to premature infants <1800 grams birthweight. |

Source: Adapted from McMaster Children's Hospital formulary

### Classification of children's formulas
Feeds are tailored to 1 to 10 years

Polymeric (intact protein)
Semi-elemental (partially hydrolyzed protein)
Amino acid based

Nutrient analysis per 100 mL

| PEDIATRICS (1–10 YR) | | | | | |
|---|---|---|---|---|---|
| FEED | Kcal | Protein grams | Fat source | mOsm/ kg H$_2$O | Indications for use |
| VIVONEX PEDIATRIC Novartis | 80 | 2.4 | Coconut, soybean 68% MCT | 360 | 1 packet powder + 220 mL water = 250 mL formula. Elemental low-fat formula for fat malabsorption 68% MCT. |
| PEDIASURE Ross | 100 | 3.0 | Safflower, soy MCT, sunflower | 310 | Sole source of nutrition or supplement, oral/tube feed. Gluten and lactose free (20% MCT). |
| PEDIASURE PLUS with fiber Ross | 150 | 4.2 | Safflower, soy, MCT, sunflower | 345 | High calorie (1.5 kcal/mL). Oral/tube feed. Lactose and gluten free (20% MCT, 0.75 g fiber/100 mL FOS = 0.35 g/100 mL). |
| NUTREN JR Nestle | 100 | 3 | Soy, MCT, canola, soy lecithin | 350 | Sole source nutrition or supplement, oral/tube feed, (20% MCT, 80% LCT), lactose and gluten free. |

(continued)

**PEDIATRICS (1–10 YR)**

| FEED | Kcal | Protein grams | Fat source | mOsm/ kg H$_2$O | Indications for use |
|---|---|---|---|---|---|
| NUTREN JR + fiber Nestle | 100 | 3 | Soy, MCT, canola, soy lecithin | 350 | Supplement/tube feed, (20% MCT, 80% LCT), lactose and gluten free, 0.36 g pea fiber and 0.22 g FOS/ inulin per 100 mL. |
| PEPTAMEN JR Nestle | 100 | 3 | MCT, soy, canola | 360 | Partially hydrolyzed protein (60% MCT, 100% whey peptides). |
| NEOCATE JR (unflavored) Nutricia | 100 | 3 | Coconut, canola, safflower | 607 | Amino acid-based formula for allergy, protein intolerance, malabsorption. Tropical fruit flavor available. |

Source: Adapted from McMaster Children's Hospital formulary

## Classification of formulas for children over 10 years of age

These feeds are designed for adult use. They are used for children older than 10 years of age. In consultation with the Dietitian they can be used in younger children. Use high-protein feeds with caution with adolescents in ICU with very high energy requirements.

Polymeric (intact protein)
Semi-elemental (partially hydrolyzed protein)
Amino acid based

**PEDIATRICS (10+ YR)**

| FEED | Kcal | Protein grams | Fat source | mOsm/ kg H$_2$O | Indications for use |
|---|---|---|---|---|---|
| JEVITY 1 CAL Ross | 106 | 4.4 | Sunflower, canola safflower, MCT | 310 | Isotonic, fiber containing formula for tube feeding. 1.4 g fiber per 100 mL. Lactose and gluten free. |
| RESOURCE 2.0 Novartis | 200 | 9.0 | Canola, MCT | 790 | High nitrogen, calorically dense for fluid restriction. Oral supplement/tube feed. |
| ENSURE Ross | 106 | 4.0 | Safflower, corn sunflower, canola, | 455 | Oral supplement/tube feed. Lactose and gluten free. Vanilla, strawberry, chocolate. NOT ODB covered. (Ensure with fiber is ODB covered.) |

**PEDIATRICS (10+YR)**

| FEED | Kcal | Protein grams | Fat source | mOsm/ kg H$_2$O | Indications for use |
|---|---|---|---|---|---|
| ENSURE PLUS Ross | 150 | 5.7 | Safflower, canola, sunflower, corn | 540 | Oral supplement. Calorically dense, high protein for fluid restrictions. Lactose/ gluten free. Strawberry, chocolate, vanilla, butter pecan. |
| ENSURE HP Ross | 96 | 5.1 | Safflower, corn sunflower, canola | 546 | High protein supplement/tube feed. Lactose and gluten free. Van/choc/straw |

**Adolescents or pediatrics > 10 years old**

| FEED | Kcal | Protein grams | Fat source | mOsm/ kg H$_2$O | Indications for use |
|---|---|---|---|---|---|
| JEVITY 1.5 Ross | 150 | 6.8 | Canola, MCT, corn | 525 | High nitrogen, calorically dense for fluid restriction/elevated energy needs. Tube or oral feed. 19% of fat as MCT. 1.2 g fiber per 100 mL. Lactose and gluten free. FOS 1.0 g. |
| ISOSOURCE VHN Novartis | 100 | 6.2 | Canola, MCT, soy | 300 | High nitrogen, isotonic. Tube or oral feed. 50% of fat as MCT. 1.0 g fiber per 100 mL. Lactose and gluten free. |
| OXEPA Rossw | 150 | 62.5 | Canola, MCT, sardine and borage oils, soy lecithin | 535 | Low CHO, calorically dense tube feed for modulating inflammation in the critically ill on mechanical ventilation. Contains EPA&GLA. 25% of fat as MCT. Lactose and gluten free. |
| PERATIVE Ross | 130 | 6.7 | Canola, MCT, corn, lecithin | 385 | For metabolically stressed patients, ie, burns, wounds. Partially hydrolyzed protein. 40% of fat as MCT. Tube/ oral feed. Lactose and gluten free. |

*(continued)*

| FEED | Kcal | Protein grams | Fat source | mOsm/ kg H$_2$O | Indications for use |
|------|------|---------------|------------|-----------------|---------------------|
| PEPTAMEN Nestle | 100 | 4.0 | Coconut, palm, soybean, 70% MCT | 380 | Elemental diet for impaired GI function/ malabsorption. Oral and tube. 100% whey protein. 70% MCT. Vanilla flavor. |
| PEPTMEN 1.5 Nestle | 150 | 6.8 | Coconut, palm, soybean, 70% MCT | 550 | High calorie diet for impaired GI function/ malabsorption. 100% whey protein. Vanilla flavor. 70% MCT. |
| NEPRO Ross | 200 | 7.0 | Safflower, soy lecithin, canola | 665 | Acute or chronic renal failure requiring dialysis. Oral supplement or tube feed. Vanilla. |
| SUPLENA Ross | 200 | 3.0 | Safflower, soy, soy lecithin | 600 | Low protein for chronic/acute renal failure patient not on dialysis. Oral/tube feed. |

Source: Adapted from McMaster Children's Hospital formulary

# References

Stutphen JL, Abad-Sinden A. Enteral nutrition. In: Walker WA, Durie PR, Hamilton JR, et al., eds. Pediatric gastroenterology disease: pathophysiology, diagnosis and management. St. MO: Mosby-Year Book; 1996:1884–903.

Wilson SE. Pediatric enteral feeding. In: Grand RJ, Stutphen JL, Dietz WH, eds. Pediatric nutrition theory and practice. Boston: Butterworth-Heinemann; 1987:771–86.

Wilson SE, Dietz WH, Grand RJ. An algorithm for pediatric enteral alimentation. Pediatr Ann 1987;16:233–40.

Zeman FJ. Clinical nutrition and dietetics, 2nd edition. General principles of nutritional care. 1991:117–46.

Bockus S. Trouble shooting your tube feedings: solutions for the tube feeding dilemmas from verifying correct placement to determining the causes of diarrhea. Am J Nursing 1991;91(5):24–8.

# C. Parenteral Nutrition

Kevan Jacobson
Diana Calligan

## Introduction

Parenteral nutrition (PN), total parenteral nutrition (TPN), or hyperalimentation (hyperal) are interchangeable terms for IV nutrition administered to patients who are unable to meet caloric needs through enteral feeding. Three to five days without successful enteral nutrition is usually sufficient indication for instituting PN in the PICU. PN may be started earlier if one anticipates that the GI tract will be unusable for greater than 5 days.

## Indications

The following are some indications for initiation of PN.

> Low birth weight infants
> Surgical gastrointestinal disorders
>
> * Gastroschesis
> * Omphalocele
> * TEF
> * Multiple intestinal atresias
>
> Intractable diarrhea and/or vomiting
> Short bowel syndrome
> Severe malabsorption
> Severe pancreatitis
> Inflammatory bowel disease
> Intestinal pseudo-obstruction/prolonged ileus
> Postop with moderate/severely malnourished patients*
> Gut ischemia or poor gut perfusion

Hypermetabolic states when enteral nutrition is unlikely for >3 days

- Trauma
- Burns

Marrow and organ transplantation
Chemotherapy/radiation/mucositis/radiation enteritis
FTT (if gut not working)

*Note: proceed with caution to prevent refeeding syndrome whereby anabolic processes cause an increase and rapid cellular uptake of nutrients that can lead to profound hypophosphatemia, hypomagnesemia, hypokalemia, sodium and fluid retention with subsequent cardiac and respiratory complications.

Children at risk for refeeding syndrome

- Acute weight loss of >10% in the past 1 to 2 months
- Kwashiorkor or marasmus
- Underfeeding/fasting >14 days
- Protein-calorie malnutrition
- Anorexia nervosa
- Prolonged IV hydration with insufficient calories and protein

There are many guidelines for nutritional support of children at risk for refeeding syndrome. Principles are outlined below:

- Initiate hypocaloric feeds at approximately 80% of basal requirements
- Provide multivitamin and mineral supplements
- Monitor serum electrolytes, phosphorous, magnesium, calcium, and glucose every 12–24 hours.
- Increase calories 10% to 25% per day

## Composition

PN is composed of an amino acid dextrose solution and a lipid solution. It can be infused as a 3-in-1 solution (amino acid, dextrose and lipid together) or a 3-in-2 solution (lipids in a separate solution).

Amino acid solutions contain:

- Protein
- Dextrose
- Standard vitamins (lipid- and water-soluble)
- Vitamin K may be added to solutions for teens
- Trace elements (zinc, copper, chromium, manganese, magnesium)
- Selenium and iodine may be added in some institutions

Lipids can be given as 20% or 30%:

- In North America, only soybean-based intravenous fat emulsions are available at this time

## Methods of Delivery

PN can be delivered by either peripheral or central administration.

Peripheral route

- Short-term use (less than 10 days)
- Increased incidence of phlebitis
- Short life span of peripheral vein
- Can administer only up to 10% (12.5% in younger pts) dextrose solution (osmolarity <1100 mOsm/L)
- Total nutritional needs often cannot be met

Central (including PICC line)

- Long-term use
- Can administer up to 25% dextrose solution
- Nutritional needs can be fully met

## Complications

Sepsis
Thrombosis
Electrolyte imbalances

Hyperlipidemia
Hyperglycemia
Rebound hypoglycemia
Cholestasis
Fatty infiltration of the liver
Damage to hepatocytes
Cirrhosis of the liver
Lipid deposition in the lung—especially in context of postop
    hearts + ARDS
Refeeding syndrome (outlined previously)

## Management of Complications

| Sepsis | Antibiotics, may require line removal |
|---|---|
| Thrombosis | May require line removal, anticoagulation |
| Hyperlipidemia—poor lipid clearance—gross lipemia, elevated TG and cholesterol | Decrease lipids by 50% and repeat lipemic profile |
| Hyperglycemia | ↓ concentration of glucose infusion, insulin infusion may be required |
| Rebound hypoglycemia—occurs when Aminosyn infusion is stopped without weaning, especially in infants | Wean Aminosyn infusion by 50% during last hour of infusion or add dextrose containing maintenance IVF |
| Cholestasis—↑ conjugated bilirubin | Stimulate bile flow via enteral feeds, cycling TPN and ursodeoxycholic acid (Ursodiol) Remove Cu/Mn, with cholestasis |
| $CO_2$ retention with high glucose infusion rate | Reduce glucose infusion |

During suspected or proven sepsis, thrombocytopenia, acidosis, and hyperbilirubinemia, lipid infusion should be decreased to 0.5 to 1.0 g/kg/day or stopped until the child improves.

# Stepwise Approach to PN

How to calculate PN (see Table 1 for explanation)

1. Determine whether fluid requirements will restrict the ability to deliver caloric needs. Determination of caloric requirements in critically ill patients is outlined earlier in this chapter.

2. Calculate lipid requirements starting with 0.5 to 2 g/kg/day and increase as shown in table. Then determine volume of lipid (20% = 2g/10 mL). Subtract this volume from the total fluid requirements to calculate volume of Aminosyn. Determine calories: 20% lipid provides 2 kcal/mL, or 1 g of lipid provides 10 kcal.

3. Calculate dextrose requirements: start with 5% to 7.5% dextrose in infants, 10% or higher for patients 1 year increase by 2.5% dextrose/day as tolerated. Dextrose should routinely be increased to provide 40% to 60% of total calories. However, often fluid restriction limits the amount of glucose that can be given. Determine the mmol concentration of glucose (0.2 g = 1 mmol) and the % dextrose (g/total volume). Determine calories: 1 mmol of dextrose provides 0.67 kcal, or 1 g of dextrose provides 3.4 kcal.

4. Calculate protein requirements starting with table on next page and increase as shown in table. Determine protein calories: 1 g provides 5.7 kcal.

5. Determine electrolytes, vitamins, and trace element requirements as shown in the table.

6. Monitor weight daily.

7. Blood glucose: check daily after starting or changing infusion rate or glucose concentration.

8. Serum electrolytes, BUN, and creatinine daily for 2 days after starting or changing infusion rate or composition, then twice/week.

9. Check total bili, ALT, Alk Phos, INR, and PTT initially and then weekly.

10. Serum triglyceride and cholesterol initially and when changing quantity of fat, then weekly.

11. Note: frequency of blood work may vary according to the clinical situation and protocol of the particular institution.

*Table 1*
## Stepwise Approach to TPN

| Fat | |
|---|---|
| 20–30% | For infants, start at 2 g/kg/d and increase by 0.5 to 1.0 g/kg/d to a max. of 3.5 g/kg/d |
| 20% = 0.21 g fat/mL or 2 kcal/mL | For older infants/children, start with 1–2 g/kg/d and increase by 0.5 g/kg/d to a max. of 60% of total calories |

| Protein | |
|---|---|
| 1 g = 4 kcal | For infants, start at 2–2.5 g/kg/d and increase by 0.5 g/kg/d to a max. of 3.5 g/kg/d |
| Older infants/children | For older infants/children, start with 1 g/kg/d and increase by 0.5 g/kg/d to reach estimated requirements |

| Dextrose | |
|---|---|
| CVL: start 15%, not to exceed 25% | 1 mmol dextrose solution = 0.2 g dextrose |
| Peripheral line: start 7.5%, not to exceed 10% because of high osmolality (D10W = 505 mOsm/kg) | % dextrose solution = grams of dextrose/volume of solution |
| Maximum dextrose dose: Infants and children 10–14 mg/kg/min | Ref. Values for dextrose: (increase by D2.5W) |
| adolescents 5–8.5 mg/kg/min | 5%    = 250 mmol/L  = 50 g |
| | 7.5%  = 375 mmol/L  = 75 g |
| | 10%   = 500 mmol/L  = 100 g |
| | 12.5% = 675 mmol/L  = 125 g |
| | 15%   = 750 mmol/L  = 150 g |
| | 20%   = 1000 mmol/L = 200 g |

| Calculate energy provided | |
|---|---|
| Fat | 10% lipid = 1.07 kcal/mL |
| Protein | 20% lipid = 2 kcal/mL |
| Dextrose | 1 g = 4 kcal |
| | 1 mmol = 0.67 kcal, or 1 g = 3.4 kcal (IV dextrose is in the monohydrated form, reducing its caloric yield from 4 kcal/g in the parenteral form to 3.4 kcal/g) |

| Lytes/minerals | <10 kg (mmol/kg) | >10 kg (mmol/kg) |
|---|---|---|
| Na | 2–3 | 1.5 |
| K | 2–3 | 1.5 |
| $PO_4^{3-}$ | 1 | 0.25 |
| Ca | 1 | 0.25 |
| Mg | 0.25 | 0.13 |

Sum Ca/P not to exceed 20 mmol/liter

Maximum K (Central TPN—100 mmol/L; Peripheral TPN—40 mmol/L

| Vitamins (MVI Peds or Adults) | |
|---|---|
| <1 kg | 1.5 mL |
| 1–3 kg | 3.25 mL |
| 3–40 kg | 5.0 mL |
| >40 kg | 10 mL + 0.2 mg vit K (adult) |

| Trace elements (varies by institution) | |
|---|---|
| <3 kg | Neo 1 mL/kg max 3 mL |
| 3–40 kg | Peds 1 mL/kg |
| >40 kg | Adults 2.1 mL/d |

# References

Kerner JA. Parenteral nutrition. In: Walker WA, Durie PR, Hamilton JR, et al., eds. Pediatric gastroenterology disease: pathophysiology, diagnosis and management. St. MO: Mosby-Year Book; 1996:1904–51.

Pencharz P, Zlotkin S et al. HSC Handbook—guidelines for the administration of parenteral nutrition, 9th ed., Saint Louis: C. V. Mosby; 1997.

ODA-OHA nutrition care manual. Don Mills (ON): The Association; 1989.

# Chapter 16

# Endocrine

## A. Adrenal Insufficiency

Seth D Marks

Adrenal insufficiency (AI) is a state of glucocorticoid and/or mineralocorticoid deficiency. Adrenal crisis describes a potentially fatal state of acute AI with overwhelming metabolic and circulatory disturbances.

## Key Principles

- AI can present with vague symptoms mandating a high level of clinical suspicion to diagnose.
- Adrenal crisis occurs most commonly, given major physiological stress such as fever, critical illness, trauma, or surgery.
- Fluid resuscitation and corticosteroid replacement is central to the management of adrenal crisis.
- The biochemistry of AI is characterized by hyponatremia, hyperkalemia, and hypoglycemia.

## Pathophysiology

- Cortisol is produced by the adrenal glands under the stimulation of adrenocorticotropin hormone (ACTH) from the pituitary gland, itself stimulated by corticotropin-releasing hormone (CRH) from the hypothalamus.
- Cortisol is important for cell function including metabolism, wound healing, catecholamine action, and vascular tone and permeability.

- In the normal state, cortisol levels rise during acute critical illness secondary to increased activation of the hypothalamic-pituitary-adrenal axis.
- Primary AI results from failure of the adrenal glands to produce cortisol.
- Secondary AI results from failed stimulation of the adrenal glands by the pituitary or hypothalamus.

# Etiology

## Primary Adrenal Insufficiency

- Autoimmune [Addison's disease, autoimmune polyglandular syndrome (APS) type I or II]
- Congenital adrenal hyperplasia (CAH)
- Adrenal hemorrhage or infarct (eg, Waterhouse-Friderichsen syndrome)
- Infectious (eg, tuberculosis, HIV)
- Infiltrative (eg, amyloidoses, metastatic carcinoma)
- Adrenoleukodystrophy
- Smith-Lemli-Opitz syndrome
- Mitochondrial disorder
- Adrenal dysgenesis (eg, congenital adrenal hypoplasia, ACTH unresponsiveness, steroidogenic factor-1 mutation)
- Medication (eg, etomidate, ketoconazole)

# Secondary Adrenal Insufficiency

- Intercurrent illness, trauma, or surgery in patient with underlying primary AI
- Hypopituitarism
- CNS tumor or radiation
- Glucocorticoid withdrawal or ongoing therapy (corticosteroid therapy, including inhaled corticosteroids, for underlying medical illnesses, eg, inflammatory bowel disease, asthma)

# Clinical Features

- Weight loss, muscle weakness, fatigue, anorexia, abdominal pain, nausea, emesis, confusion, depression, fever
- Salt craving and hyperpigmentation in primary AI
- Hypotension, dehydration, shock—constituting the so-called "adrenal crisis"

- Hypoglycemia, hyponatremia, hyperkalemia, hypercalcemia, metabolic acidosis, increased plasma renin, neutropenia, eosinophilia
- Initiation of thyroid replacement for hypothyroidism may precipitate an adrenal crisis in a patient with previously undiagnosed AI

**Levels of Cortisol**

The symptoms of chronic AI can be non specific; therefore a high index of suspicion is required.

- AI or adrenal crisis should be considered in hemodynamically unstable patients who do not respond to standard therapy especially with documented hyponatremia, hyperkalemia, and hypoglycemia.
- A random cortisol level <85 nmol/L indicates absolute AI in non-critically ill patients.
- The appropriate or "normal" serum cortisol level in response to critical illness is controversial. Given an ACTH stimulation test, the baseline cortisol levels and the incremental increases at 30 and 60 minutes may be useful, and have both been used to guide therapy and assess prognosis in critically ill patients.

  - Traditionally, a cortisol level of at least 500–550 nmol/L, or 700 nmol/L in some studies, at baseline or following ACTH stimulation testing has been considered adequate in critically ill patients.
  - Higher cortisol levels generally reflect more severe illness.
  - A baseline cortisol level greater than 935 nmol/L and an increase <250 nmol/L with ACTH stimulation testing have both been shown to be associated with poor outcome in septic shock.
  - Relative adrenal insufficiency (RAI) refers to an apparent "normal" or even elevated baseline cortisol level but an inadequate increase of <250 nmol/L with ACTH stimulation testing. Some studies have shown RAI to be associated with a poor prognosis, and therefore warranting treatment, but the significance of RAI is still debatable.

# Investigations

- Collect blood work prior to initiating corticosteroid treatment.
- Serum sodium, potassium, chloride, bicarbonate, glucose, BUN, creatinine, calcium, CBC, blood gas, cortisol, renin, ACTH.

- Frequent (hourly initially) bedside glucose monitoring.
- 17-Hydoxyprogesterone (especially in newborn), anti-adrenal antibodies, coagulation profile, blood culture.
- ACTH stimulation test. The use of 1 mcg versus 250 mcg is contentious.
- Free cortisol, when available, may reflect adrenal status better than total cortisol.
- Adrenal ultrasound, CT/MRI brain.
- Auto immune adrenalitis (Addison's) and APS I or II are associated with other auto immune diseases (eg, hypothyroidism, type 1 diabetes mellitus, hypoparathyroidism), and should be investigated as appropriate after initial acute management.

## Treatment

- Corticosteroid, fluid, and salt replacement are the mainstays of both acute and chronic treatment.
- Short-term side effects of excess corticosteroid include hyperglycemia, hypertension, immunosuppression, poor wound healing, and psychosis.
- The serum cortisol level used to diagnosis AI and to therefore initiate therapy is controversial (see Clinical Features—Levels of Cortisol above).
- The diagnosis of RAI and the need to treat is controversial but has been shown to improve outcome in some studies.

### Acute

- Resuscitation with intravenous normal saline (NS) as clinically indicated.
- Dextrose should be included in ongoing intravenous fluid (eg, D5NS, D10NS) to address risk of hypoglycemia.
- Hydrocortisone 50–100 mg/m$^2$ IV or IM once; then 50–100 mg/m$^2$/day IV or IM divided q.i.d. (200–300 mg/day in adults).
- Additional mineralocorticoid replacement is not usually required in the acute adrenal crisis, but some authorities do recommend it.
- Any significant hyponatremia ($<$130 mmol/L) should be corrected slowly at a rate no greater than 0.5 mmol/L per hour unless neurologic symptoms such as seizures are present (see SIADH, section F of this chapter and Hyponatremia, Chapter 12).
- Treat hyperkalemia and hypoglycemia as indicated (see Chapter 12, "Intravenous Fluid and Electrolyte Management" and section B of this chapter).

# Chronic

- Oral corticosteroid replacement with hydrocortisone 8–25 mg/m²/day divided t.i.d. depending on underlying etiology. Prednisolone or prednisone equivalent may be used at between 5:1 to 15:1 relative potency to hydrocortisone (eg, 1 mg/m²/day) divided b.i.d.
- Mineralocorticoid replacement with fludrocortisone (Florinef) 0.05 to 0.3 mg daily.
- Patients should wear medical alert identification.
- Intercurrent illness management

  - Patients on long-term corticosteroid therapy for underlying AI should double or triple their maintenance dose to achieve "stress" doses during significant intercurrent illness (eg, fever).
  - Patients that are not tolerating oral intake require IV or IM corticosteroid.
  - Adjustment in the fludrocortisone is not required.

# References

Torrey SP. Recognition and management of adrenal emergencies. Emerg Med Clin North Am 2005;23:687–702.

Beishuizen A, Thijs LG. Relative adrenal failure in intensive care: an identifiable problem requiring treatment? Best Pract Res Clin Endocrinol Metab 2001;15:513–31.

Widmer IE, Puder JJ, Konig C et al. Cortisol response in relation to the severity of stress and illness. J Clin Endocrinol Metab 2005;90:4579–86.

Ten S, New M, Maclaren N. Clinical review 130: Addison's disease 2001. J Clin Endocrinol Metab 2001;86:2909–22.

Perry R, Kecha O, Paquette J, Huot C, et al. Primary adrenal insufficiency in children: twenty years experience at the Sainte-Justine Hospital, Montreal. J Clin Endocrinol Metab 2005;90:3243–50.

Oelkers W. Adrenal insufficiency. N Engl J Med 1996;335:1206–12.

Absalom A, Pledger D, Kong A. Adrenocortical function in critically ill patients 24 h after a single dose of etomidate. Anaesthesia 1999;54:861–7.

Todd GR, Acerini CL, Ross-Russell R, Zahra S, Warner JT, McCance D. Survey of adrenal crisis associated with inhaled corticosteroids in the United Kingdom. Arch Dis Child 2002;87:457–61.

Cooper MS, Stewart PM. Corticosteroid insufficiency in acutely ill patients. N Engl J Med 2003;348:727–34.

Annane D, Sebille V, Troche G, Raphael JC, Gajdos P, Bellissant E. A 3-level prognostic classification in septic shock based on cortisol levels and cortisol response to corticotropin. JAMA 2000;283:1038–45.

Ligtenberg JJ, Zijlstra JG. The relative adrenal insufficiency syndrome revisited: which patients will benefit from low-dose steroids? Curr Opin Crit Care 2004;10:456–60.

Hamrahian AH, Oseni TS, Arafah BM. Measurements of serum free cortisol in critically ill patients. N Engl J Med 2004;350:1629–38.

Coursin DB, Wood KE. Corticosteroid supplementation for adrenal insufficiency. JAMA 2002;287:236–40.

Annane D, Sebille V, Charpentier C, et al. Effect of treatment with low doses of hydrocortisone and fludrocortisone on mortality in patients with septic shock. JAMA 2002;288:862–71.

Gonzalez H, Nardi O, Annane D. Relative adrenal failure in the ICU: an identifiable problem requiring treatment. Crit Care Clin 2006;22:105–18.

Sterns RH, Riggs JE, Schochet SS Jr. Osmotic demyelination syndrome following correction of hyponatremia. N Engl J Med 1986;314:1535–42.

Albanese A, Hindmarsh P, Stanhope R. Management of hyponatraemia in patients with acute cerebral insults. Arch Dis Child 2001;85:246–51.

Vachharajani TJ, Zaman F, Abreo KD. Hyponatremia in critically ill patients. J Intensive Care Med 2003;18:3–8.

Crown A, Lightman S. Why is the management of glucocorticoid deficiency still controversial: a review of the literature. Clin Endocrinol (Oxf) 2005;63:483–92.

Punthakee Z, Legault L, Polychronakos C. Prednisolone in the treatment of adrenal insufficiency: a re-evaluation of relative potency. J Pediatr 2003;143:402–5.

Compendium of Pharmaceuticals and Specialties: The Canadian Drug Reference for Health Professionals. Ottawa: Canadian Pharmacists Association; 2006.

# B. Hypoglycemia

## Karen McAssey

The precise definition of hypoglycemia in childhood remains controversial. Symptoms of insulin-induced hypoglycemia are reported at a plasma glucose of 3.3 mmol/L (60 mg/dL) or less and impairment of CNS function at a plasma glucose of 2.8 mmol/L (50 mg/dL). Whole blood glucose values may be 10–15% less than plasma glucose values. For diagnostic purposes, hypoglycemia will be defined as a whole blood glucose less than 2.2 mmol/L (40 mg/dL).

## Key Principles

- Children with hypoglycemia may be asymptomatic or may present with severe central nervous system (CNS) and cardiorespiratory dysfunction. Every acutely ill child should be evaluated for hypoglycemia, particularly if presenting history includes decreased oral intake.
- Prolonged or repeated hypoglycemia in childhood may cause irreversible brain damage and permanently impair neurologic development.
- When the diagnosis of hypoglycemia is suspected, always obtain "critical" laboratory blood specimens before treatment with intravenous dextrose is begun, to confirm the diagnosis with a laboratory plasma glucose and to evaluate the etiology of hypoglycemia.
- Since children are particularly sensitive to hypoglycemia, tight glycemic control for pediatric critical illness is controversial and not supported by evidence at this time.

## Pathophysiology

- In the fed state, glucose supply is plentiful, insulin levels are high and guides glucose flux toward glycogen synthesis. Excess glucose is converted to acetyl CoA, which enters fatty acid oxidation synthesis and is stored as fat.

- Fasting adaptation initially involves glycogenolysis. The hormonal balance shifts with a decrease in insulin and rise in glucagon and epinephrine.
- As glycogen stores are depleted, gluconeogenesis is active with increasing cortisol and growth hormone levels.
- To prevent excessive breakdown of muscle, fatty acid oxidation and ketogenesis are favored. Lipolysis is triggered by secretion of the counter-regulatory hormones (glucagon, epinephrine, cortisol, growth hormone) and removal of the inhibitory effect of insulin.
- Almost all hypoglycemia in childhood occurs during fasting, when these adaptive mechanisms (glycogenolysis, gluconeogenesis, and/or fatty acid oxidation and ketogenesis) fail to maintain normal glucose homeostasis.

# Etiology

Hyperinsulinism:

- Transient—newborn infant either of a diabetic mother, small for gestational age or asphyxiated, preterm with inadequate intake, erythroblastosis fetalis; exogenous insulin, oral hypoglycemic agent
- Persistent—genetic defects of beta cell regulation (persistent hypoglycemic hyperinsulinism of infancy), islet cell adenoma

Defects in glycogenolysis:

- Limited/depleted glycogen stores—small for gestational age and premature newborn
- Inability to mobilize glycogen stores—enzyme deficiency or inhibition of enzyme activity (glycogen storage disease), growth hormone deficiency

Defects in gluconeogenesis:

- Enzyme deficiency or inhibition of enzyme activity (galactosemia, fructose intolerance)
- Alcohol intoxication, salicylate intoxication, beta blockers
- Liver failure
- Inborn errors of amino or organic acid metabolism, growth hormone (GH deficiency), or cortisol deficiency

In childhood idiopathic ketotic (substrate deficient) hypoglycemia, easily depleted glycogen stores, in combination with inadequate production of glucose through gluconeogenesis, contribute to hypoglycemia.

Defects in ketone production (fatty acid oxidation):

- Inadequate fat stores—SGA and preterm newborns, malnutrition, anorexia
- Inborn errors of fatty acid oxidation

Increased glucose utilization concurrent with impaired fasting adaptation:

- Infection, fever
- Acute brain injury: seizure, encephalitis, trauma, hemorrhage, hypoxia
- Circulatory disease: hypoxemia, hypotension, septic shock

## Clinical Features

### Autonomic Nervous System Activation

- Tachycardia, palpitations
- Tremor, jitteriness
- Anxiety
- Pallor
- Hunger, nausea, vomiting
- Perspiration
- Weakness

### Neuroglycopenia

- Headache
- Dizziness
- Incoordination, ataxia
- Lethargy
- Seizure, hemiparesis
- Confusion, irritability
- Coma

## Investigations

- Capillary blood glucose at presentation.
- Confirm hypoglycemia with laboratory plasma glucose value.
- Obtain critical (archival) sample immediately before therapeutic intervention.
- Collect the first urine void during or following hypoglycemia for urine ketones, organic acids and toxicology screen as indicated.

| Basic bloodwork | Volume of blood and collection tube required |
|---|---|
| Glucose, blood gas (venous or arterial) | Standard blood tubes |
| Electrolytes, liver function tests | |
| Complete blood count | |
|   Critical Sample | |
|   • Insulin, cortisol, growth hormone | |
|   • Free fatty acids, beta-hydroxybutyrate | |
|   • C peptide | • 8 mL serum (2 red top) tubes |
|   • Total and free carnitine, acylcarnitine profile | |
|   • Ammonia | • 2 mL plasma (green top) tube on ice |
|   • Lactate on ice | • 1–2 mL EDTA (grey top) tube |

## Prolonged Fast

- An elective diagnostic fast is considered for some children with hypoglycemia within a controlled setting with appropriate supervision and monitoring.
- The duration of fast depends on the child's age and normal feeding patterns.
- During the fast, plasma concentrations of glucose, ketone bodies, and insulin are serially monitored. Plasma concentrations of growth hormone and cortisol are obtained at the time of hypoglycemia.

## Treatment

- Assess and manage ABCs according to PALS guidelines.
- IV access and blood work (including critical sample).
- If child is asymptomatic or mildly symptomatic and able to tolerate oral fluids then give glucose-containing drink (3–4 ounces of formula or juice). If hypoglycemia does not improve in 10–15 minutes then parental glucose is required.
- Infuse an intravenous bolus of dextrose for moderate to severe hypoglycemia to provide 0.5–1 g/kg of dextrose (2.5–5 mL/kg of D10W, 1–2 mL/kg of D25W, or 0.5–1 mL/kg of D50W).

- Following intravenous bolus, provide a continuous infusion of a dextrose-containing solution to provide glucose at 6–9 mg/kg/minute (usually a minimum of D10W).
- Monitor blood glucose every 15–30 minutes until stable between 4.0 and 6.7 mmol/L
- If hypoglycemia does not resolve, then increase dextrose infusion to provide 10–15 mg/kg/minute. A dextrose requirement above 10 mg/kg/minute is very suspicious for hyperinsulinism. Continue to monitor blood glucose.

---

The rate of infusion (mg/kg/minute) can be calculated as follows:

(% dextrose in solution × 10 × rate of infusion (mL/hr)) ÷ (60 × weight in kg)

---

- *Persistent Hypoglycemia:* Additional treatment options (particularly for hyperinsulinism):
- Glucagon 0.5–1 mg IV/IM/SC or a continuous infusion of 1–2 mg/day
- Diazoxide 5–15 mg/kg/day PO divided q8h
- Hydrocortisone 5–6 mg/kg/day IV divided q6h
- Octreotide 2–10 mcg/kg/day divided q6–12h
- If a diagnosis of hyperinsulinemia is suspected, Glucagon administration (glucagon challenge test) at the time of hypoglycemia can be therapeutic and provides useful diagnostic information about glycogen stores. A clear glycemic response above 1 to 2 mmol/L increase in plasma glucose following intravenous or intramuscular injection of glucagon (0.03 mg/kg) supports inappropriate sequestration of hepatic glycogen.

# References

Cornblath M, Sachwartz R, Aynsley-Green A, Lloyd JK. Hypoglycemia in infancy: the need for a rational definition. Pediatrics 1990;85:834.

Kappy MS, Bajaj L. Endocrine/metabolic emergencies in children. Adv Pediatr 2002;49:245–72.

Flykanada-Gantenbein C. Hypoglycemia in childhood: long term effects. Pediatr Endocrinol Rev 2004;(1 Suppl):530.

Warren RE, Frier BM. Hypoglycemia and cognitive function. Diabetes Obes Metab 2005;7;5:493.

Thornton PS, Finegold DN, Stanley CA, Sperling MA. Hypoglycemia in the Infant and Child. In: Sperling MA, ed. Pediatric endocrinology, 2nd ed. Pennsylvania: Saunders; 2002, p. 367.

Haymond MW, Sunehag A. Controlling the sugar bowl. Regulation of glucose homeostasis in children. Endocrinol Metab Clin North Am 1999;28(4):663.

Darmaun D, Haymond MW, Bier DM. Metabolic aspects of fuel homeostasis in the fetus and neonate. In: DeGroot LJ, Besser M, Burger HG, et al., eds. Endocrinology. 3rd ed. Philadelphia: WB Saunders; 1995, p. 2258.

Schartz R, Tarama KA. Effects of diabetic pregnancy on the fetus and newborn. Semin Perinatol 2000;24(2):120.

Fournet JC, Junien C. The genetics of neonatal hyperinsulinism. Horm Res 2003;59(Suppl 1):30.

Sperling MA, Menon RK. Hyperinsulinemic hypoglycemia of infancy. Recent insights into ATP-sensitive potassium channels, sulfonylurea receptors, molecular mechanisms, and treatment. Endocrinol Metab Clin North Am 1999;28:695.

Hawdon JM, Weddel A, Aynsley-Green A, Ward Platt MP. Hormonal and metabolic response to hypoglycaemia in small for gestational age infants. Arch Dis Child 1993;68:3:269.

Chen YT, Burchell A. Glycogen storage diseases. In: Scriver CR, Beaudet AL, Sly WS, Valle D, eds. The metabolic and molecular bases of inherited disease. 7th ed. New York: McGraw Hill; 1995, p. 935.

Van den Berghe, G. Disorders of gluconeogenesis. J Inherit Metab Dis 1996;19:470.

Laron Z. Hypoglycemia due to hormone deficiencies. J Pediatr Endocrinol Metab 1998;11(Suppl 1):117.

Lteif AN, Schwenk WF. Hypoglycemia in infants and children. Endocrinol Metab Clin North Am 1999;28:619.

Taroni F, Uziel G. Fatty acid mitochondrial beta-oxidation and hypoglycaemia in children. Curr Opin Neurol 1996;9:477.

Losek JD: Hypoglycemia and the ABC'S (sugar) of pediatric resuscitation. Ann Emerg Med 2000;35:43.

Verrotti A, Fusilli P, Pallotta R, et al. Hypoglycemia in childhood: a clinical approach. J Pediatr Endocrinol Metab 1998;11(Suppl 1):147.

Service FJ. Hypoglycemia disorders. N Engl J Med 1995;332:1144.

Kane C, Lindley KJ, Johnson PR, et al. Therapy for persistent hyper-insulinemic hypoglycemia of infancy. Understanding the responsiveness of beta cells to diazoxide and somatostatin. J Clin Invest 1997;100:1888.

Ehara A, Takahashi M, Nobumoto K, et al. Successful control of persistent hyperinsulinemic hypoglycemia of infancy with a high dextrin formula. Acta Paediatr Jpn 1998;40:293.

Thornton PS, Alter CA, Katz LE, et al. Short- and long-term use of octreotide in the treatment of congenital hyperinsulinism. J Pediatr 1993;123:637.

Aynsley-Green A, Hussain K, Hall J, et al. Practical management of hyperinsulinism in infancy. Arch Dis Child Fetal Neonatal Ed 2000;82:F98.

# C. Thyroid Storm

## Karen McAssey

Thyroid storm is an extreme and life-threatening hypermetabolic state involving multiple organ systems that occurs when the effects of free thyroid hormone abruptly increase in an individual with hyperthyroidism. Thyroid storm is the most severe state of thyrotoxicosis.

## Key Principles

- Thyroid storm can develop in patients with long-standing untreated hyperthyroidism. More commonly it is precipitated by an acute event.
- Careful management in the intensive care unit (ICU) is essential. Mortality rate in thyroid storm is significant. Rapid diagnosis and aggressive treatment is critical.
- Salicylates interfere with protein binding and may lead to increased levels of free thyroid hormone. Use acetaminophen for fever.
- One to two percent of infants born to mothers with Graves' disease will develop neonatal thyrotoxicosis secondary to transplacental passage of maternal TSH receptor stimulating antibodies.

## Pathophysiology

- Graves' disease is the most common cause of childhood thyrotoxicosis and therefore most cases of thyroid storm in children occur with underlying Graves' disease. Graves' disease occurs more often in adolescents.
- Other causes of thyrotoxicosis associated with thyroid storm include McCune-Albright syndrome with autonomous thyroid function, hyperfunctioning thyroid nodule, or multinodular goiter.
- Thyroid storm occurs with an abrupt relative rise in free thyroid hormone levels. This may be associated with a decline in binding proteins. Beta-adrenergic receptor activation may also contribute.

- Free thyroid hormone may have a direct sympathomimetic effect related to its structural similarity to catecholamines.
- The clinical findings in thyroid storm relate to the grossly exaggerated effects of thyroid hormone.

## Etiology

Thyroid storm is often precipitated by one of the following conditions in an individual with thyrotoxicosis:

- Infection
- Thyroid or nonthyroidal surgery
- General trauma
- Acute iodine load
- Withdrawal of antithyroid medication, noncompliance
- Exogenous thyroid hormone ingestion
- Diabetic ketoacidosis

## Differential Diagnosis

- Drug intoxication or withdrawal
- Septic shock
- Malignant hyperthermia
- Hypertensive encephalopathy
- Pheochromocytoma
- Anxiety disorder/panic disorder

## Clinical Features

- Fever
- Sweating
- Vomiting, diarrhea
- Jaundice
- Weight loss
- Tachycardia, congestive heart failure
- Cardiac arrhythmia
- Tachypnea
- Agitation, delirium, psychosis
- Seizures, coma
- Goiter, exophthalmos

## Investigations

- Thyroid storm is a clinical diagnosis. Laboratory results will support this diagnosis but treatment should not be delayed while awaiting laboratory confirmation.

- Usual findings will include elevated free thyroxine (T4) and/or triiodothyronine (T3) and with a suppressed thyroid-stimulating hormone (TSH). TSH will be elevated if the etiology is TSH hypersecretion.
- TSH receptor stimulating antibodies will be elevated in Graves' disease.
- Serum glucose, blood gas (VBG/ABG), electrolytes, calcium, urea and creatinine, liver enzymes
- Complete blood count (CBC)
- If there is evidence of infection, obtain appropriate cultures
- ECG, cardiac monitor
- Chest X-ray

## Treatment

- Assess and manage ABCs according to PALS guidelines.
- Treat fever with antipyretics, cooling blankets, ice packs.
- Identify and treat precipitating illness.
- Specific therapy directed toward the thyroid gland includes several medications that act via complimentary mechanisms.
- **Beta blockers** are used to control adrenergic hyperactivity. Propranolol additionally decreases peripheral conversion of T4 to active T3. Congestive heart failure and asthma are contraindications for the use of beta blockers.

  - PO/NG: 2–4 mg/kg/day divided q 6–8 hours
  - IV: 0.01–0.02 mg/kg IV
  - Repeat as needed every 15 minutes to usual maximum of 5 mg/dose

- **Thionamides** [Propylthiouracil (PTU) or methimazole] inhibit oxidation of iodide and block synthesis of newly formed thyroid hormone. These medications are unable to affect the release of preformed hormone from the thyroid gland. PTU but not methimazole will decrease peripheral conversion of T4 to active T3. Methimazole has a longer duration of action. Both medications can be suspended in liquid for rectal administration.

  - PTU 10–20 mg/kg/day PO/NG/PR divided q 6–8 hours
  - OR Methimazole 0.5–1 mg/kg/day PO/NG/PR divided q 8–12 hours

- **Iodine** in large doses blocks the release of T3 and T4 from the thyroid, inhibits the release of preformed hormone, and renders the gland less vascular. The administration of iodine should be delayed for at least one hour after thionamide administration to prevent the iodine from being used as a substrate for new hormone synthesis. Iodinated radio contrast agents (iopanoic acid) likely achieve a similar effect. There is only limited experience with their use in children.

- Lugol's solution (5% iodine and 10% potassium iodide): Children and adults: 1 mL PO/NG q8h, infants: 1–3 drops PO/NG q8h.
- SSKI (saturated solution of potassium iodide, 1 g/mL): Children and adults: 6–10 drops PO/NG q8h, infants: 1–5 drops PO/NG q8h.

- **Glucocorticoids** reduce peripheral conversion of T4 to active T3. Glucocorticoid treatment is particularly important if coexisting adrenal insufficiency is suspected.

  - Hydrocortisone 16–20 mg/kg/day IV divided q6 hours
  - **OR** dexamethasone 0.2–0.6 mg/kg/day divided q6 hours

# References

Burch HB, Wartofsky L. Life threatening thyrotoxicosis. Thyroid storm. Endorinol Metab Clin North Am 1993;22:263–77.

McKeown NJ, Tews MC, Gossain VV, Shah SM. Hyperthyroidism. Emerg Med Clin N Am 2005;23:669–85.

Fisher DA. Disorders of the thyroid in the newborn and infant. In: Sperling MA, ed. Pediatric endocrinology. 2nd ed. Pennsylvania: Saunders; 2002, pp. 161–85.

Aiello DP, DuPlessis AJ, Pattishall EG. Thyroid storm. Presenting with coma and seizures in a 3-year-old girl. Clin Pediatr (Phila) 1989;28:571–4.

Dabon-Almirante CLM, Surks MI. Clinical and laboratory diagnosis of thyrotoxicosis. Endocrin Metabol Clin North Am 1998;27:25–35.

Wynne AG, Gharib H, Scheithauer BW, et al. Hyperthyroidism due to inappropriate secretion of thyrotropin in 10 patients. Am J Med 1992;92:15–24.

Takasu N, Oshiro C, Akamine H, et al. Thyroid stimulating antibody and TSH binding inhibitor immunoglobulin in 277 Graves' patients and 686 normal subjects. J Endocrinol Invest 1997;20:452–61.

Feely J, Penden N. Use of beta-adrenoceptor blocking drugs in hyperthyroidism. Drugs 1984;27:425–46.

Azizi F. The safety and efficacy of antithyroid drugs. Expert Opin Drug Saf 2006;5:107–16.

Walter RM, Bartle WR. Rectal administration of propylthiouracil in the treatment of Graves' disease. Am J Med 1990;88:69.

Wolff J, Chaikoff IL, Goldberg RC, Meier JR. The temporary nature of the inhibitor action of excess iodide on organic iodine synthesis in the normal thyroid. Endocrinology 1949;45:504.

Han YY, Sun WZ. An evidence-based review on the use of corticosteroids in peri-operative and critical care. Acta Anaesthesiol Sin 2002;40:71–9.

# D. Sick Euthyroid Syndrome

## Seth D Marks

Sick euthyroid syndrome (SES), also known as nonthyroidal illness, euthyroid sick syndrome, low T3 syndrome, or low T3-low T4 syndrome, is a disturbance of the hypothalamic-pituitary-thyroid axis that can occur during critical illness and result in altered thyroid hormone levels.

## Key Principles

- SES can occur in a variety of clinical settings and is common in critically ill patients.
- Serum biochemistry demonstrates low tri-iodothyronine (T3), increased reverse T3 (rT3), normal or low thyroxine (T4), and normal or low thyrotropin (TSH).
- SES's effect on recovery and the need to treat is controversial. Generally, treatment is not recommended.

## Pathophysiology

- Decreased type 1 iodothyronine 5'-monodeiodinase enzyme activity results in decreased peripheral conversion of T4 to T3 and decreased metabolism of rT3.
- Alteration in hypothalamic and pituitary function results in decreased release of thyrotropin releasing hormone (TRH) and TSH.
- Elevated levels of cytokines, like interleukin-6 (IL-6) and interleukin-1 (IL-1), and decreased levels of leptin may also play a role in the pathophysiology of SES.
- Dopamine administration, cardiopulmonary bypass, and liver disease can accentuate SES.

## Etiology

- It is controversial whether SES is an adaptive or maladaptive response to illness.

# Clinical Features

- SES has been documented in many clinical settings including starvation, critical illness, surgery, sepsis, cardiovascular illness, burns, malignancy, liver disease, and renal failure.
- SES may be associated with a prolonged recovery in critically ill patients and be predictive of morbidity and mortality.
- Low T3, increased rT3, normal to low T4, and normal to low TSH.
- Initial biochemical findings are followed by a recovery phase marked by increased levels of TSH, which may rise above baseline and/or the upper limits of normal, and then a delayed increase in T3 and T4.

# Investigations

- Serum TSH, free T4, T3 index, and rT3.
- Arguably, investigations should not be routinely performed in critically ill patients since the presence of SES is not unexpected and treatment is not recommended.

# Treatment

- Treatment of SES has not been proven to significantly improve clinically relevant outcomes. Therefore, treatment is not recommended. This is somewhat controversial.

# References

Peeters RP, Wouters PJ, Kaptein E, et al. Reduced activation and increased inactivation of thyroid hormone in tissues of critically ill patients. J Clin Endocrinol Metab 2003;88:3202–11.

Fliers E, Guldenaar SE, Wiersinga WM, Swaab DF. Decreased hypothalamic thyrotropin-releasing hormone gene expression in patients with nonthyroidal illness. J Clin Endocrinol Metab 1997;82:4032–6.

Davies PH, Black EG, Sheppard MC, Franklyn JA. Relation between serum interleukin-6 and thyroid hormone concentrations in 270 hospital in-patients with non-thyroidal illness. Clin Endocrinol (Oxf) 1996;44:199–205.

Hashimoto H, Igarashi N, Yachie A, Miyawaki T, Sato T. The relationship between serum levels of interleukin-6 and thyroid hormone in children with acute respiratory infection. J Clin Endocrinol Metab 1994;78:288–91.

Legradi G, Emerson CH, Ahima RS, Flier JS, Lechan RM. Leptin prevents fasting-induced suppression of prothyrotropin-releasing hormone messenger ribonucleic acid in neurons of the hypothalamic paraventricular nucleus. Endocrinology 1997;138:2569–76.

Yu J, Koenig RJ. Regulation of hepatocyte thyroxine 5'-deiodinase by T3 and nuclear receptor coactivators as a model of the sick euthyroid syndrome. J Biol Chem 2000;275:38296–301.

Murzi B, Iervasi G, Masini S, et al. Thyroid hormones homeostasis in pediatric patients during and after cardiopulmonary bypass. Ann Thorac Surg 1995;59:481–5.

Van den Berghe G, de Zegher F, Lauwers P. Dopamine and the sick euthyroid syndrome in critical illness. Clin Endocrinol (Oxf) 1994;41:731–7.

Van den Berghe G, de Zegher F. Anterior pituitary function during critical illness and dopamine treatment. Crit Care Med 1996;24:1580–90.

Bettendorf M, Schmidt KG, Tiefenbacher U, et al. Transient secondary hypothyroidism in children after cardiac surgery. Pediatr Res 1997;41:375–9.

Zucker AR, Chernow B, Fields AI, et al. Thyroid function in critically ill children. J Pediatr 1985;107:552–4.

Uzel N, Neyzi O. Thyroid function in critically ill infants with infections. Pediatr Infect Dis 1986;5:516–9.

Joosten KF, de Kleijn ED, Westerterp M, et al. Endocrine and metabolic responses in children with meningococcal sepsis: striking differences between survivors and nonsurvivors. J Clin Endocrinol Metab 2000;85:3746–53.

Allen DB, Dietrich KA, Zimmerman JJ. Thyroid hormone metabolism and level of illness severity in pediatric cardiac surgery patients. J Pediatr 1989;114:59–62.

Bartalena L, Martino E, Brandi LS, et al. Lack of nocturnal serum thyrotropin surge after surgery. J Clin Endocrinol Metab 1990;70:293–6.

Bettendorf M, Schmidt KG, Grulich-Henn J, Ulmer HE, Heinrich UE. Triiodothyronine treatment in children after cardiac surgery: a double-blind, randomised, placebo-controlled study. Lancet 2000;356:529–34.

Chowdhury D, Ojamaa K, Parnell VA, et al. A prospective randomized clinical study of thyroid hormone treatment after operations for complex congenital heart disease. J Thorac Cardiovasc Surg 2001;122:1023–5.

Mainwaring RD, Lamberti JJ, Nelson JC, et al. Effects of triiodothyronine supplementation following modified Fontan procedure. Cardiol Young 1997;7:194–200.

Mainwaring RD, Nelson JC. Supplementation of thyroid hormone in children undergoing cardiac surgery. Cardiol Young 2001;12:211–7.

Portman MA, Fearneyhough C, Ning XH, et al. Triiodothyronine repletion in infants during cardiopulmonary bypass for congenital heart disease. J Thorac Cardiovasc Surg 2000;120:604–8.

Stathatos N, Levetan C, Burman KD, Wartofsky L. The controversy of the treatment of critically ill patients with thyroid hormone. Best Pract Res Clin Endocrinol Metabol 2001;15:465–78.

# E. Diabetes Insipidus

## Seth D Marks

Diabetes insipidus (DI) is characterized by polyuria with inappropriately dilute urine, hypernatremia, serum hyperosmolality, and dehydration resulting from arginine vasopressin (AVP) deficiency (central DI) or resistance (nephrogenic DI).

## Key Principles

---

- Morbidity and mortality in DI is secondary to dehydration and/or electrolyte imbalances.
- Close monitoring of fluid balance and electrolytes is imperative.
- Rapid electrolyte or fluid correction can lead to hyponatremia, seizures, cerebral edema, and neurologic sequelae.
- Correct the hypernatremia slowly. Aim to decrease serum sodium at a rate no greater than 0.5 mmol/L per hour.

---

## Pathophysiology

- AVP is normally secreted by the posterior pituitary in response to increased plasma osmolality, and acts upon the renal collecting ducts to increase water permeability and reabsorption.
- Central DI is secondary to deficient AVP production.
- Nephrogenic DI is secondary to renal resistance to AVP.
- Both central and nephrogenic DI result in decreased free water retention.

## Etiology

### Central Diabetes Insipidus

- Idiopathic
- CNS tumor (eg, craniopharyngioma, dysgerminoma, optic glioma, leukemia, metastases)

- Congenital midbrain malformations (eg, septo-optic dysplasia, absent or ectopic posterior pituitary, absent or small anterior pituitary, thickened pituitary stalk)
- Genetic (autosomal dominant, autosomal recessive, X-linked recessive)
- Head trauma
- Neurosurgery (see Chapter 10A)
- Infiltrative (eg, histiocytosis X, granulomatosis, sarcoidosis)
- Infectious (eg, meningitis, encephalitis, congenital cytomegalovirus, toxoplasmosis, tuberculosis)
- Autoimmune
- Central DI may be isolated or occur in association with other hypothalamic-pituitary hormone deficiencies. Therefore, clinical suspicion of other pituitary hormone deficiencies is prudent.

## Nephrogenic Diabetes Insipidus

- Genetic (X-linked recessive, autosomal recessive, autosomal dominant)
- Drugs (eg, amphotericin, cisplatin, lithium, tetracycline)
- Electrolyte abnormalities (eg, hypokalemia, hypercalcemia)
- Renal disease (eg, obstructive uropathy, renal tubular acidosis, renal failure)
- Systemic disease (eg, sickle cell disease, Sjögren syndrome, sarcoidosis)

*We focus in the remainder of this section on central and not nephrogenic DI.*

## Clinical Features

- Polyuria (>2–4 ml/kg/hour), nocturia, polydipsia with preference for cold water
- Dehydration, hypovolemic shock
- Irritability, confusion, lethargy, seizure
- Hypotension, tachycardia
- Weight loss
- Fever
- Onset is usually sudden
- Infants with DI—require more vigilance to diagnose as they may present with vague symptoms including poor feeding, emesis, failure to thrive, and irritability
- Hypernatremia (>145 mmol/l), plasma hyperosmolality (>300 mmol/kg), urine hypoosmolality (<300 mmol/kg, specific gravity <1.005)

- Neurosurgery may be followed by a "triple phase response":
  - An initial short period of polyuria secondary to DI, lasting for hours to a few days, may result from the acute swelling of the vasopressin neurons and fiber tracts.
  - Followed by a fluid retention phase secondary to the syndrome of inappropriate secretion of antidiuretic hormone (SIADH) (see section of this chapter), lasting for hours to several days,
  - Followed again by transient or permanent DI.

- In the initial postoperative setting, aggressive intraoperative fluid expansion may lead to appropriate subsequent hypo-osmolar polyuria that masquerades as DI.
- Coexisting adrenal insufficiency, which can decrease free water clearance, can mask DI until glucocorticoid replacement is initiated.

## Investigations

- Serum sodium (Na), potassium (K), chloride (Cl), bicarbonate ($HCO_3$), glucose, calcium (Ca), urea (U), creatinine (Cr), and osmolality.
- Urine specific gravity, osmolality, and electrolytes.
- Frequent, often hourly, repeated laboratory investigations are required especially in early management.

## Water Deprivation Test

- Should only be performed under a controlled setting with appropriate supervision and monitoring.
- Various protocols all with the aim of assessing the concentrating abilities of the urine under the condition of dehydration.
- Start deprivation test in the morning.
- Baseline and hourly serum sodium, serum osmolality, urine osmolality, and specific gravity.
- Baseline and hourly vitals, weight and urine output.
- Stop deprivation test if excessive weight loss (>5%).
- DI excluded by normal plasma osmolality (285–295 mmol/kg) and increased urine osmolality >750 mmol/kg with water deprivation.
- In DI, serum osmolality will rise with continued polyuria and low urine osmolality and specific gravity.

- Can distinguish between central DI and nephrogenic DI after positive water deprivation test by assessing response to desmopressin acetate (DDAVP). DDAVP therapy will increase the urine osmolality in central DI but not in nephrogenic DI.
- MRI of the pituitary and hypothalamus.

# Treatment

## Acute

- Initial resuscitation with normal saline (NS) as required if hemodynamically unstable (see Chapter 5, "Resuscitation").
- Use hypotonic saline (eg, 0.45 NS, 0.2 NS) after initial resuscitation.
- Initial fluid volume should equal urine output and insensible losses. The calculation of insensible losses is controversial but estimates include 400 mL/m$^2$/day or 30–35 mL/kg/day.
- The intravenous fluid rate and solution requirements are dynamic and should be adjusted according to clinical status, urine output, and serum and urine electrolytes and osmolality. Large volumes may be required.

---

- The Na deficit or requirement can be calculated:

$$[Na]_{deficit} = \text{total body water estimate (eg, 0.6)} \times \text{weight (kg)} \times ([Na]_{desired} - [Na]_{actual})$$

- The effect of 1 L of intravenous fluid solution on the serum Na can be calculated and therefore aid at setting an appropriate intravenous fluid rate:

$$\text{Serum } [Na]_{change} = [Na]_{solution} - [Na]_{serum} / [\text{total body water estimate (eg, 0.6)} \times \text{weight (kg)}] + 1$$

---

- Aim for a slow and cautious correction of the hypernatremia. The rate of the serum sodium correction should not exceed 0.5 mmol/L per hour.
- More rapid correction (1 mmol/L per hour) may be safe and may even decrease morbidity in acute onset hypernatremia, but if the rate of onset of the hypernatremia is longer than a matter of hours, or is unknown, then it is prudent to correct the sodium more slowly.

- Close clinical and biochemical monitoring is imperative including frequent monitoring of fluid input, fluid output, serum electrolytes and osmolality, and urine electrolytes and osmolality.
- Excessive dextrose concentrations in the intravenous fluids should be avoided to prevent glucosuria and osmotic diuresis.
- When clinically stable and if developmentally appropriate, oral fluids are preferred over intravenous as patient can control intake more accurately based on thirst.
- *Postoperative management* of a patient with known or new-onset DI can be complex.

    - Iatrogenic water overload and dilutional hyponatremia is a common complication in postoperative NPO patients with DI on intravenous fluids and DDVAP.
    - Intravenous fluid volume should be conservative and matched to urine output, insensible losses, and clinical fluid status.
    - DDAVP should be used cautiously in this setting due to the significant risk of dilutional hyponatremia. Generally, DDAVP should be administered only with the onset of significant polyuria. A low dose vasopressin infusion with cautious fluid restriction can also be considered for inpatients and postoperative patients and should be titrated to urine output <2 mL/kg/hour but not anuria.
    - Fluid intake should be managed orally as early as possible.

## Chronic

- The goal of ongoing outpatient therapy is to limit polyuria.
- Nasal or oral DDAVP is the mainstay of therapy.
- Patients should have free access to water and drink according to thirst.
- Problems arise when access to water is limited (eg, infants, elderly, or bedridden patients), the central thirst center is not intact, or in contrast when excess water is ingested beyond symptoms of thirst.

## DDAVP (Desmopressin Acetate)

- Synthetic analogue of AVP.
- DDAVP is best used under the guidance of a physician with expertise in its use to minimize the risk of dilutional hyponatremia.
- Usual maintenance dose is 5 to 40 mcg/day intranasal divided once to three times per day.

- Nasal spray preparation delivers 10 mcg of DDAVP per spray. Nasal doses less than 10 mcg require the rhinyle preparation.
- Dose effectiveness of nasal preparations can be altered by nasal congestion.
- Accuracy of nasal dosing can be difficult and interpersonal delivery may differ. If possible, for consistency, have the patient or parent deliver the nasal dose in an inpatient with previously diagnosed DI.
- IV or SC dose is approximately 10% of intranasal dose. A dose of 0.4 mcg once a day is a reasonable initial parenteral dose in children.
- Oral dose is approximately 10–20 times the intranasal dose divided two to three times per day. Oral response may be less reliable than nasal.
- Consider allowing patient to "break through" with increased urine output (>2 mL/kg/hour for 1 to 2 hours) prior to giving next dose of DDAVP to avoid dilutional hyponatremia.
- Side effects include nasal irritation and congestion with the nasal preparations, headache, nausea, flushing, abdominal pain, and hypertension. Side effects are dose-dependent.

# References

Donoghue MB, Latimer ME, Pillsbury HL, Hertzog JH. Hyponatremic seizure in a child using desmopressin for nocturnal enuresis. Arch Pediatr Adolesc Med 1998;152:290–2.

Williford SL, Bernstein SA. Intranasal desmopressin-induced hyponatremia. Pharmacotherapy 1996;16:66–74.

Adrogue HJ, Madias NE. Hypernatremia. N Engl J Med 2000;342:1493–9.

Weiss-Guillet EM, Takala J, Jakob SM. Diagnosis and management of electrolyte emergencies. Best Pract Res Clin Endocrinol Metab 2003;17:623–51.

Saborio P, Tipton GA, Chan JC. Diabetes insipidus. Pediatr Rev 2000;21:122–9.

Robertson GL. Antidiuretic hormone. Normal and disordered function. Endocrinol Metab Clin North Am 2001;30:671–94, vii.

Cheetham T, Baylis PH. Diabetes insipidus in children: pathophysiology, diagnosis and management. Paediatr Drugs 2002;4:785–96.

Maghnie M, Cosi G, Genovese E, et al. Central diabetes insipidus in children and young adults. N Engl J Med 2000;343:998–1007.

Dashe AM, Cramm RE, Crist CA, Habener JF, Solomon DH. A water deprivation test for the differential diagnosis of polyuria. JAMA 1963;185:699–703.

Lindsay RS, Seckl JR, Padfield PL. The triple-phase response—problems of water balance after pituitary surgery. Postgrad Med J 1995;71:439–41.

Ikkos D, Luft R, Olivecrona H. Hypophysectomy in man: effect on water excretion during the first two postoperative months. J Clin Endocrinol Metab 1955;15:553–67.

Albanese A, Hindmarsh P, Stanhope R. Management of hyponatraemia in patients with acute cerebral insults. Arch Dis Child 2001;85:246–51.

Lipsett MB, Maclean JP, West CD, Li MC, Pearson OH. An analysis of the polyuria induced by hypophysectomy in man. J Clin Endocrinol Metab 1956;16:183–95.

Kamoi K, Tamura T, Tanaka K, Ishibashi M, Yamaji T. Hyponatremia and osmoregulation of thirst and vasopressin secretion in patients with adrenal insufficiency. J Clin Endocrinol Metab 1993;77:1584–8.

Kleeman CR, Czaczkes JW, Cutler R. Mechanisms of impaired water excretion in adrenal and pituitary insufficiency. IV. antidiuretic hormone in primary and secondary adrenal insufficiency. J Clin Invest 1964;43:1641–8.

Reynolds RM, Padfield PL, Seckl JR. Disorders of sodium balance. BMJ 2006;332:702–5.

Reeves WB, Bichet DG, Andreoli TE. Posterior pituitary and water metabolism. Wilson JD, Foster DW, Kronenberg HM, Larsen PR (eds). Williams Textbook of Endocrinology. Philadelphia: W.B. Saunders Company, 1998: 341–87.

Sterns RH. Hypernatremia in the intensive care unit: instant quality—just add water. Crit Care Med 1999;27:1041–2.

Taylor D, Durward A. Pouring salt on troubled waters. Arch Dis Child 2004;89:411–4.

Hatherill M. Rubbing salt in the wound. Arch Dis Child 2004;89:414–8.

Adrogue HJ, Madias NE. Aiding fluid prescription for the dysnatremias. Intensive Care Med 1997;23:309–16.

Wise-Faberowski L, Soriano SG, Ferrari L, et al. Perioperative management of diabetes insipidus in children. J Neurosurg Anesthesiol 2004;16:220–5.

Tommasino C. Fluids and the neurosurgical patient. Anesthesiol Clin North America 2002;20:329–46.

Robson WL, Leung AK. Hyponatremia in children treated with desmopressin. Arch Pediatr Adolesc Med 1998;152:930–1.

Compendium of Pharmaceuticals and Specialties—The Canadian Drug Reference for Health Professionals. Ottawa: Canadian Pharmacists Association, 2006.

Dashe AM, Kleeman CR, Czaczkes JW, Rubinoff H, Spears I. Synthetic vasopressin nasal spray in the treatment of diabetes insipidus. JAMA 1964;190:1069–71.

# F. Syndrome of Inappropriate Antidiuretic Hormone

## Seth D Marks

Syndrome of inappropriate antidiuretic hormone (SIADH) is characterized by oliguria with hyponatremia, serum hypo-osmolality, urine hyperosmolality, and euvolemia or mild hypervolemia resulting from inappropriate release or excess activity of arginine vasopressin (AVP or ADH).

## Key Principles

- Close monitoring of fluid balance and electrolytes is imperative.
- Rapid electrolyte correction may lead to central pontine myelinosis and neurologic sequelae.
- Correct the hyponatremia slowly. Aim to increase the serum sodium at a rate no greater than 0.5 mmol/L per hour.
- Faster correction may be needed in the setting of neurologic deterioration.

## Pathophysiology

- AVP is normally secreted by the posterior pituitary in response to increased plasma osmolality and acts upon the renal collecting ducts to increase water permeability and reabsorption.
- SIADH is secondary to inappropriately elevated nonosmotic stimulated secretion of AVP that results in increased free water retention.

## Etiology

Critically ill children are at significant risk of SIADH secondary to the etiologies listed below

- CNS tumors
- Neurosurgery

- Head trauma
- Respiratory illness (eg, pneumonia, asthma, bronchiolitis, positive pressure ventilation)
- Infection (eg, meningitis, encephalitis, tuberculosis)
- Hydrocephalus
- Drugs (eg, vincristine, cyclophosphamide, carbamazepine, tricyclic antidepressants, selective serotonin reuptake inhibitors, morphine, NSAIDS, Ecstasy)
- Neoplasm (eg, small cell lung carcinoma, neuroblastoma)
- Major surgery especially spinal surgery
- Emesis, pain, physiologic stress, and hypoxia

## Clinical Features

- Decreased urine output
- Euvolemia or mild hypervolemia
- Headache, muscle cramps, nausea, emesis, irritability, confusion, seizure, coma, respiratory arrest, cerebral edema
- The severity of symptoms may be related to the degree of hyponatremia and rate of serum Na decrease
- Hyponatremia (<135 mmo/L, usually <125 mmol/L), plasma hypoosmolality (<280 mmol/L), urine hyperosmolality (urine osmolality > plasma osmolality, specific gravity >1.020, urine Na >20 mmol/L)
- Decreased serum uric acid and urea
- Often transient

## Differential

- Cerebral salt wasting (CSW)—likely caused by excess atrial natriuretic peptide (ANP). CSW's role is not as well recognized as SIADH, but is likely important in some patients with central nervous system disease. Like SIADH, CSW presents with hyponatremia and urine hyperosmolality. However, CSW is characterized by significant polyuria and hypovolemia secondary to sodium losses in the urine. CSW is treated with aggressive fluid resuscitation with isotonic or hypertonic saline.

## Investigations

- Serum sodium (Na), potassium (K), chloride (Cl), bicarbonate ($HCO_3$), glucose, urea (U), creatinine (Cr), uric acid, and osmolality
- Urine specific gravity, osmolality, electrolytes

- Frequent, often hourly, repeated laboratory investigations are required especially in early management
- MRI/CT head as indicated
- Rule out hypothyroidism and adrenal insufficiency

# Treatment

- Fluid restriction: aim for a negative water balance.
- Fluid intake should be less than insensible losses and urine output. The calculation of insensible losses is controversial but estimates include 400 mL/m$^2$/day or 30–35 mL/kg/day.
- Use normal saline (NS, 154 mEq/L of Na) solution. If serum Na <120 mmol/L can consider using hypertonic saline (eg, 3% NaCl, 513 mEq/L of Na).
- If significant neurologic sequelae or deterioration present then give 3% NaCl 0.5 to 2 mL/kg over 1 hour and repeat if necessary. Each 1 mL/kg of 3% NaCl should raise serum Na level by approximately 1 mmol/L. In addition, furosemide may also be used in this scenario (see Chapter 23, "Pharmacology").
- Aim for a slow cautious correction of the hyponatremia. The immediate goal is not a normal serum Na. The rate of serum Na correction should not exceed 8–12 mmol/l per 24 hours.

---

- The Na deficit or requirement can be calculated:

$$[Na]_{deficit} = \text{total body water estimate (eg, 0.6)} \times \text{weight (kg)} \times ([Na]_{desired} - [Na]_{actual})$$

- The effect of 1 L of intravenous fluid solution on the serum Na can be calculated and therefore aid at setting an appropriate intravenous fluid rate:

$$\text{Serum } [Na]_{change} = [Na]_{solution} - [Na]_{serum} / \text{[total body water estimate: } 0.6 \times \text{weight (kg)]} + 1$$

---

- Close clinical and biochemical monitoring is imperative including frequent monitoring of fluid input, fluid output, serum electrolytes and osmolality, and urine electrolytes and osmolality.
- Chronic long-term maintenance therapy may be possible with the cautious use of demeclocycline if fluid restriction alone is not effective.

## Comparative Characteristics of SIADH, CSW, and DI

|  | SIADH | CSW | DI |
|---|---|---|---|
| Hydration status | euvolemia or mild hypervolemia | hypovolemia | hypovolemia |
| Urine output | decreased | increased | increased |
| Serum [Na] | decreased | decreased | increased |
| Serum osmolality | decreased | decreased | increased |
| Urine [Na] | increased | increased ++ | decreased |
| Urine osmolality | increased | increased | decreased |

CSW, cerebral salt wasting; DI, diabetes insipidus; SIADH, syndrome of inappropriate antidiuretic hormone.

# References

Sterns RH, Riggs JE, Schochet SS Jr. Osmotic demyelination syndrome following correction of hyponatremia. N Engl J Med 1986;314:1535–42.

Albanese A, Hindmarsh P, Stanhope R. Management of hyponatraemia in patients with acute cerebral insults. Arch Dis Child 2001;85:246–51.

Moritz ML, Ayus JC. Disorders of water metabolism in children: hyponatremia and hypernatremia. Pediatr Rev 2002;23:371–80.

Moritz ML, Ayus JC. Prevention of hospital-acquired hyponatremia: a case for using isotonic saline. Pediatrics 2003;111:227–30.

Robertson GL. Antidiuretic hormone. Normal and disordered function. Endocrinol Metab Clin North Am 2001;30:671–94, vii.

Baylis PH. The syndrome of inappropriate antidiuretic hormone secretion. Int J Biochem Cell Biol 2003;35:1495–9.

Janicic N, Verbalis JG. Evaluation and management of hypo-osmolality in hospitalized patients. Endocrinol Metab Clin North Am 2003;32:459–81, vii.

Arieff AI. Management of hyponatraemia. BMJ 1993;307:305–8.

Arieff AI, Ayus JC, Fraser CL. Hyponatraemia and death or permanent brain damage in healthy children. BMJ 1992;304:1218–22.

Bhalla P, Eaton FE, Coulter JB, Amegavie FL, Sills JA, Abernethy LJ. Lesson of the week: hyponatraemic seizures and excessive intake of hypotonic fluids in young children. BMJ 1999;319:1554–7.

Adrogue HJ, Madias NE. Hyponatremia. N Engl J Med 2000;342:1581–9.

Cole CD, Gottfried ON, Liu JK, Couldwell WT. Hyponatremia in the neurosurgical patient: diagnosis and management. Neurosurg Focus 2004;16:E9.

Reynolds RM, Seckl JR. Hyponatraemia for the clinical endocrinologist. Clin Endocrinol (Oxf) 2005;63:366–74.

Vachharajani TJ, Zaman F, Abreo KD. Hyponatremia in critically ill patients. J Intensive Care Med 2003;18:3–8.

Arieff AI, Llach F, Massry SG. Neurological manifestations and morbidity of hyponatremia: correlation with brain water and electrolytes. Medicine (Baltimore) 1976;55:121–9.

Milionis HJ, Liamis GL, Elisaf MS. The hyponatremic patient: a systematic approach to laboratory diagnosis. CMAJ 2002;166:1056–62.

Bussmann C, Bast T, Rating D. Hyponatraemia in children with acute CNS disease: SIADH or cerebral salt wasting? Childs Nerv Syst 2001;17:58–62; discussion 63.

Berger TM, Kistler W, Berendes E, Raufhake C, Walter M. Hyponatremia in a pediatric stroke patient: syndrome of inappropriate antidiuretic hormone secretion or cerebral salt wasting? Crit Care Med 2002;30:792–5.

Taylor D, Durward A. Pouring salt on troubled waters. Arch Dis Child 2004;89:411–4.

Hatherill M. Rubbing salt in the wound. Arch Dis Child 2004;89:414–8.

Decaux G, Waterlot Y, Genette F, Mockel J. Treatment of the syndrome of inappropriate secretion of antidiuretic hormone with furosemide. N Engl J Med 1981;304:329–30.

Adrogue HJ, Madias NE. Aiding fluid prescription for the dysnatremias. Intensive Care Med 1997;23:309–16.

Forrest JN Jr, Cox M, Hong C, Morrison G, Bia M, Singer I. Superiority of demeclocycline over lithium in the treatment of chronic syndrome of inappropriate secretion of antidiuretic hormone. N Engl J Med 1978;298:173–7.

# G. Calcium Disorders

Karen McAssey

## Key Principles

- Without adequate PTH or vitamin D, calcium levels always fall.
- It is critical to obtain a PTH level at a time of hypocalcemia in order for the PTH value to be interpreted. A child with hypocalcemia and a low serum PTH level has hypoparathyroidism. An elevated PTH level indicates an appropriate compensatory response or resistance to PTH (pseudohypoparathyroidism).
- Monitor IV site carefully to avoid extravasation burns.
- Never bolus intravenous calcium to correct hypocalcemia except for life-threatening emergencies.

## Major Physiology

- Total serum calcium is divided into three fractions: approximately 40% is bound to albumin, about 15% is bound to organic and inorganic anions, and 45% exists as the physiologically active ionized calcium.
- The major hormones affecting serum calcium levels are parathyroid hormone (PTH), vitamin D, and to a lesser extent calcitonin.
- Gut, kidney, and bone are key sites of action in the interplay of these hormones.
- The calcium sensing receptor (CaSR) is a membrane protein that binds ionized calcium, triggering the release of PTH in response to minute changes in the calcium level.
- The release of PTH from the parathyroid glands increases the serum calcium level. PTH acts on bone to mobilize calcium and phosphate. In the kidneys, PTH stimulates tubular calcium reabsorption and inhibits phosphate reabsorption.
- Vitamin D is initially formed in the skin and then hydroxylated twice, first in the liver and then in the kidney. PTH stimulates renal $1\alpha$ hydroxylase converting 25 hydroxyvitamin D to the more active 1,25 dihydroxyvitamin D (calcitriol).

- The main activity of vitamin D is to enhance intestinal absorption of calcium and phosphate. Secondarily, vitamin D enhances the activity of PTH in the kidney.
- Calcitonin is synthesized and released from the parafollicular cells of the thyroid gland. The exact role and importance of calcitonin on calcium homeostasis is uncertain. When calcium levels are increased, calcitonin levels rise and decrease calcium resorption from bone.

# Hypocalcemia

The definition of hypocalcemia is age-dependent. Total serum calcium concentration in preterm infants below 1.8 mmol/L, in term infants below 2.0 mmol/L, and in children or adolescents below 2.2 mmol/L constitutes hypocalcemia. If hypoalbuminemia is present, total serum calcium measurement may be falsely low. Measure ionized calcium if serum albumin or pH is abnormal.

# Etiology

## Early Neonatal (within first 48–72 hours):

- Prematurity/small for gestational age
- Birth asphyxia
- Sepsis
- Iatrogenic—exchange transfusion
- Infant of a diabetic mother
- Maternal hypercalcemia/hyperparathyroidism

## Late Neonatal (3–7 days of life):

- Congenital hypoparathyroidism (transient or permanent, including parathyroid aplasia or hypoplasia in 22q11.2 deletion (Velocardiofacial or DiGeorge syndrome)
- Pseudohypoparathyroidism
- High phosphate formula or cow's milk intake
- Magnesium deficiency
- Severe infantile osteopetrosis

## Children and Adolescents:

- Aquired Hypoparathyroidism
- Autoimmune (isolated, type 1 polyglandular syndrome)
- Postsurgical
- Chronic magnesium deficiency
- Infiltration (iron overload, Wilson's disease)
- Vitamin D deficiency
- "Hungry bone" syndrome following treatment for vitamin D deficiency
- Pseudohypoparathyroidism
- Hyperphosphatemia
- Chronic renal failure
- Pancreatitis
- Respiratory alkalosis
- Medications, eg, furosemide, pamidronate

## Clinical Features

- Tetany
- Circumoral numbness
- Paresthesias of the hands and feet
- Hyperreflexia
- Muscle weakness
- Seizure, confusion
- Laryngospasm
- Chvostek's sign (twitching of the circumoral muscles caused by tapping over the ipsilateral facial nerve).
- Trousseau's sign (carpal spasm when maintaining a blood pressure cuff 20 mm Hg above systolic blood pressure for 3 minutes)
- Arrhythmias (Prolonged QTc interval)
- Infants may have nonspecific signs of lethargy, vomiting, or poor feeding
- Infants or children may be asymptomatic

## Investigations

- Total and/or ionized calcium
- Phosphate, magnesium, alkaline phosphatase, blood gas, albumin or total protein, creatinine, liver function tests
- 25 hydroxy vitamin D, 1,25 dihydroxy vitamin D, PTH
- ECG monitoring
- In general, the plasma calcium falls by 0.2 mmol/L for every 10 g/L fall in the plasma albumin concentration. The measured

plasma calcium can be corrected by hypoalbuminemia according to the following calculation

$$\text{Corrected Calcium} = \text{Measured total calcium} + (0.02 \times (40 - [\text{albumin}]))$$

## Treatment

- Intravenous calcium should be reserved for symptomatic or severe hypocalcemia. Most mild hypocalcemia can be managed with optimal dietary calcium intake and an oral calcium supplement if needed.
- Oral calcium is available in many preparations including calcium carbonate, calcium gluconate, calcium phosphate, calcium citrate, and calcium lactate. Differences in chemical solubility between preparations are not usually clinically significant. A divided dose regimen (3–4 times daily) with meals provides superior absorption.
- Oral calcium intake should reach 100 mg elemental calcium/kg/day.
- If peripheral intravenous calcium is required, use calcium gluconate diluted to 0.04 mmol/mL. (Add 10 mL of 10% calcium gluconate to 40 mL normal saline.)
- Most pediatric hypocalcemia will respond well to a continuous infusion of 0.05 mmol/kg/hour.
- For seizures or arrhythmia start continuous infusion with 0.1 mmol/kg/hour.
- Intravenous bolus of calcium should be reserved for life-threatening cases under the guidance of a pediatric intensivist.
- Intravenous calcium chloride can also be used; however, some authors discourage its use because of associated metabolic acidosis.
- Follow plasma calcium levels q 4 hours while patient is on a calcium infusion. Intravenous calcium infusion may be adjusted as needed to maintain serum calcium in the low normal range (total calcium $\geq 2.0$ mmol/L) while the primary cause of hypocalcemia is under investigation.
- All individuals receiving intravenous calcium must be on a cardiac monitor.
- All intravenous sites must be monitored carefully to avoid subcutaneous tissue burns.
- Never mix calcium with fluids containing phosphate or bicarbonate.
- Never give calcium intramuscularly or subcutaneously.
- If hypoparathyroidism or prolonged need for intravenous calcium is suspected, start vitamin D metabolite, either $1,25$ $(OH)^2$ vitamin D or $1\alpha$ (OH) vitamin D.

# Hypercalcemia

Hypercalcemia exists when total serum calcium is greater than 2.75 mmol/L in a child or adolescent.

# Key Principles

> • Effective management of hypercalcemia begins with rehydration using normal saline. Hypercalcemia impairs renal concentrating ability leading to polyuria and causes mental status changes diminishing the sensation of thirst.

# Etiology

- Immobilization
- Malignancy: Bony metastases, production of PTH-related protein (PTHrP)
- Hypervitaminosis D: Nutritional, granulomatous disease (sarcoidosis, histoplasmosis, tuberculosis)
- Hyperparathyroidism: Sporadic, familial: multiple endocrine neoplasia, secondary/tertiary (renal failure)
- Familial hypocalciuric hypercalcemia (FHH)
- Medications—Lithium, thiazide diuretic, vitamin A, alkali
- Endocrine—Hyperthyroidism, Addison's disease, pheochromocytoma
- Idiopathic infantile hypercalcemia is often transient and considered as part of Williams syndrome

## Clinical Features

- Polyuria
- Polydipsia
- Anorexia, nausea, vomiting
- Constipation
- Abdominal pain
- Muscle weakness
- Altered level of consciousness
- Dehydration
- Shortened QTc interval on ECG
- Nephrocalcinosis and renal calculi on ultrasound

## Investigations

- Total and ionized calcium, phosphate, urea, creatinine, PTH, 25(OH) vitamin D, 1,25(OH)$^2$ vitamin D
- Urine calcium and creatinine
- When clinically indicated include: TSH, free T4 and/or free T3, serum cortisol, ACTH, FISH for the elastin gene (Williams syndrome), urinary catecholamines

## Treatment

- There are currently a number of available approaches for correcting hypercalcemia. The choice of therapy depends on the cause and severity of this condition.
- Almost all patients will benefit from a low calcium diet with high fluid intake.
- Patients with familial hypocalciuric hypercalcemia, an autosomal dominantly inherited inactivating mutation of the calcium-sensing receptor, often have mild hypercalcemia that is asymptomatic and does not require treatment.
- Urinary calcium excretion can be increased by intravenous saline administration to restore and expand the extracellular fluid volume. Provide 0.9% normal saline at a minimum of twice maintenance and adjusted to maintain a urine output of >2 mL/kg/hour.
- Once fluid repletion has been achieved furosemide may be considered to further increase urinary calcium excretion. This requires careful monitoring of hypokalemia, hypomagnesemia, and volume depletion.
- Bone resorption can be inhibited by administration of a bisphosphonate or calcitonin.
- Calcitonin 4 IU/kg can be administered subcutaneously to lower serum calcium levels by 0.3–0.5 mmol/L within 4–6 hours if the patient is calcitonin sensitive. Calcitonin 4–8 IU/kg can be repeated in 6–12 hours for a maximum of 2 doses.
- Bisphosphonate therapy is more effective than saline or calcitonin in patients with severe hypercalcemia. Bisphosphonates act to lower serum calcium levels in 2–4 days with a sustained response over 2–4 weeks. Bisphosphonates are the treatment of choice in malignancy-associated hypercalcemia. Pamidronate 1 mg/kg to a maximum of 90 mg is administered intravenously over 4 hours. Zoledronic acid 4 mg intravenous over a minimum of 15 minutes has been used in adults but specific pediatric dosing is currently unavailable.

- Intestinal absorption of calcium can be reduced by administration of glucocorticoids. This approach may be helpful in cases where increased calcitriol production is responsible for hypercalcemia (granulomatous disease, lymphoma).
- Dialysis is generally reserved for patients with severe hypercalcemia and renal insufficiency in whom aggressive fluid hydration is contraindicated.

# References

Heaney RP, Weaver CM. Calcium and vitamin D. Endocrinol Metab Clin North Am 2003;32:181–94.

Fukugawa M, Kurokawa K. Calcium homeostasis and imbalance. Nephron 2002;92:41–5.

Silverman SL. Calcitonin. Endocrinol Metabol Clin North Am 2003;32:273–84.

Sarko J. Bone and mineral metabolism. Emerg Med Clin North Am 2005;23:703–21.

Guise TA, Mundy GR. Clinical review 69: evaluation of hypocalcemia in children and adults. J Clin Endocrinol Metab 1995;80:1473–8.

Ladenson JH, Lewis JW, Boyd JC. Failure of total calcium corrected for protein, albumin and pH to correctly assess free calcium status. J Clin Endocrinol Met 1978;46:986.

Singh J, Moghal N, Pearce SHS, Cheetham T. The investigation of hypocalcemia and rickets. Arch Dis Child 2003;88:403–7.

Tiras U, Erdeve O, Karabulut AA, et al. Debridement via collagenase application in two neonates. Pediatr Dermatol 2005;22:472–5.

Venkataraman PS, Tsang RC, Chen IW, Sperling MA. Pathogenesis of early neonatal hypocalcemia: studies of serum calcitonin, gastrin, and plasma glucagon. J Pediatr 1987;110:599.

Banerjee S, Mimouni FB, Mehta R, et al. Lower whole blood ionized magnesium concentrations in hypocalcemic infants of gestational diabetic mothers. Magnes Res 2003;16:127.

Kaplan EL, Burrington JD, Klementschitsch P, et al. Primary hyperparathyroidism, pregnancy, and neonatal hypocalcemia. Surgery 1984;96:717.

Steffenshrud S. Parathyroids: the forgotten glands. Neonatal Netw 2000;19:9–16.

Perez E, Sullivan KE. Chromosome 22q11.2 deletion syndrome (DiGeorge and velocardiofacial syndromes). Curr Opin Pediatr 2002;14:678–83.

Specker BL, Tsang RC, Ho ML, et al. Low serum calcium and high parathyroid hormone levels in neonates fed 'humanized' cow's milk-based formula. Am J Dis Child 1991;145:941.

Pearce SH, Cheetham TD. Autoimmune polyendocrinopathy syndrome type 1: treat with kid gloves. Clin Endocrinol (Oxf). 2001;54:433–5.

Root AW, Diamond FB. Disorders of calcium metabolism in the child and adolescent. In: Sperling MA, ed. Pediatric Endocrinology. 2nd ed. Pennsylvania: Saunders; 2002:629.

Ahmed MA, Martinez A, Mariam S, Whitehouse W. Chvostek's sign and hypocalcaemia in children with seizures. Seizure 2004;13:217–22.

Rubin, LP. Disorders of calcium and phosporus metabolism. In: Taeusch, HW, Ballard, RA, eds. Avery's Diseases of the Newborn, 7th ed. Philadelphia: WB Saunders; 1998:1189.

Ladhani S, Srinivasan L, Buchanan C, Allgrove J. Presentation of vitamin D deficiency. Arch Dis Child 2004;89:781–4.

Heaney RP. Calcium supplements: practical considerations. Osteoporos Int 1991;1:65–71.

Tohme JF, Bilezikian JP. Diagnosis and treatment of hypocalcemic emergencies. The Endocrinologist 1996;6:10.

Hosking DJ, Cowley A, Bucknall CA. Rehydration in the treatment of severe hypercalcaemia. Q J Med 1981;50:473.

Langman CB. Hypercalcemic syndromes in infants and children. In: Favus MJ, ed. Primer on the Metabolic Bone Diseases and Disorders of Mineral Metabolism. 4th ed. Philadelphia: Lippincott Williams & Wilkins; 1999:219–23.

Bilezikian JP. Management of hypercalcemia. J Clin Endocrinol Metab 1993;77:1445.

Law WM Jr, Heath H III. Familial benign hypercalcemia (hypocalciuric hypercalcemia)—clinical and pathogenetic studies in 21 families. Ann Intern Med 1985;102:511.

Body JJ. Hypercalcemia of malignancy. Semin Nephrol 2004;24:48.

Mathur M, Sykes JA, Saxona VR, et al. Treatment of acute lymphoblastic leukemia induced extreme hypercalcemia with pamidronate and calcitonin. Prediatric Critical Care Medicine 2003;4:252.

Deftos LJ, First BP. Calcitonin as a drug. Ann Intern Med 1981;95:192.

Pecherstorfer M, Brenner K, Zojer N. Current management strategies for hypercalcemia. Treat Endocrinol 2003;2:273–92.

Berenson JR. Treatment of hypercalcemia of malignancy with bisphosphonates. Semin Oncol 2002;29:12.

Major, P. The use of zoledronic acid, a novel, highly potent bisphosphonate, for the treatment of hypercalcemia of malignancy. Oncologist 2002;7:481.

Sandler LM, Winearls CG, Fraher LJ, et al. Studies of the hypercalcemia of sarcoidosis: effect of steroids and exogenous vitamin D3 on the circulating concentration of 1,25 dihydroxy vitamin D3. Q J Med 1984;53:165.

# H. Diabetic Ketoacidosis (DKA)

## Karen McAssey

Definition: Diabetic ketoacidosis is a state of relative or absolute insulin deficiency, aggravated by an excess of the counter-regulatory hormones glucagon, epinephrine, growth hormone and cortisol. Clinically, it is recognized in a child with newly diagnosed or established diabetes who develops

- hyperglycemia (serum glucose >11 mmol/L),
- ketosis (ketones in urine or serum), and
- metabolic acidosis (serum pH <7.3 and/or bicarbonate <15 mmol/L

## Key Principles

- Treat vascular decompensation with normal saline (0.9% NaCl) 10–20 mL/kg to correct shock, repeated as necessary to expand intravascular space.
- Sodium bicarbonate therapy is not recommended for treatment of acidosis.
- Do not give a bolus of insulin.
- Begin potassium replacement early. Serum potassium will decrease during treatment because of urinary losses and intracellular movement of potassium during correction of acidosis.
- Clinically significant cerebral edema (CE) occurs in 0.3–1% of episodes of DKA. The etiology of CE remains unproven and the ideal treatment is debated in the literature. Most commonly it occurs within 4–12 hours of initiating therapy but may occur at the onset of DKA or later. CE is the leading cause of DKA-related deaths and neurologic impairment in children.

## Pathophysiology

Insulin deficiency, together with counter-regulatory hormone excess, results in exaggerated hepatic glucose production and decreased peripheral glucose uptake in muscle and adipose tissue—culminating in hyperglycemia.

- Hyperglycemia results in osmotic diuresis with electrolyte loss (potassium, sodium, chloride, phosphate, and magnesium), dehydration, decreased glomerular filtration, and hyperosmolarity.
- Low insulin concentrations and concomitant stress hormone elevation stimulates lipolysis. The oxidation of free fatty acids generates ketone bodies (acetoacetic and β-hydroxybutyric acid). Overwhelming metabolic acidosis is compounded by lactic acidosis from poor tissue perfusion.
- Worsening acidosis and dehydration trigger further production of stress hormones perpetuating the cycle of progressive metabolic decompensation.
- Intestinal ileus from acidosis causes abdominal pain and vomiting.
- Vomiting compromises oral fluid intake, worsening dehydration and lactic acidosis.
- Dehydration may reduce renal function diminishing the clearance of ketones and glucose.

## Etiology

- New-onset type 1 diabetes where early signs and symptoms of hyperglycemia are unrecognized
- Insulin omission (deliberate or accidental)
- Infection, sepsis, surgery, trauma
- Risk of DKA is increased in young children at the onset of type 1 diabetes and in children with poor metabolic control or previous episodes of DKA
- Cerebral Edema
- DKA is associated with a low mortality rate in the PICU ranging from 0.15% to 0.3%.
- Primary causes of mortality in DKA in order of frequency:

  - Cerebral edema with subsequent herniation (57–87% of deaths)
  - Hypokalemia
  - Hyperkalemia
  - Hypoglycemia

    - Decompensated (hypovolemic) shock with subsequent SIRS response
- Cerbral edema in DKA is associated with the following:

  - low initial serum bicarbonate at presentation
  - higher BUN on presentation
  - higher serum glucose on presentation
  - bicarbonate administration

- new diagnosis of diabetes
- young age (<5 years)
- longer interval between onset of disease and therapy
- Unproven but assumed associations for cerebral edema include the following:

  - volume of fluid administration, higher rates of fluid administration
  - rate of decrease in serum osmolality, serum glucose
  - hypotonic fluid administration

# Clinical Features

- Shock
- Hypotension
- Dehydration
- Confusion, irritability, lethargy
- Deep sighing respiration (Kussmaul breathing), acetone breath
- Polyuria, nocturia
- Polydipsia
- Anorexia, malaise, weight loss
- Vomiting, abdominal pain
- Ketosis
- Metabolic acidosis
- Clinical assessment of dehydration severity correlates poorly with actual percentage dehydration. Assume a 5% dehydration in most cases.
  Do not depend on urine output to assess degree of dehydration as it will be normal or increased secondary to obligate osmotic diuresis from glycosuria. Urine output will be decreased only in very severe dehydration.

# Investigations

- Capillary glucose immediately and every 1 hour
- Serum glucose, venous blood gas, sodium, potassium, chloride, bicarbonate, urea, creatinine, osmolality immediately and 1 hour after IV fluid initiated and then every 2–4 hours
- Urine ketones, glucose immediately and with every void (every 4 hours if catheterized)
- A CBC
- If there is evidence of infection obtain appropriate cultures
- ECG

- Note "hyponatremia" is often secondary to hyperglycemia
- Therefore perform a correction on serum values obtained as follows:
  - Corrected Sodium = [(glucose (mmol/L) × 1.5)] ÷ 5.5 + measured sodium (mmol/L)
  - Anion gap = sodium − (chloride + bicarbonate). Normal values are 12 ± 2 mmol/L

# Treatment

- Assess and manage ABCs according to PALS guidelines.
- Many protocols and guidelines exist and may vary between institutions; the attached guideline is modified from an Ontario Ministry of Health consensus protocol.
- Replace fluid and electrolyte deficits.
- Sodium bicarbonate should be reserved only for symptomatic hyperkalemia.
- If needed, first treat incipient hypotension/shock with initial bolus volume expansion.
- Then calculate rate of IV fluid to rehydrate evenly over 48 hours. This is usually accomplished with a total fluid intake (including insulin infusion) of 3.5–5 mL/kg/hour.
- The sodium content of the fluid may need to be increased if serum corrected sodium is low or the measured serum sodium does not rise appropriately as the glucose declines. Calculation of effective osmolality may be a helpful guide to fluid and electrolyte therapy.
- Start low dose insulin infusion of 0.1 units/kg/hour (25 units of regular insulin in 250 mL of normal saline) after initial volume expansion.
- The starting potassium concentration after initial volume expansion should be 40 mEq/L. If child is hypokalemic, start potassium replacement immediately. If potassium is >5.5 mEq/L, defer potassium replacement until renal function is assessed.
- If the blood glucose concentration declines quickly or decreases too low before DKA has resolved, increase the amount of glucose administered. Do not decrease the insulin infusion.
- Treatment of cerebral edema must be initiated as soon as it is suspected (see below).

# Monitoring

- Continuous cardiorespiratory monitor (with ECG tracing).
- Pediatric DKA flow sheet.
- Hourly documentation of heart rate, respiratory rate, and blood pressure.
- Hourly documentation of accurate fluid intake and output and calculation of fluid balance minimum every 4 hours.
- Cerebral edema is likely underrecognized; close hourly neurologic observations are crucial to detect warning signs or symptoms of cerebral edema.
- Children with severe DKA (suspect with: depressed level of consciousness, circulatory compromise, significant acidosis), or those at highest risk for cerebral edema (age <5 years, new-onset diabetes) should be considered immediately for treatment in a pediatric intensive care unit.

# References

Dunger DB, Sperling MA, Acerini CL, Bohn DJ, Daneman D, Danne TPA, et al. European Society for Paediatric Endocrinology/Lawson Wilkins Pediatric Endocrine Society consensus statement on diabetic ketoacidosis in children and adolescents. Pediatrics 2004;113:e133–40.

Wolfsorf J, Craig ME, Daneman D, et al. International Society for Pediatric and Adolescent Diabetes. Clinical Practice Guidelines 2006–2007. Pediatric Diabetes 2007;8:28–42.

Assal JP, Aoki TT, Manzano FM, Kozak GP. Metabolic effects of sodium bicarbonate in management of diabetic ketoacidosis. Diabetes 1974;23:405–11.

Lever E, Jaspan JB. Sodium bicarbonate therapy in severe diabetic ketoacidosis. Am J Med 1983;75:263–8.

Wolfsdorf J, Glaser N, Sperling MA. Diabetic ketoacidosis in infants, children, and adolescents. A consensus statement from the American Diabetes Assiciation. Diabetes Care 2006;29:1150–9.

Lindsay R, Bolte RG. The use of an insulin bolus in low-dose insulin infusion for pediatric diabetic ketoacidosis. Pediatr Emerg Care 1989;5:77–9.

Defronzo RA, Felig P, Ferrannini E, Wahren J. Effect of graded doses in insulin on splanchnic and peripheral potassium metabolism in man. Am J Physiol. 1980;238:E421–7.

Glaser N, Barnett P, McCaslin I, et al. Risk factors for cerebral edema in children with diabetic ketoacidosis. The Pediatric Emergency Medicine Collaborative Research Committee of the American Academy of Peditrics. N Engl J Med 2001;344:264–9.

Edge JA, Hawkins MM, Winter DL, Dunger DB. The risk and outcome of cerebral oedema developing during diabetic ketoacidosis. Arch Dis Child 2001;85:16–22.

Rosenbloom AL. Intracerebral crises during treatment of diabetic ketoacidosis. Diabetes Care 1990;13:22–33.

Bello FA. Cerebral edema in diabetic ketoacidosis in children. Lancet 1990; 336:64.

Lawrence SE, Cummings EA, Gadboury I, et al. Population based study of incidence and risk factors for cerebral edema in pediatric diabetic ketoacidosis. J Pediatr 2005;146(5):688–92.

Krane E. Cerebral edema in diabetic ketoacidosis. J Pediatrics 1989;114:166–8.

Hoffman WH, Steinhart CM, el Gammal T, et al. Cranial CT in children and adolescents with diabetic ketoacidosis. AJNR 1988;9:733–9.

Gerich JE, Lorenzi M, Bier DM, et al. Prevention of human diabetic ketoacidosis by somatostatin. Evidence for an essential role of glucagon. N Engl J Med 1975;292:985–9.

Shade D, Eaton RP. Glucagon regulation of plasma ketone body concentration in human diabetes. J Clin Invest 1975;56:1340–4.

Gustavson SM, Chu CA, Nishizawa M, et al. Glucagon's actions are modified by the combination of epinephrine and gluconeogenic precursor infusion. Am J Physiol Endocrinol Metab 2003;285:E534–44.

Fukao T, Lopaschuk GD, Mitchell GA. Pathways and control of ketone body metabolism: on the fringe of lipid biochemistry. Prostaglandins Leukot Essent Fatty Acids 2004;70:243–51.

Brink SJ. Diabetic ketoacidosis. Acta Paediatr Suppl 1999;88:14–24.

Rewers A, Klingensmith G, Davis C, et al. Predictors of acute complication in children with type 1 diabetes. JAMA 2002;287:2511–8.

Koves IH, Neutze J, Donath S, et al. The accuracy of clinical assessment of dehydration during diabetic ketoacidosis in childhood. Diabetes Care 2004;27:2485–7.

Katz MA. Hypoglycemia-induced hyponatremia-calculation of expected serum sodium depression. N Engl J Med 1973;289:843–3.

Harris GD, Fiordalisi I, Harris WL, Mosovich LL, Finberg L. Minimizing the risk of brain herniation during treatment of diabetic ketoacidemia; a retrospective and prospective study. J Pediatr 1990;117:22–31.

Roberts MD, Slover RH, Chase HP. Diabetic ketoacidosis with intracerebral complications. Pediatr Diabetes 2001;2:109–114.

Curtis JR, Bohn D, Daneman D. Use of hypertonic saline in the treatment of cerebral edema in diabetic ketoacidosis (DKA). Pediatr Diabetes 2001;191–4.

# Chapter 17

# Hematology/Oncology

## A. Hematology Considerations for the PICU

Isaac Odame

### Anemia

Anemia is defined as hemoglobin concentration more than 2SD below mean for age-specific normal population.

## Causes:

1. *Reduced RBC and Hb production*
   Nutritional deficiencies
   - Iron deficiency
   - Folic acid and vitamin $B_{12}$ deficiency

   Hypoplastic and aplastic anemias
   - Diamond-Blackfan syndrome
   - Fanconi's anemia
   - Transient erythroblastopenia of childhood
   - Aplastic anemia
   - Infections: parvovirus, EBV, CMV, HHV-6
   - Malignancy

   Abnormal hemoglobin or heme synthesis
   - Thalassemia syndromes
   - Lead poisoning
   - Sideroblastic anemia

   Anemia of chronic disorders

2. *Increased RBC destruction*
   Membrane defects

- Spherocytosis
- Elliptocytosis
- Pyknocytosis

Enzyme defects
- G6PD
- Pyruvate kinase

Hemoglobinopathies
- Sickle cell disorders
- Unstable hemoglobins

Immune-mediated hemolysis
- Autoimmune hemolytic anemia
- Alloimmune hemolytic anemia
- Infections
- Drugs
- Inflammatory/collagen disorders
- Malignancy

Microangiopathic anemias
- Disseminated intravascular coagulation (DIC)
- Hemolytic-uremic syndrome (HUS)
- Cavernous hemangiomas (Kasabach-Merritt syndrome)

3. *Blood loss*

Acute
- Severe trauma

Chronic
- Gastrointestinal: Meckel's diverticulum, peptic ulcer, inflammatory bowel disorder

Pulmonary
- Idiopathic pulmonary hemosiderosis

Generalized bleeding
- Inherited bleeding disorders

Anemia is a common clinical problem in ICU patients. Factors that may be responsible for anemia in critically ill patients include:

- Blood loss
  - Secondary to frequent laboratory blood sampling
  - Overt or occult gastrointestinal blood loss from stress-related gastritis or tissue trauma from gastric suctioning
  - Surgical procedures preceding ICU admission
  - Trauma preceding admission to ICU
- Bone marrow suppression
  - Secondary to renal failure, chronic disease, or inflammation

- Decreased iron availability combined with blunted response to erythropoietin
- Nutritional deficiencies

## Investigation:

### Initial tests

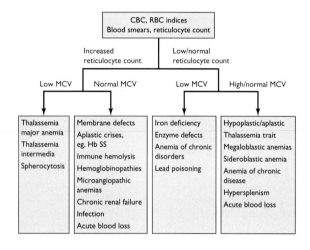

## Future Investigations

| Serum bilirubin, haptoglobin, hemopexin | Serum iron, TIBC, ferritin | RBC folate |
|---|---|---|
| Coomb's test, cold agglutinins | Free erythrocyte protoporphyrin | Serum vitamin B$_{12}$ |
| Hb analysis | Hb analysis | Bone marrow aspirate |
| CGPD, Pyruvate kinase | Lead level | Parvovirus serology |
| Osmotic fragility | | |
| Heinz body preparation | | |

# Hematological Emergencies Associated with Anemia

I. Sudden blood loss
   - Severe trauma
   - Requires supportive measures including blood transfusion to correct shock, hypoxia, and cardiac failure

II. Severe hemolysis
   A. G6PD deficiency with oxidative stress
   - Ingestion of (specific) drugs
   - G6PD test may be normal because of marked reticulocytosis and predominant young erythrocytes
   - Supportive management; avoid offending drugs

   B. Immune hemolysis
   1. Autoimmune hemolysis
   - Usually IgG-mediated hemolysis—Coomb's test positive
   - Laboratory investigation to determine specific antibody
   - Transfusion of incompatible blood should be avoided if possible
   - Use of steroids and IV immunoglobulin of benefit
   - PRBC transfusion only when anemia is severe and life-threatening—by slow transfusion
   - Splenectomy in very severe cases

   2. Alloimmune hemolysis
   - Hemolytic disease of the newborn
     - antibodies to D, E, c, Kell antigens
   - Blood group incompatibility, eg, ABO

   3. Microangiopathy
   - DIC
   - Commonly associated with infections
   - Accompanying coagulopathy and thrombocytopenia
   - Management is supportive with treatment of underlying cause
   - Use of     PRBC
                    FFP
                    Platelet concentrate
   C. Hemolytic-uremic syndrome
   - Erythrocyte fragmentation and thrombocytopenia is associated with acute renal failure
   - Management—Treat acute renal failure
   - Transfusion is supportive

III.  Sickle cell anemia

> Affected patients are usually of African, Afro-Caribbean, Mediterranean, Indian, and Middle Eastern descent.

*Infections*
- Second most common cause of mortality in patients with sickle cell disease.
- Common organisms: pneumococcus, Haemophilus influenza, meningococcus, and salmonella.
- Sites of infection: septicemia, pneumonia, osteomyelitis.
- Antibiotic prophylaxis (PenV) from age 2–4 months reduces early mortality in sickle cell patients.
- Vaccination: pneumococcal, Haemophilus influenza, meningococcal vaccines should be given.
- Treatment: prompt use of antibiotics during febrile episodes while cultures are awaited due to increased susceptibility to severe sepsis. Use of third-generation cephalosporin is recommended. IV clindamycin can be given if patient is significantly allergic to beta-lactam antibiotics (eg, anaphylaxis or serum sickness). Clindamycin alone should not be used if meningitis is suspected. IV vancomycin should be added if the child is severely ill.

  Empirical therapy when meningitis is *not* suspected:
  > Give IV cefotaxime until cultures are sterile or clinical status improves. IV clindamycin could be used if the patient has significant beta-lactam allergies (as stated before).

  Empirical therapy in sickle cell disease patient with suspected meningitis:
  > Give IV ceftriaxone plus vancomycin. In the case of significant beta-lactam allergy, rifampicin can be given in place of ceftriaxone. Antibiotics may be changed when culture sensitivity results become available.

  Empirical treatment in patients with respiratory symptoms:
  > Should include a macrolide or azolide (eg, erythromycin, azithromycin) because of the high suspicion of mycoplasma infection.

*Acute Chest Syndrome*
- Most common cause of mortality.
- New radiological findings associated with chest pain, tachypnea, and hypoxemia.
- Manage by:
  - $O_2$ supplementation
  - Antibiotics—IV third-generation cephalosporin + macrolide as broad-spectrum coverage of respiratory pathogens (see under "Infection")

- PRBC transfusion to Hb 100–110 g/L
- Respiratory therapy (incentive spirometry, chest physiotherapy)
- Bronchodilators for patients with reactive airway disease

> In severe cases:
> Mechanical ventilation
> Exchange blood transfusion to keep HbS <30%
> IV dexamethasone
> Inhaled nitric oxide 1–10 ppm
> ECMO

## Splenic Sequestration

- Third most common cause of mortality in early life.
- Sudden anemia (Hb at least 20 g/L below baseline steady state) with splenic enlargement.
- May be severe in the first year of life, presenting with circulatory collapse.
- Managed by urgent PRBC transfusion to steady state Hb level (max. 100 g/L), as higher Hb level (increased blood viscosity) increases risk of vaso-occlusion.
- Recurrence should be prevented by splenectomy (for patients >2 years old) or chronic blood transfusion to maintain Hb S level <30% (for patients <2 years old).

## Aplastic Crises

- Anemia with low reticulocyte count.
- Usually associated with infection, particularly parvovirus B19.
- Managed by PRBC transfusion and supportive care.

## Central Nervous System Crises

- Incidence: 5–10%.
- Cerebral infarction.
- Cerebral hemorrhage may occur.
- Propensity to recur.
- Management: Chronic transfusion program to reduce risk of recurrence (Hb <30%).
- Chronic blood transfusion in patients with increased transcranial ICA or MCA velocity >200 cm/s (by Doppler) has demonstrated efficacy in primary stroke prevention.
- Hydroxyurea therapy may be effective, but not yet proven by randomized studies.
- If child is febrile, investigate for infection including meningitis and treat as outlined under "Infection."
- CT without contrast to exclude intracranial hemorrhage.

- MRI and MRA should be done to diagnose infarction.
- For diagnosed CVA, perform RBC exchange transfusion to target Hb of 100 g/L and Hb S <30%.

*Vaso-occlusive (Painful) Crises*
- Most common clinical problem in sickle cell disease.
- Precipitating factors include: dehydration, infection, and exposure to the cold.
- Management: IV fluids     150% maintenance, with close monitoring of fluid balance to avoid fluid overload.

      Analgesics     Acetaminophen with codeine—mild-moderate crisis

          NSAIDS ± acetaminophen

          Morphine—severe crisis.

          For pain crisis lasting more than 24–48 hours in children older than 6 years, consider PCA pump for patient-controlled analgesia.

      Hydroxyurea     Long-term treatment for decreasing pain rate in patients who have frequent and severe vaso-occlusive crises.

*Priapism*
- Two clinical forms: scattered episodes and stuttering pattern.
- Severe or prolonged events (longer than 2 hours) require prompt medical intervention.
- None of the many treatments attempted have had controlled assessment.
- Management     IV morphine if severe painful priapism

          IV hydration

          Oral pseudoephedrine

Severe and prolonged priapism.
     Urology consultation: penile aspiration and irrigation of corpora cavernosa with adrenaline
     Exchange blood transfusion (to HbS <30%) may be considered if no detumescence after 12 hours.
     Surgery (Winter shunt) can be undertaken in intractable cases.

# Neutropenia

Neutrophil count varies with age.
**Definition:** Absolute neutrophil count (ANC) $<1.5 \times 10^9$/L
Severe neutropenia (ANC $<0.5 \times 10^9$/L) is associated with markedly increased risk of bacterial and fungal infections. Febrile episodes should be treated promptly with empirical antimicrobial agents according to institutional protocols.

## Causes

I.  **Acquired**
    Infection
    Malignancies
    Drugs
    Radiation
    Hypersplenism
    Immune
    Aplastic anemia
    Vitamin $B_{12}$ and
    folate deficiency

II. **Congenital**—rare
    Cyclic neutropenia
    Chronic benign neutropenia
    Severe congenital neutropenia
    (Kostmann syndrome)
    Fanconi's anemia
    Shwachman-Diamond
    syndrome
    Metabolic disorders
    (eg, organic acidurias)
    Osteopetrosis

Specific treatment with granulocyte colony stimulating factor (G-CSF) may be indicated (higher doses may be required for severe congenital neutropenia). Intravenous gamma globulin therapy may be useful in immune-mediated neutropenia.

# Thrombocytopenia

Definition: Platelet count $<150 \times 10^9$/L
Highest risk of life-threatening bleeds at counts $<10 \times 10^9$/L (higher in thrombocytopenia resulting from impaired production than from increased peripheral destruction).

## Causes

I.  **Acquired**
    Idiopathic thrombocy-
    topenic purpura (ITP)

    Neonatal alloimmune
    thrombocytopenia (NAIT)

II. **Congenital/Inherited**—rare
    Thrombocytopenia with absent
    radii syndrome (TAR)
    Wiskott-Aldrich syndrome
    Fanconi's anemia
    Familial thrombocytopenia

Microangiopathy
- DIC
- HUS
- Cavernous hemangioma
  (Kasabach-Merritt syndrome)

Infection

Drugs

Malignancy

Autoimmune disorders (eg, SLE)

Hypersplenism

Radiation

Aplastic anemia

**General Treatment for Thrombocytopenia**
- Supportive treatment with platelet transfusion is indicated in severe thrombocytopenia (generally not useful in ITP).
- Treat underlying cause.

## Some Specific Causes of Thrombocytopenia

### ITP

Immune-mediated thrombocytopenia is not associated with drugs or evidence of disease. It is generally a benign disorder with incidence of ICH <1%.

Treatment

- In an emergency, and life-threatening bleeding, platelet transfusions are necessary. However, they often do not stabilize the count.

CNS or life-threatening bleeding:

- Emergency splenectomy ± craniotomy with massive platelet transfusion
    IV gamma globulin (IVIG) and IV methylprednisolone

### Acute ITP

- Platelet count >20 × 10⁹/L—observe only
- Steroids—Prednisone 0.4 mg/kg/day for 7 days, taper over 2–3 weeks
- IVIG infusion. Repeat if platelet <30 × 10⁹/L after first infusion
- Anti-D immunoglobulin (only useful for Rh (D) + patients) 50μ g/kg IV

**Chronic ITP**
- Intermittent treatment with steroid, anti-D, or IVIG
- Splenectomy
- Consider use of rituximab

# Neonatal Alloimmune Thrombocytopenia (NAIT)

Transplacental maternal antibodies against platelet-specific antigens (usually HPA-1a) cause destruction of fetal platelets and in utero bleeding.

Increased risk of ICH with fetal platelet count <50 $\times$ 10$^9$/L.

Treatment
    Prenatal
- Maternal immunosuppression with IVIG 1 g/kg weekly for 6–8 weeks before delivery
- Intrauterine transfusion with washed irradiated maternal platelets or HPA-1a negative platelets
- Delivery by caesarean section to be considered

    Postnatal
- If severe: transfusion of washed irradiated maternal platelets or random HPA-1a negative platelets

# Transfusion of Blood Components

1. *Red Cell Concentrate/Packed RBC (PRBC)*

| Common indications: | Symptomatic anemia |
| --- | --- |
| | Bleeding |
| | Neonatal exchange transfusion (reconstituted with FFP) |

Typed and cross-matched PRBC preferred where possible. Unless in situations of acute blood loss or shock, PRBC should be infused no faster than 2–3 mL/kg/hr (10 mL/kg over 3–4 hours) to prevent the complication of congestive heart failure.

*Transfusion thresholds for critically ill patients:*

There is a high level of evidence from randomized trials in both adults (TRIC), children (TRIPICU) and newborns (PINT) that a restrictive strategy of red cell transfusion (lowest thresholds of 70 g/L to maintain Hb at 70–90 g/L) as effective and possibly superior (particularly in the less acutely ill) to a liberal transfusion strategy. However, optimal Hb concentrations in critically ill patients are yet to be determined.

Transfusion volume can be calculated by using this formula:

$$\text{Vol. of PRBC (mL)} = \text{EBV (mL)} \times \frac{\text{Desired Hct} - \text{Actual Hct}}{\text{Hct of PRBC}}$$

EBV — estimated blood volume (Neonate: weight (kg) $\times$ 100 mL; 1 mo – 10 yrs: weight (kg) $\times$ 80 mL; >10 yrs: weight (kg) $\times$ 70 mL)

Hct of PRBC is 0.55–0.65

## Exchange transfusion:

Single-volume exchange = Actual Hct $\times$ EBV
(A single-volume exchange usually lowers Hb S 30% or less.)

Double-volume exchange = 2 $\times$ (actual Hct $\times$ EBV)
(A double-volume exchange usually lowers Hb S to about 10% level.)

## Selection of RBC concentrate in sickle cell disease:

Simple transfusion in emergency (eg, sequestration or aplastic crisis): Use RBCs up to 14 days old, cross-matched for Rh and Kell antigens.

Exchange transfusion (eg, CVA or acute chest syndrome): Use RBCs, leucocyte-reduced, matched for Rh and Kell antigens and sickle-negative. May be reconstituted to a desired Hct of 0.45–0.56.

Leucocyte-depleted PRBC reduces the risk of nonhemolytic febrile transfusion reactions and CMV transmission.

Irradiated blood products should be transfused to prevent graft vs host disease in the following situations: hemopoietic stem cell or organ transplantation, intensive chemotherapy, congenital immunodeficiency states, intrauterine transfusions, and transfusions in preterm babies.

CMV-negative products are indicated for preterm babies and CMV-negative recipients of hemopoietic stem cell or solid organ transplants.

2. *Platelet Concentrate*
   Common indications:
   - Bleeding from thrombocytopenia or platelet function defect
   - Prevention of bleeding in thrombocytopenic patients especially prior to surgery
     - Bleeding complications are rare with platelet counts >10 $\times$ 10$^9$/L

- Platelet count $>50 \times 10^9$/L recommended for minor surgery and $>100 \times 10^9$/L for major surgery
- Clinical observations have demonstrated that in the absence of other hemostatic defects, platelet counts of $10 \times 0^9$/L or lower can provide adequate hemostasis for insertion of central venous lines and chest tubes, and for lumbar punctures.
- Consensus on these levels have not yet been achieved.

Give 4 units/m² or 1 unit/5 kg body weight or 10 mL/kg (in neonates)

3. *Fresh Frozen Plasma (FFP)*
   Has all clotting factors.
   Common indications: DIC
       TTP (plasma exchange preferred)
       Vitamin K deficiency with active bleeding
       Urgent reversal of warfarin
   Give 10–15 mL/kg; repeat doses as required

4. *Cryoprecipitate*
   Rich in F VIII, vWF and fibrinogen.
   Common indications: Hypofibrinogenemia
       Rarely in von Willebrand disease and hemophilia A (only if concentrate is unavailable)

# Complications of Blood Product Transfusions

## Common

Volume overload
Allergic reaction (hives)
Febrile nonhemolytic reaction

## Rare

### Infection

- Acute bacterial particularly with platelet concentrates (1:10,000 morbidity)
- HIV (1:1,930,000)
- Hepatitis B (1:130,000), Hepatitis C (1:500,000), Hepatitis A (very rare)
- HTLV (virtually zero with leukodepletion)
- Syphilis (very rare)

- CMV
- Acute or delayed hemolysis
- Anaphylaxis due to IgA deficiency
- Acute respiratory failure
- Graft-versus-host disease

## *Massive Blood Transfusion*

Usually defined as the need to transfuse one to two times the patient's normal blood volume (ie, newborns 80 mL/kg, to 60–70 mL/kg in teenage).

Potential complications include:

- Dilutional thrombocytopenia: Most common cause of bleeding after large volume RBC transfusion. Should be treated with platelet concentrate.
- Coagulopathy: From dilution of coagulation factors should be corrected with FFP after correction of thrombocytopenia.
- Citrate toxicity: May result in hypocalcemia if profound. More likely to occur in patients with hepatic disease or dysfunction as citrate metabolism is primarily hepatic. Treatment is with IV calcium administration.
- Hypothermia: This is avoided by warming all blood products and fluid to body temperature.
- Acid-base imbalance: Most commonly metabolic alkalosis as citrate and lactate are converted to bicarbonate by the liver following an initial state of acidosis.
- Hyperkalemia: Occurs because potassium concentration in stored blood increases steadily with time. Large amounts of blood given at a high rate of delivery are required to result in hyperkalemia, as the concentration of potassium is usually <4 mmol per unit of blood.
- Massive blood transfusion has been implicated as a risk factor for acute lung injury (TRALI) and severe acute respiratory syndrome (ARDS).

## References

Cohen AR, Norris CF, Smith-Whitney K. Transfusion therapy for sickle cell disease. In: Capon SM, Chambers LA, eds. New Directions in Pediatric Hematology. Bethesda, MD: American Association of Blood Banks, 1996;39–85.

DeLoughery TG, Liebler JM, Simmonds V, et al. Invasive line placement in critically ill patients: do hemostatic defects matter? Transfusion 1996;36:827–831.

Fink MP. Pathophysiology of intensive care unit-acquired anemia. Critical Care 2004;8(Suppl 2):S9–10.

Hebert PC, Wells G, Blajchman MA, et al. A multicenter, randomized, controlled clinical trial of transfusion requirements in critical care. N Engl J Med 1999;340:409–417.

Howard SC, Gajjar A, Ribeiro RC, et al. Safety of lumbar puncture for children with acute lymphoblastic leukemia and thrombocytopenia. JAMA 2000;284:2222–4.

Kirpalani H, Whyte RK, Andersen C, et al. The premature infants in need of transfusion (PINT) study: a randomized, controlled trial of a restrictive (low) versus liberal (high) transfusion threshold for extremely low birth weight infants. J Pediatr 2006 Sep;149(3):301–7.

Lacroix J, Hébert PC, Hutchinson JS, et al. Transfusion strategies for patients in pediatric intensive care units. Pediatric Acute Lung Injury and Sepsis Investigators Network. N Engl J Med 2007 Apr 19;356(16):1609–19.

Nathan DG, Orkin SH, Ginsburg D, Look TM, eds. Nathan and Oski's hematology of infancy and childhood, 6th edition. Philadelphia, PA: W. B. Saunders Company; 2003.

National Institutes of Health Publication. The Management of Sickle Cell Disease, 4th edition. No. 02-2117. Bethesda, Maryland: National Institutes of Health Publication; 2002.

# B. Coagulation Disorders

Anthony K C Chan
Isaac Odame

## Tests of Coagulation

1. **Prothrombin time (PT):** Measures overall efficiency of the extrinsic pathway: fibrinogen, FII, FV, FVII, FX.

    **INR** (international normalized ratio): PT ratio normalized to standard human reference thromboplastin. Used for monitoring anticoagulant therapy.

2. **Activated partial thromboplastin time (APTT):** Measures overall efficiency of the intrinsic pathway: fibrinogen, FII, FV, FVIII, FIX, FX, FXI, FXII, prekallikrein, HMWK.

3. **Thrombin time (TT):** Measures conversion of fibrinogen to fibrin.

4. **FDP and D-dimers:** FDP produced by lysis of fibrinogen and non–cross-linked fibrin; D-dimers produced by lysis of cross-linked fibrin in clot.

5. **Specific factor assay:** Used to establish hemophilia, von Willebrand disease, and other congenital factor deficiencies.

6. **Inhibitor screen:** Used to establish whether a prolonged APTT is due to a circulating anticoagulant (inhibitor) or factor deficiency. APTT is repeated with 50:50 mixtures of patient plasma and normal plasma. APTT remains prolonged in the presence of a circulating anticoagulant.

## Interpretation of Results

1. **PT-long,** APTT-normal, TT-normal, Platelet count-normal
    FVII deficiency
    Early oral anticoagulation

2. **APTT-long,** PT-normal, TT-normal, Platelet count-normal
    Congential deficiencies or defects of intrinsic pathway: FVIII, FIX, FXI, FXII, prekallikrein, HMWK
    von Willebrand disease (APTT can be normal in von Willebrand disease.)
    Heparin administration/contamination from central venous line (Discard from CVL may not be able to ensure no heparin contamination.)
    Circulating anticoagulant

3. **PT-long, APTT-long,** TT-normal, Platelet count-normal
   Vitamin K deficiency (PT more prolonged)
   Oral anticoagulant administration (PT more prolonged)
   Liver disease
   Deficiencies of prothrombin, FV, FX
4. **PT-long, APTT-long, TT-long,** Platelet count-normal
   Heparin administration
   Hypo- and dysfibrinogenemia
   Liver disease
   Hyperfibrinolysis
5. **PT-long, APTT-long, Platelet count-low**
   Acute disseminated intravascular coagulation (DIC)
   Massive transfusion of stored blood
   Liver disease, acute liver necrosis, chronic liver disease

# Prothrombotic States

1. **Inherited thrombotic risks**
   Family history of thrombosis and strokes
   Protein C deficiency
   Protein S deficiency
   Antithrombin deficiency
   Activated protein C resistance/factor V Leiden
   Prothrombin mutations
   Hyperhomocysteinemia, C677T MTHFR polymorphism
   Plasminogen abnormalities
   Dysfibrinogenemia
2. **Acquired thrombotic risks**
   Endothelial damage: Indwelling vascular catheters, surgery, trauma, hypertension, and hyperlipidemia
   Hyperviscosity: Sickle cell disease, polycythemia
   Antiphospholipid syndromes: SLE, postinfection, and pregnancy
   Platelet activation: Thrombotic thrombocytopenic purpura (TTP), heparin-induced thrombocytopenia (HIT), oral contraceptives, thrombocytosis
   Drugs (eg, L-asparaginase)
   Infection
   Malignancies
   Renal disease, nephrotic syndrome
   Liver disease
   Inflammatory disease
   Diabetes
   Paroxysmal nocturnal hemoglobinuria (PNH)

## Investigation

**Imaging:**     Venogram (not sensitive for jugular vein thrombosis)

Ultrasonography: Compression or duplex (not sensitive for intrathoracic vessels)

Pulmonary embolism: CXR, ventilation/perfusion scan, spiral CT scan, MRI, MR angiography (MRA)

D-dimer test (There is no study to verify the sensitivity and specificity of D-dimer in the diagnosis of DVT in children.)

Pulmonary angiography (invasive)

Strokes: MRI, MRA, MRV, CT, angiography (invasive), transcranial Doppler

**Laboratory:**

Look for and exclude acquired and congenital causes.

Coagulation studies

Nonspecific inhibitor, lupus anticoagulant, anticardiolipin antibodies

Protein C & S, antithrombin

Activated protein C resistance

Factor V Leiden, prothrombin 20210 mutation

Total plasma homocysteine

Lipoprotein (a)

Fibrinogen

FVIII, FIX, and FXI

## Treatment of Thromboses

### a)   Unfractionated heparin (UFH)

- For DVT and PE
- Initial loading dose 75 U/kg IV bolus (omitted in circumstances that the bleeding risk seems to be high) followed by 28 U/kg/hr by continuous infusion in patients <1 year old, or 20 U/kg/hr in patients 1 year old. Monitor APTT every 6 hours until therapeutic range (1.5–2.5 times baseline correlating to an anti-Factor Xa level of 0.35–0.7 U/mL; please note the therapeutic anti-Factor Xa level for UFH is different from LMWH) has been achieved. Thereafter, monitor APTT and platelet count daily and adjust dose.
- Effect can be reversed with protamine sulphate 1 mg per 100 units heparin. (Consider half-life of heparin to calculate dose of protamine.)

b) **Low-molecular weight heparin (LMWH)**

- Longer half-life, more specific anti-Xa activity and less anti-IIa activity, more predictable dose/response ratio, less heparin-induced thrombocytopenia, more costly.
- Doses vary with preparation.
- Enoxaparin 1 mg/kg/dose q12h SC in patients >2 month old, or 1.5 mg/kg/dose q12h in patients <2 months old. Prophylactic doses are half the doses for full anticoagulation.
- Monitoring of LMWH therapy: anti-Xa activity (4 hours post dose).

  Therapeutic range: 0.5–1.0 units/mL for full anticoagulation
  
  0.1–0.3 units/mL for prophylactic treatment

- Effect can be reversed (100% anti-IIa, approximately 60% anti-Xa) by protamine 1 mg for 1 mg enoxaparin (consider half-life to calculate dose).

c) **Warfarin**

- For long-term anticoagulation.
- Give together with heparin until INR is within the therapeutic range for 2 consecutive days, then discontinue heparin.
- Loading dose 0.1–0.2 mg/kg/day PO (maximum 5 mg) day, followed by 25–100% loading dose on days 2–5 depending on INR. Subsequently, dose is adjusted to maintain target INR of 2–3.
- Beware of drug interaction with warfarin, effect of dietary intake of vitamin K, and intercurrent illness.
- Effect can be reversed with vitamin K administration or IV fresh frozen plasma (10–15 mL/kg).

d) **Thrombolytic therapy**

| | |
|---|---|
| **Indications:** | Arterial occlusions (eg, following cardiac catheterization) |
| | Pulmonary embolism (PE)—massive PE; PE unresponsive to heparin therapy |
| | Threat of organ or limb viability |
| | Extensive deep venous thrombosis |
| **Contraindications:** | Active bleeding |
| | General surgery <10 days before |
| | Neurosurgery <3 weeks before |
| | Hypertension |
| | AV malformation |
| | Severe trauma (recent) |

**Thrombolytic therapy in children must be undertaken and monitored by medical personnel with experience in this area.**

### Tissue plasminogen activator (t-PA)

Admit to ICU or designated area for thrombolytic therapy.

Start or continue heparin infusion at 10 U/kg/hour. Do not administer heparin bolus.

Give t-PA as infusion at 0.5 mg/kg/hour for 6 hours.

Re-evaluate—Return of pulses and BP (arterial thrombus) and radiographic investigations after 6 hours of t-PA.

Do plasminogen levels. If plasminogen is low, give FFP 20 mL/kg IV 8 hourly. In neonate and young infants, consider giving FFP before administration of FFP even when fibrinogen is normal to decrease risk of bleeding.

| **Monitoring:** | APTT, PT (INR), Platelet count and Fibrinogen—4 hours post-initiation of therapy, then every 6–8 hours thereafter |
| --- | --- |
| | Plasminogen level—if no response after 6 hours of t-PA |
| | D-dimers test—to assess ongoing thrombolysis |
| | Fibrinogen >1.0 g/L (infusion of cryoprecipitate 1 U/5kg), Platelets >100 × 10⁹/L |

**Streptokinase is not recommended in children and urokinase may be difficult to obtain.**

## Inherited Abnormalities of Coagulation Factors

1. **Factor VIII deficiency (Hemophilia A)**
   X-linked recessive disorder
   About 30% of cases are spontaneous mutations
   Diagnosis in the newborn not problematic as FVIII:C levels are within adult range at birth

   | **Classification:** | Mild—FVIII:C >=5–40% |
   | --- | --- |
   | | Moderate—FVIII:C 1–<=50% |
   | | Severe—FVII:C <1%, at least 50% of hemophiliacs |

## Treatment of Bleeding Episodes

**DDAVP (desmopressin acetate)**  Mild hemophiliacs should be treated with DDAVP 0.3 µg/kg in 10–20 mL NS infused over 20 minutes whenever possible (beware of hyponatremia as a complication and advice on fluid restriction).

FVIII:C level rises to 2–4 times basal levels.

Response diminishes with continued use >3–4 days.

Thus, even mild hemophiliacs require factor replacement for prolonged postsurgical hemostasis or severe bleeding.

## FVIII Concentrates

Recombinant FVIII concentrates (eg, Kogenate FS or recombinate) preferred to reduce risk of infection. (Currently, only recombinant factor VIII concentrates are used in Canada.)

FVIII:C level rose by a mean 2% per 1 U of FVIII/kg with half-life of 8–12 hours. (Recovery is usually lower in younger children, and thus it is important to demonstrate the FVIII:C level attained in severe bleeding such as head injury.)

Dose schedule depends on clinical situation.

Intermittent dosing is q12h after the initial dose.

Special considerations apply to management of patients with inhibitors (Table 1).

Continuous infusion may be required postsurgically or following life-threatening bleeds: 50–60 U/kg loading dose followed by 3–4 U/kg/hour.

### 2. Factor IX deficiency (Hemophilia B, Christmas disease)

X-linked recessive; clinically indistinguishable from hemophilia A.

F IX is vitamin K-dependent and gestationally reduced at birth.

It is therefore difficult to diagnose mild hemophilia B in the newborn due to potential overlap with normal range (severely affected neonates easy to identify).

### Treatment

F IX concentrates (F IX:C raised by 1% for each unit F IX concentrate/kg with half-life of 18–24 hours). The recovery is usually lower with the use of recombinant factor IX concentrate and as such the dose required should be multiplied by a factor of 1.4.

*Table I*
## Management of Patients with Inhibitors

**FVIII inhibitors** will develop in 6–10% of patients on replacement therapy

| **Genetic factors:** | FVIII gene mutation—inversion of intron 22, larger deletion of Factor VIII gene |
| | Ethnic group—more common in blacks |
| | Sibling having inhibitors |

## Treatment
    Activated prothrombin complex concentrates (APCC) for non-critical bleeds
    Feiba, Autoplex
    Human FVIII concentrates—2–3 times higher for critical hemorrhage
    Porcine FVIII concentrate
    Recombinant FVIIa
    A pediatric hematologist with experience in hemophilia care should always be consulted in such situations

Avoid concurrent use of antifibrinolytic agents

| Indications | Desired FVIII:C (%) | Desired FIX:C (%) |
| --- | --- | --- |
| Early hemarthrosis | 30 | 30 |
| Mucosal bleeds unresponsive to tranexamic acid | | |
| Established hematoma | 50 | 50 |
| Life-threatening bleed | 80–100 | 80 |
| Intracranial hemorrhage | | |
| Major trauma with bleed | | |
| Surgery | | |
| Potential airway obstruction | | |
| Overtreating is preferable to undertreating | | |

### 3. Von Willebrand Disease

Von Willebrand factor (vWF) is a large and highly complex molecule with two major functions:

1) Mediates platelet adhesion to subendothelium
2) Functions as a carrier protein for F VIII:C

## Classification:

**Type I:** Partial quantitative deficiency
**Type II:** Qualitative defect of vWF that affects platelet or FVIII binding (ie, abnormal vWF)
**Type III:** Virtual absent of vWF

**Laboratory:** Ristocetin cofactor activity $< 1$

## Treatment

**Type I:** DDAVP 0.3 µg/kg in NS at a concentration of 0.5 µg/mL over 20 minutes (maximum 240 µg)
**Type II:** Since the native vWF is abnormal, this renders the use of DDAVP possibly inappropriate or ineffective in this subset of patients
**Type III:** Unresponsive to DDAVP

Type III and most type II patients should be treated with F VIII concentrate rich in HMW multimers such as Humate-P (heat-inactivated vWF-enriched concentrate).

Cryoprecipitate through containing the entire FVIII-vWF should be avoided because it is not virucidally treated. The therapy of hemophilia and vWD should be guided by a hematologist.

## Prophylaxis for Immobilized Patient   There is no data to support routine thromboprophylaxis in immobilized pediatric patients at the present time. The decision has to be individualized depending on the following:

1. Any history of previous thrombosis.
2. Any family history of thrombosis.
3. Puberty status: The hemostatic system of a postpubertal patient can be considered to be the same as an adult and thus the risk of thrombosis in this cohort would be similar to an adult in contrast to a prepubertal patient.
4. Non-pharmacological thromboprophylaxis can be used.

5. One golden rule is not to anticoagulate a patient that has bleeding or deemed to have increased risk of bleeding because the evidence for efficacy and safety in thromboprophylaxis is scant.

## Prophylaxis for Non–Weight-Bearing Pediatric Orthopedic Patients

Thromboprophylaxis of non–weight-bearing adult orthopedic patients is standard of care with ample evidence substantiating the practice. However, there are essentially no data to guide such therapy in children. This clinical guide is of the author's opinion.

One approach to this problem is to say that there is no data in thromboprophylaxis in this age group and thus do not do it until further evidence is available. However, this approach will not be consistent with how we approach a lot of the problems in pediatric medicine. The following is our approach until further evidence is available. (See Figure 1.)

- Risk of bleeding and HIT in using LMWH for thromboprophylaxis, estimated to be less than 1%.
- Risk of thrombosis in non–weight-bearing pediatric orthopedic patient is unclear, though it does happen.

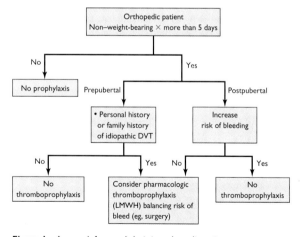

**Figure 1**    Approach for prophylaxis in orthopedic patients.

- Continue LMWH until 50% weight-bearing or up to a maximum of 6 weeks. After 6 weeks, if patient is still non–weight-bearing, one can continue with LMWH or switch the patient over to aspirin.
- Dose of enoxaparin: 0.5 mg/kg/dose (maximum 30 mg) twice a day or 0.8 mg/kg/dose (maximum 40 mg) once a day.
- Patient/parents preference should be taken into account.
- Assessment of puberty can be done according to Tanner Staging or consider postpubertal once the growth plate has closed.

## Suggested Readings

Canadian Hemophilia Society: www.hemophilia.ca

Monagle P, Chan AKC, deVeber G, Massicotte M. Andrew's thromboembolism and stroke protocol, 3rd Ed. Hamilton: BC Decker; 2006.

Monagle P, Chan AKC, Massicotte P, et al. Antithrombotic therapy in children: the seventh ACCP conference on antithrombotic and thrombolytic therapy. Chest 2004;126:(3Suppl):645S–87S.

World Federation of Hemophilia: www.wfh.org

# C. Hemophagocytic Lymphohistiocytosis (HLH)

## Carol Portwine

## Key Principles

- HLH is a rare disorder that may mimic more common ICU diseases.
- If untreated, HLH is eventually fatal.
- HLH should be considered, especially in atypical cases of presumed septic shock.

## Pathophysiology

- It is a specific disease falling within the category of histiocytic disorders. These are systemic disorders, largely confined to childhood, of cells whose function is to ingest bacteria (dendritic cells, macrophages, monocytes).
- HLH is not felt to be a truly malignant disorder, but rather one of altered biologic behavior of normal macrophages, which are phagocytic cells of the reticuloendothelial system.
- HLH is a disorder of widespread accumulation of lymphocytes and mature macrophages, with hemophagocytosis primarily involving the spleen, lymph nodes, bone marrow, liver, and cerebral spinal fluid. It is associated with defective triggering of apoptosis and reduced cytotoxic activity. Often, there is an underlying infection, lymphoma, other malignant disease, autoimmune disease, or metabolic disease.
- It is a hypercytokinemia, mainly involving proinflammatory cytokines, which mediates the clinical and laboratory findings.
- HLH is a great *chameleon of many diseases*. If not diagnosed in time, the child may have permanent disabilities or die. It may mimic septic shock with multi-organ involvement.
- There are two forms:

  - Familial or primary (related to PRF 1 and UNC13D mutations plus others as yet unclassified, and defects in STX11 have been detected in patients of Turkish origin)—heterogenous autosomal recessive

- Infection-associated or secondary—occurs sporadically

- It is clinically difficult to distinguish between familial and secondary unless there is a family history.

## Familial Form (FHL—Familial Hemophagocytic Lymphohistiocytosis)

- These patients can experience recurring episodes of life-threatening, often infection-induced, lymphohistiocyte activation.
- Annual childhood incidence is estimated at 1.2 cases per 1,000,000.
- Clinical presentation is that of a generalized disease.
- Invariably fatal if untreated.
- Seen mostly in infants and early childhood but the disease has rarely presented in early adulthood.
- Presence of a positive family history is obviously helpful, but more often than not it is lacking. Often the correct diagnosis is reached only after a second family member is affected.
- The most promising treatment is chemotherapy to get the disease under control followed by allogeneic bone marrow transplantation.

## Infection-Associated (IAHS—Infection-Associated Hemophagocytic Syndrome)

- This was first described as a response to a viral infection in an immunocompromised host. Since then it has been reported in association with various infections including viral, bacterial, fungal, and parasitic infections.
- This often, but not always, occurs in a setting of immunodeficiency.
- It can occur at any age.

## Signs and Symptoms/Investigations

This life-threatening immune disorder presents with specific clinical and laboratory findings. The diagnostic criteria for HLH are based on the recommendations of the Histiocyte Society. These are in Table 1 below:

*Table I*
**Diagnostic Guidelines for HLH
(Revised from Henter, et al. Semin Oncol
1991;18:29–33.)**

The diagnosis of HLH can be established if one of either 1 or 2 below is fulfilled.

1. A molecular diagnosis consistent with HLH.
2. Diagnostic criteria for HLH fulfilled (5 out of the 8 criteria from A and B below).

   A) Initial diagnostic criteria (to be evaluated in all patients with HLH).

Clinical Criteria

- Fever
- Splenomegaly

Laboratory Criteria

- Cytopenias (affecting at least >2 of 3 lineages in the peripheral blood):

  - Hemoglobin (<90 g/L) (In infants <4 weeks: Hgb <100 g/L)
  - Platelets (<100 × $10^9$/L)
  - Neutrophils (<1.0 × $10^9$/L)

- Hypertriglyceridemia and/or hypofibrinogenemia fasting triglycerides >3.0 mmol/L (ie, >265 mg/dL), fibrinogen ≤1.5 g/L

Histopathologic Criteria

- Hemophagocytosis in bone marrow, spleen, or lymph nodes. No evidence of malignancy.

  B) New diagnostic criteria.

- Low or absent NK-cell activity (according to local laboratory reference).
- Ferritin >500 microgram/L.
- Soluble CD25 (ie, soluble IL-2 receptor) >2400 U/mL.

Notes: The diagnosis of FHL is justified by a positive family history or disease-causing mutations in the targeted genes, and parental consanguinity is suggestive.

## Comments:

1. If hemophagocytic activity is not proven at the time of presentation, further search for hemophagocytic activity is encouraged. If the bone marrow specimen is not conclusive, material may be obtained from other organs. Serial marrow aspirates and biopsies over time may also be helpful.

2. The following findings may provide supportive evidence for the diagnosis:

   a. Spinal fluid pleocytosis (mononuclear cells) and/or elevated spinal fluid protein
   b. Histological picture of the liver resembling chronic, persistent hepatitis

3. Other abnormal clinical laboratory findings consistent with the diagnosis are cerebromeningeal symptoms, lymph node enlargement, jaundice, edema, skin rash, hepatic enzyme abnormalities, hypoproteinemia, hyponatremia, VLDL elevated, and HDL decreased.

## Management

- Without treatment, FHL is usually rapidly fatal with a median survival of about two months. The Histiocyte Society in 1994 developed a common treatment protocol (HLH-94), primarily designed for the primary, inherited disease FHL. This protocol has been moderately modified, and the present Histiocyte Society protocol is entitled HLH-2004. In general, the current drugs used for this disease include steroids, etoposide, and cyclosporin. The aim is first to achieve a clinically stable resolution and ultimately to cure by bone marrow transplantation (BMT).

- For IAHS, the goal is to get the disease in complete remission to the point where the patient can come off all therapy. If refractory to treatment, the patient may still require a bone marrow transplant as in FHL. It is important to investigate for infections as the primary cause of the HLH.

- See Figure 1 for a schematic view of the treatment plan for FHL and IAHS.

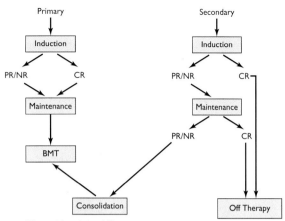

PR – partial remission; NR – no response;
CR – complete remission; BMT – bone marrow transplant

**Figure 1**    Treatment plan for HLH – primary and secondary.

# References

Filipovich A. Genetic testing for hemophagocytic lymphohistiocytosis. Histiocyte Society website. www.HistiocyteSociety.org (last accessed March 2009)

Henter J. Hemophagocytic lymphohistiocytosis (HLH): Symptoms, signs and diagnosis of a rapidly fatal childhood disease. Histiocyte Society website. www.HistiocyteSociety.org (last accessed March 2009)

Imashuku S. Advances in the management of hemophagocytic lymphohistiocytosis. Int J Hematol 2000;72(200):1–11.

Rheingold SR, Lange BJ. Histiocytoses. In: Pizzo PA, Poplack DG, eds. Principles and practice of pediatric oncology, 4th ed. Philadelphia: Lippincott Williams & Wilkins; 2002, pp. 744–6.

# D. Superior Vena Cava Syndrome (SVCS)

Carol Portwine

## Key Principles

---

- SVC syndrome can cause life-threatening airway compromise or cardiac obstruction.
- If SVC syndrome is suspected from clinical symptoms, anesthesia and PICU should be alerted immediately for airway management
- An urgent cardiology consult and echocardiogram should follow.
- Surgery should be consulted to assess for tissue diagnosis.

---

## Pathophysiology

- SVCS refers to the symptoms associated with the compression or obstruction of the superior vena cava (SVC); technically, the compression of the trachea is termed superior mediastinal syndrome (SMS). Because SMS and resulting respiratory compromise often occur with SVCS in children, the two entities have become synonymous in pediatric practice.
- Unlike in adults, the trachea and right mainstem bronchus are less rigid in a child and therefore more susceptible to compression. Moreover, the intralumenal size of the airway in a child is significantly smaller and can tolerate minimal reduction before respiratory symptoms occur. In view of the respiratory component usually seen in children, SVCS differs in pediatrics than in adults and constitutes a medical emergency.
- SMS is an uncommon but life-threatening condition in pediatrics that represents tracheal and vascular compression. It is seen at presentation in 12% of children with a malignant mediastinal mass (lymphoma, germ-cell tumors, neuroblastoma). It can also be caused by SVC obstruction, especially as seen with thrombosed indwelling central venous catheters.

## Signs and Symptoms

Presenting features are distension of the neck veins, edema above the clavicles, facial plethora, symptoms of increased intracranial pressure, orthopnea respiratory distress with retractions, stridor, wheezing, cyanosis, nasal flaring, and occasional pleural effusion. Progressive vascular compression may result in thromboembolic phenomena and fatally increased intracranial pressure.

## Investigations

- Physical exam, history, and CXR are usually sufficient to establish a diagnosis of SVCS.
- CT should be completed once the patient's airway is secured to determine cause of the SVCS and to look for other potential sites of disease amenable for biopsy if the cause is a mediastinal mass.
- A flow volume loop may help evaluate anesthetic risk.
- Echocardiogram should be completed to look at cardiac function and outflow tracts, vascular compression, SVC blood clot and blood flow, pericardial effusion, and risk of tamponade.

## Management

- The underlying management principle is to minimize risk of airway or cardiac compromise.
- Venous pressures can be decreased with bedrest, reverse Trendelenburg position, and occasionally diuresis.
- Keeping patient in a sitting position may minimize anatomic compression and improve vascular drainage.
- BLOOD CLOT: If caused by clot, surgical management may be necessary. Indwelling catheter removal should be considered if thrombosed. Anticoagulants may be required and thrombolytic therapy may be considered.
- MEDIASTINAL MASS: Emergency radiotherapy (consult radiation oncologist) or high doses steroids (dexamethasone IV 10 mg/m/day divided TID) may be necessary for empiric management prior to diagnosis. Since radiotherapy may not be on site for pediatrics, medical management with steroids is often the treatment of choice. **When initiating**

**therapy, always remember to assess for and treat tumor lysis syndrome. (See Chapter 17, "Tumor Lysis Syndrome.")**

- Do not delay making a specific diagnosis (lymph node biopsy, bone marrow, pleural tap), as not all masses will shrink with steroids. In those that do respond, a delayed biopsy may result in cell necrosis and insufficient viable tissue for pathologic diagnosis. Generally, 24 hours of therapy (and often less) is enough to render histology as uninterpretable.
- A procedure to obtain a specimen for pathology may involve significant anesthetic risks and may not be feasible. Always consider local anesthetic if possible when a readily accessible site is available for biopsy. Children with SVCS have a poor tolerance for general anesthesia because of the accompanying cardiovascular and pulmonary changes that may aggravate the SVCS. This often makes intubation impossible, and extubation may be difficult, resulting in prolonged intubation. Spontaneous respiration is generally the best method of managing the airway.
- **The least invasive option for diagnosis is always the best option.**

Emergency airway management may require the use of the following:

- Bronchoscopic placement of endotracheal tube
- Awake intubation
- Double lumen endotracheal tube
- Armored tube to stent airway

In the event of cardiac tamponade:

- Ensure airway is secure and breathing controlled.
- Use isotonic fluid resuscitation with 20 mL/kg boluses as needed.
- Position patient to relieve obstruction; exact position will vary depending on location of the tumor.
- Lower limb IVs should be used to administer drugs and fluids.
- Ensure that patient has received steroids.
- In rare cases, cardiopulmonary bypass or cardiothoracic surgery may be required as a bridge to definitive therapy.

See Figure 1 for a flow diagram to the approach and management of SVC syndrome in a child with a mediastinal mass.

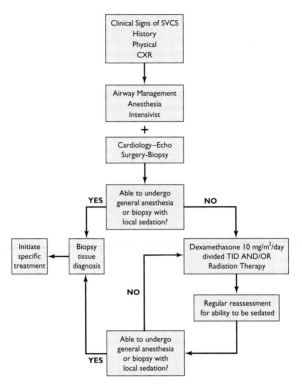

**Figure 1**    Management of patient with SVCS secondarty to mediastinal mass.

# References

Fasano R, Kent P, Valentino L. Superior vena cava thrombus treated with low-dose, peripherally administered recombinant tissue plasminogen activator in a child: Case report and review of the literature. J Pediatr Hematol Oncol 2005 Dec;27(12):692–5.

Rheingold SR, Lange BJ. Oncologic emergencies. In: Pizzo PA, Poplack DG, eds. Principles and practice of pediatric oncology, 4th ed. Philadelphia: Lippincott Williams & Wilkins; 2002, pp. 1177–80.

Yellin A, Rosen A, Reichert N, et al. Superior vena cava syndrome: the myth—the facts. Am Rev Respir Dis 1990;141(5):1114–8.

# E. Hypercalcemia in Pediatric Malignancy

## Carol Portwine

## Key Principles

> - Hypercalcemia is seen much less frequently in children (0.5–1.0%) with malignancy when compared to adults (10–20%).
> - Early diagnosis and treatment with hydration and hypocalcemic drugs can improve symptoms fairly rapidly. Unfortunately, diagnosis can be delayed because symptoms can be insidious in onset.
> - The most effective long-term treatment is appropriate management of the underlying malignancy.
> - See Chapter 16, "Calcium Disorders" for additional details.

## Introduction

Hypercalcemia is defined as a serum calcium level in excess of 3.0 mmol/L. Levels higher than 3.0 mmol/L can affect multiple organ systems. Levels exceeding 5.0 mmol/L can be fatal. Generally, symptoms begin with serum calcium levels of 3.5 mmol/L, but clinical manifestations are more closely related to the rapidity of onset as opposed to a particular level. In contrast to adults, in which hypercalemia is seen in about 20% of all patients with cancer, it is rarely present in children with malignancies (0.5–1% of all cases).

# Pathophysiology

- Calcium hemostasis is maintained by parathyroid hormone (PTH) and calcitriol. Healthy kidneys are capable of filtering calcium that is subsequently reclaimed by tubular reabsorption. Hypercalcemia occurs when the serum calcium concentration overwhelms the kidneys.
- Increased release of calcium from bones by direct destruction (ie, extensive bone metastasis).
- Secretion of humoral factors by the malignant cells (ie, parathyroid hormone-related peptide, prostaglandine E2, etc.) that cause increased bone resorption, increased renal calcium resorption, and/or decreased renal phosphate excretion.
- Immobilization.
- Hypercalcemia may cause nephrocalcinosis and irreversible damage to the kidneys.

# Signs and Symptoms

The diagnosis is often delayed because the symptoms are nonspecific and often insidious in onset.

1. Neurologic (drowsiness, lethargy, confusion, weakness, decreased deep tendon reflexes, psychotic symptoms)
2. Gastrointestinal (abdominal pain, anorexia, nausea, vomiting, constipation)
3. Renal (acute renal failure, renal calculi)
4. Cardiac (myocardial irritability, short QT interval, $\uparrow$PR interval and QRS duration, ± AV block, cardiac arrest)
5. Metabolic (hypokalemia, hypophosphatemia, hypermagnasemia, alkalosis)

# Investigations

- History of symptoms and duration:

  - Any exogenous source of calcium?
  - Any use of thiazide diuretics?
  - Any predisposition to dehydration and immobility?
  - Which may exacerbate this condition?

- Clinical status:

  - Neuromuscular
  - Neurologic

- Cardiovascular
- Renal
- Gastrointestinal

- Radiographs of areas of concern for primary or metastatic bony disease
- Serum calcium, albumin
- Ionized calcium

> Symptoms are caused by the disturbances of the ionized calcium.
> In case of hypoalbuminemia, the total calcium needs to be corrected in order to account for a changed relation of ionized to total calcium:

$$Ca_{corrected} = [(albumin_{normal} - albumin_{patient}) \times 0.8] + Ca_{patient}$$

- Sodium, potassium, phosphate, magnesium
- Blood gas
- Creatinine, urea
- PTH, 1–25-dihydroxyvitamin D
- ECG

# Management

## Prevention

Patients at risk should be informed of the symptoms to ensure early intervention. Always ensure adequate fluid intake, salt intake, nausea and vomiting control, and mobility.

## Treatment

The principles of treatment and general management include:

- Hydration and diuretics for increased renal calcium excretion
- Bisphosphonates, etc. for decreased calcium mobilization from bone
- Treatment of the underlying malignancy
- Hydration and diuresis; consult endocrine and nephrology
- If Ca <2.8–3.5 mmol/L:

  1. Hydrate with saline 3 L/m/day.
  2. Follow with loop diuretic (furosemide 1 mg/kg IV).

- If Ca >3.5 mmol/L:

  1. Hydrate until good urine flow.
  2. Loop diuretic IV (furosemide 1 mg/kg)—repeat q2h as needed to maintain good urine output.

3. Serial chemistry to watch for other metabolic complications.

Specific management includes the following options:

- Bisphosphonates inhibit osteoclast-mediated resorption of bone and reduce osteoclast viability (pamidronate 0.5–1 mg/kg IV infused over 4–6 hours). Close monitoring of serum calcium, phosphate, and magnesium levels is necessary. Note that although there are no prospective randomized trials of the use of bisphosphonates in pediatrics, they have been shown to be effective in quickly lowering calcium in the setting of malignancy.

- Calcitonin opposes the physiologic effect of PTH on bone and renal tubular calcium absorption. Initial dose is 4 IU/kg subcutaneous or intramuscular every 12 hours. After 1–2 days, dose may be increased to 8 IU/kg every 12 hours. Maximum 8 IU/kg body weight every 6 hours if the response to lower doses is unsatisfactory. Tachyphylaxis commonly occurs so the effect may last only a few days.

- Prednisone (1.5–2 mg/kg/day) will slowly reduce the serum calcium level if it is mediated by osteoclast-activating factor or calcitriol.

- To maintain normal Ca, encourage ambulation and a low Ca diet; avoid dehydration.

- The most effective long-term treatment is appropriate management of the underlying malignancy.

# References

Bajorunas DR. Clinical manifestations of cancer-related hypercalcemia. Semin Oncol 1990;17(2 Suppl 5):16–25.

Kerdudo C, Aerts I, et al. Hypercalcemia and childhood cancer. J Pediatr Hematol Oncol 2005;27:23–7.

McKay C, Furman WL. Hypercalcemia complicating childhood malignancies. Cancer 1993;72(1):256–60.

Rheingold SR, Lange BJ. Oncologic emergencies. In: Pizzo PA, Poplack DG, eds. Principles and practice of pediatric oncology, 4th ed. Philadelphia: Lippincott Williams & Wilkins; 2002, pp. 1177–80.

Ritch PS. Treatment of cancer-related hypercalcemia. Semin Oncol 1990;17(2 Suppl 5):26–33.

# F. Hyperleukocytosis

Uma Athale

## Hyperleukocytosis

Patients presenting with acute leukemia and hyperleukocytosis [very high leukemic blast count ($>/=100 \times 10^9$/L)] are at high risk of severe metabolic complications, leukostasis syndrome, and multi-organ failure. Respiratory failure, intracranial bleed, renal failure, and tumor lysis syndrome are predictors of high early mortality (20–40%).

### Incidence

12–25% of pediatric acute myeloid leukemia (AML), 9–10% of childhood acute lymphoblastic leukemia (ALL), and almost all children in the chronic phase of chronic myeloid leukemia (CML).

### Risk Factors

- Age <1 year
- Monoblastic leukemia (AML M4, M5)
- Acute promyelocytic leukemia (AML-M3), especially microgranular variant
- T-cell ALL (especially with mediastinal mass)
- Hypodiploid ALL
- 11q23 positive ALL or AML
- Philadelphia chromosome positive ALL

Leukostasis syndrome is often empirically diagnosed when patients with leukemia and hyperleukocytosis have respiratory or neurologic symptoms. They may also have signs caused by small blood vessel occlusion or coagulopathy. Leukostasis syndrome is more common in patients with AML, whereas metabolic complications (including tumor lysis syndrome) are more frequent in children with ALL.

### Pathophysiology

The pathophysiology of leukostasis syndrome is poorly understood. Although hyperleukocytosis is an important predisposing factor, leukostasis syndrome can develop at WBC counts much lower than $100 \times 10^9$/L, especially in patients with AML. Potential mechanisms of leukostasis syndrome include hyperviscosity by increased packed leukocyte volume, cellular interaction, and aggregation. In addition, leukemic blasts are not easily deformable to navigate the microvasculature. Myeloid blasts are larger than lymphoid blasts and hence patients with AML may have manifestations of leukostasis at lower blast count compared to those with ALL.

Packed red cell transfusion can increase the viscosity and worsen the leukostasis. Hence, routine red cell transfusion should be avoided in patients with hyperleukocytosis.

## Signs and Symptoms

Patient could be asymptomatic or may present with shortness of breath, tachypnea, dyspnea, hypoxia, visual problems, confusion, delirium, somnolence, coma, and death. Priapism and dactilytis have been described with hyperleukocytosis.

Clinical and radiological manifestations are similar to infectious and hemorrhagic complications in association with leukemia. Hence, a high index of suspicion is required.

**Laboratory data:** CBC, serum electrolytes, LDH, uric acid, Serum Ca, phosphorous, renal functions, LFTs, VBG, and CXR. Other imaging studies (eg, CT of head) as indicated.

Because leukemic blasts are metabolically active in vitro, the laboratory results (eg, hypoxia, hyperkalemia) may be spuriously abnormal. Similarly, blast fragments may be mistakenly counted as platelets spuriously increasing platelet count.

## Management

Supportive care and prompt leukocytoreduction are the mainstay of therapy. Medical emergency team referral or PICU admission should be considered in the presence of cardiopulmonary compromise or altered mental status.

## Supportive care:

1. Adequate fluid therapy
2. Correction of metabolic abnormalities
3. Prevention and management of tumor lysis syndrome
4. Blood and blood product transfusion: platelets, FFP for coagulopathy

Important: Avoid indiscriminate PRBC transfusion. The Hb level should not be raised >100 gm/L.

Leukocytoreduction: Prompt leukocytoreduction is absolutely essential. It can be achieved by:

1. Leukopheresis or exchange transfusion (in small babies). This effectively reduces cell burden. However, there is controversy regarding the best use of leukopheresis. There are no accepted criteria for initiation or stopping leukopheresis or monitoring. Problems with leukopheresis include need for anticoagulation, venous access, and limited availability. Further, leukopheresis has only temporizing effects.

2. Initiation of chemotherapy, especially in patients with ALL. Hydroxyurea in a dose 50–100 mg/kg/day is recommended for hyperleukocytic AML patients.

3. Radiation therapy: Cranial or renal irradiation for CNS or renal affection is not effective and not recommended.

# References

Howard SC, Ribeiro RC, Pui CH. Acute complications. In: Pui CH, ed. Childhood leukemias, 2nd ed. Cambridge: Cambridge University Press 2006, Chapter 29, pp. 709–949.

Rheingold SR, Lange BJ. Oncologic emergencies. In: Pizzo PA, Poplack DG, eds. Principle and Practice of Pediatric Oncology, 4th ed. Philadelphia: Lippincott Williams & Wilkins; 2002, pp. 1177–1203.

Porcu P, Farag F, Marcucci G, et al. Leucocytoreduction for acute leukemia. Ther Apher 2002;6:15–23.

# G. Tumor Lysis Syndrome
Uma Athale

## Definition

Tumor lysis syndrome (TLS) consists of metabolic abnormalities resulting from rapid lysis of a large number of tumor cells releasing the intracellular contents into the circulation. Hyperuricemia, hyperphosphatemia, and hyperkalemia form the classic triad of TLS.

## Timing

TLS usually manifests within 12–72 hours of initiating anticancer therapy. However, it can occur before any therapy. With remission of the cancer, there is no risk of TLS, but TLS may recur with the recurrence of disease.

## Risk Factors for TLS

- TLS occurs with cancers that have a high growth rate, large volume, or wide dissemination and that are sensitive to chemotherapy (see list below).
- Patients with high tumor burden [as reflected by hyperleukocytosis, high serum lactate dehydrogenase (LDH) levels, and/or massive organomegaly] are at high risk for TLS.
- Patients with dehydration, hyperuricemia, and renal insufficiency may develop fatal complications. Associated fever, hypoxia, and infection can complicate the management.
- TLS is common in patients with:

  1. Burkitt's lymphoma
  2. Lymphoblastic lymphoma
  3. Acute lymphoblastic leukemia (ALL), especially T-cell lineage ALL
  4. Hyperleukocytosis (WBC $>$ 100 $\times$ 10$^9$/L)
  5. Rhabdomyosarcoma

## Manifestations of TLS

The biochemical abnormalities associated with TLS include hyperuricemia, hyperphosphatemia, hyperkalemia, azotemia, and hypocalcemia. Please refer to Table 1 for details of pathophysiology and clinical manifestations.

*Table 1*

**Pathophysiology and Clinical Manifestations of Biochemical Alterations Observed in Patients with Tumor Lysis Syndrome**

| Biochemical abnormality | Pathophysiology | Clinical manifestations |
|---|---|---|
| Hyperuricemia | Uric acid, end product of purine metabolism, can precipitate in renal distal tubules and collecting ducts especially when urine pH is <5.0 | Nausea, vomiting, lethargy, agitation, somnolescence, hypertension, cloudy urine, back and joint pain, renal insufficiency |
| Hyperkalemia | Release of intracellular $K^+$. Acidosis shifts intracellular K to extra-cellular compartment, interferes with reuptake and re-utilization of K. Reduced excretion of K with renal insufficiency | Cardiac arrythmia or cardiac arrest |
| Hyperphosphatemia | Release of intracellular phosphate. Metabolic acidosis exacerbates hyperphosphatemia | Hypocalcemia, renal insufficiency |
| Hypocalcemia | When solubility product factor reaches 60 (Ca × P ≥60), calcium phosphate precipitates in microvasculature causing hypocalcemia | Cardiac arrythmia, cardiac arrest, Hypocalcemic tetany |

*(continued)*

| Biochemical abnormality | Pathophysiology | Clinical manifestations |
|---|---|---|
| Azotemia | Precipitation of uric acid crystals and calcium phosphate within renal tubules and vasculature leads to acute renal failure. Patients with massive TLS treated with allopurinol are at risk for xanthine nephropathy | Oliguria, fluid overload, pulmonary edema, cerebral edema, respiratory failure, hypoxia, and death |

## Management

- Aggressive hydration is the mainstay of therapy. It helps to dilute intravascular solutes, improves renal blood flow and glomerular filtration, and flushes precipitated solutes from renal tubules.
- However, fluid overload can lead to hyponatremia, pulmonary edema, and cerebral edema. Hence, close monitoring of fluid balance is essential.
- Secure venous access and a Foley catheter are necessary in most cases.
- Central venous monitoring may be required. For adequate urine output, mannitol and/or furosemide is often required.
- Patient should be euvolemic before the use of diuretic.
- Avoid known precipitating events (eg, avoid contrast agents during radiography: or nephrotoxic drugs).

Table 2 outlines the specific measures for prevention and management of tumor lysis syndrome.

## Indications for PICU Monitoring and/or Dialysis

- Consider PICU monitoring for patients with high risk of symptomatic tumor lysis syndrome.
- Patients with complications of preventative therapy (eg, respiratory distress secondary to fluid overload) should also be managed in a PICU.
- Dialysis is indicated if persistent and life-threatening electrolyte disturbances despite medical intervention, or in patients with oliguria. Nephrology consultation is advised if dialysis is anticipated.

*Table 2*
**Prevention and Management of Tumor Lysis Syndrome (Adopted from Howard et al.)**

| Biochemical abnormality | Intervention | Dose | Comments |
|---|---|---|---|
| Prevention of renal failure | Avoid nephrotoxic agents (eg, hyperosmolar contrast agents, NSAIDs, aminoglycosides) Resuscitate any existing shock state | N/A | N/A |
| Hydration and maintenance of renal perfusion | Fluid therapy | NS boluses if dehydrated until euvolemic then 2–4 times maintenance | Choice of fluid needs to be individualized Alkalinization of urine as below Do NOT add potassium, even if hypokalemia is present |
| | Mannitol or Furosemide | 0.5 g/kg <9 years q 6 h 15 g/m² ≥9 years q 6 h 1–2 mg/kg q 6 h | Diuretic therapy ONLY for adequately hydrated patients Use with caution |
| Hyperuricemia | Urine Alkalinization: (Aim: urine pH 6.5–7.5)   $NaHCO_3$ | 0.5–1 mEq/kg IV q4h as needed May be administered as continuous infusion with 20–100 mEq/L of IVF | Avoid over-alkalinization of urine which leads to intra-renal calcium phosphate deposit Reduce or discontinue $NaHCO_3$ if: |

| Biochemical abnormality | Intervention | Dose | Comments |
|---|---|---|---|
| | | | 1. Serum $HCO_3^-$ level ≥30 mEq/L |
| | | | 2. Urine pH >7.3 |
| | | | 3. African-American Serum uric acid level normalizes |
| | | | 4. Increase in serum phosphate, or |
| | | | 5. If patient is receiving urate oxidase |
| | Acetazolamide | 150 mg/m² PO q 6–8 h maximum 1 g/day | If the serum bicarbonate level is ≥ 30 mEq/L but urine not alkalinized with $NaHCO_3$ |
| | Allopurinol | 100–500 mg/m²/day, maximum 800 mg/day | Reduce the dose of allopurinol in presence of renal insufficiency |
| | Urate oxidase | Uricozyme 100 U/Kg Rasburicase 0.15 U/kg IV over 30 min q 12–24 h until uric acid levels normalize | Risk of allergic reactions including anaphylaxis<br>G6PD deficiency is a contraindication; in case G6PD status unknown, watch for hemolysis especially in boys, as ~10% are G6PD deficient<br>Use with caution in asthmatic patient |

(continued)

| Biochemical abnormality | Intervention | Dose | Comments |
|---|---|---|---|
| Hyperkalemia | Cation exchange resins | Sodium polystyrene sulfonate: PO/PR:0.5–1 g/kg/dose may be repeated q4–6h prn (usual maximum 30–60 g/dose) | Do not use for acute management<br>Hold potassium-containing fluids or food<br>Do NOT treat hypokalemia unless symptomatic |
| Hyperkalemia with EKG changes | NaHCO$_3$ | 0.5 mEq/kg IV push | Refer to hyperkalemia section in Chapter 12, Fluids and Electrolytes |
| | Calcium chloride | 10–20 mg/kg/dose | Urgent hemodialysis if no or transient response to medical management |
| | Dextrose/insulin | 0.5 g/kg of glucose IV with 0.1 U/kg of regular insulin | |
| Hyperphosphatemia | Aluminum hydroxide | 50–150 mg/kg/day PO divided q 6 h | Avoid over alkalinization of urine; alkaline urine reduces phosphate excretion and leads to intra-renal calcium-phosphate deposition |
| Symptomatic hypocalcemia | Calcium gluconate | 50 mg/kg IV over 10 minutes | |

NSAID = nonsteroidal anti-inflammatory drugs, IV = intravenous, PO = per orally EKG = electrocardiogram, U = units
Refer to formulary for additional dosing information.

Following are indications for either intermittent hemodialysis or continuous renal replacement therapy (CRRT):

- Renal failure
- Hyperkalemia
- Hyperphosphatemia
- Hyperuricemia
- Symptomatic hypocalcemia
- Volume overload

For details of CRRT, see Chapter 13, "Renal Replacement Therapy."

# References

Rheingold SR, Lange BJ. Oncologic emergencies. In: Pizzo PA, Poplack DG, eds. Principle and Practice of Pediatric Oncology, 4th ed. Philadelphia: Lippincott Williams & Wilkins; 2002, pp. 1177–1203.

Howard SC, Ribeiro RC, Pui CH. Acute complications. In: Pui CH, ed. Childhood Leukemias, 2nd ed. Cambridge: Cambridge University Press; 2006, Chapter 29, pp. 709–949.

Jones DP, Mahamoud H, Chesney RW. Tumor lysis syndrome: pathogenesis and management. Pedaitr Nephrol 1995;9:206–12.

Pui CH, Mahmoud HH, Wiley JM, et al. Recombinant urate oxidase for the prophylaxis or treatment of hyperuricemia in patients with leukemia or lymphoma. J Clin Oncol 2001;19:697–704.

# H. Fever and Neutropenia

Uma Athale

## Key Principles

> - **Fever:** This is defined as a single *oral* temperature of $\geq 38.3°C$ (101.0°F) **or** two oral temperatures of $\geq 38.0°C$ (100.4°F) taken one hour apart and not associated with administration of pyrogenic substances (such as blood products).
>   Axillary temperature measurements can be converted to oral temperature by adding 0.5°C. (Rectal temperature measurements can be converted to oral temperature by subtracting 0.5°C. Note that rectal temperature measurements are contraindicated in neutropenic patients.)
> - **Neutropenia:** Although neutropenia is defined as an absolute neutrophil count (ANC) of $<1.0 \times 10^9/L$, the risk of infection increases dramatically when the neutrophil count is less than $0.5 \times 10^9/L$. Hence, the term neutropenia in this chapter will be referred to as ANC $<0.5 \times 10^9/L$.
>   The afebrile neutropenic patient with an obvious focus suggestive of bacterial and/or fungal infection should be treated as other febrile neutropenic patients until the ANC recovers and infection is under control.

Infection is a major cause of significant morbidity and mortality in children on active therapy for cancer. Infections secondary to neutropenia are mainly bacterial and fungal. About half of neutropenic patients with fever have an established or occult infection and ~20% of patients with ANC $<0.1 \times 10^9/L$ have bacteremia. Symptoms or signs of infection may be minimal or absent in patients with severe neutropenia. Untreated sepsis has a high mortality; for this reason always assume that sepsis exists in the febrile neutropenic patient.

## Risk Factors

Risk factors for developing life-threatening infection in patients with fever and neutropenia:

1. Neutropenia: $<0.1 \times 10^9/L$; whether prolonged >7 days or of rapid onset

2. Absence of marrow recovery: declining ANC or absence of monocytes
3. Identified focus of infection (eg, GI, pulmonary, catheter)
4. Mucositis caused by chemotherapy, herpes simplex
5. Signs of sepsis: hypotension, rigors, altered mental status, respiratory distress
6. Unfavorable colonization: colonization with *P. aeruginosa* or *C. tropicalis*
7. Unfavorable cancer type: AML, T-cell ALL
8. Unfavorable cancer status: active or relapsed disease
9. Intense therapy: eg, high dose methotrexate or high dose Ara-C
10. Allogeneic BMT
11. Poor nutritional status: TPN increases the risk of infection

For the initial evaluation and management of patient with fever and neutropenia presenting with septic shock, please refer to Chapter 18, "Septic Shock."

## Management

After stabilization of patient, initiate broad-spectrum empiric antibiotic therapy; speed is important.

The choice of type and number of antibiotics may vary by institution. A guideline utilizing double coverage is outlined below Table 1. Monotherapy with pipracillin-tazonbactam or a fourth-generation cephalosporin is also an acceptable practice.

Neutropenic patients can have multiple infections; therefore, even in patients with known bacterial infections, antifungal therapy should be considered, as they are at risk of secondary fungal infection. A "fungal work-up" including imaging of sinuses, chest, abdomen, and pelvis should be performed. Try to do this imaging by MRI to decrease radiation dosing.

*Table 1*

**Guidelines for Initial Empiric Antibiotic Therapy for Patients with Fever and Neutropenia**

| Clinical status | Preferred antibiotics therapy for all patients | Alternative therapy for patients with [1]Penicillin allergy |
| --- | --- | --- |
| [2]Patients with fever and neutropenia | Piperacillin and gentamicin | Ceftazidime and gentamicin |

| Hemodynamically unstable patients Either at presentation, or deterioration while on therapy | | Piperacillin-tazobactam, gentamicin, and [4]vancomycin (Pip/Tazo provides adequate anaerobic coverage) | Ceftazidime, gentamicin, and [4]vancomycin, (+/- metron-idazole if anaerobic infection suspected) |
|---|---|---|---|
| When improved <u>gram +ve coverage</u> required | Evidence of skin, soft tissue, or line infection, or extensive mucositis or colonization with [3]MRSA | Piperacillin, gentamicin, and [4]vancomycin | Ceftazidime, gentamicin, and [4]vancomycin |
| When improved <u>anaerobic coverage</u> required | Perianal disease, or typhlitis, or intra-abdominal infection Dental or oral infection | Piperacillin, gentamicin, and metronidazole | Ceftazidime, gentamicin, and metronidazole |

[1] <u>Penicillin allergy</u>: Documentation of rash or hives (alone) while on penicillin is only a relative contradiction to its use. The cephalosporins or carbapenems can be used in this situation with caution. Consider ciprofloxacin as an alternative to ceftazidime in these situations.

[2] <u>Patients with renal impairment</u> will need to have the antibiotic dosage adjusted according to their creatinine clearance.

[3] <u>MRSA</u>: Methicillin resistant *S. aureus*.

[4] <u>Reassess vancomycin at 48 hours</u>. Vancomycin should not be continued beyond 48 hours unless a clinically significant resistant organism sensitive only to vancomycin is isolated. Vancomycin should not be added empirically for prolonged fever of unknown origin.

## Additional Considerations

1. Cases in which herpetic stomatitis or herpes zoster is evident, add acyclovir.
2. Patients with suspected oral and/or vaginal/perianal candidiasis, consider adding fluconazole while awaiting culture results.
3. Central venous cases in which pulmonary infection is suspected: eg, focal lesions (? *Aspergillus*) or interstitial pneumonitis

(? *Pneumocystis, Legionella, Mycoplasma*)—consider ID consultation to address further management.

4. Central venous catheter removal should be considered:

   1) when there is recurrent or persistent infection (eg, persistent positive blood culture after 2–3 days of appropriate antibacterial therapy)
   2) evidence of tunnel or periportal infection (eg, local swelling, erythema)
   3) septic emboli
   4) hypotension with catheter use
   5) a non-patent catheter

Organisms that warrant catheter removal without a trial of treatment include *S. aureus, Bacillus* species, fungi, and *Mycobacteria*.

**PICU Admission**    Patients with fever and neutropenia are at high risk for developing septic shock, and thus there should be a low threshold for referral to a medical emergency team or admission to the PICU. Indications for PICU admission include the following:

- Persistent or decompensated shock
- Patient requires 60 mL/kg of fluid resuscitation in a 12-hour period
- Deterioration or poor response to initial management of shock
- Respiratory failure or arrest
- Severe electrolyte abnormalities
- Prior history of sudden septic deterioration
- Focal or diffuse CXR abnormalities with significant tachypnea, or signs of respiratory distress

**Consultation with Infectious Disease Service**    Such consultation is recommended for cases with:

1. Consideration of alterations to the initial coverage with failure to respond
2. Positive blood culture
3. Pulmonary focus of infection
4. Hemodynamic instability
5. Transfer to the PICU
6. Consideration of antifungal therapy
7. Uncertain duration of treatment
8. Persistent fever for >4 days

## Continued Management

For continued management of patient with fever and neutropenia, please refer to Figure 1.

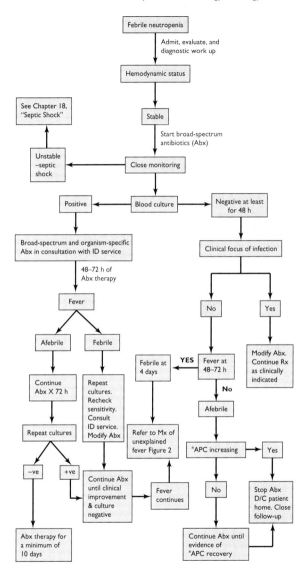

*APC = Absolute phagocyte (monocytes plus granulocytes) count

**Figure 1**   Initial management of patients with fever and neutropenia.

When fever persists >4 days while on antibiotics, consider following conditions:

1. Normal response (Some bacteremias cause fever for 3–5 days despite appropriate treatment.)
2. Non-bacterial infection (eg, viral or fungal)
3. Bacterial infection not covered by the antibacterial regimen
4. Second/new infection (eg, bacterial or fungal)
5. Inadequate drug levels
6. Infection at an avascular site (abscess or catheter infection)
7. Drug fever

At this point, re-evaluate the patient for an overt or occult focus of infection (eg, repeat blood cultures, imaging of sinuses, chest/abdomen/pelvis, if needed, preferably by MRI) and follow the guidelines for "persistent fever." (See Figure 2.)

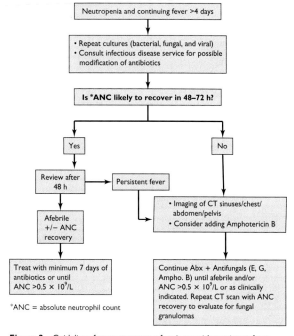

**Figure 2**  Guidelines for management of patients with persistent fever.

# References

Alexander SW, Walsh TJ, Freifeld G, Pizzo PA. Infectious complications in pediatric cancer patients. In: Pizzo PA, Poplack DG, eds. Principle and Practice of Pediatric Oncology, 4th ed. Philadelphia: Lippincott Williams & Wilkins; 2002; pp. 1177–1203.

Hughes WT, Armstrong D, Bodey GP, et al. Guidelines for the use of antimicrobial agents in neutropenic patients with cancer. Clin Infect Dis 2002;34:730–51.

Klasterskey J. Prevention of infection in neutropenic cancer patients. Curr Opin Oncol 1996;8:270–277.

McCullers JA, Shenep JL. Assessment and management of suspected infection in neutropenic patients. In: Patrick CC, ed. Clinical Management of Infections in Immunocompromised Infants and Children. Philadelphia: Lippincot Williams & Wilkins; 2001, pp. 353–87.

Pizzo PA. Current concepts: fever in immunocompromised patients. N Eng J Med 1999;341:893–900.

Pizzo PA. Management of fever in patients with cancer and treatment-induced neutropenia. N Eng J Med 1993;328:1323–31.

Shenep J. Outpatient management of the neutropenic patient with unexplained fever. Semin Pediatr Infect Dis 2000;11:105–12.

Wheelar AP, Bernard GR. Treating patients with severe sepsis. N Eng J Med 1999;340:207–14.

# I. Common Problems Related to Allogeneac Hematopoietic Stem Cell Transplantation (HSCT)

Brigitte Strahm

## Graft-versus-Host Disease

Allogenic HSCT is a high risk procedure associated with complications that may need intensive care. In addition to common medical problems like infections and organ toxicities, there are complications that are almost exclusive to the setting of allogeneic HSCT. The following section will focus on the most frequent of these HSCT-specific complications, namely Graft-versus-Host Disease and Sinusoidal Ostruction Syndrome/Veno Occlusive Disease.

Graft-versus-host disease (GVHD) is the most significant complication following allogeneic hematopoietic stem cell transplantation (HSCT). The transfer of non-histocompatible, immunocompetent donor cells into an immunoincompetent recipient results in an acute inflammatory disease that may affect skin, gastrointestinal tract, and liver. Although multiple preventive and therapeutic strategies have been developed, GVHD still remains the major limiting factor for long-term survival after HSCT. On the other hand, there is a beneficial effect of the donor immune reaction against residual malignant cells of recipient origin termed graft-versus-leukemia effect (GVL). A basic understanding of the balance between harmful (GVHD) and potentially beneficial (GVL) immune effects is crucial for a critical approach to prevention and therapy of GVHD.

## Incidence and Risk Factors

The incidence of moderate to severe (grade II–IV) GVHD in children transplanted from an HLA identical sibling is approx 35%, but may be much higher in the setting HSCT from unrelated or mismatched donors. Established risk factors for the development of GVHD are:

- HLA compatibility (matched sibling < matched unrelated < mismatched)
- Sex mismatch (female donor to male recipient ⇒ higher risk)

- Type of graft (cord blood < bone marrow < peripheral blood stem cells)
- Type of GVHD prophylaxis (T-cell depletion, intensity of immunosuppression)
- Age of recipient (younger < older)
- CMV status (negative < positive)

## Clinical Features and Grading

**Acute GVHD** is usually diagnosed within the first 100 days after HSCT. The main target organs are skin (maculopapular rash often involving the palms and soles), gastrointestinal tract (nausea; green, watery, and in severe cases, bloody diarrhea; abdominal pain), and liver (cholestatic liver disease). The organ involvement is defined by stage (Table 1), whereas the overall severity is defined by grade (Table 2).

*Table 1*
**GVHD Organ Involvement**

| Stage | Skin (surface area covered by rash) | Liver (bilirubin) | GI tract (volume of diarrhea) |
|---|---|---|---|
| 1 | < 5% | 34–50 mmol/L | 10–15 mL/kg/d or nausea |
| 2 | 25–50% | 51–102 mmol/L | 16–20 mL/kg/d |
| 3 | >50% | 103–255 mmol/L | 21–25 mL/kg/d |
| 4 | Erythroderma | 255 mmol/L | Severe abdominal pain +/− ileus |

*Table 2*
**Severity of GVHD**

| Grade | Skin (stage) | Liver (stage) | GI tract (stage) |
|---|---|---|---|
| I | 1–2 | 0 | 0 |
| II | 3 or | 1 or | 1 |
| III–IV | 4 or | 2–4 or | 2–4 |

**Chronic GVHD** is by definition diagnosed later than 100 days after HSCT. Skin involvement is very frequent (80%) and manifests as depigmentation, lichenoid papules, and dermal and subcutaneous fibrosis with alopecia. Other affected organs include mouth, eyes, nails, hair, genital organs, liver, lung, GI tract, joints, and muscles. The symptoms may resemble those of autoimmune diseases.

## Investigations

The diagnosis of acute as well as chronic GVHD is based on clinical observations. Biopsies (especially skin and gut) may be used to confirm the diagnosis. When isolated liver GVHD is suspected, liver biopsies can be helpful to rule out other causes of liver disease such as viral hepatitis and drug toxicity.

## Prophylaxis (Table 3)

The prevention of GVHD has been attempted by multiple strategies including immunosuppression of the host and in vitro or in vivo T-cell depletion of the graft. Despite a huge variety of regimes, the standard GVHD prophylaxis remains the same as established in 1986 in a large RCT including short course methotrexate and cyclosporine A. Depending on the estimated risk and the underlying disease, this regimen has been intensified or reduced in multiple ways.

## Treatment (Table 4)

**Symptomatic and supportive treatment** includes GI rest, parental alimentation, replacement of enteral fluid losses, and pain control. Prophylaxis and pre-emptive treatment of infections is crucial as viral, bacterial, and fungal infections are the major causes of death in patients with acute GVHD.

The established **first line therapy** for acute GVHD is methyl-prednisone (2 mg/kg/d) for 1–2 weeks in addition to the prophylactic regimen (usually cyclosporine). In case of a complete response, methyl-prednisone should be tapered after 1–2 weeks. The response to this initial treatment is of particular importance for the prognosis.

Failure of the initial therapy is usually defined as:

- Progression after 3 days of therapy
- No change after 7 days of therapy
- Incomplete response after 14 days of therapy

*Table 3*
**Possible Components of GVHD Prophylaxis**

| Intervention | Mechanism | Regimen | Major toxicities | Remarks |
|---|---|---|---|---|
| Short-course methotrexate | Nonspecific cytotoxic effect | 15 mg/m² d1 10 mg/m² d3/6/11 | Hepatotoxicity, mucositis | Usually combined with CsA |
| Cyclosporine A (CsA) | Calcineurin inhibitor; inhibition of T-cell function | 3 mg/kg/d ÷2 doses IV 5 mg/kg/d ÷2 doses p.o. | Renal dysfunction, hypokalemia, hypomagnesemia, tremor, hirsutism, hypertension, gingival hyperplasia | Dose-adjusted according to target trough levels (typically 100–200 ng/mL) |
| Tacrolimus | Calcineurin inhibitor; inhibition of T-cell function | 0.03 mg/kg/d c.i. | Renal dysfunction, hyperkalemia, hypomagnesemia, tremor, hypertension, nausea, diarrhea | Greater immunosuppressive potency compared to CsA, dose-adjusted according to target trough levels (typ. 10–20 ng/mL) |

*(continued)*

| Intervention | Mechanism | Regimen | Major toxicities | Remarks |
|---|---|---|---|---|
| Anti-thymocyte/anti-lymphocyte globuline (ATG) | Pan T-cell antibody, eradication of donor lymphocytes in vivo | Dose depending on specific product | Allergic reactions, profound immunosuppression | Mainly in HSCT from unrelated donors |
| CAMPATH-1H | Anti-CD52 monoclonal antibody eradication of donor lymphocytes in vivo | Variable regimens | Profound immunosuppression | Also used as "campath-in-the-bag" for in vitro T-cell depletion |
| T-cell depletion | Eradication of donor lymphocytes in vitro | n.a. | Impaired engraftment, delayed immune reconstitution, lack of GVL | Mainly in mismatched or haploidentical HSCT |
| Mycophenolate mofetil (MMF) | Blocking of T- and B-cell proliferation | 1200 mg/m$^2$/d ÷ q12h | Neutropenia, gut ulceration | Frequently used with reduced intensity conditioning regimens |
| Corticosteroids | Inhibition of T-cell proliferation and function | Variable regimens | Hypertension, hyperglycemia, etc. | Role in prevention controversial |

Table 4
**Options for Second Line Therapy in Acute GVHD**

| Intervention | Mechanism | Regimen | Major toxicities | Remarks |
|---|---|---|---|---|
| MMF<sup></sup> | Inhibition of T-cell proliferation and function | 1200 mg/m²/d ÷ q12h 1800 mg/m²/d ÷ q8h | Neutropenia, gut ulceration | |
| Daclizumab | Monoclonal anti-IL2 receptor antibody | 1 mg/kg/day iv on days 1, 4, 8, 15, and 22 | No specific toxicities | |
| Infliximab | Monoclonal anti-TNF alpha antibody | 10 mg/kg iv once weekly | No specific toxicities | Possibly greater benefit with GI involvement |
| ATG | Pan T-cell antibody, eradication of donor lymphocytes in vivo | Dose depending on specific product | Allergic reactions, profound immunosuppression | |
| Extracorporeal photophoresis | Immunomodulation by UV-A irradiation of mononuclear cells collected by apheresis and photosensitized by 8-methoxypsoralen | Starting at 3 days/week or 2 consecutive days/ week | None | Venous access must be suitable for apheresis |

Failure of the primary therapy should result in initiation of the **second line therapy**. There is no uniform approach to steroid refractory GVHD and the decision will be triggered by the type of GVHD prophylaxis received, the main organ manifestation, the toxicity profile of the potential drug, and the underlying disease. The following table will give an overview for possible strategies.

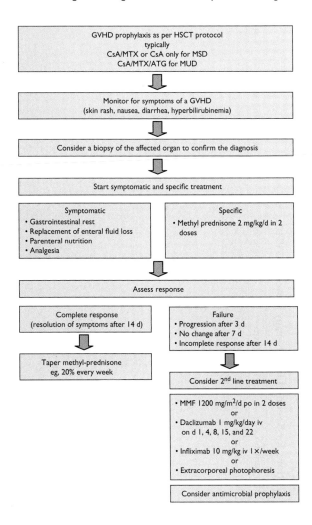

GVHD prophylaxis as per HSCT protocol
typically
CsA/MTX or CsA only for MSD
CsA/MTX/ATG for MUD

Monitor for symptoms of a GVHD
(skin rash, nausea, diarrhea, hyperbilirubinemia)

Consider a biopsy of the affected organ to confirm the diagnosis

Start symptomatic and specific treatment

| Symptomatic | Specific |
| --- | --- |
| • Gastrointestinal rest<br>• Replacement of enteral fluid loss<br>• Parenteral nutrition<br>• Analgesia | • Methyl prednisone 2 mg/kg/d in 2 doses |

Assess response

| Complete response (resolution of symptoms after 14 d) | Failure<br>• Progression after 3 d<br>• No change after 7 d<br>• Incomplete response after 14 d |
| --- | --- |

Taper methyl-prednisone
eg, 20% every week

Consider 2nd line treatment

• MMF 1200 mg/m²/d po in 2 doses
or
• Daclizumab 1 mg/kg/day iv
on d 1, 4, 8, 15, and 22
or
• Infliximab 10 mg/kg iv 1×/week
or
• Extracorporeal photophoresis

Consider antimicrobial prophylaxis

GVHD and its therapy results in a high level of immuno-suppression and patients are at risk of infections. Antimicrobial prophylaxis should be considered for these patients.

The **first line therapy** for **chronic** GVHD is based on prednisone in combination with CsA. Possibilities for **second line therapy** include ECP, MMF, tacrolimus, and thalidomide.

# Sinusoidal Obstruction Syndrome/Veno-Occlusive Disease

Sinusoidal obstruction syndrome (SOS)/veno-occlusive disease (VOD) of the liver is the term used to designate the signs and symptoms that appear early (usually within the first 3–4 weeks) after hematopoietic stem cell transplantation (HSCT) as a result of endothelial and hepatocyte damage caused by the chemo-radio-therapy of the conditioning regimen. The syndrome is character-ized by hepatomegaly frequently combined with upper quadrant pain, fluid retention, weight gain, and hyperbilirubinemia.

## Incidence and Risk Factors

The incidence of SOS after HSCT in children has been reported between 10% and 60% in different series depending on the presence of risk factors. Established risk factors are:

- Pre-existing liver disease (eg, previous hepatotoxic chemo-therapy, abdominal irradiation, viral hepatitis, iron overload).
- Conditioning regimen including busulfan, especially in combina-tion with cyclophosphamide.
- Allogeneic HSCT (vs autologous HSCT).
- 2nd HSCT/HSCT beyond the 2nd relapse.

## Clinical Features

SOS is usually diagnosed within the first 3 weeks after HSCT according to either the modified Seattle or the Baltimore criteria. Occasionally, SOS may develop later in the course of post-HSCT.

- Seattle criteria (modified): In the first 20 days after HSCT, two or more of the following:

  - Bilirubin >34.2 μmol/L (>2 mg/dl)
  - Hepatomegaly or right upper-quadrant pain
  - Weight gain (>2% basal weight)

- Baltimore criteria

1. In the first 21 days after HSCT bilirubin >34.2 μmol/L (>2 mg/dl) and at least two of the following:

   - Painful hepatomegaly
   - Ascites
   - Weight gain (>5% basal weight)

In severe cases, refractoriness to platelet transfusions, signs of progressive multi-organ failure (especially renal and pulmonary), and encephalopathy may be present. The mortality varies according to the severity of the clinical presentation and has been reported to be up to 90% in patients with severe SOS and multi-organ failure. To accept the diagnosis of SOS causes of similar clinical features as graft-versus-host-disease, infections and drug toxicity should be excluded as far as possible.

## Investigations

The following investigations may be helpful in confirming the clinical diagnosis of SOS and excluding other causes of the symptoms:

- **Ultrasound:** Gall bladder thickening, ascites, hepatomegaly, attenuated or reversed portal flow.
- **Histology:** Confirmation by classical histological changes as concentric non-thrombotic narrowing of the lumen of small intrahepatic veins. Exclusion of differential diagnoses such as graft-versus-host disease or viral hepatitis.
- **Hemodynamic study:** A hepatic venous gradient pressure of 10 mm Hg in a patient without previous liver disease is indicative of SOS (usually not feasible).

## Prophylaxis (Table 5)

Given the severity of the disease, several preventive strategies including prostaglandine E1, pentoxifyllin, ursodeoxycholic, acid and heparin have been suggested, but no single strategy has been established yet.

## Treatment (Table 6)

**Symptomatic treatment** with the goal of reducing fluid overload while maintaining the intravascular volume and urine output:

- Restriction of crystalloid fluid administration

*Table 5*
**Prophylaxis for SOS/VOD**

| Intervention | Mechanism | Evidence | Conclusion |
|---|---|---|---|
| Prostaglandine E1 | Vasodilatation, inhibition of platelet aggregation, stimulation of t-PA release | Reduction of incidence of SOS in a non-randomized trial<br>No effect and high incidence of side effects in phase I/II study | Not recommended |
| Pentoxifyllin | Increase in regional blood flow and local thrombolysis | No reduction of SOS incidence in 2 RCTs | Not recommended |
| Ursodeoxycholic acid 10–20 mg/kg/d ÷ bid | Reduction of hydrophobic bile acid | Reduction of SOS incidence in 2 RCTs, no reduction in 2 RCTs, no major side effects | Possible benefit |
| Heparin 100 U/kg/d c.i. | Anti-thrombotic activity | Non-significant reduction of SOS in meta-analysis<br>2 of 3 included RCTs suggest benefit | Possible benefit |
| Defibrotide 40–100 mg/kg/d ÷ q6h | Anti-thrombotic activity<br>Thrombolytic activity | Significant reduction of SOS in case series compared to historical controls | Possible benefit |

- Diuretics
- Red blood cell transfusion if indicated

**Specific Treatment** should be initiated as soon as the diagnosis is established as early intervention has been associated with a better outcome.

**Prior to HSCT**

Assess risk of SOS
(previous liver disease, conditioning, type of HSCT, state of disease)
Consider prophylaxis
(heparin, ursodeoxycholic acid, defibrotide)

**Early (first 3 weeks) after HSCT**

Monitor clinical signs and symptoms
(hyperbilirubinemia, hepatomegaly, fluid retention, weight gain)

Accept clinical diagnosis of SOS,
if clinical signs are present (Seattle/Baltimore criteria)
and differential diagnoses are unlikely

| DD: GVHD | DD: viral hepatitis | DD: drug toxicity |
|---|---|---|
| • timepoint in course of HSCT (SOS earlier vs GVHD later)<br>• engraftment<br>• involvement of other organs (skin rash, diarrhea) | • liver function tests (SOS ↑ vs hepatitis ↑↑)<br>• screening for viral infections | • evaluate medications (azoles, MTX, CsA etc.) |

Consider additional investigations

| Abdominal ultrasound | Liver biopsy |
|---|---|
| (hepatomegaly, ascites, gall bladder wall thickening, attenuated or inversed portal flow) | Histological confirmation/exclusion of other pathologies<br>High risk procedure usually reserved for atypical cases |

Initiate symptomatic and specific treatment without delay

| Symptomatic | Specific |
|---|---|
| • fluid restriction<br>• diuretics<br>• maintenance of intravascular volume (RBC transfusions)<br>• others (analgesia, ventilation, dialysis) as indicated | Defibrotide 25 mg/kg/d √q6h or Defibrotide 15–60 mg/kg/d √q6h |

*Table 6*
## Treatment of SOS/VOD

| Intervention | Mechanism | Evidence | Conclusion |
| --- | --- | --- | --- |
| Recombinant humanized tissue plasminogen activator (rh tPA) | Thrombolytic activity | Low response rate and significant side effects (severe bleeding) in case series | Not recommended |
| Defibrotide 25 mg/kg/d ÷ q6h (sickkids) 15–60 mg/kg/d ÷ q6h (UKF)* | Anti-thrombotic activity Thrombolytic activity | Response rate of 36–75% in three case series, no severe side effects | Most promising and safe approach |

*The optimal dosing remains to be determined. Although several studies use incremental dosing, there is no pharmacological or clinical rational.

# References

Storb R, et al. Methotrexate and cyclosporine compared with cyclosporine alone for prophylaxis of acute graft versus host disease after marrow transplantation for leukemia. N Engl J Med 1986;314(12):729–35.

Nash RA, et al. Phase 3 study comparing methotrexate and tacrolimus with methotrexate and cyclosporine for prophylaxis of acute graft-versus-host disease after marrow transplantation from unrelated donors. Blood 2000;96(6):2062–8.

Bacigalupo A. Antilymphocyte/thymocyte globulin for graft versus host disease prophylaxis: efficacy and side effects. Bone Marrow Transplant 2005;35(3):225–31.

Hale G, et al. Improving the outcome of bone marrow transplantation by using CD52 monoclonal antibodies to prevent graft-versus-host disease and graft rejection. Blood 1998;92(12):4581–90.

Basara N, et al. Mycophenolate mofetil for the treatment of acute and chronic GVHD in bone marrow transplant patients. Bone Marrow Transplant 1998;22(1):61–5.

Basara N, et al. Mycophenolate mofetil in the treatment of acute and chronic GVHD in hematopoietic stem cell transplant patients: four years of experience. Transplant Proc 2001;33(3):2121–3.

Baudard M, et al. Mycophenolate mofetil for the treatment of acute and chronic GVHD is effective and well tolerated but induces a high risk of infectious complications: a series of 21 BM or PBSC transplant patients. Bone Marrow Transplant 2002;30(5):287–95.

Kiehl MG, et al. Mycophenolate mofetil in stem cell transplant patients in relation to plasma level of active metabolite. Clin Biochem 2000;33(3):203–8.

Przepiorka D, et al. Daclizumab, a humanized anti-interleukin-2 receptor alpha chain antibody, for treatment of acute graft-versus-host disease. Blood 2000;95(1):83–9.

Srinivasan R, et al. Improved survival in steroid-refractory acute graft versus host disease after non-myeloablative allogeneic transplantation using a daclizumab-based strategy with comprehensive infection prophylaxis. Br J Haematol 2004;124(6):777–86.

Teachey DT, Bickert B, Bunin N. Daclizumab for children with corticosteroid refractory graft-versus-host disease. Bone Marrow Transplant 2006;37(1): 95–9.

Couriel D, et al. Tumor necrosis factor-alpha blockade for the treatment of acute GVHD. Blood 2004;104(3):649–54.

Patriarca F, et al. Infliximab treatment for steroid-refractory acute graft-versus-host disease. Haematologica 2004;89(11):1352–9.

MacMillan ML, et al. Early antithymocyte globulin therapy improves survival in patients with steroid-resistant acute graft-versus-host disease. Biol Blood Marrow Transplant 2002;8(1):40–6.

Tagliabue A, et al. Favourable response to antithymocyte globulin therapy in resistant acute graft-versus-host disease. Bone Marrow Transplant 2005;36(5):459.

Kanold J, et al. Update on extracorporeal photochemotherapy for graft-versus-host disease treatment. Bone Marrow Transplant 2005;35(Suppl 1):S69–71.

McDonald GB, et al. Venocclusive disease of the liver after bone marrow transplantation: diagnosis, incidence, and predisposing factors. Hepatology 1984;4(1):116–22.

Jones RJ, et al. Venoocclusive disease of the liver following bone marrow transplantation. Transplantation 1987;44(6):778–83.

Gluckman E. et al. Use of prostaglandin E1 for prevention of liver venoocclusive disease in leukaemic patients treated by allogeneic bone marrow transplantation. Br J Haematol 1990;74(3):277–81.

Bearman SI, et al. A phase I/II study of prostaglandin E1 for the prevention of hepatic venocclusive disease after bone marrow transplantation. Br J Haematol 1993;84(4):724–30.

Attal M, et al. Prevention of regimen-related toxicities after bone marrow transplantation by pentoxifylline: a prospective, randomized trial. Blood 1993;82(3):732–6.

Clift RA, et al. A randomized controlled trial of pentoxifylline for the prevention of regimen-related toxicities in patients undergoing allogeneic marrow transplantation. Blood 1993;82(7):2025–30.

Essell JH, et al. Ursodiol prophylaxis against hepatic complications of allogeneic bone marrow transplantation. A randomized, double-blind, placebo-controlled trial. Ann Intern Med 1998;128(12 Pt 1):975–81.

Ohashi K, et al. The Japanese multicenter open randomized trial of ursodeoxycholic acid prophylaxis for hepatic veno-occlusive disease after stem cell transplantation. Am J Hematol 2000;64(1):32–8.

Park SH, et al. A randomized trial of heparin plus ursodiol vs. heparin alone to prevent hepatic veno-occlusive disease after hematopoietic stem cell transplantation. Bone Marrow Transplant 2002;29(2):137–43.

Ruutu T, et al. Ursodeoxycholic acid for the prevention of hepatic complications in allogeneic stem cell transplantation. Blood 2002;100(6):1977–83.

Imran H, et al. Use of prophylactic anticoagulation and the risk of hepatic veno-occlusive disease in patients undergoing hematopoietic stem cell transplantation: a systematic review and meta-analysis. Bone Marrow Transplant 2006;37(7):677–86.

Chalandon Y, et al. Prevention of veno-occlusive disease with defibrotide after allogeneic stem cell transplantation. Biol Blood Marrow Transplant 2004;10(5):347–54.

Bearman SI, et al. Treatment of hepatic venocclusive disease with recombinant human tissue plasminogen activator and heparin in 42 marrow transplant patients. Blood 1997;89(5):1501–6.

Chopra R, et al. Defibrotide for the treatment of hepatic veno-occlusive disease: results of the European compassionate-use study. Br J Haematol 2000;111(4):1122–9.

Corbacioglu S., et al. Defibrotide in the treatment of children with veno-occlusive disease (VOD): a retrospective multicentre study demonstrates therapeutic efficacy upon early intervention. Bone Marrow Transplant 2004;33(2):189–95.

Richardson PG, et al. Multi-institutional use of defibrotide in 88 patients after stem cell transplantation with severe veno-occlusive disease and multisystem organ failure: response without significant toxicity in a high-risk population and factors predictive of outcome. Blood 2002;100(13):4337–43.

# Chapter 18

# Infection

## A. Septic Shock

Lennox Huang

### Key Principles

- Assess and manage ABCs according to PALS/ACCM guidelines.
- Early rapid fluid resuscitation is associated with improved outcomes.
- Do not delay treatment in order to obtain diagnosis.
- Inotropic therapy should be reserved for shock that is refractory to multiple fluid boluses.
- Clinical endpoints include improvement in vital signs, and peripheral and end-organ perfusion.
- Biochemical endpoints may include serum lactate, metabolic acid/base balance, and central venous $O_2$ saturation.
- Both clinical and biochemical therapeutic endpoints should be used to assess efficacy of therapy.
- Attempt to identify and treat focus of infection.

### Background

- Sepsis is the fourth most common reason for admission to a pediatric hospital in the United States.
- Severe sepsis and septic shock forms a leading cause of death in children.
- Overall associated pediatric mortality rate of 8–10%.
- Mortality is higher in certain subpopulations, notably post-bone marrow transplant.

- Mortality increases with each additional organ system affected.
- Early aggressive fluid resuscitation and early empiric antibiotic therapy improve outcome from septic shock.
- Septic shock may present with either a normal, high, or low cardiac output.
- A high suspicion for sepsis in children with abnormal vital signs is key to early recognition and treatment.

## Major Physiology/Pathophysiology

Shock is defined as inadequate oxygen delivery to meet metabolic needs. Septic shock results from a complex cascade of inflammatory mediators initiated by an infectious etiology. In this chapter, the section "Sepsis and Bacteremia" deals with initiating insults for septic shock.

Pathophysiology begins at the micro-cellular level with a multitude of mediators involved in the systemic inflammatory response syndrome (SIRS), and ends with varying degrees of multi-organ dysfunction (MODS) and failure. Actions of and interactions between specific mediators is complex and remains controversial. Table 1 lists some of the mediators implicated in septic shock.

*Table 1*
**Mediators and Systems Involved in Septic Shock**

| |
|---|
| Arachidonic acid metabolites (leukotrienes, prostaglandins, thromboxanes) |
| Cytokines: TNF-alpha, IL-1, 2, 6, 10 |
| Complement system |
| Coagulation cascade |
| Fibrinolytic system |
| Catecholamines |
| Glucocorticoids |
| Prekallikrein |
| Bradykinin |
| Histamines |
| Beta-endorphins |
| Enkephalins |
| Adrenocorticoid hormone |
| Circulating myocardial depressant factor(s) |

- At a microvascular level, systemic inflammation leads to the following:

  - Vasodilatation and vasoconstriction
  - Endothelial damage
  - Microthrombi
  - Capillary leak

- End organs are affected in the following way:

  - Poor perfusion
  - Ischemia
  - Direct depression (eg, myocardial depressant factor)

## Differential Diagnosis

Consider all other etiologies for shock—see Chapter 5, "Shock."

The following diagnoses may closely mimic septic shock in initial presentation:

- Adrenal insufficiency—see Chapter 16.
- Hemophagocytic lymphohistiocytosis—see Chapter 17.
- Critical aortic stenosis—see Chapter 8A Cardiac Assessment of Patients with Suspected Heart Disease (pre-cardiac surgery).
- Pancreatitis—see Chapter 14.
- Fulminant hepatic failure—see Chapter 14.
- Inborn errors of metabolism—see Chapter 19.

Note that excessive fluid management may worsen cardiogenic shock.

## Clinical Features

Septic shock is diagnosed clinically by a combination of:

1) Patient risk factors for sepsis (eg, age, burns, severe head injury, cancer, congenital or acquired immunodeficiency)
2) Physical exam—fever, altered vital signs (tachycardia, tachypnea, wide pulse pressure, hypotension), altered end organ (eg, mental status, urine output) or peripheral perfusion (poor capillary refill)
3) Laboratory data—white count, acidosis, positive blood cultures

Table 7 lists reference values for the identification of septic shock. Early/warm septic shock is often subtle in clinical presentation (hyperdynamic circulation, high cardiac output, vasodilated, wide pulse pressures). Late/cold septic shock is more obvious. Many end organs can be affected by septic shock (Table 3).

*Table 2*
**Alterations in Vital Signs**

|  | Early septic shock | Late septic shock |
| --- | --- | --- |
| Heart rate | Tachycardia | Tachycardia or bradycardia |
| Respiratory rate | Tachypnea | Tachypnea or apnea |
| Blood pressure | Wide or normal | Low |

*Table 3*
**End Organs Potentially Affected in Septic Shock**

| Organ system | Clinical manifestations |
| --- | --- |
| Brain | Altered mental status |
| Kidney | Acute renal failure with oliguria or anuria Urine output can be used to monitor effectiveness of resuscitative efforts |
| Pulmonary | Hypoxia and hypercapnia—from shunt and from poor cardiac output ARDS develops in up to 40% of patients |
| Cardiac | Poor cardiac output in late stages of septic shock |
| Splanchnic | Malabsorption and ileus Pancreatitis Hepatic dysfunction |
| Hematologic | DIC may develop in up to 40% of patients resulting in thrombosis or hemorrhage |

*Table 4*
**Investigations**

| Blood gas | Provides a measure of tissue perfusion, cardiac function, and guides resuscitation |
| --- | --- |
| Serum lactate | Persistent lactic academia is linked with poor prognosis in adult studies |
| CBC | Abnormal leukocyte count for age is part of defining criteria for sepsis Platelets may increase as an acute phase reactant or decrease if DIC is present |

(continued)

| Electrolytes | Altered by capillary leak, renal dysfunction, fluid resuscitation |
| Serum glucose | Hypoglycemia may be early indicator of sepsis in infants and neonates; hyperglycemia in septic shock is associated with poor outcome |
| Liver enzymes | Elevated transaminases are an early sign of liver involvement |
| Coagulation studies | May be abnormal from poor end-organ perfusion or DIC |
| Cultures | Blood cultures may be negative in up to 30% of patients with septic shock. Remember urine and tracheal cultures as well Cultures should be repeated if patient is persistently febrile or has initially positive cultures |
| Lumbar puncture | If patient is hemodynamically stable |
| Cortisol level | For vasopressor-resistant shock, may use random cortisol level or cortisol stimulation test |
| Procalcitonin | May be a marker for bacterial sepsis; elevated levels correlated with poor outcome |
| Chest X-ray | Should routinely be performed for patients with septic shock |
| Echocardiogram | May help guide choice of inotropic or vasopressor support (see Tables 5 and 6) |
| Other | Additional imaging for the nidus of infection may be needed after initial resuscitation |

## Management

*Definitive airway management:*

- Perform early intubation or noninvasive positive pressure ventilation even in absence of respiratory distress—delays may lead to crash intubations.
- Mechanical ventilation can diminish metabolic demands by removing work of breathing.
- Always use lung-protective strategies in mechanical ventilation.

*Vascular access and monitoring:*

- Central venous access is essential for vasopressors, CVP, and $SCVO_2$ monitoring.

  - Low $SVO_2$ <65 $SCVO_2$ <70 may indicate incomplete resuscitation or myocardial involvement.
  - High $SVO_2$ >80 often seen in septic shock.
  - Normal or high $SVO_2$ does not necessarily indicate adequate resuscitation.

- A large-bore IV is necessary for rapid fluid administration.
- Swan-Ganz catheters do not improve outcome in the pediatric population and are not routinely used.
- Central or peripheral arterial line for continuous pressure monitoring if patient requires inotropic or vasopressor therapy.
- Oscillometric, noninvasive blood pressure measurements are inaccurate in shock states.
- Place Foley catheter to follow urine output.

*Fluid management:*

- Massive isotonic fluids boluses are often needed early in management.
- In the setting of continued vascular leak, continued fluid resuscitation is required.
- Administer 20 mL/kg boluses as needed every 15 minutes—may require up to 200 mL/kg initially.
- Fluids should be titrated to a combination of heart rate, blood pressure, perfusion, and central venous pressure.
- There is no difference in patient outcomes between isotonic crystalloid versus colloid solutions for acute resuscitation.

*Early goal-directed therapy (EGDT):*

- Defined as the titration of resuscitation to physiologic and biochemical endpoints reflecting cardiac output.
- Studies in adults utilized a set protocol for patients presenting to the emergency department.
- Key protocol components of adult EGDT protocols include:

  - Early invasive central venous monitoring, arterial catheterization, urine catheterization.
  - Initial rapid fluid resuscitation to a CVP target.
  - Inotropic support according to mean arterial pressure.
  - Blood transfusion to a hemoglobin of 100 g/L.
  - Activated protein C for patients without contraindications.

- An adult trial of EGDT has demonstrated lower mortality for patients managed with EGDT.
- Earlier pediatric studies have supported individual components of EGDT, but have not protocolized it to the same extent.

*Empiric antibiotics:*

- Should be administered within an hour of recognition of septic shock.
- Delay in antibiotic administration is associated with increased mortality.
- Antibiotics should not be delayed for prolonged attempts at obtaining blood cultures or other diagnostic investigations.
- Antibiotic choice should be tailored to the specific clinical situation.

*Sodium bicarbonate:*

- Do not use simply to correct lactic acidosis.
- No evidence to support its use in improving hemodynamics or vasopressor effectiveness.
- May worsen intracellular acidosis.
- May be effective for pH lower than 7.15.

*Vasopressors and inotropes (Tables 5 and 6):*

- Should be considered after adequate fluid resuscitation.
- Require central venous access for safe and consistent delivery.
- Infusions should be titrated to maintain low-normal blood pressure.
- Supranormal blood pressures increase afterload and may negatively impact cardiac output.
- There is inadequate randomized controlled trial evidence regarding the optimal choice of inotropes and vasopressors for pediatric septic shock.
- Infusions should be tailored to the specific clinical and physiologic scenario. Table 4 matches potential physiologic states with suggested inotropic or vasopressor therapy.

*Blood products:*

- Optimal level of hemoglobin is yet to be determined:

  - the following guideline is based on a combination of non-randomized human and animal studies as well as consensus agreement.

*Table 5*
**Septic Shock Physiology and Choice of Inotropic or Vasopressor Therapy**

| Physiologic state | Initial therapy | Secondary therapy |
|---|---|---|
| ↓ CO + ↑ SVR | Fluid resuscitation | Inodilator or inotrope + vasodilator eg, milrinone Or milrinone + norepinephrine Or nitroprusside + epinephrine or norepinephrine |
| ↑ CO + ↓ SVR | Fluid resuscitation | Vasopressor eg, high dose dopamine, epinephrine, or norepinephrine |
| ↓ CO + ↓ SVR | Fluid resuscitation | Inotrope or inodilator + vasopressor eg, high dose dopamine, epinephrine Or milrinone + norepinephrine Or nitroprusside + norepinephrine or epinephrine |

CO—Cardiac Output
SVR—Systemic Vascular Resistance

- Consider packed cell transfusion if patient is in a shock state and has a hemoglobin <100 g/L.
- Patients may tolerate lower levels (70–90 g/L) when stabilized.

*Steroids:*

- Indication: Catecholamine-resistant shock and suspected adrenal insufficiency

  - Random cortisol level ≤18 µg/dL (496 nmol/L), or
  - Cortisol-stimulation test level ≤9 µg/dL (248 nmol/L)

- High dose steroids are not supported by literature.
- Low or stress dose steroids may have role in septic shock.

*Table 6*
## Vasopressor and Inotrope Use in Septic Shock

| | |
|---|---|
| Dopamine | Indication: to improve cardiac output + blood pressure<br>Often used as early first line therapy<br>Consider starting with norepinephrine or epinephrine in patients under 6 months of age<br>If patient is in severe decompensated shock, consider starting with norepinephrine or epinephrine<br>If doses >10 mcg/kg/min are needed for prolonged periods, consider switching to norepinephrine and adding milrinone<br>No role for routine renal dose dopamine |
| Epinephrine | Indication: to improve cardiac output + blood pressure<br>High doses can compromise peripheral perfusion + result in tissue necrosis<br>Can decrease splanchnic perfusion<br>Increases myocardial oxygen demand |
| Norepinephrine | Indication: to improve blood pressure, smaller inotropic effect<br>More potent vasopressor than dopamine<br>Favorable splanchnic flow distribution<br>First line therapy in adults to treat blood pressure refractory to fluid resuscitation |
| Milrinone | Indication: to improve cardiac output + tissue perfusion without chronotropy<br>Frequently used in combination with a vasopressor agent (eg, norepinephrine) for patients with low cardiac output determined by low $SVO_2$, physical exam, or echocardiogram<br>Do not use loading dose in hemodynamically unstable patients |
| Vasopressin | Indication: catecholamine refractory vasodilatory shock<br>Evidence for pediatric use is unclear |
| Dobutamine | Indication: to improve cardiac output<br>Use is often precluded secondary to tachyphylaxis |
| Phenylephrine | Indication: refractory vasodilatory shock<br>May decrease stroke volume<br>Evidence for pediatric use is unclear |

- Steroids may be administered intermittently or as a continuous infusion.
- Dexamethasone or hydrocortisone are steroids of choice for stress dosing.
- Routine empiric use is controversial in pediatric patients.
- Consider empiric use in patients on recent systemic steroid therapy.

*Activated protein C:*

- Rates of hemorrhagic complications exceed potential benefit in pediatric patients.
- Not recommended for use in pediatric patients.

*Continuous renal replacement therapy (CRRT):*

- May be required for MODS resulting in oliguric renal failure,
- CRRT has been shown to be beneficial for patients with septic shock and oliguria.
- Early use of CRRT to modify the inflammatory response is controversial. Some practitioners suggest that continuous veno-venous hemofiltration (CVVH) without dialysis may be beneficial when initiated early in septic shock. Randomized, controlled data is lacking for both adult and pediatric patients.
- See Chapter 13, in "Renal Replacement Therapy," for additional details.

*Nutrition:*

- Start nutrition early.
- Enteral nutrition is preferred.

*Table 7*
## Reference Values for Pediatric Septic Shock

| Age | Normal heart rate | Upper limit resting respiratory rate | Lower limit of systolic BP | Abnormal leukocyte count |
|---|---|---|---|---|
| Newborn | 180–100 | >50 | 60 | >34 |
| 1 mo–1 yr | 180–90 | >34 | 70 | >17.5 or <5 |
| 2–5 yr | 140–80 | >22 | 70 + age × 2 | >15.5 or <6 |
| 6–12 yrs | 130–60 | >18 | 70 + age × 2 | >13.5 or <4.5 |
| >13 yrs | 100-60 | >14 | 90 | >11 or <4.5 |

Modified from Goldstein, et al. Pediatr Crit Care Med 2005

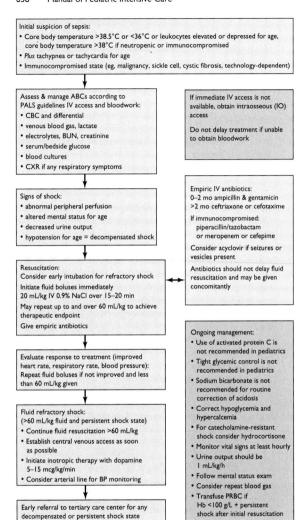

**Figure 1**   Septic shock flowchart.
Modified from Pediatric Critical Care Network (Ontario). Clinical practice guideline: Septic shock. 2006.

- Septic ileus may interfere with enteral nutrition early in the course of disease.
- Overall nutritional requirements are high in septic shock.
- Over-feeding is associated with poor outcomes.
- Insufficient evidence to recommend immunonutrition.

*Glycemic control:*

- Hyperglycemia is associated with poor outcomes.
- Tight glycemic control is recommended in adult population as part of the surviving sepsis campaign.
- Associated with improved mortality/morbidity in adult ICUs but not recommended for pediatric ICU population.
- Retrospective review suggests that it may benefit subgroup of pediatric burn patients by decreasing number of infections.

*ECMO:*

- Criteria for extracorporeal support vary between centers.
- According to ESLO registry data, there is 76% survival in neonates, and some centers are up to 80%.
- 50% survival for all other pediatric patients.
- See "Extracorporeal Life Support in the PICU (ECMO)" in Chapter 8 for additional details.

*Therapeutic endpoints of resuscitation:*

- Clinical—improved vital signs, perfusion
- $SVO_2$—may be used in patients without cyanotic heart disease
- A-V $O_2$ difference
  - Trends in lactate

# References

Annane D, Bellisant E, Bollaert PE, et al. Corticosteroids for treating severe sepsis and septic shock. Cochrane Database Syst Rev 2004;(1):CD002243.

Branco RG, Garcia PC, Piva JP, et al. Glucose level and risk of mortality in pediatric septic shock. Pediatr Crit Care Med 2005 Jul;6(4):470–2.

Carcillo JA, Fields AI. Clinical practice parameters for hemodynamic support of pediatric and neonatal patients in septic shock. Crit Care Med 2002;30(6)1365–78.

Carcillo JA, Davis AL, Zaritsky A. Role of early fluid resuscitation in pediatric septic shock. JAMA 1991;266:1242–5.

Goldstein B, et al. International pediatric sepsis consensus conference: definitions for sepsis and organ dysfunction in pediatrics. Pediatr Crit Care Med 2005(6)1:2–8.

Ham Y, Carcillo JA, Dragotta M, et al. Early reversal of pediatric-neonatal septic shock by community physicians is associated with improved outcome. Pediatr 2003(112):4:793–9.

Lodha R, Vivekanandhan S, Sarthi M, Kabra SK. Serial circulating vasopressin levels in children with septic shock. Pediatr Crit Care Med 2006 Mar 28; 2006 May;7(3):220–4.

Huang L. Pediatric Critical Care Network (Ontario). Clinical practice guideline: Septic shock.  2006. Available at: www.criticall.com

Saladino R. Management of septic shock in the pediatric emergency department in 2004. Clin Ped Emerg Med 2004;5:20–7.

# B. Toxic Shock Syndrome (TSS)

Anupma Wadhwa

## Key Principles

- Characterized by acute onset of fever, hypotension, renal failure, and multi-system organ involvement.
- Caused by toxin-producing *Staphylococcus* aureus or group A streptococcus.
- Both forms can be associated with an invasive infection (pneumonia, osteomyelitis, endocarditis) or no identifiable focus.

## Staphylococcal TSS

Staphylococcal TSS typically presents with profuse watery diarrhea, vomiting, erythroderma, conjunctival injection, and myalgias. The presence of a foreign body at the site of infection is common. This can be menstrual or non-menstrual related. Risk of recurrences exists. (See Table 1.)

*Table 1*
### Definition of Staphylococcal TSS

**Major criteria** *(all required)*
1. Fever $>/= 38.8°C$
2. Hypotension (orthostatic or shock)
3. Rash (erythroderma then desquamation)

**Minor criteria** *(any 3 required)*
1. Gastrointestinal—vomiting or diarrhea
2. Muscular—severe myalgia or CPK $>/= 2×$ normal
3. Mucous membranes—vaginal, oropharyngeal, or conjunctival hyperemia
4. Renal—BUN or Cr $>/= 2×$ normal, or U/A with $>5$ WBC/hpf
5. Hepatic—bili, AST, ALT $>/= 2×$ normal
6. Hematologic—platelets $<100×10^9/L$
7. Central nervous system—altered level of consciousness noted when fever and hypotension are absent

**Additional criteria**
1. Absence of other explanations
2. Blood cultures negative (except for *S. aureus*)

## Streptococcal TSS

Streptococcal TSS is typically more insidious in onset, and has a scarlatiniform rash. Evidence of soft tissue infection (abscess, necrotizing fasciitis—a spreading erythema overlying a swollen extremity with skin-tissue crepitus) with severe increasing pain is common. Increased risk exists in patients with varicella zoster infection. Managing hypotension associated with streptococcal TSS is more difficult than staphylococcal and results in greater morbidity and mortality. (See Table 2.)

*Table 2*
**Definition of Streptococcal TSS**

Hypotension or shock ($<5^{th}$ percentile for age), plus any two of the following:
1. Scarlet fever rash—may desquamate
2. Hepatic abnormalities—bili, AST, ALT $>/= 2\times$ normal
3. Renal insufficiency—BUN or Cr $>/= 2\times$ normal
4. Disseminated intravascular coagulopathy
5. ARDS
6. Soft-tissue necrosis—necrotizing fasciitis, gangrene

Definite case: Group A streptococcus isolated from a normally sterile site
Probable case: Group A streptococcus isolated from a non-sterile body site

## Treatment

- Similar management is recommended for both streptococcal and staphylococcal TSS.
- Initial stabilization and ongoing management of organ failure. (See Chapter 5, in "Shock.")
- Airway and breathing control as needed.
- Significant fluid resuscitation is often required and should be titrated to clinical and biochemical endpoints (eg, heart rate, perfusion, urine output, acid-base balance).
- Identification and drainage of site of infection, debridement of infected tissue, and/or appropriate tension release of compartment syndromes (necrotizing fasciitis); removal of foreign bodies.
- Consult pediatric gynecology in cases involving vaginal foreign bodies.
- Initial antibiotic coverage: cefazolin AND clindamycin.

- Immune globulin intravenous (IGIV) considered for infection refractory to several hours of aggressive therapy, presence of an undrainable focus, or persistent oliguria with pulmonary edema (1 g/kg q24h for 2 days or 2 g/kg IV as a single dose).
- Cefazolin may be changed to penicillin (for streptococcal TSS) or cloxacillin (for staphylococcal TSS) when the diagnosis is confirmed.
- Duration is generally 10–14 days or longer depending on the initial focus of infection.

## References

American Academy of Pediatrics. Toxic shock syndrome. In: Pickering LK, ed. Red book: 2006 report of the committee on infectious diseases, 27th ed. Elk Grove Village, IL: American Academy of Pediatrics; 2006; pp. 660–5.

Kaul R, McGeer A, Norrby-Teglund A, et al. Intravenous immunoglobulin therapy for streptococcal toxic shock syndrome: a comparative observational study. Clin Infect Dis 1999;28(4):800–7.

# C. Bacterial Meningitis

## Anupma Wadhwa

## Definition

Bacterial meningitis is inflammation of the membranes surrounding the brain and spinal cord due to bacterial infection.

## Key Principles

- Manage septic shock as needed.
- Prompt empiric antibiotic therapy is associated with improved outcomes.
- Anticipate alterations of mental status with raised intracranial pressure.
- Consider steroids for before or with the first dose of antibiotics.
- Chemoprophylaxis for contacts if *H. influenza* or *N. meningitides* meningitis.

## Pathogenesis

Bacteria reach the central nervous system either by hematogenous spread or direct extension from contiguous site. In neonates, pathogens are acquired by non-sterile maternal genital secretions. In infants and children, many of the causative organisms have colonized the upper respiratory tract. After bacterial invasion, an intense inflammatory response occurs, contributing to cerebral edema and increased intracranial pressure.

## Etiology

### Risk Factors for Bacterial Meningitis

- Immunocompromised host:

  - malignancy
  - malnutrition
  - HIV
  - asplenia
  - terminal complement deficiency
  - immunoglobulin deficiency
  - chronic diseases (eg, diabetes, chronic renal failure)

*Table 1*
**Etiology Affected by the Patient's Age**

| Patient age | Etiologic agent to consider |
| --- | --- |
| Neonate | Group B streptococcus, gram negative enteric bacilli, Listeria monocytogenes, Staphylococcus sp, Enterococcus sp, Viridians group streptococci |
| Infant, children <5 years old | S. pneumoniae, N. meningitides, H. influenza type b (non-immunized) |
| Children >5 years old, adolescents | S. pneumoniae, N. meningitides |

- Breaches of the CSF space including foreign material implants:

  - Congenital: Dermal sinus or dural defect
  - Penetrating head injury, neurosurgical procedures, CSF leaks
  - Ventriculoperitoneal shunt (*Staphylococcal* species and gram negative bacilli)
  - Cochlear implants (*S. pneumoniae*)

## Clinical Features

- Fever, neck stiffness, mental status changes
- Kernig and Brudzinski signs present in less than 5% of patients
- Seizures (more commonly seen with *S. pneumoniae* and *H. influenza*)
- Petechiae and purpura (seen with any, but more commonly seen in *N. meningitides*)

Signs and symptoms are often more subtle in infants (fever only, irritability, lethargy, difficulty feeding, apnea, seizures, bulging fontanel, rash).

## Diagnosis/Investigations

- CBC, electrolytes, serum glucose, blood culture
- If focal neurological signs, papilledema, or cardiovascular instability are present may be indicative of increased intracranial pressure. In these cases, it is advisable to obtain neuroimaging prior to lumbar puncture to avoid possible herniation.
- Lumbar puncture:

  - White blood cell count with differential
  - Glucose, protein

- Gram stain, culture
- Hold tube for further tests if the above results are suggestive, for example:

  - Acid fast bacilli stain and mycobacterial culture
  - Viral culture, HSV PCR, enterovirus PCR

Bacterial meningitis typically has CSF pleocytosis, predominant neutrophils (although lymphocytes may predominate early), low CSF glucose, and increased protein. CSF-to-serum glucose ratio is 0.6 or lower in neonates and 0.4 or lower in children >2 months of age. A traumatic tap where blood is introduced into the spinal fluid should be interpreted with caution—calculations to supposedly "correct" are fraught. It is advisable to treat and await cultures.

# Management

Not all patients with meningitis require ICU admission; it may depend on local facilities.

Criteria for PICU admission include but are not limited to the following:

- Septic shock
- Altered mental status
- End organ failure
- Critical electrolyte imbalances

Treat septic shock first. (See Chapter 5.)

Fluid restriction should be reserved for patients with evidence of SIADH. (See Chapter 16.) Note that for neonates and younger infants, SIADH is more often discussed than seen.

Anticipate and manage increased intracranial pressure—similar to management of closed head injury (Chapter 20). The overall goal is to maintain adequate cerebral perfusion.

- Ensure airway is secure.
- Perform serial neurologic examinations including Glasgow coma scale.
- Use minimal external stimulation.
- Provide isotonic intravenous fluids.
- Use antipyretic agents.
- Elevate head of the bed to 30°.
- Hyperventilation should be reserved for active cerebral herniation.
- Provide osmol therapy with hypertonic saline or mannitol.

- Barbiturate therapy may be necessary in extreme cases.
- Control and prevention of seizures (anticonvulsants).

Empiric antibiotic therapy regimens are selected to cover the most likely organisms (Table 2). Therapy should be modified when culture and sensitivity results are known.

*Table 2*
**Empiric Antibiotic Therapy**

| Patient group | Empiric antibiotic |
| --- | --- |
| Neonate up to 3 weeks of age | Ampicillin and aminoglycoside or cefotaxime |
| Neonate with late onset sepsis *(need to include anti-staphyloccal coverage)* | Vancomycin and cefotaxime +/− aminoglycoside |
| Children >1 month of age | Vancomycin and cefotaxime |
| Penetrating trauma, post-neurosurgery, CSF shunt | Vancomycin and ceftazidime or meropenem |
| Basilar skull fracture | Vancomycin and cefotaxime |

Evidence has shown benefit with dexamethasone in adults with pneumococcal meningitis. Clinical benefit has been demonstrated in children primarily with *H. influenza* meningitis. Benefit is less evident with pneumococcal meningitis. Because dexamethasone can decrease antibiotic penetration into the CNS, concerns have been raised with its use potentially impeding eradication of resistant pneumococcal strains. Current recommendation is to use dexamethasone in children with *H. influenza* meningitis. Dexamethasone may be considered in pneumococcal meningitis after considering the risks and benefits. However, because benefit from steroids is greatest when given early, these considerations are often tricky. We suggest the following:

- Dexamethasone suggested dosing regimen: 1 mg/kg/day div q6h × 4 days
- First dose given before or with the first dose of antibiotics

Chemoprophylaxis to contacts should be administered in cases of *H. influenza* or *N. meningitides* meningitis.

## Complications

- Cerebral edema
- Septic shock

- Disseminated intravascular coagulation
- Hyponatremia
- Sensorineural hearing loss
- Seizures
- Subdural effusions
- Subdural empyema (rare but should be suspected with prolonged fever and irritability)
- Brain abscess, hydrocephalus, hemorrhage, infarction (rare)

## Prognosis

- The mortality rate for bacterial meningitis in children is 4–10%.
- Seizures that occur or persist after the fourth day of treatment are more likely to be associated with neurological sequelae.
- Hearing impairment is the most common neurological sequelae and occurs in 10% of patients.
- Neuromotor, learning disabilities, and speech and behavioral problems develop in 10% of children.

## References

Chavez-Bueno S, McCracken GH. Bacterial meningitis in children. Pediatr Clin N Am 2005;52:795–810.

De Gans J, van de Beek D. Dexamethasone as adjunctive therapy in bacterial meningitis. N Engl J Med 2002;347:1549–56.

Tunkel AR, Hartman BJ, Kaplan SL, et al. Practice guidelines for the management of bacterial meningitis. Clin Infect Dis 2004;39:1267–84.

# D. Encephalitis

## Anupma Wadhwa

## Definition

Encephalitis is encephalopathy (altered state of consciousness) with CSF pleocytosis (5 or more cells) plus one or more of the following

- fever
- seizure
- focal neurological findings
- compatible EEG
- abnormal diagnostic imaging (CT, MRI)

## Key Principles

- Presentation is highly variable; encephalitis should be considered for any patient presenting to the PICU with altered mental status.
- Exclude reversible and treatable causes of altered mental status.
- Once diagnosis is established, management is primarily supportive.

## Common Etiologic Agents

No organism identified in >50% of cases.

- Enteroviruses (eg, coxsackie, polio)
- Arboviruses (eg, West Nile, St. Louis encephalitis)
- Herpes viruses (HSV, EBV, HHV 6)
- Influenza
- Mycoplasma pneumonia
- Mycobacterium tuberculosis
- Bartonella hensalae
- Borellia burgdoferi

Many other infectious agents have been implicated.

# Clinical Features

- Typically presents acutely with high fever, altered consciousness, and focal neurological symptoms (seizures, cranial nerve palsies, bizarre behavior, ataxia).
- Exposure history: travel, outdoor camping, insect bites, contact with animals, TB, and other ill contacts.
- Mortality varies according to etiology and subsequent management.
- Children under a year of age generally have higher mortality and morbidity associated with encephalitis.

# Differential Diagnosis

- Purulent meningitis
- Aseptic meningitis
- Febrile delirium (associated with bacteremia, infective endocarditis, shigellosis, and typhoid fever)
- Hypoglycemia
- Uremic or hepatic encephalopathy
- Inborn errors of metabolism
- Drug ingestion
- Reye syndrome
- Mass lesions (tumor, abscess)
- Subarachnoid hemorrhage
- Acute multiple sclerosis

# Investigations

Tests required are based on clinical scenario and test availability. At minimum, a lumbar puncture and radiographic imaging is needed to rule out other treatable causes of altered mental status. Table 1 outlines a suggested diagnostic evaluation.

*Table 1*
**Suggested Diagnostic Evaluation**

| Blood tests | • CBC, electrolytes, creatinine, glucose, blood culture |
|---|---|
| Paired serology *acute and then convalescent in 2–4 weeks* | • West Nile, Mycoplasma, Bartonella, Lyme<br>• Hold 3–5 cc for possible future tests |

| CSF studies | • Protein, glucose, cell count<br>*In encephalitis, elevated protein,*<br>*normal glucose, pleocytosis with*<br>*predominant lymphocytosis are*<br>*typically seen.*<br>• Viral culture<br>• Bacterial culture and gram stain<br>• Mycobacterial culture and AFB stain<br>• Mycoplasma, HSV, enterovirus PCR<br>  if available<br>• Hold 1–2 cc for possible future<br>  tests |
| NP swab | • Influenza, other respiratory viruses |
| Throat swab | • Mycoplasma PCR if available |
| Stool | • Viral culture (enterovirus) |
| Imaging | • Head CT or MRI |
| Other | • EEG |

## Management

- Close monitoring of vital signs and fluid status.
- Initiate IV antibacterials (eg, ceftriaxone) until bacterial etiology has been excluded.
- Although HSV is not the most common etiologic agent, it is reasonable to begin acyclovir as empiric treatment while awaiting test results (45–60 mg/kg/day IV div q8).
- PICU admission may be necessary depending on the clinical presentation.
- Monitor and prepare to treat the following complications:

  - Seizures (See "Seizures and Status Epilepticus" in Chapter 9.)
  - Cerebral edema
  - Coma (See "Coma and Altered Mental States" in Chapter 9.)
  - Hyperpyrexia
  - Respiratory insufficiency
  - Fluid and electrolyte abnormalities
  - Aspiration pneumonitis
  - Cardiac decompensation
  - Gastrointestinal bleeding
  - Disseminated intravascular coagulation
  - Cardiopulmonary arrest of central origin

Consult infectious diseases and neurology for other specific treatment considerations.

## Prognosis

- Known risk of recurrence in HSV encephalitis.
- Spectrum of illness: short benign illness to severe sequelae and death.
- May completely recover after weeks of depressed consciousness.
- Children with apparently benign illness can progressively deteriorate over weeks to months after hospital discharge. Follow-up is therefore extremely important.

## References

Ford-Jones EL, MacGregor D, Richardson S, et al. Acute childhood encephalitis and meningoencephalitis: diagnosis and management. Paediatr Child Health 1998 Jan/Feb;3(1):33–40.

Kolski H, Ford-Jones EL, Richardson S, et al. Etiology of acute childhood encephalitis at The Hospital for Sick Children, Toronto, 1994–1995. Clin Infect Dis 1998;26:398–409.

# E. Pneumonia

Anupma Wadhwa

## Key Principles

- Early anticipatory cardiopulmonary support is fundamental to ICU management.
- Initiate broad empiric therapy according to the clinical picture presented.
- When possible, narrow antibiotic therapy if etiology is determined.

## Definition

Pneumonia is the presence of fever, acute respiratory symptoms, or both, plus evidence of parenchymal infiltrates on chest radiography.

## Etiology

Streptococcus pneumoniae is the most common bacterial cause of childhood community-acquired pneumonia. Viruses are the most common infectious cause found in young children (eg, RSV, parainfluenza, influenza). An etiology is not found in an estimated 20–60% of cases. Age is a helpful predictor of likely pathogens. Table 1 lists common bacterial causes of pneumonia grouped by age.

*Table 1*
**Etiologic Causes of Community-Acquired Pneumonia by Age Group**

| Age | Bacterial etiologic agents |
| --- | --- |
| <2 weeks | Group B streptococcus<br>Listeria monocytogenes<br>Gram negative enteric bacilli<br>Staphylococcus aureus |
| 2 weeks–3 months | Streptococcus pneumonia<br>Staphylococcus aureus<br>Haemophilus influenzae type b<br>Chlamydia trachomatis |

*(continued)*

| Age | Bacterial etiologic agents |
| --- | --- |
| Over 3 months | Streptococcus pneumonia<br>Staphylococcus aureus<br>Haemophilus influenza type b<br>Mycoplasma pneumoniae |
| Other agents to consider | Mycobacterium tuberculosis (any age)<br>Bordetella pertussis (<1 year old or<br>>10 years old) |

## Clinical Presentation

Children: high fever, tachypnea, difficulty breathing, cough, post-tussive vomiting

Neonates: fever, tachypnea, decreased activity, poor feeding, agitation may be an indicator for hypoxia; apnea often a feature, especially with bordetella

## Physical Signs

- Signs of progression and respiratory distress: nasal flaring, intercostal retractions, cyanosis, grunting, rising heart rate, irregular breathing.
- Auscultation may show classical bronchial breathing, inspiratory crackles, and decreased percussion notes. Combinations of dullness to percussion, and focal diminished breath sounds may indicate an effusion.
- Lower lobe pneumonia may have associated abdominal pain; upper lobe pneumonia may have associated meningismus.

## Diagnosis

Diagnosis is based on clinical presentation and chest X-ray findings if obtained.

## Differential Diagnosis

- Asthma: wheezing, response to bronchodilators, can predispose to pneumonia
- Congestive heart failure: hepatosplenomegaly, cardiomegaly, murmur, added third or fourth heart sounds, poor perfusion
- Foreign body aspiration: history of observed choking episode, chest X-ray appearance

- Aspiration pneumonitis: chemical injury caused by inhalation of sterile gastric contents (generally complication of anesthesia for surgical procedures)

## Chest Imaging

### Chest X-ray

Indications for chest X-ray include:

- Respiratory distress
- Age <2 months
- Unclear diagnosis—always suspect foreign body aspiration (obtain comparison inspired to expired films for ball-valving)
- Suspicion of pleural effusion
- 48 hours of antibiotics without improvement
- Worsening symptoms in critically ill patients
- Mechanical ventilation

Radiographic findings often lag behind the clinical picture; clinical correlation is always needed. Chest X-ray is insensitive in differentiating between patients with bacterial and non-bacterial pneumonia. The pattern, however, can provide a clue toward possible etiologies:

- Lobar pattern: bacterial infections (eg, S. pneumoniae, H. influenzae type B)
- Diffuse pattern: viral pneumonia, chlamydia, mycoplasma, tuberculosis, disseminated fungal disease
- Para-pneumonic effusions: S. pneumoniae, H. influenzae type b, Group A Streptococcus, S. aureus, tuberculosis*

*Tuberculosis can have protean appearances on chest X-ray: hilar adenopathy, peripheral pneumonia, atelectasis, hyperaeration, multifocal-diffuse pattern, para-pneumonic effusion.

### Chest Ultrasound

May be indicated in para-pneumonic effusion.

### Chest CT

May be indicated in severe progressive pneumonia, pneumonia in immunocompromised host, or para-pneumonic effusion.

## Diagnostic Work-up

- CBC with differential
- Blood culture (positive in 10% of cases)
- Nasopharyngeal specimen for viral studies
- Sputum or deep endotracheal suction specimens for gram stain and culture

If pleural effusion, consider diagnostic thoracentesis (pleural fluid culture positive in 17% of cases). If severe progressive pneumonia, bronchoalveolar lavage or lung biopsy specimens for culture may be indicated.

Other tests depending on clinical suspicion:

- PPD, gastric aspirates, or induced sputum for mycobacterial stain and culture (TB)
- Serology (Mycoplasma pneumoniae, Chlamydia pneumoniae, Q fever, psittacosis)
- Nasopharyngeal specimen for Chlamydia trachomatis, and Bordetella pertussis culture and PCR
- Urine for Legionella antigen
- Respiratory specimen (eg, BAL) for fungal stain and culture (Pneumocystis jiroveci, Histoplasma, Blastomyces, Coccidioides, Cryptococcus)

## Other Tests to Consider

- Electrolytes if severely ill (SIADH), dehydrated or requiring IV fluids
- LP if suspect meningitis (fever, irritability, obtundation, lethargy, meningismus)

## Management

- Assess adequacy of breathing
- Pulse oximetry or arterial blood gas
- Administer supplemental oxygen if oxygen saturation $<92\%$ or $PO_2$ $<65$ mm Hg
- Monitor at least q4hours with pulse oximetry
- Early noninvasive mechanical ventilation for moderate to severe distress
- Intubation for progressive respiratory failure

- Pneumonia may lead to ARDS; see Chapter 6 in "Acute Respiratory Distress Syndrome" for management of ARDS
- Minimal handling of an ill child may reduce metabolic and oxygen requirements
- Consider bronchodilators for wheezing and suspected reactive airways
- Use antipyretics and analgesics

## Empiric Antibiotic Choices (Tables 2 and 3)

Oral antibiotic treatment is safe and effective if tolerated by patient.

IV indicated if poor oral absorption (eg, vomiting) or severe signs and symptoms are present.

*Table 2*
### Empiric Antibiotic Choice Based on Suspected Etiologies

| | |
|---|---|
| S. pneumoniae, S. aureus, H. influenza (community-acquired pneumonia) | Amoxicillin-clavulanate or Cefuroxime or Cefotaxime |
| Mycoplasma or Chlamydia | Macrolide |
| Methicillin resistant S. aureus (hospital acquired or high incidence in the community) | Vancomycin |
| Legionella | Quinolone or macrolide |
| Pneumocystis jiroveci suspected (underlying immune deficiency, elevated LDH, hypoxia) | Co-trimoxazole +/− steroids |
| Mycobacterium tuberculosis | Isoniazid, pyrazinamide, rifampin, and ethambutol |

*Table 3*
### Empiric Antibiotic Choice Based on Clinical Scenarios

| | |
|---|---|
| Aspiration pneumonia (pharyngeal flora, anaerobes, gram negative rods in chronically ill patients) | Penicillin or clindamycin and gentamicin |

*(continued)*

| Pneumonia associated with cystic fibrosis (S. aureus, H. influenza, Pseudomonas, Burkholderia) | Piperacillin and gentamicin (where possible, based on patient's sputum culture results) |
| --- | --- |
| Immunocompromised host or malignancy (any organism, in particular S. aureus, Pseudomonas, gram negative enteric bacilli, Aspergillus, other mycoses, cytomegalovirus, other viruses) | Piperacillin/tazobactam $+/-$ antifungal (eg, amphotericin) $+/-$ antiviral |

# Not Improving after 48 Hours

Consider:
- Appropriateness of antibiotic choice and dose
- Lung complication such as abscess or empyema
- Host issues such as immunocompromised or cystic fibrosis

If persistently febrile, consider metastatic foci (osteomyelitis or septic arthritis, especially with S. aureus).

# Follow-up

Chest X-ray abnormalities can persist for 8 to 12 weeks after the acute illness. Repeat chest X-ray suggested for patients with lobar collapse, apparent round pneumonia (rule out tumor mass), or for continuing symptoms.

# Special Considerations

1. **Para-pneumonic effusion or empyema**
   If chest X-ray suggests pleural effusion, perform chest ultrasound to confirm and assess for loculations.
   Chest CT may be of benefit if surgical management is planned. Surgical or interventional radiology consultation for chest tube with fibrinolytics or video-assisted thoracopic surgery if loculated.
2. **Aspiration pneumonia**
   An infectious process caused by inhalation of oropharyngeal secretions that are colonized by pathogenic bacteria (as differentiated from aspiration pneumonitis) leading to pneumonia in the dependent lung segments. Table 4 lists features of aspiration pneumonia vs pneumonitis.

*Table 4*
**Comparison of Aspiration Pneumonia with Aspiration Pneumonitis**

| Feature | Aspiration pneumonia | Aspiration pneumonitis |
|---|---|---|
| Mechanism | Aspiration of colonized oropharyngeal secretions | Aspiration of sterile gastric contents |
| Pathophysiologic process | Acute pulmonary inflammatory response to bacteria | Acute lung injury from acidic gastric material |
| Bacteriologic findings | Pharyngeal flora, anaerobes, gram negative rods in chronically ill patients | Initially sterile, with subsequent bacterial infection possible |
| Predisposing factors | Dysphagia, neuromuscular defect | Marked depressed level of consciousness, post-anesthesia |
| Clinical features | Tachypnea, cough, signs of pneumonia, infiltrate in dependent bronchopulmonary segment | May range from no symptoms, to marked respiratory distress 2 to 5 hours after aspiration |
| Management | Antibiotics targeted at pharyngeal flora may be of benefit; however, clinical judgment necessary as no good prospective studies available | Consider antibiotics if symptoms last >48 hours or use of antacids |

3. **Ventilator-associated pneumonia**

   Nosocomial pneumonia is found in mechanically ventilated patients and develops >48 hours after initiation of mechanical ventilation.

   Endotracheal aspirates from these patients commonly grow Pseudomonas aeruginosa, enteric gram negative bacilli, and S. aureus.

Endotracheal aspirate cultures are sensitive but not specific for VAP.

Diagnosis based on clinical criteria including worsening respiratory status, change in sputum, chest X-ray change, fever, leukocytosis or leukopenia, positive BAL or endotracheal aspirate culture with pus cells seen on gram stain.

See "Nosocomial Infections in the PICU" in Chapter 18 for additional management.

# References

Balfour-Lynn IM, Abrahamson E, Cohen G, et al. BTS guidelines for the management of pleural infection in children. Thorax 2005;60:1–21.

Elward AM. Pediatric ventilator-associated pneumonia. Pediatr Infect Dis J 2003;22:443–6.

Fisher RG, Boyce TG. Pneumonia syndromes. In: Fisher RG, Boyce TG, eds. Moffet's Pediatric Infectious Diseases: A Problem-Oriented Approach, 4th ed. Philadelphia: Lippincott Williams and Wilkins; 2005, pp. 174–218.

Marik PE. Aspiration pneumonitis and aspiration pneumonia. N Engl J Med 2001;665–71.

McIntosh K. Community-acquired pneumonia in children. N Engl J Med 2002;346:429–37.

# F. Sepsis and Bacteremia
## Anupma Wadhwa

## Key Principles

> - Sepsis and bacteremia are common reasons for admission to the PICU, and common complications in the PICU.
> - Early recognition and empiric treatment is necessary to avoid progression to septic shock.

## Terminology

Bacteremia is bacteria in the blood, generally evidenced by a positive blood culture.

Systemic inflammatory response syndrome (SIRS) is clinically recognized by the presence of two or more of the following:

- tachycardia
- tachypnea
- leukocytosis or leukopenia
- abnormal temperature (hyper or hypothermia)

SIRS is not always caused by bacterial infection. It may be triggered by entities such as major blood loss and burns.

Sepsis: SIRS caused by infection.

Severe sepsis: sepsis plus evidence of organ dysfunction, hypotension, or hypoperfusion.

## Etiology

Many bacteria can cause bacteremia and sepsis. Age and predisposing host conditions provide a clue toward possible etiologic agents. (See Tables 1 and 2.)

*Table 1*

## Etiologic Agents for Bacteremia by Age

| Age | Most common etiologic agents |
| --- | --- |
| 0–30 days | Group B streptococcus, E. coli, other gram negative enteric bacilli, Listeria monocytogenes, S. aureus, Enterococcus (consider herpes simplex virus infection) |
| 1–3 months | Organisms seen in both neonates or older children |
| 3 months–5 years | S. pneumoniae, N. meningitidis, Salmonella spp., group A. streptococcus, S. aureus, H. influenzae |
| >5 years | N. meningitidis, S. aureus, S. pneumoniae |

*Table 2*

## Etiologic Agents for Bacteremia Based on Predisposing Risk Factors

| Predisposing condition | Etiologic agents to consider |
| --- | --- |
| Intravascular device | S. epidermidis, S. aureus, Candida species |
| Hematologic malignancy, neutropenia | Organisms seen related to intravascular devices as well as gram negative enteric bacilli, Pseudomonas aeruginosa |
| Prior therapy with broad-spectrum antibiotics | Resistant gram negative bacilli, Candida species |
| Splenic dysfunction | Encapsulated bacteria (S. pneumoniae, N. meningitidis, H. influenzae) |
| Immunologic disorders | *Antibody deficiency:* pyogenic bacteria (S. pneumoniae, S. aureus, group A streptococcus, N. meningitides) *Terminal complement deficiency:* N. meningitides *Chronic granulomatous disease:* S. aureus, Serratia marcescens |

# Clinical Features

Positive blood cultures are present in the following various clinical scenarios.

- Contaminated blood cultures are estimated to occur in 2–25% of pediatric blood cultures:

  - Coagulase negative staphylococcus, Bacillus species, Propionibacterium, and Corynebacterium species are often contaminants in patients without predisposing conditions (eg, not neutropenic, no central venous catheter)

- Occult (unsuspected) bacteremia:

  - Occurs in infants and toddlers
  - Usual presentation is high fever and high peripheral white blood cell count
  - Often observed as outpatients

- Bacteremia with focal infection:

  - Bacteremia presumed secondary to a focal infection (eg, pneumonia, meningitis, septic arthritis, cellulitis)

- Bacteremia related to central venous lines:

  - Common source of bacteremia in immunocompromised hosts

- Presumed sepsis:

  - Fever, toxic appearance, disseminated intravascular coagulation

- Severe sepsis or septic shock

  - Rapid course, hypotension, hypoperfusion

# Investigations

Based on severity of clinical presentation, may include:

- CBC with differential
- Blood cross and type
- Electrolytes
- BUN, creatinine
- Liver function tests
- Glucose
- Calcium
- Fibrinogen, PT, PTT
- Arterial blood gas

Blood culture:

- Two sets, separated by time and site, are ideal if feasible.
- If central line is present, one set from each lumen and one peripheral culture.
- If persistently positive blood cultures, search for occult focus (eg, endocarditis).

Culture other possible sources of infection (eg, urine, CSF).

## Treatment

Recognize and promptly treat the signs and symptoms of shock. (See "Septic Shock" in Chapter 18.)

- Early goal-directed therapy:

  - Support and maintain circulation
  - Counteract hypoxemia and impaired tissue oxygenation
  - Frequently reassess and anticipate issues that lead to progression of shock
  - Identify source of infection, drain infection if applicable
  - Begin empiric antibiotic therapy

- Choice of antibiotic depends on local resistance patterns (eg, consider empiric coverage with vancomycin in areas with high rates of methicillin resistant S. aureus) and predisposing host factors.
- Early consultation with an ID specialist is recommended.
- Once sensitivities are known, therapy can be changed if necessary.
- Table 3 lists suggested empiric antibiotic regimens.

*Table 3*
**Suggested Empiric Antibiotic Therapy Based on Age**

| Age | Empiric therapy |
| --- | --- |
| 0–30 days | Ampicillin plus cefotaxime or ceftriaxone or gentamicin (consider acyclovir) |
| 1–3 months | Ampicillin plus cefotaxime or ceftriaxone or gentamicin |
| >3 months | Cefotaxime or ceftriaxone; for high-risk cases add vancomycin |

1. Consider addition of vancomycin if there are high rates of MRSA in your unit. Reassess vancomycin after 48 hours.

# What to Do If Bacteremia in Presence of Long Lines

Although the safest advice would be to remove all long lines, this is not so straightforward in young infants and children. Ultimately, the decision needs to be balanced in the clinical circumstances for each child. For example, the issue of ease of potential access versus risk of ongoing invasion from a potentially infected catheter site, versus the need for access for hemodynamic stability—all need to be traded off.

However, some guidelines can be suggested. Remove lines with some urgency if:

- No clinical improvement has been gained despite therapy for 48 hours; or, continuing positive cultures are obtained.
- Serious complications develop: endocarditis, endovasculitis, septic emboli, ongoing consumption of platelets, tunnel infection.
- Highly invasive or virulent organism is present: S. aureus, fungi, gram negative and not in shock.

Consider trial of therapy to eradicate source, leaving line in situ, and repeat cultures in 48 hours if:

- A local infection exists at the insertion site.
- Peripheral culture is positive in face of central culture negativity.
- Patient has a fever but is not systemically ill.
- Coagulase negative staphylococcus (CONS).

# References

Fisher RG, Boyce TG. Sepsis and bacteremia. In: Fisher RG, Boyce TG, eds. Moffet's Pediatric Infectious Diseases: A Problem-Oriented Approach, 4th ed. Philadelphia: Lippincott Williams and Wilkins; 2005, pp. 354–7.

Melendez E, Bachur R. Advances in the emergency management of pediatric sepsis. Curr Opin Pediatr 2006;18:245–53.

Mernel LA, Far BM, Sherertz RJ. Guidelines for the management of intravascular-related infections. Clin Infect Dis 2001;32:1249–72.

# G. Necrotizing Fasciitis/ Necrotizing Soft Tissue Infections

## C Hui

## Key Principles

- All necrotizing soft tissue infections require the same management.
- A high index of suspicion is required.
- The clinical syndrome can progress rapidly; frequent reassessment is essential.
- Early surgical management is crucial.
- Do not delay surgical management with imaging, laboratory studies, or antimicrobial therapy.
- Change antimicrobial therapy based on local and national epidemiology. (Add vancomycin if concerned about CA-MRSA.)

## Definitions

Necrotizing fasciitis is in the continuum of necrotizing soft tissue infection (NSTI) which includes necrotizing fasciitis, gas gangrene/anaerobic cellulitis, progressive bacterial synergistic gangrene, and synergistic necrotizing cellulitis. It can be difficult to classify the infection to one anatomic layer (dermis, subcutaneous tissue, superficial fascia, deep fascia, muscle) and multiple components may be involved; however, the pathophysiology, clinical presentation, and management of NSTIs are similar. The most important distinction is whether a necrotizing component is present. It is a clinical diagnosis.

Necrotizing fasciitis I

- anaerobic, mixed infection

Necrotizing fasciitis II

- group A streptococci (GAS) alone or in combination with other pathogens
- M protein elaborates pyrogenic exotoxin A

Associated with the recent epidemic of community-acquired methicillin-resistant *Staphylococcus aureus* (CA-MRSA) infections, there have been reports of CA-MRSA necrotizing fasciitis. Although CA-MRSA infection is widespread in the United States, increasing numbers are occurring in Canada. Knowledge of national, provincial, and local epidemiology of infectious organisms and their resistance is important in the management of all infections.

The identified risk factors for CA-MRSA skin and soft-tissue infection (infection, not necessarily NSTI) are:

- Household contact with proven CA-MRSA
- Children
- Day-care contacts of hospitalized patients with MRSA
- Men who have sex with men
- Soldiers
- Incarcerated persons
- Athletes, particularly those involved in contact sports
- Native Americans
- Pacific Islanders
- Persons with a previous CA-MRSA infection
- Intravenous drug users

## Diagnosis

### Clinical Presentation   Requires a high index of suspicion

- Initially can present as a soft tissue infection. Frequent reassessment is **crucial.** Clinical picture may change rapidly.
- Mostly present in extremities, surgical sites, and perineum

  - Swelling, erythema, warmth, pain, fever

- Classic/later presentation: sensitivity is low (<50%); specificity is good

  - Discolored skin, blisters/bullae, crepitus, **pain disproportionate to clinical appearance**, hypesthesia, tachycardia, hypotension/shock, subcutaneous gas (polymicrobial/anaerobic infection)
  - Progressing to cutaneous gangrene with anesthesia

### Risk Factors

- Primary varicella infection: ~60 times increased risk
- Minor trauma
- Immunosuppression
- Diabetes mellitus
- Parenteral drug abuse

## Laboratory Parameters

- Inflammatory parameters and white blood count (wbc) appear high; hyponatremia and organ dysfunction may also be present.
- Laboratory-based scores appear promising, but require prospective validation, especially in a pediatric population.

## Imaging

- Subcutaneous gas on plain radiographs is specific, but not sensitive for NSTI. NF II typically does not elaborate gas.
- MRI or CT appears to be sensitive but not specific for NSTI. Enhancement may represent inflammation of subcutaneous layers, but not necrosis. These imaging modalities may assist in delineating the extent of involvement, especially when the infection skips areas.
- Imaging should not delay definitive management.

## Complications

- Compartment syndrome
- Toxic shock syndrome
- Mortality rate >30%

## Management

- Immediate surgical assessment with surgical exploration for diagnosis and operative management is required.

    - All necrotic tissue must be resected until healthy, viable, bleeding tissue is present at the excision border.
    - Multiple surgical explorations may be required.

- Supportive and close-monitored care in the intensive care unit is recommended as multi-organ failure is not uncommon.
- Empiric antimicrobials (2–6 weeks, depending on clinical course):

    - Clindamycin is employed to decrease the protein synthesis (toxin), has a long post-antimicrobial effect, and is not affected by inoculum size, in addition to anaerobic activity.
        - Pipercillin/tazobactam and clindamycin: Consider adding an aminoglycoside if it is polymicrobial gram negative bacteria.

- High-dose penicillin, clindamycin, and an aminoglycoside.
- Clindamycin and cefazolin—**only** if suspecting methicillin-sensitive *Staphylococcus aureus* (MSSA) or GAS.
- Add vancomycin if concerned with CA-MRSA.
- Prolonged antimicrobial therapy should be guided by culture and sensitivity results.

## Adjuvant Therapy

- Polyclonal IGIV in the setting of toxic shock (see toxic shock management)
- Hyperbaric oxygen

  - Literature is not clear on benefit.
  - Potential benefit of hyperbaric oxygen needs to be weighed against risks of patient transfer and lack of the ability to monitor the patient adequately.

## Prophylaxis

- Many public health departments require immediate reporting of invasive group A streptococcal disease.
- There is increased risk of contacts developing invasive group A streptococcal disease, yet there is little evidence for efficacy of prophylaxis; decisions surrounding prophylaxis should be made in conjunction with the local public health department and infectious diseases consultants.
- The AAP Red Book 2006 suggests that prophylaxis be considered only to household contacts who are greater than 65 years of age or are at high risk of death (ie, HIV, varicella, diabetes).

# References

Anaya DA, Dellinger EP. Necrotizing soft-tissue infection: diagnosis and management. Clin Infect Dis 2007;44:705–10.

Barton M, Hawkes, M, Moore D, et al. Guidelines for the prevention and management of community-acquired methicillin-resistant Staphylococcus aureus: a perspective for Canadian health care practitioners. Can J Infect Dis Med Microbiol 2006;17:(Suppl C):4C–24C.

Infectious diseases and immunization committee, Canadian Paediatric Society. Community-associated methicillin-resistant Staphylococcus aureus: implications for the care of children. Pediatr Child Health 2007;12(4):323–4.

www.car-r.ca

Daum RS. Skin and soft-tissue infections caused by methicillin-resistant Staphylococcus aureus. N Engl J Med 2007;357:380–90.

McHenry CR, Piotrowski JJ, Petrinic D, Malangoni MA. Determinants of mortality for necrotizing soft-tissue infections. Ann Surg 1995;221:558–63.

Wong CH, Khin LW, et al. The LRINEC (Laboratory Risk Indicator for Necrotizing Fasciitis) score: a tool for distinguishing necrotizing fasciitis from other soft tissue infections. Crit Care Med 2004 July;32(7):1535–41.

American Academy of Pediatrics. Group A streptococcal infections. In: Pickering LK, Baker CJ, Long SS, McMillan JA, eds. Red Book: 2006 Report of the Committee on Infectious Diseases, 27th ed. Elk Grove Village, IL: American Academy of Pediatrics; 2006; p. 617.

# H. The Immunocompromised Patient

A Desirée La Beaud
Philip Toltzis

## Introduction

Infection in the immunocompromised host is becoming an increasingly common admitting diagnosis to pediatric intensive care units. These patients can be critically ill and warrant specialized care. A basic understanding of common immune deficits and likely infecting pathogens can improve the care and prognosis for these children.

## Key Principles

- Primary immunodeficiency is a state in which the host's immune system is dysfunctional from an inherited or genetic defect. Examples include X-linked agammaglobinemia and chronic granulomatous disease.
- Secondary immunodeficiency is a state in which the host's intact immune system has been altered and rendered dysfunctional by external factors, either by infection, as in HIV infection, or medication, as in cancer and transplant patients.

## Pathophysiology

The immune system's functions are to prevent infection and to protect against autoimmunity and malignancy. It has four primary components: humoral immunity (B cell derived antibody), cell-mediated immunity (T cell immunity), the phagocytic system (neutrophils and macrophages), and the complement system (Table 1).

## Etiology of Infection

The etiology of many infections in immunocompromised hosts is the same as those in immunocompetent hosts. For example, immunodeficient children will contract the same

*Table 1*

**Immune System Components, Function, and Related Immune Diseases**

| Immune system component | Primary component function | Diseases with component defect |
|---|---|---|
| Phagocytes | Chemotaxis to site of infection, ingestion, and intracellular killing of bacteria and fungi | Neutropenia (congenital or acquired) Chronic granulomatous disease Leukocyte adhesion deficiency Chediak-Higashi syndrome |
| B cells | Antibody production | X-linked agammaglobinemia Common variable immunodeficiency IgA deficiency IgG subclass deficiencies Hyper IgM |
| T cells | Cytokine production, targeted B cell activation and antibody production to specific antigen | DiGeorge syndrome HIV/AIDS Cyclosporine |
| Combined B and T cells | Adaptive immunity | Severe combined immunodeficiency Wiskott-Aldrich syndrome Ataxia telangiectasia Hyper IgE |
| Complement | Lysis of infected cells and microorganisms | Component deficiencies Properdin deficiency Mannose binding lectin deficiency |

respiratory viruses in the winter and may have many of the same minor bacterial infections, such as otitis media, as children with a competent immune system. Because of their underlying immune deficiencies, however, these children are at higher risk of serious illness from common infections than their immunocompetent counterparts. Additionally, they may have specific infections caused by organisms of low intrinsic pathogenicity as a consequence of their immune deficits.

a) **By defect**

Defects in each of the immune system components produce characteristic infections, although overlap exists in microbiologic causes (Table 2).

*Table 2*
**Characteristic Disease Presentations and Microbiologic Pathogens (most common in bold type) in Specific Immune Component Defects**

| Immune system defect | Disease presentation | Likely microbiologic pathogen |
|---|---|---|
| Phagocytes | Recurrent skin, soft tissue, and bone infections Deep tissue abscesses | **Bacterial: Staphylococcus aureus,** Staphylococcus epidermidis, **Pseudomonas aeruginosa,** E. coli, Klebsiella pneumoniae, Corynebacterium JK, Alpha hemolytic streptococcus, **Serratia marcescens,** Nocardia **Fungal: Candida species, Aspergillus species,** Mucor, Fusarium, Alternaria |
| B cells | Recurrent sinopulmonary infections | **Bacteria: Streptococcus pneumoniae,** Staphylococcus aureus, Hemophilus influenzae, Pseudomonas aeruginosa, Campylobacter fetus, Neisseria meningitidis, Mycoplasma hominis, Ureaplasma urealyticum, Salmonella species **Viruses: Enteroviruses,** Rotavirus **Protozoa:** Giardia lamblia |

(continued)

| Immune system defect | Disease presentation | Likely microbiologic pathogen |
|---|---|---|
| T cells | Recurrent viral and fungal (intracellular organisms) infections | **Viral: Herpes simplex virus, Cytomegalovirus, varicella-zoster virus,** Epstein-Barr virus, measles, polyomaviruses JC and BK<br>**Fungal: Candida albicans, Pneumocystis jiroveci,** Cryptococcus neoformans, Histoplasma capsulatum, Coccidioides immitis, Aspergillus fumigatus<br>**Bacterial:** Listeria monocytogenes, Salmonella, Legionella, Nocardia,<br>**Atypical mycobacteria, Mycobacterium tuberculosis,** Mycobacterium bovis<br>**Protozoal:** Cryptosporidium parvum, Toxoplasma gondii |
| Complement | Recurrent severe infections | **Bacterial: Neisseria meningitidis, Neisseria gonorrhoeae,** Streptococcus pyogenes, Streptococcus pneumoniae, Staphylococcus aureus, Hemophilus influenzae |

b) **By host**

Both primary and secondary immunodeficient patients may have one or more immune component defects resulting in the infections detailed above.

## Primary immunodeficiency:

Primary immunodeficiency patients will have specific infections related to their specific defect. For example, patients with chronic granulomatous disease often have infections due to *Staphylococcus aureus, Serratia,* and *Aspergillus* because their neutrophils are unable to kill catalase positive organisms.

# Secondary immunodeficiency:

a) **HIV**—HIV patients may have recurrent bacterial infections with encapsulated organisms such as *Streptococcus pneumoniae* and *Salmonella*, secondary to HIV-related humoral immunity dysfunction. Those with severe depression of CD4 counts will be at risk for opportunistic infections, such as *Pneumocystis jiroveci* and cytomegalovirus infections.

b) **Cancer**—Although many arms of the immune system are altered dysfunctional in the cancer patient, the most important is the severe neutropenia that accompanies most chemotherapy. Cancer drugs further cause cell death and ulcerations along mucous membranes, diminishing the integrity of anatomical barriers in the pharynx and gastrointestinal tract and increasing the risk of invasion by colonizing flora. Moreover, most patients receiving cancer chemotherapy have an implanted central venous catheter, which represents a potential nidus of blood stream infection. Gram positive bacterial infections, such as coagulase-negative staphylococci, *Staphylococcus aureus*, and *Streptococcus pneumoniae*, are common, but gram negative bacterial infections, such as *Pseudomonas aeruginosa*, *Klebsiella* species, and *E. coli*, can also cause severe infection in these patients. Additionally, these patients are at risk for severe manifestations of rare infections, including disseminated varicella, *Aspergillus* pneumonia, ecthyma gangrenosum, *Pneumocystis jiroveci* pneumonia (PJP), and *Candida* sepsis.

c) **Transplant**—Certain immunodeficient patients, such as transplant recipients, may have characteristic infections temporally related to their immunodeficient state.

**Bone Marrow Transplantation (BMT):** In BMT, patients can have infections in the pretransplant, pre-engraftment, and post-engraftment periods (Table 3). Infections in the pretransplant period are usually localized to the skin, soft tissues, or urinary tract. Bacteremia is the most common infection in the pre-engraftment period, when the patient is profoundly neutropenic. As in the patient receiving conventional cancer chemotherapy, the organisms frequently disseminate from contaminated indwelling catheters or translocate across damaged mucous membranes. Post-engraftment infections occur during the period of lost host cell-mediated immunity resulting from immunosuppressive drugs and insufficient

*Table 3*

**Bone Marrow Transplant Patient Infections According to Transplant Timing and Host Immune Deficit**

| Bone marrow transplant period | Host immune deficits | Likely microbiologic pathogen |
|---|---|---|
| Pretransplant | Neutropenia Anatomic barrier | **Bacterial:** Facultative gram negative bacilli, gram positive cocci |
| Pre-engraftment (0–30 days) | Neutropenia Anatomic barrier | **Bacterial:** Facultative gram positive bacteria, enteric facultative gram negative bacteria **Fungal:** *Candida* and *Aspergillus* **Viral:** HSV, respiratory viruses |
| Post-engraftment (30–100 days) | Slowly recovering humoral and cell-mediated immunity | **Viral:** CMV, EBV, VZV, Adenovirus **Opportunistic:** *Pneumocystis jiroveci, Toxoplasma gondii* **Bacterial:** Gram positive cocci, enteric gram negative bacilli |

donor immunity, and manifest as opportunistic infections, including PJP.

**Solid Organ Transplantation (SOT):** As one progresses through solid organ transplantation, early immune defects and related infections are primarily secondary to surgery and indwelling catheters, whereas later in the transplantation course (1–6 months), immunosuppressive drug therapy targeting T cell function puts patients at risk for opportunistic infections (Table 4). Infections occurring at least 6 months after transplantation are usually caused by typical community acquired pathogens, although prolonged immunosuppression does increase the risk for infections due to EBV and *Aspergillus*.

*Table 4*
**Solid Organ Transplant Patient Infections According to Transplant Timing and Host Immune Deficit**

| Timing of transplant | Host deficits | Likely microbiologic pathogen |
|---|---|---|
| Early (0–30 days) | Anatomic barrier (surgical complication, indwelling lines) | **Bacterial:** All commensals (gram negative enterics, gram positives) **Fungal:** *Candida* **Viral:** HSV, respiratory viruses |
| Middle (1–6 months) | Medication-induced cell-mediated immunity dysfunction | **Viral:** CMV, EBV, VZV **Opportunistic:** *Pneumocystis jiroveci, Toxoplasma gondii* **Bacterial:** *Pseudomonas aeruginosa*, gram negative enterics |
| Late (>6 months) | Slowly recovering humoral and cell-mediated immunity | ***Community acquired infections* Viral:** EBV, VZV **Bacterial:** *Pseudomonas aeruginosa*, gram negative enterics **Fungal:** Aspergillus |

## Investigations

Immunosuppressed patients admitted to the PICU warrant investigations specific to their admitting complaint, in addition to a small list of general laboratory tests: CBC/diff, ESR, CRP, complete chemistry, and microbiologic cultures (see below).

**Blood cultures:** Peripheral blood cultures should be drawn on all immunocompromised patients with fever and/or signs of significant illness on admission to the ICU.

**Indwelling lines:** Peripheral blood cultures in addition to cultures from indwelling vascular devices should be drawn. In situations where only one culture can be obtained, blood culture from the vascular device is preferred. Whether or not to culture each port of an indwelling device is controversial, but when possible, is likely good practice. Patients with indwelling catheters should have their catheter sites examined and any expressible purulent drainage around the site should be sent for gram stain and culture. Patients with an obvious tunnel infection, embolic phenomena, vascular compromise, or sepsis should have the line removed, if possible, and the catheter tip should be sent for gram stain and culture.

**Pulmonary infections:**   In patients with clinical signs and symptoms of respiratory disease, a CXR should be obtained. Significant pulmonary or pleural disease may necessitate a Computed Tomography (CT) scan to clarify diagnosis and guide therapy. Patients requiring intubation should have an endotracheal tube gram stain and culture sent at the time of intubation or soon after. Respiratory antigen panels on nasal swabs can be sent to quickly identify common childhood viral pathogens. Significant pleural fluid should be drained via thoracentesis and sent for standard tests including pH, glucose, LD, protein, cell counts, cytology, bacterial gram stain and culture, fungal stain and culture, AFB smear and culture, and viral culture. Bronchoscopy should be entertained in those patients in whom PCP pneumonia, mycobacterial disease, or CMV infection is highly suspected.

**CNS infection:**   CNS infection in the immunocompromised host may present only with fever, so ICU physicians need to have a high index of suspicion for this important diagnosis. Any immunocompromised host with neurologic symptomatology or signs needs a thorough neurologic evaluation, including head CT and lumbar puncture with opening pressure. Those with intracranial devices should have the device accessed and fluid sent for culture when possible. CSF should be sent for protein, glucose, cell counts with differentials, and bacterial gram stain and culture. Patients with HIV and those with severe immune compromise should have cryptococcal antigen, fungal stain and culture, and AFB smear and culture sent. Those presenting with encephalopathy or seizures should also have viral studies sent including HSV PCR, enteroviral PCR, and arboviral studies (during warm months).

**Diarrhea:**   Immunocompromised patients with diarrhea on admission, especially those with HIV, should have stool studies sent, including stool culture for SSYCE, rotavirus antigen, ova and parasite studies, and giardia antigen. Those who have recently (within the last month) taken antibiotics or chemotherapeutic agents should also have stool sent for *C. difficile* toxin. CMV, which can cause a significant colitis in transplant patients and in those with HIV, is diagnosed by colonic biopsy.

**Urinary tract infections:** Urinalysis and urine culture should be done on all immunocompromised patients presenting to the ICU, especially in those with known history of UTI. Both bacterial and fungal pathogens will be detected via routine culture.

**Sinusitis:** Although sinusitis can be a cause of fever in these patients, other causes should be evaluated before extensive evaluation of the sinuses takes place. The finding of sinus opacification and air-fluid levels on sinus CT is diagnostic. It may be necessary in an immunocompromised patient with a history of chronic sinusitis or one with severe acute sinusitis to undergo sinus aspiration to obtain bacterial, fungal, and AFB cultures in order to direct therapy.

When targeting specific groups of microorganisms, the following tips can be used.

**Bacteria:** Aerobic and anaerobic blood cultures and standard urine cultures will detect most bacterial pathogens. Fastidious or unusual bacteria can be grown with prolonged incubation time, such as common for MTB and NTM. Sputum culture and BAL are sufficient for most bacterial pulmonary pathogens. With *Legionella* species, addition of urinary antigen test is helpful. Gram stains and AFB smears for *Mycobacterium tuberculosis* should be performed.

**Fungi:** Most *Candida* species will be detected on standard blood and urine cultures. Respiratory failure secondary to *Pneumocystis jiroveci* can be detected via direct fluorescence antibody or silver stain from induced sputum or BAL. *Cryptococcus neoformans* can be detected by checking cryptococcal antigen in serum or CSF that is more sensitive than CSF India ink and culture. Endemic fungi infections, such as *Histoplasma capsulatum,* can be detected by tissue stain and culture or by fungal antibody serologies. Mold infections (*Aspergillus* species, *Fusarium* species, *Scedosporium* species, others) may be detected in fungal cultures of sputum and blood, BAL, and biopsy. Galactomannan antigenemia mainly detects *Aspergillus*.

**Viruses:** Many respiratory and community viruses can be detected by antigen panels or viral culture of suspected lesions, nasopharynx, throat, urine, and stool. HSV readily grows within 48 hours, whereas adenovirus and VZV require 4–5 days of incubation. CMV can be detected by antigen detection, CMV PCR, and shell vial from BAL or urine viral culture. Viruses that do not grow in culture and require PCR detection or serological evidence of infection include EBV, parvovirus, HHV-6, 7, and 8, the hepatitis viruses, and the polyomaviruses BK and JC.

**Protozoa:** *Cryptosporidium parvum* and Giardia lamblia can be detected via direct visualization of stool cysts, or more commonly stool antigen tests. *Toxoplasma gondii* can be detected by cyst staining of tissue, PCR, or serology (IgM often negative; 90% of toxoplasmosis disease in intensive care hosts is reactivation).

## Clinical Features and Targeted Therapies

Immunocompromised patients admitted to the PICU may present with localized infections, such as pneumonia, or systemic involvement, including septic shock. Most patients warrant empiric broad antimicrobial coverage to cover gram positive and gram negative pathogens. Empiric viral and fungal coverage is dependent on the clinical suspicion, presentation, and underlying immune deficit. Specific immunocompromised states and their initial empiric antibiotic regimens are detailed below.

**HIV:** With the availability of highly active antiretroviral therapy in developed nations and the rate of maternal-to-child transmission of HIV decreasing to <2%, childhood HIV infection is becoming less common. Still, an appreciation of pediatric HIV infection and its associated opportunistic infections remains important for two reasons: (1) successful outcome of many of the complicating infections requires early diagnosis and treatment, and (2) the identification of an opportunistic pathogen typical of pediatric HIV disease in a previously healthy child may lead to the diagnosis of the underlying HIV infection itself.

Respiratory infections are the most common cause of morbidity and mortality among HIV-positive children, and *Pneumocystis jiroveci*-induced respiratory failure is often the presenting sign of their HIV infection. Patients frequently present to PICUs in respiratory failure during the first year of life, usually between 2 and 6 months of age. Respiratory failure secondary to PJP or other pathogens continues to be the most frequent reason for PICU admission among all children. Coinfection of PJP and CMV with bacterial pathogens is common. Gram negative bacterial pneumonia has also been shown to be a major cause of acute respiratory failure in these patients. Septic shock is the second most common admitting diagnosis of HIV-infected children to PICUs.

Adolescent HIV-infected patients who have acquired their disease through drug use or sexual activity present to PICUs with opportunistic infections typical of HIV-infected adults, including fungal diseases (systemic and central nervous system) and mycobacterial disease. Respiratory failure in these patients can also be secondary to PJP, but may be due to lymphocytic interstitial pneumonitis, which can cause both acute and chronic respiratory compromise (Table 5).

*Table 5*
**Clinical Presentation, Likely Pathogens, and Empiric Therapy of Infections in HIV Patients**

| Clinical presentation | Organisms | Empiric treatment |
|---|---|---|
| Respiratory failure | *Pneumocystis jiroveci*, with or without bacterial or viral coinfection | Trimethoprim/ Sulfamethoxazole and steroids |
| Sepsis | **Bacterial:** Wide spectrum of both gram positive and gram negative organisms | Piperacillin/ Tazobacam or Meropenem, +/− Vancomycin Narrow spectrum as feasible after susceptibility testing |
| | **Fungal:** *Candida albicans, Cryptococcus neoformans Aspergillus* species | Empiric therapy dependent on grade of immunosuppression |
| Gram negative bacteremia | *Pseudomonas aeruginosa, Salmonella* species, *E. coli* | Piperacillin/ Tazobacam or Meropenem Narrow spectrum as feasible after susceptibility testing |

*(continued)*

| Clinical presentation | Organisms | Empiric treatment |
|---|---|---|
| Pneumonia | **Bacterial:** *Streptococcus pneumoniae, Hemophilus influenzae, Staphylococcus aureus* | Third generation cephalosporin, +/− Vancomycin Narrow spectrum as feasible after susceptibility testing |
| | **Viral:** RSV, influenza, parainfluenza, adenovirus, CMV | |
| | **Mycobacterial:** *Mycobacterium tuberculosis,* nontuberculous mycobacteria | Specific TB regimen |
| Meningitis/ Encephalitis | **Bacterial:** *Streptococcus pneumoniae, Neisseria meningiditis, Hemophilus influenzae* | Third generation cephalosporin, +/− Vancomycin Narrow spectrum as feasible after susceptibility testing |
| | **Fungal:** *Cryptococcus neoformans, Aspergillus species, Candida albicans,* | Empiric therapy dependent on grade of immunosuppression and clinical suspicion |
| | **Protozoa:** *Toxoplasma gondii* | Pyrimethamine plus sulfadiazine |

**Neutropenia:** Empiric broad-spectrum antibacterial therapy should be initiated immediately after appropriate cultures have been obtained in the neutropenic patient with fever or other signs or symptoms of infection. To cover for gram positive and gram negative bacterial infections, including *Pseudomonas aeruginosa,* a carbapenem, ceftazidime, cefepime, and/or anti-pseudomonal penicillin (for example, piperacillin/

tazobactam) should be started. Addition of an aminoglycoside and/or vancomycin depends on risk factors. Antimicrobial coverage with amphotericin B should be added if shock develops in the course of neutropenia, or if fever remains at day 5 of antimicrobial therapy. If *Aspergillus* is detected, voriconazole has been shown to have superior efficacy over amphotericin.

**BMT:** During the pre-engraftment period, the therapeutic approach is the same as in the patient with neutropenia from conventional chemotherapy (see above). During the post-engraftment period, broad-spectrum antibacterial coverage, including anti-pseudomonal drugs, should be administered while comprehensively searching for opportunistic pathogens. Targeted therapy is dependent on the pathogen detected.

**SOT:** During the early period (0–30 days), infections are likely related to surgical complications, and should empirically cover gram positive skin organisms and other possible sources of surgical infection depending on location of surgery. For example, vancomycin and piperacillin/tazobactam would be a good drug combination for an infection during the early period in a kidney transplant recipient. The use of vancomycin is dependent on the severity of host infection and the likelihood of hospital- or community-acquired methicillin-resistant *Staphylococcus aureus*. During the middle period (1–6 months) broad-spectrum coverage, including pseudomonal coverage, should accompany a comprehensive search for opportunistic pathogens. Targeted therapy should depend on the pathogen that is detected. Infections during the late period (>6 months) are usually caused by typical community-acquired pathogens. Patients should have empiric broad-spectrum antibiotic coverage, and if the clinical suspicion is high, additional empiric antiviral and antifungal, particularly *Aspergillus*, coverage should be added.

## Pitfalls of Therapy

Although antimicrobial drugs are generally safe, all drugs have side effects. Severely ill immunocompromised patients in the PICU setting are at risk for suffering a number of potentially severe antimicrobial drug toxicities (Table 6).

*Table 6*

## Commonly Used Antimicrobial Drugs in the PICU and Their Side Effects

| Antimicrobial drug | Drug toxicities |
| --- | --- |
| Beta lactam drugs: penicillins, cephalosporins, monolactams, carbapenems | Rash, leukopenia, platelet dysfunction, interstitial nephritis, GI toxicity, phlebitis, seizures, anaphylaxis, serum sickness |
| Aminoglycosides | Ototoxicity, nephrotoxicity, anaphylaxis (rare), neuromuscular blockade |
| Macrolides | GI toxicity, drug interactions (competitively inhibits other cytochrome p450 drug metabolism) |
| Vancomycin | Red Man's syndrome, ototoxicity, hypotension, phlebitis, renal toxicity (rare) |
| Metronidazole | Seizures, ataxia, encephalopathy, peripheral neuropathy, disulfuram reaction |
| Fluoroquinolones | Tendonitis, phototoxicity, GI toxicity, headache, seizures, confusion |
| Tetracyclines | Tooth discoloration, phototoxicity, GI toxicity, pseudotumor cerebri, hepatotoxicity |
| Sulfonamides/Trimethoprim | Rash, Steven Johnson syndrome, GI toxicity, pancreatitis, anemia, thrombocytopenia |
| Linezolid | Anemia, thrombocytopenia, leucopenia, GI toxicity, rash |
| Amphotericin B | Electrolyte disturbance, nephrotoxicity, agranulocytosis, hepatotoxicity, infusion reaction, anemia, headache |
| Voriconazole | Abnormal vision, GI toxicity, hepatotoxicity |
| Acyclovir | GI toxicity, nephrotoxicity, seizures, leucopenia, thrombocytopenia |

# References

Bonilla FA, Geha RS. Update on primary immunodeficiency diseases. J Allergy Clin Immunol 2006;117:S435–41.

Kleigman RM. Practical strategies in pediatric diagnosis and therapy, 2nd ed. Philly: W.B. Saunders Co; 2004.

Michaels MG, Green M. Infections in immunocompromised persons. Nelson textbook of pediatrics. Philly: Saunders; 2004.

Steele RW. Infection in the immunocompromised host. Pediatr Infect Dis 1985;4:309–14.

Dykewicz CA. Summary of the guidelines for preventing opportunistic infections among hematopoietic stem cell transplant recipients. Clin Infect Dis 2001;33:139–44.

O'Grady NP, Barie PS, Bartlett JG, et al. Practice guidelines for evaluating new fever in critically ill adult patients. Task force of the society of critical care medicine and the infectious diseases society of America. Clin Infect Dis 1998;26:1042–59.

Gea-Banacloche JC, Opal SM, Jorgensen J, et al. Sepsis associated with immunosuppressive medications: an evidence-based review. Crit Care Med 2004;32:S578–90.

Guay LA, Musoke P, Fleming T, et al. Intrapartum and neonatal single-dose nevirapine compared with zidovudine for prevention of mother-to-child transmission of HIV-1 in Kampala, Uganda: HIVNET 012 randomised trial. Lancet 1999;354:795–802.

Wilkinson JD, Greenwald BM. The acquired immunodeficiency syndrome: impact on the pediatric intensive care unit. Crit Care Clin 1988;4:831–44.

Hatherill M. Sepsis predisposition in children with human immunodeficiency virus. Pediatr Crit Care Med 2005;6:S92–8.

Notterman DA. Pediatric AIDS and critical care. Crit Care Med 1993;21:S319–21.

Cooper S, Lyall H, Walters S, et al. Children with human immunodeficiency virus admitted to a paediatric intensive care unit in the United Kingdom over a 10-year period. Intensive Care Med 2004;30:113–8.

Vernon DD, Holzman BH, Lewis P, et al. Respiratory failure in children with acquired immunodeficiency syndrome and acquired immunodeficiency syndrome-related complex. Pediatrics 1988;82:223–8.

Benson CA, Kaplan JE, Masur H, et al. Treating opportunistic infections among HIV-exposed and infected children: recommendations from CDC, the National Institutes of Health, and the Infectious Diseases Society of America. MMWR Recomm Rep 2004;53:1–112.

Hughes WT, Armstrong D, Bodey GP, et al. 2002 guidelines for the use of antimicrobial agents in neutropenic patients with cancer. Clin Infect Dis 2002;34:730–51.

# I. Nosocomial Infections in the PICU

Philip Toltzis

## Introduction

Nosocomial (hospital-acquired) infections are a prominent cause of morbidity and mortality among hospitalized patients, and they add tens of billions of dollars to health care costs in the United States each year. Nosocomial infections occur 5–10 times more frequently among ICU patients compared with those cared for on the routine ward. The incidence of nosocomial infections specifically in pediatric ICUs is variable depending on the nature of the patient population; on average, approximately 5% of children admitted to a PICU will acquire an infection while there.

## Key Principles

- An infection is categorized as "nosocomial" if signs and symptoms begin >48 hours after admission. The infection is presumed to be community-acquired if the onset occurs prior to this. These criteria follow the guidelines of the Centers for Disease Control and Prevention (CDC) and National Nosocomial Infection Surveillance (NNIS) system (recently renamed the National Safety Healthcare Network [NSHN]).
- Many community-acquired infections have incubation periods exceeding 48 hours, and occasionally a hospital-acquired pathogen can produce symptoms very shortly after hospital admission.
- The key sites of nosocomial infections in ICU patients are the blood stream, lungs, urinary tract, surgical wound, and gastrointestinal tract. Among adult patients, the urinary tract usually ranks as the most common site of nosocomial infection, likely a result of the high use of bladder catheters in this population. In most surveys of PICUs, the bloodstream is the most common site of nosocomial infection, followed by the lungs.
- The spectrum of microorganisms that cause nosocomial infections depends on the site of infection and is similar in adults and children (Table 1).

*Table 1*
## Organisms Most Frequently Implicated in Nosocomial Infections in the PICU

| Infected site | Organism class | Most common species |
|---|---|---|
| Blood stream | Gram positive bacteria | Coagulase-negative staphylococci, *S. aureus*, Enterococcus spp. |
| | Gram negative bacteria | Enteric (from the family Enterobacteriaceae): *E. coli*, *Klebsiella*, *Enterobacter*, *Serratia*, *Citrobacter* |
| | | Non-enteric (derived from the environment): *Pseudomonas*, *Acinetobacter* |
| | Fungus | *Candida* |
| Lungs | Bacteria (most commonly occurring in the context of ventilator-associated pneumonia) | *S. aureus*, *Pseudomonas* |
| | Virus (frequently detected in non-ventilated children) | RSV, parainfluenza, influenza |
| Urinary tract | Gram negative bacteria | Enteric: *E. coli*, *Klebsiella*, *Enterobacter*, *Serratia*, *Citrobacter* |
| | | Non-enteric: *Pseudomonas* |
| | Gram positive bacteria | Enterococcus spp., coagulase-negative staphylococci, *S. aureus* |
| | Fungus | *Candida* |

*(continued)*

| Infected site | Organism class | Most common species |
|---|---|---|
| Gastrointestinal tract | Bacteria | *C. difficile* |
| | Virus | Rotavirus, Calicivirus, and other enteric viral pathogens |

# Pathophysiology

- Patients admitted to the ICU rapidly become colonized in the nasopharynx and gastrointestinal tract with organisms not usually found in high numbers in healthy subjects.
- This is partially explained by exposure to resident bacteria that are transmitted to the patient through the hands of caregivers.
- Populations of these organisms then expand after the patient is administered antibiotics to which they are resistant, a frequent scenario in the ICU.
- Critical illness, in and of itself, promotes colonization by these "hospital" pathogens. Critically ill patients become colonized by gram negative bacteria in their throats within a couple of days of ICU admission, for example, while less ill patients and caregivers, exposed to the same environment for the same duration of time, do not.
- Colonization by hospital organisms is a prelude to invasion. Often, the organisms invade the critically ill patient by traveling along a plastic device that extends from a normally colonized space to a normally sterile one.
- Nosocomial blood stream infections are most frequent in the patient with a central venous catheter, nosocomial pneumonias occur in patients on a mechanical ventilator with an endotracheal tube, and nosocomial urinary tract infections occur most commonly in patients with a Foley catheter in place.
- The risk of nosocomial infections in the patient with invasive devices is cumulative over time.
- Consequently, removal of such devices at the earliest possible time is key in the prevention of nosocomial infection.
- Less commonly, invasion of microorganisms occurs through "translocation," a process by which the bacteria or fungi enter the bloodstream through a mucosal surface in the setting of serious illness.

# Clinical Features

The cardinal sign of a nosocomial infection is a new onset fever in a previously afebrile hospitalized patient. Severe nosocomial infections may occur in the absence of fever, however. Moreover, there are multiple causes of fever in the PICU patient that are not related to infections (Table 2). Although atelectasis frequently is cited as a cause of non-infectious fevers in the ICU, the association between atelectasis and fever has not been well established.

Clinical features of nosocomial infections at specific sites are as follows.

## Nosocomial Primary Blood Stream Infections (BSIs)

"Primary BSIs" are episodes of bacteremia or fungemia in which there is no evidence of infection in a solid organ (the lungs or urinary tract, for example). The vast majority of primary BSIs result from contamination of the intravascular portion of a central venous or arterial catheter. Serum proteins deposit rapidly on the plastic of these catheters shortly after their insertion. Microorganisms become established on this proteinacious coat either by traveling down the internal or external surface of the catheter from the skin, or via translocation from the pharynx or gastrointestinal tract. Several agents that typically cause primary BSIs, particularly coagulase-negative staphylococci and *Candida* species, produce a biofilm that further embeds the organisms on the catheter, protecting them from clearance by the immune system and antibiotics. Although occasionally purulence or erythema at the catheter exit site is associated with catheter related BSIs, more

*Table 2*
**Causes of Non-infectious Fevers in the ICU**

| Children and adults | Primarily adults |
|---|---|
| Atelectasis | Stroke |
| Drug fever | Myocardial infarction |
| Post-transfusion fever | Ischemic bowel |
| Aspiration | Pulmonary embolus |
| Blood clot (vascular, intracranial, retroperitoneal) | Adrenal insufficiency |
| Neoplasm | |
| Pancreatitis | |

commonly there are no signs other than fever or hypothermia. Catheter-associated BSIs may occasionally be severe enough to cause overt sepsis.

## Nosocomial Pneumonia

Bacterial nosocomial pneumonia almost always occurs in the intubated patient (in this setting, it is referred to as "ventilator-associated pneumonia (VAP)." The bacteria enter the lungs when the patient aspirates upper airway secretions, often mixed with regurgitant gastric fluid, around the endotracheal tube, carrying bacteria into the lower respiratory tract. The diagnosis of VAP frequently is difficult to detect with certainty, since most patients on mechanical ventilators have pre-existing cardiopulmonary dysfunction with an abnormal chest radiograph and pulmonary mechanics. Accordingly, the CDC has proposed the following signs and symptoms to establish a provisionary diagnosis of VAP:

- New onset fever or hypothermia
- Change in volume or character of tracheal secretions (particularly thickness, with purulence documented by finding many neutrophils on Gram stain)
- A new infiltrate on chest radiograph that persists for >48 hours
- Worsening respiratory status, usually manifested by a requirement for increased mechanical ventilatory support
- Leukopenia (<4000 cells/mm$^3$) or leukocytosis (>12,000 cells/mm$^3$)

## Nosocomial Urinary Tract Infection

Nosocomial UTIs usually occur in the patient with a Foley catheter in place. Frequently the signs and symptoms of community-acquired UTI, such as frequency or pain on urination, are difficult to solicit in the critically ill child.

## Surgical Wound Infection

The diagnosis of surgical wound infection is established virtually exclusively by inspection of the wound. The wound usually becomes purulent and often foul smelling, with erythema and induration around the edges and increased tenderness to palpation.

## Gastrointestinal Tract

Nosocomial GI tract infections usually are heralded by new-onset diarrhea. Constipation or abdominal distension and pain may occur as well. Severe cases of *C. difficile* colitis are associated with leukocytosis, sepsis, toxic megacolon, and intestinal perforation.

# Investigations

## Primary BSI

To diagnose primary BSI in the patient with a central venous or arterial catheter, most authorities recommend obtaining at least one blood culture through each port of the indwelling catheter and one from a peripheral vein. The catheter is implicated as the source of the infection if there is 5–10-fold higher bacterial concentration from the catheter-derived blood compared with that obtained from the periphery, as documented by quantitative blood cultures. In practice, quantitative blood cultures are cumbersome to perform and frequently unavailable. In these situations, one may use time-to-blood-culture-positivity as a surrogate: central venous catheter blood cultures that are positive >2–3 hours before peripheral-vein derived blood, as determined by the automated blood culture systems used by many hospitals, implicates the catheter as the source of the infection. In practice, particularly in pediatrics, often only through-the-catheter blood cultures are obtained. When these become positive, particularly with coagulase-negative staphylococci, distinguishing whether the blood culture indicates a true bacteremia or a contamination becomes essentially impossible. If the catheter is removed, sending the intravascular portion in a dry, sterile container for semiquantitative culture, an assay performed by most large hospitals, can establish true catheter-related BSI, albeit retrospectively.

## VAP

Establishing the diagnosis of VAP is very difficult. Although in practice many clinicians will submit tracheal aspirates from the endotracheal tube for qualitative microbiology, this test has very poor predictive value for lower tract infection. In really troublesome cases, invasive approaches may be necessary: A more reliable approach is to obtain lower respiratory tract specimens through fiber-optic bronchoscopy (either with a protected brush specimen or with a bronchoalveolar lavage) and then subjecting the specimen to quantitative cultures. The diagnosis can also be secured by isolating the organism from pleural fluid or from a lung biopsy. Isolation of a pathogenic organism from a blood culture in the intubated patient with a new infiltrate is presumptive evidence of VAP but, given the multiple other possible sources of a positive blood culture in the PICU patient, is not definitive.

## Surgical Wound Infection

The diagnosis of a surgical wound infection is established through inspection of the wound. Culture of wounds that appear clean on examination may yield mixed bacterial flora that have no pathogenic importance; thus, culture of a well-appearing wound may yield confusing or misleading results. If the site appears infected, culture of the wound may help guide therapy if the sample yields heavy growth of a single pathogen.

## Gastrointestinal Tract

Most hospitals are able to test stool specimens for *C. difficile*, usually by assaying for the toxins elaborated by the organism. Excretion of *C. difficile* toxin is uneven and detection may require testing 2–3 samples. Rotavirus stool detection kits also are commercially available and widely employed. Caliciviruses and other enteric viral pathogens are not detectable by most non-research laboratories. *Salmonella, Shigella, Yersinia, Campylobacter,* pathogenic *E. coli,* and intestinal parasites are rarely implicated in nosocomial diarrhea and should be tested only under specific circumstances (for example, after contact with a known source).

## **Management**

The principles for treating nosocomial infections in the PICU are as follows:

- The requirement for immediate antibiotics depends upon the severity of illness and stability of the patient. Not all nosocomial fevers in the ICU require immediate antibiotics.
- If immediate therapy is warranted, cover the most likely organisms (Table 1). Most regimens include combinations of anti-staphylococcal drugs and antibiotics providing broad activity against enteric and non-enteric gram negative bacteria.
- Narrow the spectrum of antibiotics once culture and susceptibility testing is complete.

- Continue antibiotics for a maximum of 14 days unless there is an abscess or other purulent collection left undrained. There are no data justifying a more prolonged antibiotic course, even in the very ill patient.
- Remove plastic devices whenever possible.
- If a surgical wound is infected, consider suture removal and debridement.
- Consider empiric antifungal drugs if fever remains unresponsive to antibiotics and the patient has one or more of the following:

    - Poor or worsening clinical stability
    - Prolonged prior exposure to antibacterial agents
    - Prolonged central venous or Foley catheterization
    - Recent history of abdominal perforation
    - T-lymphocyte dysfunction

Nosocomial pathogens in many ICUs have become resistant to commonly employed antibiotics. The clinician should consult the hospital microbiology laboratory to get an accurate assessment of the most common resistant phenotypes in a given unit. The most frequently encountered antibiotic resistant organisms and their therapies are listed in Table 3.

*Table 3*
**Commonly Encountered Resistance Phenotypes among Nosocomial Pathogens the PICU[1]**

| Organism | Resistance pattern | Alternatives |
| --- | --- | --- |
| *S. aureus* | Methicillin (MRSA) | Vancomycin Linezolid Daptomycin |
| Coagulase-negative staph species including S. epidermidis | β-lactams some vancomycin resistance reported | Vancomycin Linezolid |
| Enterococcus | β-lactams/aminoglycoside | Vancomycin +/− aminoglycoside |
| | Vancomycin (VRE) | Linezolid Daptomycin |

(continued)

| Organism | Resistance pattern | Alternatives |
|---|---|---|
| Gram negative bacilli | A wide variety of β-lactams (both early and late generation), +/− aminoglycosides, +/− quinolones | Consider a carbepenem or cefepime, plus amikacin as initial therapy and narrow as able; substitution or addition of a quinolone[2] may be necessary |
| Candida | Fluconazole | Amphotericin B Echinocandin Newer triazole (eg, voriconazole) |

[1]Consultation with an infectious diseases specialist is strongly advised when these organisms are isolated or suspected.
[2]Quinolones are not labeled for use in children <18 years.

# References

Coffin SE, Zaoutis TE. Infection control, hospital epidemiology, and patient safety. Infect Dis Clin North Am 2005;19(3):647–65.

Richards MJ, Edwards JR, Culver DH, Gaynes RP. Nosocomial infections in pediatric intensive care units in the United States. National Nosocomial Infections Surveillance System. Pediatrics 1999;103(4):e39.

Richards MJ, Edwards JR, Culver DH, Gaynes RP. Nosocomial infections in medical intensive care units in the United States. National Nosocomial Infections Surveillance System. Crit Care Med 1999;27(5):887–92.

Safdar N, Maki DG. The pathogenesis of catheter-related bloodstream infection with noncuffed short-term central venous catheters. Intensive Care Med 2004;30(1):62–7.

Costa SF, Miceli MH, Anaissie EJ. Mucosa or skin as source of coagulase-negative staphylococcal bacteraemia? Lancet Infect Dis 2004;4(5):278–86.

Chastre J, Fagon JY. Ventilator-associated pneumonia. Am J Respir Crit Care Med 2002;165(7):867–903.

Starr J. Clostridium difficile associated diarrhoea: diagnosis and treatment. Bmj 2005;331(7515):498–501.

Maki DG, Weise CE, Sarafin HW. A semiquantitative culture method for identifying intravenous-catheter-related infection. N Engl J Med 1977; 296(23):1305–9.

Jourdain B, Novara A, Joly-Guillou ML, et al. Role of quantitative cultures of endotracheal aspirates in the diagnosis of nosocomial pneumonia. Am J Respir Crit Care Med 1995;152(1):241–6.

O'Grady NP, Barie PS, Bartlett JG, et al. Practice guidelines for evaluating new fever in critically ill adult patients. Task Force of the Society of Critical Care Medicine and the Infectious Diseases Society of America. Clin Infect Dis 1998;26(5):1042–59.

# Chapter 19

# Inborn Errors of Metabolism

Aneal Khan
Murray Potter

## Introduction

- We highlight some of the major issues in the intensive management of children presenting with an inborn error of metabolism (IEM).
- The focus is not on a differential of metabolic disorders, but on the clinical presentations associated complications, and immediate actions.
- While the number of metabolic diseases exceeds 400, the body's responses are few.

## Major Manifestations

The main presentations are:

- neurologic disease (encephalopathy, seizures, hypotonia).
- movement disorders.
- hepatocellular disease.
- hypoglycemia.
- cardiomyopathy.

## Other Manifestations

- Children and adults can also present with a psychiatric disturbance.
- There can be a symptom-free interval before decompensations occur. The presentation can be indistinguishable from a catastrophic illness due to other causes such as drug intoxications, severe nutritional deficiencies often triggered and

commensurate with intercurrent illness, dehydration, vomiting, poor tolerance to certain foods (such as protein), and in the newborn, adaptation to extrauterine life.

## Clinical Suspicion for an IEM

- The presenting symptoms of metabolic disorders are often nonspecific or are similar to or masked by acquired illnesses.
- Always consider and evaluate non-IEM causes and IEM causes of a presentation simultaneously.
- In particular, nutritional deficiencies or ingestion of certain drugs can mimic IEM. An example is encephalopathy due to lead intoxication exacerbated by anemia.
- A toxicologic screen including an alcohol level, particularly in an adolescent, may prove to be informative.
- Non-IEM causes will not be exhaustively reviewed or included in differentials in this section. Metabolic disorders should always be considered in any individual for which no clear cause of the illness is identified, particularly in newborn infants, in any child with a pattern of recurrent illness of the same variety, when the child is not improving despite adequate supportive measures or if the child has become ill after an initial symptom-free period.
- In a child, any change in the level of consciousness, whether or not accompanied by focal neurological signs, seizures, strokes or intracranial hypertension, acute onset of psychiatric disturbances or movement disorders should prompt consideration of an IEM. Also consider an IEM with a family history of a previous child presenting with the same symptoms or an unexplained death, especially if the parents are consanguineous.

## Investigations

- It's important to emphasize that there is no such thing as a "comprehensive metabolic screen." With hundreds of disorders, no single test strategy is adequate.
- What is often offered as a metabolic screen in some centers includes urine $\alpha$-ketoacids, ketones, reducing substances, sulfites and an amino acid screen. Only a limited number of conditions can be screened for these tests, and in some cases, such as for maple syrup urine disease, amino acids levels in plasma are more sensitive than those in urine.

- In some jurisdictions with expanded newborn screening, samples for diagnostic studies may have already been taken before discharge.
- By the limited clinical nature in which metabolic diseases can present, a clinical diagnosis may not be possible even in the hands of an experienced practitioner.
- A comprehensive laboratory evaluation is essential at the time of the decompensation.
- In the neonatal intensive care unit (NICU), family history and history of death in children can sometimes lead to directed investigations, but in virtually all cases, the diagnosis is initially unknown.
- In children admitted to the pediatric intensive care unit (PICU), there is often an established diagnosis with the child having a decompensation of their metabolic illness.

## Overall Management Principles

A few general principles apply when managing patients in the intensive care setting. The principles can be applied in almost any setting:

1. Support and stabilize the patient.
2. Restore homeostasis and treat the cause of the decompensation.
3. Remove the accumulated toxin.
4. Provide nutritional support.
5. Provide adjunct therapies (if applicable).

    - Always consult a physician experienced in managing metabolic disorders early in the course regarding special therapies or management issues.
    - The management is truly multidisciplinary, and can involve different medical specialists not only to determine the extent of the decompensation, but to evaluate for features which may help in determining the final outcome and management.

For an additional detailed review, please see Preitsch et al., in the Journal of Inherited Metabolic Disease, 2002.

## Specific Treatment Principles

IEMs are genetic disorders that in most cases result in a defective enzyme that does not allow a normal reaction to occur. Using an analogy of a urea cycle defect, think of a blockage in the water nozzle at the end of a garden hose in which the pressure has built up, there is a leak and the water hose is ready to burst. The accumulation of water pressure before the block is the danger. In metabolic disease, the danger is intoxication from substrate accumulation (eg ammonia). This "substrate intoxication" can be removed by turning down the main water supply (ie, protein-free diet), soaking up the leaked water with a sponge (ie, giving drugs), coupling the hose to a working hose (ie, dialysis), and perhaps hand-watering the plants (ie, provide essential amino acids or energy) until the cause of the whole problem is fixed.

- ABCs The first principle is to support and stabilize the patient, always ensure general measures are taken—airway, respiration, circulation, oxygenation and fluids.
- Fluids should involve adequate electrolytes, replacement of fluid deficits and compensate for ongoing losses.
- In almost all cases, glucose serves as an adequate energy source to reverse catabolism.
- Prevent hypoglycemia: The glucose infusion rate should provide at least 8 to 10 mg/kg/min. In general this involves using a 10% dextrose solution at 150% maintenance, but higher rates, even requiring the use of insulin to control hyperglycemia, may be necessary. A useful goal is to maintain a blood sugar of at least 4 to 5 mmol/L based on physiologic levels (Kalhan and Peter-Wohl, 2000).
- Reverse catabolism: is achieved when ketones are no longer formed measured either through a urine dipstick for ketones or blood ketone measurement.

## Stabilize electrolyte status

- The sodium chloride concentration should reflect clinical needs. In a patient who is hypotensive or who has moderate to severe dehydration, 0.9% NaCl would generally be preferred. Depending on the size of the child, the volume of fluid to be infused and the total daily amount of NaCl to be replaced, and the supply of Na from medications (such as Na benzoate), the 10% dextrose can be mixed with a range of NaCl between 0.2 0.9%.
- Potassium can be added as needed.
- Bicarbonate is often not added initially unless there is severe acidosis since the provision of fluids will often lead to

improvement and the acidosis can be monitored during the initial hours of management to see if bicarbonate is necessary. We generally do not give bicarbonate unless the serum/plasma levels fall below 15 to 17 mEq/L.

- Plasma osmolarity should be kept >300 mOsmol/L and any signs of cerebral edema should be treated.

## Removal of toxic intermediates

- If the IEM has led to accumulation of toxic substances, such as ammonium, immediate action must be taken to remove and prevent the accumulation of the toxin (Jouvet et al., 2001).
- Reducing toxin accumulation often involves reversing a catabolic state, for example by giving an intravenous glucose infusion, and eliminating sources of the toxin, such as reducing or eliminati protein from the diet in a patient who is hyperammonemic.
- Toxin removal can involve giving a medication that will remove the toxin by using an alternate pathway (Scaglia et al., 2004) or by direct removal of the toxin, such as with dialysis.
- Toxins typically requiring removal include ammonium, amino acids such as leucine. Toxins are small molecules and easily diffusible, which make dialysis an ideal route for rapid toxin removal.
- Nutritional support must be provided at the onset, since often lack of nutrition is a contributing factor to the decompensation.
- The main decisions to make are whether to use parenteral or enteral feeding. Enteral feeding should be used whenever possible.
- Decisions on the composition of nutrients involve considering:

  - Does one use a normal diet, high carbohydrate diet (such as in glycogen storage disease)
  - Fat-limited diet (such as in fatty acid oxidation disorders)
  - Restriction of a specific carbohydrate (such as galactose in galactosemia)
  - A protein-limited diet (such as in urea cycle defects)

## Specific agents to consider

- Sodium benzoate, sodium phenylacetate, sodium phenylbutyrate are indispensable for urea cycle disorders.
- Nitisinone is vital to the treatment of type I tyrosinemia

- N-carbamylglutamate has shown superb results in select causes of hyperammonemia (Gebhardt et al., 2005).
- Vitamin $B_6$ is essential in pyridoxine-dependant seizures.

The number of adjunct therapies, either speculated or proven to work in certain inborn errors of metabolism is beyond the scope of this brief and any use of these therapies must be initiated after consultation with a specialist experienced in their use.

# Approaches to Specific Presentations

### 1. Presentation dominated by encephalopathy

- Initial laboratory work-up should include blood gas, electrolytes, glucose, ammonia, lactate, liver enzymes and functional tests, quantitative amino acids, urine ketones (urinalysis), reducing substances and urine organic acids.
- Additional studies may be indicated if the further specific presentations are also present such as hypoglycemia (discussed below), lactic acidosis (lactate-to-pyruvate ratio in blood and CSF) and hyperammonemia (urine amino acids).
- Neuroimaging is crucial T1- and T2-weighted images to look for structural changes and myelination, MRS to look at lactate, NAA, choline and creatine signals, and diffusion-weighted imaging to look at recent ischemic events. Neuroimaging can serve not only as a diagnostic tools, but to evaluate the extent of organ damage in diseases such as maple syrup urine disease that can lead to cerebral edema.
- In premature and newborn infants, total and free carnitine levels may be low and may not serve a diagnostic purpose. When these studies are performed, they should be accompanied by a plasma or whole-blood acyl-carnitine profile (not just an acyl-carnitine level). Although not the preferred sample source, blood-spot acyl-carnitines can be used if no other source is readily available.
- Pyruvate levels are not useful unless the lactate is elevated. Serum fatty acid and ketone bodies are also not useful unless the child his hypoglycemic.
- A metabolic specialist should be consulted before CSF studies are undertaken to provide recommendations for testing and sample handling. For example, comparing CSF-to-plasma glycine levels is not of use if they are sampled too far apart.
- Testing for folinic-acid responsive seizures requires specialized handling of samples and arrangements for the sample to

be shipped to labs in other centers. Having said this, any CSF sample should test for the requisite glucose, protein, amino acids and pyruvate if indicated.

## a. Presentation with metabolic acidosis (pH <7.35, $HCO_3$ <4, $pCO_2$ usually <40)

- Clinically rapid, deep breathing (Kussmaul), respiratory distress are seen.
- Severe acidosis (pH <7.20) may require bicarbonate treatment: give [0.15 × weight (kg) × base deficit] mmol bicarb intravenously.
- Elevated anion gap ($Na-Cl-HCO_3$): Lactic acidosis (see below), ketoacidosis (see below), organic acidosis.
- Measure pyruvate (calculate lactate/pyruvate or L/P), plasma ketones, urinary organic acids (UOA), carnitine, acylcarnitines.
- Organic acidopathies usually have a diagnostic UOA and/or acylcarnitine profile and low carnitine and/or low free-to-total carnitine ratio.
- Empiric therapy for organic acidopathies includes stopping protein intake, providing intravenous glucose as above to a level to reduce urine ketones to zero and providing calories using intravenous lipids at 1–2 mg/kg/day.
- Methyl-malonic acidemia can often be accompanied a megaloblastic anemia and elevated plasma total homocysteine levels. Empiric therepy with vitamin B12 1 mg IV may need to be initiated before diagnostic studies are complete.

### i) Presentation with lactic acidosis (>2.2 mmol/L):

- Most frequently from tissue hypoxia (shock, heart failure/CHD, pulmonary disease, skin ischemia, gut ischemia, renal failure), also called "type A" lactic acidosis.
- Since "type A" lactic acidosis is by far more common, all factors that may cause lactic acidosis that are not metabolic should first be considered and managed before the lactic acidosis can be considered due to an inborn error of metabolism.
- This excludes a lactic acidosis that is typical for a decompensation in a patient with an existing diagnosis (such as in mitochondrial disorders).
- A detailed clinical evaluation is more important tha obtaining a lactate-to-pyruvate ratio however, "type A" lactic acidosis generally presents with a lactate >5 mmol/L, an elevated L/P ratio (>20) in type A, and rapid resolution

by treating the underlying cause (ie, surgery for midgut volvulus).

- Common primary metabolic causes of lactic acidosis with increased L/P are mitochondrial electron transport chain (ETC) enzyme deficiencies while pyruvate dehydrogenase (PDH) deficiency and pyruvate carboxylase (PC) deficiency have a normal L/P.
- Occasionally CSF lactate (+/− pyruvate) are helpful.
- Although often regarded, but not proven, some physicians consider using a "mitochondrial cocktail" consisting of thiamine (50 mg IV load, then 10–25 mg/d), biotin (20 mg load, then 10 mg/day).
- PC deficiency may be secondary to a biotin defect, also called multiple carboxylase deficiency (biotinidase or holocarboxylase synthetase deficiency).
- Gluconeogenic, fatty acid oxidation and organic acid metabolism defects may cause a secondary lactic acidosis, but laboratory manifestations will be characteristic.

### ii) A presentation with a ketoacidosis:

- Results from many nonmetabolic causes (DKA, catabolic state) and secondary metabolic causes (MSUD, organic acidopathies, GSD, gluconeogenic defects).
- Primary ketone utilization disorders are rare.

### b. A presentation with a normal anion gap (bicarb loss, hyperchloremia)

- Many metabolic disorders can produce a renal tubular acidosis (galactosemia, hereditary fructose intolerance, hepatorenal tyrosinemia, cystinosis, GSD I, Fanconi-Bickel syndrome, congenital lactic acidosis, Wilson disease, Vitamin D dependency, osteopetrosis, Lowe syndrome).

### c. Presentation with hypoglycemia (plasma glucose <2.5 mmol/L)

- Differential: includes endocrine (insulin excess, counter-regulatory hormone deficiency) versus glucose "overutilization" (fatty acid oxidation disorder and ketone, glycogen, galactose, fructose or gluconeogenic disorder). This "overutilization" occurs when normal alternative sources of glucose or other energy molecules are unavailable.
- Critical samples: a major pitfall in the evaluation of hypoglycemia is the failure to obtain critical samples while the patient is hypoglycemic before initiating therapy. Diagnostic work-up

is much more difficult "after-the-fact" and may involve fasting the child to induce another hypoglycemic state.

- This does not mean the treatment should be delayed until results are obtained, but rather that samples are collected, as soon as possible and the intervention is given immediately. If sample collection will delay treatment, the primary objective is to treat the patient first.

- Samples considered obligatory include plasma free fatty acids, plasma beta-hydroxybutyrate, plasma glucose, lactate, uric acid, acyl-carnitine profile, urine organic acids (catherized if necessary), urine dipstick for ketones, insulin, cortisol, and growth hormone.

- If possible, additional studies at or after the even can include a TSH, free and total carnitines, and plasma creatine kinase.

- The response to certain methods to correct the hypoglycemia can often be helpful. For example, in glycogen storage disease type Ia, glucagon will not improve the blood sugar and will often worsen the lactic acidosis and plasma uric acid level.

- Emergency treatment: after critical sample is obtained treat with glucose bolus (0.5 g/kg: 1 mL/kg of D50W, 2 mL/kg of D25W, or 5 mL/kg of D10W) followed by glucose infusion to keep glucose in normal range (start at 8 mg/kg/min).

- Frequent monitoring of glucose and electrolytes is necessary.

- If a fatty acid oxidation defect is possible (Diagnostic clue: lack of urine or plasma ketones), providing fats either enterally, and especially intravenously, can worsen the situation and may be catastrophic. Therefore, in a patient with hypoglycemia in whom an inborn error of metabolism is suspect, fats should be withheld until a fatty acid oxidation defect is excluded.

- Specific metabolic work-up: urine organic acids (UOA), UMS, PAA, carnitine, urate, triglycerides, acylcarnitines, consider pyruvate and galactosemia screen.

- Metabolic Disorders: Hormonal response to hypoglycemia will be normal (low insulin, normal/high cortisol), except in glutamate dehydrogenase hyperactivity, which has hyperinsulinism and hyperammonemia. Main acute treatment for all the metabolic disorders is to supply glucose (see above).

- Hypoketotic hypoglycemia. Elevated free fatty acids (increased FFA/ketone ratio).

- Fatty acid oxidation disorders (including carnitine cycle disorders): Specific diagnosis often suggested by UOA and

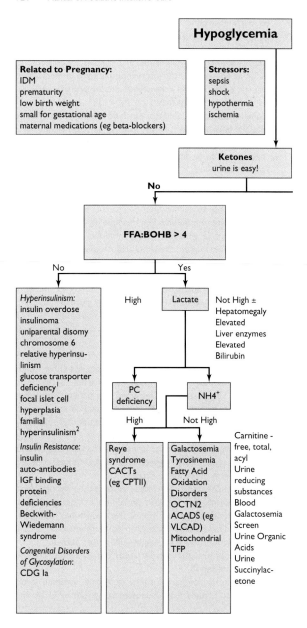

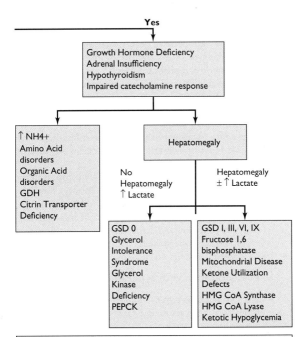

**Mechanical:**
intravenous malfunction
inadequate feeds
abrupt withdrawal of glucose infusion
post exchange transfusion

**Yes**

Growth Hormone Deficiency
Adrenal Insufficiency
Hypothyroidism
Impaired catecholamine response

↑ NH4+
Amino Acid disorders
Organic Acid disorders
GDH
Citrin Transporter Deficiency

Hepatomegaly

No Hepatomegaly ↑ Lactate

Hepatomegaly ± ↑ Lactate

GSD 0
Glycerol Intolerance Syndrome
Glycerol Kinase Deficiency
PEPCK

GSD I, III, VI, IX
Fructose 1,6 bisphosphatase
Mitochondrial Disease
Ketone Utilization Defects
HMG CoA Synthase
HMG CoA Lyase
Ketotic Hypoglycemia

**Abbreviations:** ACADs (acyl-CoA dehydrogenase deficiencies), BOHB (beta-hydroxy butyrate), CACTs (carnitine/acyl-carnitine translocase) deficiency, CDG (congenital disorders of glycosylation), CPT (carnitine palmitoyl-transferase), FFA (free fatty acid), GDH (glutamate dehydrogenase), GSD (glycogen storage disease), HADH (3-hydroxyacl-CoA dehydrogenase) HMG (hydroxy-methyl glutaryl), IDM (infant of diabetic mother), IGF (insulin-like growth factor), OCTN (organic catonic transporter), PC (pyruvate carboxylase), PEPCK (phophenol pyruvate carboxykinase), SGA (small for gestational age), TFP (trifunctional protein), VLCAD (very long chain acyl-CoA dehydrogenase). Consider mutations in genes (1) *GLUT1*, *GLUT 4* and (2) *ABCC8*, *KCNJ11*, *GLUD1*, *GCK*, and *HADHSC*.

**This flowchart is a guide and not a diagnostic algorithm.**

carnitine results, but may require acylcarnitine analysis. Other treatment involves supplying carnitine (IV or oral) while reducing dietary fat. Certain disorders also have significant muscle (rhabdomyolysis), cardiac (cardiomyopathy/arrhythmias), and liver pathology (acute fatty liver, cirrhosis/fibrosis) that may require special monitoring or treatment.

- Ketone utilization defects: HMG-CoA synthase deficiency may also show signs of liver dysfunction (fatty liver) while HMG-CoA lyase deficiency has acidosis and a diagnostic UOA profile. Other treatment includes limiting dietary fat and correcting acidosis (may require bicarbonate) for synthase and lyase deficiencies, respectively.
- Ketotic hypoglycemia. Normal/elevated FFA (normal FFA/ketone ratio).
- Glycogen storage diseases (GSD), especially types I and III. Type VI, some type IX and glycogen synthase deficiency may also present with hypoglycemia. Type I and III have hepatomegaly, elevated triglycerides and abnormal liver enzymes while type I will also have elevated lactate and urate. Some type III, VI and IX also have muscle involvement and elevated CK. Treatment is glucose.
- Galactosemia, fructose metabolism disorders: Usually positive for urine reducing substances. Further details are covered under "Hepatic disease" below.
- Gluconeogenic disorders (includes GSD I, fructose metabolism disorders, and PEP carboxykinase deficiency): Have elevated lactate (and pyruvate, therefore normal L/P ratio).
- Other metabolic disorders: many metabolic disorders, particularly organic acid and some amino acid disorders, also include variable hypoglycemia in their presentation. Most have diagnostic findings on UOA and plasma AA analysis.

### d. Presentatation with hyperammonemia

- Differential: includes urea cycle disorders (UCD) and organic acidopathies. Incorrect sample handling often leads to factitious elevations in ammonia.
- Emergency treatment: levels >100 umol/L (with symptoms) or >300 umol/L require treatment, but consider long-term neurological outcome prior to starting.
- First line therapy is hemodialysis, especially for greatly elevated ammonia levels and if pharmacologic therapy does not achieve significant decrease in ammonia within 8 hours.
- Consider other forms of dialysis (CVVHD, peritoneal) only if hemodialysis not available. Ammonium is a small, easily

diffusible molecule distributed in total body water, making other forms of ammonium removal, such as peritoneal dialysis, or blood exchange simply insufficient to remove toxin (Chan et al., 2002; Jouvet et al., 2005).

- Pharmacologic therapy should be initiated immediately with IV sodium benzoate/phenylacetate (250 mg each/kg), arginine (600 mg/kg) in D10W given as a bolus over 1 hour followed by the same amount given as an infusion over 24 hours.
- Consider an anti-emetic if there is persistent vomiting.
- Maintain nutrition to suppress catabolism: begin intravenous lipids as soon as possible, add 0.5 g/kg/day protein after first 24 hours.
- Careful monitoring of Na (hypernatremia) and K (hypokalemia) required.
- Combined, early and aggressive therapy in an encephalopathic child, for example by initiating hemodialysis rather than waiting for nutritional or pharmacologic therapy to work, may provide a better outcome in disorders where recovery should be possible, such as in maple syrup urine disease (Jouvet et al., 2001).
- In some situations, such as neonatal OTC deficiency in boys, chances are no amount of therapy is going to change the nearly universal lethal outcome. (Nassogne et al., 2005).
- Specific metabolic work-up: ammonia (repeat), plasma AA, UOA (including orotic acid), UMS (including amino acid screen), acylcarnitines.

Metabolic disorders:

- Abnormal urine organic acids. Orotic acid may be elevated in many of the UCDs, particularly OTC deficiency.
- Organic acidopathies: Usually have acidosis and/or a diagnostic urine organic acid profile. Occasionally acylcarnitine analysis is helpful. Many elevated organic acids inhibit key enzymes in the urea cycle, leading to hyperammonemia. Conversely, hyperammonemia can inhibit HMG CoA lyase, which can give a organic acid profile that mimics that enzyme deficiency.
- Abnormal plasma amino acids. Glutamine is generally increased with hyperammonemia.
- CPS or NAGS deficiency: reduced citrulline (normal orotic acid). The emergency treatment of CPS deficiency requires less arginine (200 mg/kg), otherwise treat as above. NAGS deficiency responds to administration of NAG (N-acetyl-glutamate), or the analog carbamyl-glutamate.

- OTC deficiency: reduced citrulline (elevated orotic acid). The emergency treatment requires less arginine (200 mg/kg), otherwise treat as above.
- Citrullinemia: greatly elevated citrulline, treat as above.
- Arginosuccinic aciduria: elevated arginosuccinic acid (also in urine). The emergency treatment usually requires arginine only (600 mg/kg bolus plus infusion).
- Argininemia: elevated arginine. Presents with growth delay, spastic diplegia and cognitive difficulties and rarely as hyperammonemic encephalopathy.

### e. **PRESENTATION** with no specific biochemical abnormalities on initial screen:

- UOA, PAA, carnitine and acylcarnitines should be performed on all encephalopathic patients that do not fit into the above categories.
- Maple syrup urine disease (MSUD)—Ketones usually elevated. PAA and UOA diagnostic. Some forms are thiamine responsive.
- Non-ketotic Hyperglycinemia (NKH)—Often have difficult to control seizures. Simultaneously drawn CSF and plasma AA show elevated CSF/plasma glycine, but valproate therapy makes interpretation difficult.
- Stroke (clinical, neuroimaging)—Homocystinemia (CBS, MTHFR, cobalamin defects), organic acidopathies (MMA, PA, IVA, GA I and II), OTC deficiency, mitochondrial (MELAS), CDG (Ia), Fabry. Consider empiric therapy is vitamin B12 1 mg IV, pyridoxine 100 to 200 mg IV.

### 2. **Presentation Dominated by Hepatic Disease**

Because of the high metabolic activity of the liver, metabolic disorders often have liver involvement. Conversely, specific metabolic defects are uncommon causes of most liver disorders.

Some common categories of liver dysfunction with the associated metabolic disorders are listed below. A more detailed review and approach is available in other resources (Saudubray and Charpentier) with the following focusing on conditions that require urgent attention:

- The commonest and most important disorders in the newborn period to consider: galactosemia, hereditary fructose intolerance and hepatorenal tyrosinemia.
- In endemic areas, hepatorenal tyrosinemia may be part of newborn screening.

- With galactosemia, it is important to send for diagnostic studies, starting with a blood galactosemia screen, before a blood transfusion is given. In fact, in the newborn nursery, it is useful to consider sending a galactosemia screen before any red blood cell transfusion.
- Negative urine-reducing substances are not reassuring if the child is not on a diet containing lactose or galactose.
- Galactosemia may also present as *Escherichea coli* sepsis.
- The initial management is straightforward and involves placing the child on a soy-protein formula. The reason is not for the soy protein, but because most commercial soy formulas do not contain lactose or galactose.
- Hereditary fructose intolerance is managed by a fructose-free diet.
- Medications and any sweetened product should be searched for as causes of fructose.
- In almost all cases of hepatorenal tyrosinemia, there will be a hyperchloremic renal tubular acidosis. This can be evaluated with a blood chloride level.
- Specific screening is through urine succinyl-acetones.
- In early childhood, hepatocellular disease can present in storage disorders such as Niemann-Pick type C, Wolman disease, peroxisomal diseases, Wilson disease and others. The evaluation of these latter condition requires specialized testing and can be referred to a metabolic specialist.

Initial laboratory work-up should include: blood gas, electrolytes, glucose, ammonia, lactate, liver enzymes (AST, ALT, GGT, ALP) and functional tests (albumin, coagulation tests, bilirubin), urine ketones (urinalysis) and reducing substances.

### 3. Presentation Involving Cardiomyopathy

- Inborn errors presenting as cardiomyopathy are generally of two types: hypertrophic and dilated.
- In general, storage disorders (in particular, Pompe disease, Fabry disease, and Hurler syndrome), some of the mitochondrial myopathies (such as tRNA mutations), and Danon disease present with a hypertrophic cardiomyopathy.
- When systolic function is impaired (dilated cardiomyopathy) the differential is broader and includes fatty acid oxidation defects, mitochondrial disorders, co-enzyme Q10 deficiency, Barth syndrome, carnitine transport disorders, glycogen storage disorders, congenital disorders of glycosylation and organic acidopathies.

- Cardiomyopathy may not be the cardinal manifestation, but may be a serious complication of certain inborn errors and carry a poor prognosis such as cardiomyopathy in propionic acidemia.
- Compared to cardiomyopathies due to contractile protein mutations, in virtually all cases of metabolic cardiomyopathy, there will be other associated features that can point to the diagnosis.
- The immediate management of the cardiomyopathy involves general principles of cardiac management; however, it is important to consider whether there is an underlying cause, such as a fatty acid oxidation defect.
- Initial blood work should include a plasma CK level, free, total and acyl-carnitines, urine organic acids and a urine mucopolysaccharide and oligosaccharide screen. Further investigations may require specialized arrangements through the metabolic lab and the metabolic physician can help in directing the evaluation.

## What to Do in the Event of Death

- Should the patient die or death be imminent, it may still be useful to collect samples for diagnostic testing. This can serve multiple purposes.
- It may not change the outcome of the child presenting, but may provide the family an answer as to the underlying condition.
- Since all inborn errors of metabolism are genetic disorders, there can be implications for siblings, future pregnancies and other family members.
- Prenatal diagnosis can be available in a large number of metabolic disorders, but since there is no prenatal screening test for inborn errors, a prerequisite is knowing the diagnosis.
- An attempt should be made to collect at least 3 mL of plasma frozen, 3 mL of whole blood (if necessary via a cardiac puncture) into an EDTA tube sent to the molecular genetics lab for DNA extraction, 5 mL of urine frozen, 1 mL of CSF frozen and a skin biopsy sent for fibroblast culture.
- The skin biopsy should be performed as close to the time of death as possible to ensure viability, but in cases where the death may have occurred previously, fibroblasts may still be cultured on a biopsy taken 1 to 2 days after death.
- Muscle and liver biopsies may be necessary on fresh tissue immediately flash frozen and stored at −70°C.
- Tissue collection needs to be performed in conjunction with discussing with the family the importance of fresh versus postmortem samples.

- Although not ideal, samples may be collected within a few hours of death with the expectation that the sample may not be useful.
- A full "metabolic autopsy," in the absence of identifiable patterns of a metabolic disorder or differential, rarely provides an answer.
- Samples collected after consultation with a specialist may still be more useful than a shotgun approach.
- A general autopsy can still be important to establish the actual cause of death and any related comorbidities.

Abbreviations: AA (amino acids), CBS (cystathionine beta-synthetase), CDG (congenital disorders of glycosylation), CK (creatine kinase), CSF (cerebrospinal fluid), FFA (free fatty acid), GA (glutaric aciduria), GSD (glycogen storage disease), IVA (isovaleric acidemia), MMA (methyl-malonic acidemia), MTHFR (methyle-tetrahydrofolate reductase deficiency), OTC (ornithine transcarbamoylase), PA (propionic acidemia), UOA (urine organic acids).

# References

Chan WK, But WM, Law CW. Ammonia detoxification by continuous venovenous haemofiltration in an infant with urea cycle defect. Hong Kong 2002;8:207–10.

Gebhardt B, Dittrich S, Parbel S, et al. N-carbamylglutamate protects patients with decompensated propionic aciduria from hyperammonaemia. J Inherit Metab Dis 2005;28:241–4.

Jouvet P, Hubert P, Saudubray JM, et al. Kinetic modeling of plasma leucine levels during continuous venovenous extracorporeal removal therapy in neonates with maple syrup urine disease. Pediatr Res 2005;58:278–82.

Jouvet P, Jugie M, Rabier D, et al. Combined nutritional support and continuous extracorporeal removal therapy in the severe acute phase of maple syrup urine disease. Intensive Care Med 2001;27:1798–806.

Kalhan S, Peter-Wohl S. Hypoglycemia: what is it for the neonate? Am J Perinatol 2000;17:11–8.

Morton DH, Strauss KA, Robinson DL, et al. Diagnosis and treatment of maple syrup urine disease: a study of 36 patients Pediatrics 2002;109:999–1008.

Nassogne MC, Heron B, Touati G, et al. Urea cycle defects: management and outcome. J Inherit Metab Dis 2005;28:407–14.

Prietsch V, Lindner M, Zschocke J, et al. Emergency management of inherited metabolic diseases. 2002;25:531.

Saudubray JM, Charpentier C. Clinical Phenotypes: Diagnosis/Algorithms. In Scriver CR, Beaudet AL, Sly WS Scriver's OMMBID. The Online Metabolic and Molecular Bases of Inherited Disease. 2001–2006. McGraw-Hill, Health Professions Division. New York. http://genetics.accessmedicine.com/.

Scaglia F, Carter S, O'Brien WE, Lee B. Effect of alternative pathway therapy on branched chain amino acid metabolism in urea cycle disorder patients. Mol Genet Metab 2004;81(Suppl 1)S79–85.

## Chapter 20

# Trauma

## A. Pediatric Trauma

Jennifer Kilgar
J Mark Walton
Lennox Huang

### Introduction

Trauma is responsible for more than half of all childhood deaths in North America. Injury is also responsible for considerable morbidity and permanent disability. Initial care for the pediatric trauma patient requires a rapid, organized approach to assess and manage injuries. A standard organized approach with a team ready to resuscitate the incoming trauma patient is essential. The pediatric trauma score is helpful in guiding the level of care required for a pediatric trauma patient and is correlated with outcome (Table 1).

*Table 1*
**Pediatric Trauma Score (PTS): Maximum Is +12, Minimum Is −6, PTS <9 = Referral to a Pediatric Trauma Center**

| Score factor | +2 | +1 | −1 |
|---|---|---|---|
| Weight | >20 kg | 10–20 kg | <10 kg |
| Airway | Normal | Oral or nasal airway | Intubated or tracheostomy |
| Systolic blood pressure | >90 mm Hg good peripheral pulse | 50–90 mm Hg palpable carotids/ femorals | <50 mm Hg weak pulse |

| Level of consciousness | Awake | Decreased level of consciousness | Loss of consciousness |
|---|---|---|---|
| Open wound | None | Minor | Major/ penetrating |
| Fractures | None | Minor/single/ closed | Major/open/ multiple |

Adapted from J Trauma 1987:28:425–9

## Key Principles

> - A child's anatomy and physiology causes them to respond to traumatic force differently than an adult.
> - Management of airway and breathing followed by circulation should be the initial focus of caring for pediatric trauma patients.
> - After initial stabilization, consider transfer to a pediatric trauma center for further evaluation and management.

## General Considerations

Differences in children versus adults in trauma:

1. Neurologic: CNS injuries are the most common single system injury in children and the leading etiology of traumatic death in pediatric patients.

   - There is a smaller subarachnoid space with less cushioning, resulting in an increased shearing force with a more damaging head injury. Children are more likely to have injury characterized by diffuse edema when compared to adults.
   - There is a greater passive flexion of cervical spine when the subject is placed upon a spine board. Because children have incomplete calcification of vertebrae, spinal cord injury without radiologic abnormality (SCIWORA) may occur.

2. Anatomical differences in the airway, which gives rise to specific problems:

- A large tongue and tonsils and small midface make it more difficult to visualize the larynx.
- A smaller airway, the larynx being higher and more anterior in the neck, and the vocal cords being more angled all make it more difficult to visualize the larynx.
- The smallest part of the airway is at the cricoid ring; uncuffed endotracheal tubes should be used in newborns, but may also be used in young children.
- Due to the short length of airway, there is an increased chance of a right mainstem bronchus intubation.

3. Musculoskeletal characteristics:

- Children have a more flexible skeleton with a higher cartilage:bone ratio; it is more likely to have an underlying organ damage without evidence of overlying fracture (eg, pulmonary contusion without rib fracture).
- Abdominal solid organs are more prone to injury in children because of a paucity of abdominal musculature.

4. Compactness:

- With the smaller total body mass and multiple organs more closely located, there is increased incidence of multiple organ injury.

5. Greater relative surface area:

- There is an increased heat loss with consequent risk of hypothermia.

6. Cardiovascular characteristics:

- Stroke volume relatively fixed; cardiac output increased by tachycardia; bradycardia less well tolerated.
- The first apparent hemodynamic sign of significant blood loss in a child is usually tachycardia, not hypotension.

# Factors Pointing to Possible Increased Seriousness of Injury

## History

i) Loss of consciousness
ii) Significant neurological symptoms or signs, such as severe headache, seizure, focal neurological deficit

iii) Significant mechanism of injury: pedestrian vs vehicle, serious injury or death of others involved, fall from greater than three times body height

## Physical Exam

i) Decreased level of consciousness
ii) Respiratory or hemodynamic instability
iii) Significant focal neurological signs (eg, pupil inequality; external cranial bleeding from ears, nose, etc.; focal paresis, etc.)
iv) Penetrating injury
v) Burns greater than 10% BSA (See "Acute Management of the Pediatric Burn" in Chapter 20.)
vi) Abdominal wall bruising

# The Advanced Trauma Life Support (ATLS) Approach

A—Airway assessment and maintenance with C-spine control
B—Breathing and ventilation
C—Circulation and control of hemorrhage
D—Disability: neurologic status
E—Exposure and environmental control: undress but prevent hypothermia

## Airway

- Look for facial trauma.
- Listen (for stridor).
- Feel near face and nose for evidence of air movement.
- Position head in sniffing position plus chin lift or jaw thrust without compromising C-spine stabilization.
- Assume C-spine injury until otherwise proven, and apply rigid pediatric-sized cervical collar. C-collar may be removed for intubation with a second person applying in-line neck stabilization.
- Initially start with 100% oxygen and rapidly wean if airway and breathing are secure, or continue to pre-oxygenate for intubation.

### Endotracheal Intubation

- For GCS <8 or for any patient not maintaining or in danger of not maintaining airway during transport.
- Clear oropharynx of debris.

- All trauma patients should be assumed to have a full stomach, and rapid-sequence intubation technique should be followed. (See "Airway Management" in Chapter 5.)
- For patients with head injury, intravenous lidocaine should be added to the induction to prevent ICP spikes; avoid ketamine for sedation.
- Avoid succinylcholine in crush injury.
- Nasotracheal intubation is contraindicated in facial fracture or basal skull fracture.
- Blind nasotracheal intubation is contraindicated in apnea.

## Surgical Airway Management
- Cricothyroidotomy when intubation has failed and the airway cannot be controlled with bag-valve-mask ventilation (extremely rarely needed).
- Needle cricothyroidotomy with needle jet insufflation provides adequate oxygenation but not ventilation; results in progressive hypercarbia. (See Chapter 22.)
- Surgical cricothyroidotomy should be performed by a surgeon experienced with pediatric airways.

# Breathing
- Hypoventilation and/or hypoxia is the most common cause of cardiac arrest in children.
- Carefully assess:

  - Respiratory rate, subcostal indrawing, accessory muscle use, nasal flare, central cyanosis-oxygen saturations, expiratory grunting, inspiratory or expiratory stridor, wheezing, and breath sounds

- Look for evidence of pneumothorax: chest pain, respiratory distress, hypoxemia, hyper-resonance on percussion, decreased breath sounds to the same side.
- If a tension pneumothorax is present, patient may have distended neck veins, tracheal shift, and hypotension.
- Patients with hemothorax may have decreased breath sounds with dullness to percussion.
- Needle and/or tube thoracostomy should be performed for suspected tension pneumothorax or any cardiopulmonary compromise. (See Chapter 22.)
- Insertion of needle thoracostomy regardless of a positive or negative result generally requires a follow-up chest tube as lung injury may have occurred during procedure.

## Circulation and Access

- Assess hemodynamic status using heart rate, pulses, blood pressure, and perfusion.
- Look for signs of blood loss: external bleeding, pallor, abnormal abdominal distension. (See "Shock" in Chapter and Table 1.)
- Obtain 2 large-bore peripheral IVs, ideally in upper extremities.
- After 2 failed attempts or 90 seconds, consider intra-osseous access. (See Chapter 22.)
- Central venous access only after initial stabilization. (See Chapter 22.)
- Obtain initial labs with IV access:

  - Send blood for type and cross-match (the most important blood work), CBC, PTT, INR, electrolytes, and amylase.
  - Many institutions group these labs together as a trauma panel.
  - Consider toxicologic or pregnancy screens for appropriate patients.

- If hypotensive on presentation, call for O-negative blood or O-positive blood for males immediately and start crystalloid boluses and draw blood for cross-match.
- Full equilibration of hemoglobin after an acute loss takes hours, but an actively bleeding patient will show a drop in hemoglobin almost immediately.
- Trauma patients presenting with anemia should be assumed to have a significant blood loss.
- Hemorrhagic shock should be treated primarily with blood products and definitive surgery if necessary.
- For rapid fluid resuscitation in hypotensive trauma patient, consider use of Level 1 infusor.

  - Requires large-bore IV or central line; do not use with intra-osseous.
  - Used in children >20 kg.

## Fluid Resuscitation for Shock (See "Shock" in Chapter 5.)

- Initial resuscitation with isotonic crystalloid bolus at 20 cc/kg; repeat as needed until hemodynamic status improves.
- Packed red blood cells should be given for suspected hemorrhagic shock 10–15 mL/kg warmed type-specific or O-negative PRBC, and consult surgery.
- Estimated blood volume:

- • Infants: 80 mL/kg
- • Children–teens: 70 mL/kg
- • Adults: 5 L

- • Acute replacement of >50% of blood volume = massive blood transfusion and implies need for platelet and factor replacement as well as monitoring of acid base status, ionized calcium.
- • table 2 lists clinical signs associated with blood loss in pediatric patients

## Disability

After initial ABC evaluation and management, continue to assess disability (neurologic status, level of consciousness).

Pupillary response and size: Level of consciousness (See "Coma and Altered Mental States" in Chapter 9.)

A—Alert
V—Responds to verbal stimuli
P—Responds to painful stimuli
U—Unresponsive to any stimulus

## Exposure

- • Undress completely.
- • Prevent hypothermia (blankets, heaters, lamps, warmed IV fluids, warmed inhaled gases).

*Table 2*
## Clinical Signs of Blood Loss in a Child

| Percent of blood volume lost | <15% (class I) | 15–30% (class II) | 30–40% (class III) | >40% (class IV) |
|---|---|---|---|---|
| CNS | Normal | Irritable, confused, lethargic | Decreased level of consciousness | Unconscious/ comatose |
| Cardiovascular | Normal/ borderline tachycardic | Tachycardia | Tachycardia, hypotension | Hypotension, cardiopulmonary arrest |
| Cutaneous | Normal | Cool | Cool, poor perfusion with increased capillary refill | Pale, cold |
| Renal | Normal | May have slightly decreased urine output | Oliguric | Anuric |

## Further Adjuncts to Primary Survey

- Electrocardiographic (ECG) monitoring
- $O_2$ saturation monitor
- Urinary catheter after rectal/genitalia exam (contraindications: blood at meatus, perineal ecchymosis, blood in scrotum, pelvic fracture, high-riding or nonpalpable prostate)
- Urine for R & M
- Gastric catheterization: nasogastric OR orogastric if nasogastric contraindicated (basal skull fracture-cribiform plate fracture suspected)
- X-rays: AP chest, AP pelvis, lateral C-spine (If abnormal is helpful, negative does not rule out neck injury.)

## Secondary Survey

Complete history and physical examination, including vital signs reassessment and pediatric Glasgow Coma Scale. Log roll patient off backboard to assess for obvious neck and back injury—this is often combined with external examination of rectum and digital rectal exam if indicated.

History:
A—Allergies
M—Medications
P—Past medical history
L—Last meal
E—Events/environment of trauma event

## **Imaging Techniques for Assessment**

- Plain X-rays: chest X-ray, pelvis X-ray, cervical spine X-ray lateral, AP and odontoid view, axial skeleton and extremities
- Ultrasound: useful for documentation of free fluid in abdomen
- CT scan: uncontrasted for cranial trauma, C-spine evaluation if plain radiographs inadequate

    - IV contrasted CT for abdomen and pelvis if indicated
    - Enteral contrast is controversial but primarily used for suspected intestinal injury

- Retrograde cystogram: useful for ruptured bladder
- Retrograde urethrogram: useful for ruptured urethra, sometimes seen in pelvic trauma
- Angiogram: useful for pelvic trauma with hypotension and major vessel injury in thorax

# Specific Injuries

## Thoracic Injuries

- Rib fractures

  - Rib fractures in young children generally indicate significant traumatic force.
  - The presence of a rib fracture should lead to a higher suspicion of internal organ injuries.
  - Rib fractures in infants and young children should also increase suspicion for abuse. (See "Emergent Presentations of Child Abuse" in Chapter 20.)
  - Flail chest—occurs when multiple rib fractures disrupt a large segment of chest wall.

    - Usually seen with significant pulmonary contusion
    - Physical findings: paradoxical movement of the chest wall, respiratory distress, diminished breath sounds, possible hemopneumothorax
    - Management: supplemental oxygen, analgesia, respiratory support including intubation and mechanical ventilation

- Simple pneumothorax—results from leak of air from lungs after rib fractures

  - Physical findings: often difficult to elicit in children, diminished breath sounds, tender chest wall
  - Management: chest tube for large pneumothoraces

- Tension pneumothorax—life-threatening because of kinking of the large veins with compression and shift of the mediastinum with resulting cardiorespiratory compromise

  - Physical findings: absent or diminished breath sounds, hyper-resonance to percussion and tracheal shift, classic signs may not be present in pediatric patients
  - Management: needle thoracentesis followed by chest tube

- Massive hemothorax—usually secondary to penetrating trauma or blunt trauma to a major vascular structure

  - Physical findings: absent or diminished breath sounds, dullness to percussion, flat neck veins
  - Management: chest tube, possible thoracotomy; in penetrating trauma with absent vital signs, possible emergency room thoracotomy; resuscitation for hemorrhagic shock

- Cardiovascular injury and tamponade—rare injuries usually because of mobility of the mediastinum

  - Aortic arch injuries: rare and usually occur at ligamentum arteriosum insertion on descending aorta—often fatal and need to be repaired in a cardiac unit
  - Cardiac contusion: occurs secondary to blunt anterior chest trauma and is seen more commonly in adolescence

    - Diagnosed with assistance of elevated CK-MB fraction and EKG

- Open pneumothorax—sucking chest wound, usually from penetrating chest injuries

  - Management (immediate): cover wound with impervious dressing tape on three sides; place chest tube either through wound or adjacent to it
  - Management (subsequent): prepare for the operating room

- Tracheobronchial injuries—These present with persistent pneumothorax (massive air leak) despite two and three chest tubes

  - Will need bronchoscopy and possible thoracotomy for repair if involving trachea or major bronchi

- Diaphragmatic rupture—can occur from penetrating injuries but also from significant blunt trauma to the upper abdomen or lower chest

  - More common on the left then on the right diaphragm (4:1 ratio)
  - Pass NG to prior to chest X-ray—this may show NG tube in the left hemithorax
  - Sometimes presents late with an abnormal chest X-ray
  - Management: midline laparotomy for repair and assessment of other injuries such as spleen kidney and liver

- Esophageal rupture—rare in blunt trauma, occasionally in penetrating trauma

  - May occur after endoscopy or dilatation procedures
  - Diagnosis: crepitus (subcutaneous emphysema) in the cervical region on physical exam

    - Mediastinal air on chest X-ray

- Traumatic asphyxia—occurs secondary to severe compression injury to the thorax that results in sudden compression of the superior vena cava

- Manifested by multiple petechiae in the upper part of the body as well as the conjunctiva and possibly within the brain
- Usually not associated with serious injury, but one must always check for intrathoracic injury

## Abdominal Injuries

- Intravenous enhanced CT scan

  - Use of oral contrast is controversial as it introduces delays in resuscitation and aspiration events have been reported.
  - Oral contrast is most useful in the setting of suspected hollow viscus injury (eg, seat belt sign).

- Portable bedside ultrasound

  - Focused assessment with sonography for trauma (FAST) is a validated component of adult trauma resuscitation.
  - Pediatric FAST is beginning to be implemented in some centers but has not gained widespread acceptance.

- Diagnostic peritoneal lavage (DPL)

  - Used much less commonly in children than adults
  - Possibly useful for intestinal perforation diagnosis as with seat belt injuries

- Frequency of organ injury, in descending order

  - Blunt trauma: spleen, kidney, liver, pancreas, bladder
  - Penetrating trauma: intestine, liver, vascular, spleen, kidney, pancreas, bladder

- Indications for laparotomy

  - Blunt trauma: ongoing hemodynamic instability, blood replacement greater than half the blood volume, pneumoperitoneum, signs of hollow viscus injury
  - Penetrating injuries: all gunshot injuries, selective with most stab wounds

- Splenic injury

  - Use spleen-conserving approach most often to minimize overwhelming post-splenectomy sepsis associated with left renal injury
  - Physical signs: left upper quadrant pain, shoulder pain, possible hemodynamic instability

- Management: bed rest, NPO, IV rehydration, transfusion as needed, surgery if unstable or if ongoing losses requiring transfusion of 40 cc per kg PRBC (50% of blood volume)

- Liver injuries

  - Less commonly injured than spleen, can be more serious than splenic injury if the inferior vena cava or hepatic veins are injured, associated with a right kidney injury
  - Physical signs: associate with bruises or abrasion of the skin in the upper abdomen
  - May present in shock
  - Management: fluid resuscitation, CT scan for definition of injury
  - Surgery for ongoing bleeding or unrelenting hypotension

- Intestinal injuries

  - Secondary to handle bar, seat belt
  - Mechanism: sheering/deceleration, compression, devascularization
  - Sites:
    - duodenum; duodenal hematoma associated with pancreatic injury
    - small bowel: primary repair
    - colon: possible primary repair or colostomy
    - rectal: colostomy
    - with seat belt injuries, consider lumbar spine injury

- Pancreatic and biliary injuries

  - Extra-hepatic biliary injuries are extremely rare.
  - Pancreatic injuries are secondary to penetrating or blunt trauma and can lead to pancreatitis and pseudocyst formation; always do serial serum amylase and lipase in significant abdominal trauma. (See "Pancreatitis" in Chapter 14.)

- Pelvic trauma

  - Usually secondary to severe blunt trauma.
  - Physical signs: abrasions, large bruises and possibly soft tissue disruptions in the lower abdomen, manual compression of the pelvis will possibly reveal instability.
  - Look for blood in the urethral meatus, perineal bruising (urethral disruption).
  - Look for lower limb motor nerve injury.

- Pelvic fractures may lead to major hemodynamic instability and require early external fixation.

- Renal injuries

  - Second most common organ injured in blunt trauma.
  - Usually associated with other injuries.
  - Physical signs: abrasions, costovertebral angle tenderness.
  - Consult a pediatric urologist for definitive management.

- Bladder injuries

  - Usually secondary to extensive pelvic trauma, which is usually extraperitoneal.
  - Intraperitoneal ruptured is often secondary to blunt trauma with a full bladder.
  - Extraperitoneal can be treated non-operatively with bladder drainage.

- Urethral injury

  - Usually secondary to the straddle injury or pelvic trauma
  - Physical signs: blood at the urethral meatus, perineal bruising
  - Diagnosed with urethrogram; avoid passing a urinary catheter

- Ureteral injuries: more commonly secondary to penetrating than blunt trauma
- Genital injuries: more common in males and mostly occur to the penis

## Spinal Injury

- Cervical spine injuries:

  - Due to relatively large cranial mass, young children injure present with upper cervical spine more commonly than lower cervical spine.
  - Even with negative radiographs, spinal cord injury may still be present. If patient complains of neck pain, numbness, or tingling, leave patient in cervical collar. (See "Assessment of Pediatric Cervical Spine Injury in Trauma" in Chapter 20.)
  - Pediatric patients are at risk for SCIWORA due to ligamentous injuries that are not visualized on plain radiographs.

- Thoracolumbar spine injuries:

  - Patients with back pain should be assumed to have a spinal injury until proven otherwise.

- Flexion distraction type injury in motor vehicle crashes is associated with lap belt use, may cause a lumbar spine fracture also known as a Chance fracture.
  - Associated with hollow viscus injury, neurological deficit
  - Avoid further injury by stabilizing spine; obtain orthopedic consult

## Musculoskeletal Injuries

- Principles:

  - Large volumes of blood can be lost from fractures at sites such as the femur, tibia, and pelvis.
  - Always check for distal pulses in case of vascular injury (ie, supracondylar fracture).
  - If absent pulses, reduce fracture/deformity and reassess.
  - Watch subsequently for the signs of compartment syndrome.
  - Always check for disruption of skin over fracture site (ie, compound or open fracture).
  - Dress wound, start intravenous cefazolin, and check tetanus status.
  - Stabilize and splint the fracture, especially for transportation.

- Complications

  - Vascular injury compromising soft tissue circulation
  - Vascular process compromising bone healing/perfusion (eg, following epiphyseal fractures in the proximal femur)
  - Injury to surrounding structures by bony fragment (eg, pelvic fracture resulting in bladder laceration)

## Head Injury

- See "Traumatic Head Injury" in Chapter 20.

## Burns

- See "Acute Management of the Pediatric Burn" in Chapter 20.

### Pediatric Trauma Team (PTT)

Trauma management requires a multidisciplinary team involving surgery, pediatrics, the emergency room physician, nursing, respiratory therapy, and social work.

PTT should be called prior to arrival of the trauma by a standard paging fan-out.

## Pediatric Glasgow Coma Scale

| | | |
|---|---|---|
| **Eye Opening** | Spontaneous | 4 |
| | To voice | 3 |
| | To pain | 2 |
| | None | 1 |
| **Verbal Response** | Oriented | 5 |
| (over 5 years) | Confused | 4 |
| | Inappropriate words | 3 |
| | Nonspecific sounds | 2 |
| | None | 1 |
| (2–5 years) | Appropriate words | 5 |
| | Inappropriate words | 4 |
| | Cries and/or screams | 3 |
| | Grunts | 2 |
| | None | 1 |
| (0–23 months) | Smiles/Coos/Cries appropriately | 5 |
| | Cries/Inconsolable | 4 |
| | Inappropriate cry | 3 |
| | Persistent cry/grunting | 2 |
| | None | 1 |
| **Motor Response** | Obeys command | 6 |
| (over 5 years) | Localizes pain | 5 |
| | Withdraw (pain) | 4 |
| | Flexor posturing (pain) | 3 |
| | Extensor posturing (pain) | 2 |
| | None | 1 |
| (up to 5 years) | Obeys command | 6 |
| | Localizes pain | 5 |
| | Withdraw (pain) | 4 |
| | Flexor posturing (pain) | 3 |
| | Extensor posturing (pain) | 2 |
| | None | 1 |

The trauma team leader (TTL) is a physician designated prior to the trauma who:

- is in charge of the management and directs the priorities of the resuscitation.
- coordinates but should not be involved in hands-on procedures.

- should be trained in Pediatric Advanced Life Support (PALS) as well as Advanced Trauma Life Support (ATLS).
- can be either a surgeon or a pediatrician.

PTT members (suggested)

- pediatric staff general surgeon and surgery resident
- pediatric intensivist or staff pediatrician
- senior pediatric resident
- emergency room physician
- three nurses (one to chart and two to assist with hands-on resuscitation)
- respiratory therapist to assist with airway management
- radiology technologist
- social worker/chaplain (for family support)

# References

Tepas JJ, Fallat ME, Moriarty TM. Trauma. In: APLS: The pediatric emergency resource, 4th ed. Boston: Jones and Bartlett Publishers; 2004. pp. 268–319.

Lau ST, Brisseau GF. Evaluation, stabilization and initial management after multiple trauma. In: Pediatric critical care, 3rd ed. Philadelphia: Mosby Elsevier; 2006. pp. 1579–85.

Emergency Paediatrics Section, Canadian Paediatric Society (CPS). Management of children with head trauma—Position statement. Canadian Medical Association Journal 1990;142(9):949–52. Reaffirmed 2002.

Soudack M, Epelman M, Maor R, et al. Experience with focused abdominal sonography for trauma (FAST) in 313 pediatric patients. J Clin Ultrasound 2004 Feb;32(2):53–61.

Tepas JJ 3rd, Mollitt DL, Talbert JL, Bryant M. The pediatric trauma score as a predictor of injury severity in the injured child. J Pediatr Surg 1987 Jan;22(1):14–8.

The Pediatric Trauma Score as a Predictor of Injury Severity: An Objective Assessment

Tepas, Joseph J. III; Ramenofsky, Max L.; Mollitt, Daniel L.; Gans, Bruce M.; Discala, Carla

The Journal of Trauma. 28(4):425–429, April 1988.

# B. Traumatic Head Injury

Andrew Latchman

## Key Principles

> - Identify complications of head trauma.
> - Prevent secondary brain injury.
> - Prevent hypoxia.
> - Maintain blood pressure.
> - Avoid fluid overload.
> - Avoid hyperglycemia.
> - Manage intracranial pressure (ICP).

Head injuries account for 75% of all pediatric trauma admissions and 70% of all pediatric trauma-related deaths.

Traumatic brain injuries (TBIs) are divided into two subcategories:

(1) primary injury, which occurs at the moment of trauma, and
(2) secondary injury, which occurs after the trauma.

Primary injuries can be focal injuries (eg, skull fractures, intracranial hematomas, lacerations, contusions, penetrating wounds), or they can be diffuse as in diffuse axonal injury.

Secondary injuries are attributable to ongoing cellular damage most often due to hypotension and hypoxia.

The following conditions should be considered as a primary differential diagnosis or co-existent morbidities in the patient with altered LOC and suspected TBI:

- Seizure/post-ictal state
- Medication/substance abuse/overdose
- Non-traumatic hemorrhage [eg, arteriovenous malformations (AVM)]
- Hypoglycemia
- Electrolyte derangement
- Decompensation cardiorespiratory status
- Atypical migraine

## Pertinent History

This should be taken directly from the patient, if possible, and any witnesses.

- Time of injury
- Mechanism of injury
- Loss of consciousness (time)
- How patient arrived at hospital (ie, got up after injury, remained supine)
- Any progressive irritability or lethargy
- Episodes of nausea or vomiting
- Photophobia or phonophobia
- Evidence of post-traumatic seizure
- Any numbness, tingling, or weakness
- History of seizures or bleeding diathesis
- Presence of headache or neck pain
- Presence of amnesia

## Classification of Severity of Head Injury

The criteria below can be used as a guide to determine the severity of a child's head injury. Aside from the Glasgow Coma Scale (GCS) (table 1), no one criterion is an absolute indication of severity. The following signs and symptoms should be used as a guide for management, in conjunction with the patient's overall clinical status as well as the mechanism of injury. The remainder of the chapter will deal with the management of severe TBI.

### Mild

- Glasgow Coma Scale Score of 14–15
- Asymptomatic
- Mild headache
- 3 or fewer episodes of vomiting
- Loss of consciousness for <5 minutes
- Post-traumatic amnesia <15 minutes

### Moderate

- Glasgow Coma Scale score of 9–13
- Loss of consciousness for 5 minutes or more
- Progressive lethargy
- Progressive headache

- Vomiting protracted (>3 times) or associated with other symptoms
- Post-traumatic amnesia >15 minutes
- Post-traumatic seizure
- Multiple traumas
- Serious facial injury
- Signs of basal skull fracture
- Possible penetrating injury or depressed skull fracture
- Suspected child abuse

*Table 1*
## Glasgow Coma Scale

|  | Verbal child | Nonverbal child |
| --- | --- | --- |
| Best Motor (4) | No eye opening (1) | No eye opening (1) |
|  | Eye opening to pain (2) | Eye opens to pain (2) |
|  | Eye opening to verbal command (3) | Eye opens to speech (3) |
|  | Eye opening spontaneously (4) | Eye opens spontaneously (4) |
| Best Verbal Response (5) | No verbal response (1) | No verbal response (1) |
|  | Incomprehensible sounds (2) | Infant moans to pain (2) |
|  | Inappropriate words (3) | Infant cries to pain (3) |
|  | Confused (4) | Infant is irritable (4) |
|  | Oriented (5) | Infant coos or babbles (5) |
| Best Motor Response (6) | No response (1) | No response (1) |
|  | Flexion to pain (decerebrate) (2) | Flexion to pain (2) |
|  | Extension to pain (decorticate) (3) | Extension to pain (3) |
|  | Withdrawal to pain (4) | Withdrawal to pain (4) |
|  | Localization to pain (5) | Infant withdraws from touch (5) |
|  | Obeys commands (6) | Infant moves spontaneously (6) |

## Severe

- Glasgow Coma Scale of 8 or less or decrease of 2 points not clearly caused by seizures, drugs, or decrease cerebral perfusion
- Focal neurological signs
- Penetrating skull injury
- Palpable depressed skull fracture
- Compound skull fracture

# Management of Severe Head Injury

Many patients with TBI may also have other injuries associated with the initial trauma; a management algorithm is presented in a stepwise approach according to ATLS.

## Airway and Breathing

- In adults, hypoxia ($PaO_2$ <60–65 or $SpO_2$ <90%) is associated with worse neurological outcome in patients with severe head injury. Although the small numbers of pediatric studies thus far have not shown a strong independent link, the avoidance of hypoxia in pediatric patients with severe head injury is strongly recommended.
- Airway support can be accomplished through bag-valve-mask ventilation or endotracheal intubation. Standard indications for intubation include GCS <8, inability to maintain an adequate airway, hypoxemia not corrected by supplemental oxygen, and respiratory failure.
- Endotracheal intubation, if available, is the most effective maneuver for maintaining the airway; however, it can be a difficult skill especially in the non-hospital setting and in smaller patients. Studies have shown no difference in neurological outcome in patients whose airway was maintained by bag-valve-mask ventilation versus endotracheal intubation. The most important element is to prevent secondary brain injury from hypoxemia.
- If intubation is attempted, cerebral protective measures, C-spine protection, and pre-medication with lidocaine should be employed.

## Circulation

- Hypotension (defined as systolic blood pressure less than that the 5th percentile for age), see Chapter 4, "Cardiovascular Monitoring," associated with increased mortality and morbidity in the head-injured patient. Systolic blood pressures less than $(2 \times \text{age} + 70)$ must be identified and rapidly corrected with fluid therapy.

- Hypotension in pediatrics is a relatively late sign and represents a decompensated shock state, and generally occurs after significant blood loss or airway compromise. Although conservative fluid administration of isotonic fluids to avoid exacerbation of cerebral edema is appropriate, this should not come at the cost of under-volume resuscitating patients. Fluid resuscitation is indicated for patients with signs of decreased perfusion, even in the presence of normal blood pressure. Signs of decreased perfusion include diminished peripheral and central pulses, increased capillary refill time, tachycardia, and decreased urine output ($<1$ cc/kg/hr).

- In the presence of hypotension, fluid therapy consists of 20 cc/kg of crystalloid fluid (either NS or ringer's lactate) as rapidly as possible; if hypotension persists, a repeat bolus is given.

- If after the second bolus the hypotension has not resolved, a third bolus is started and one must consider the administration of blood products (10 cc/kg or more of PRBC), especially in the patient with multiple trauma.

- An isolated head injury will not result in hypotension and secondary injuries must be sought. In the presence of hypotension and a normal heart rate, spinal shock must be considered. In this case, after adequate fluid resuscitation vasopressors are employed to maintain blood pressure.

- The avoidance of hyperglycemia is important in minimizing secondary brain injury; however, it should not come at the cost of risking hypoglycemia, especially in the neonate or young infant.

## Neurological Assessment

- Evaluation of neurological status is essential in the treatment of severe TBI. Rapid and repeated evaluations every 5–10 minutes initially of pupillary response, Glasgow Coma Scale score as well as examinations for evidence of focal neurological signs (focal seizures, asymmetrical pupillary dilatation, unilateral weakness) are essential in appropriate management.

- For status epilepticus due to severe TBI, refer to "Seizures and Status Epilepticus" in Chapter 9.

- Seizures result in increased metabolic demands and may aggravate secondary brain injury in severe TBI.

- Seizures should be treated initially with benzodiazepine (lorazepam 0.1 mg/kg) followed by a loading dose of phenytoin, phenobarbital, or carbamazepine.
- Prophylaxis for seizures may be indicated for the prevention of early post-traumatic seizures (PTS) (<7 days) in severe TBI with either phenytoin, carbamazepine, or phenobarbital. After 7 days, the use of prophylactic anti-seizure medication does not reduce the risk of late PTS.

# Intracranial Pressure (ICP)

In the absence of intracranial monitoring, signs of increased intracranial pressure include:

- Decreasing GCS score
- Abnormality or changes in pupillary size and reaction to light
- Cushing's response (hypertension, bradycardia [tachycardia early on], and respiratory abnormalities)
- Papilledema
- Focal seizures or focal neurological deficit
- Abnormal CT scan
- Midline shift
- Absence of basal cisterns
- Diffuse axonal injury
- Compression of ventricles

## Indications for Intracranial Pressure Monitoring

See Chapter 10 for more details.

- Severe head injury (GCS <8)
- Conscious patients with traumatic mass lesions at risk of neurological deterioration
- Patients for whom serial neurological exams are not possible due to sedation, neuromuscular blockade, or anesthesia

## Management of Increased ICP

There have been several approaches to the management of increased ICP. Two main approaches include CPP (cerebral perfusion pressure) and ICP targeted approaches. Studies have supported using CPP; however, in the adult population, there have been concerns with higher rates of complication in the CPP group. There is very little evidence to support the role of CPP in pediatric patients; however, studies consistently show an increased mortality in patients with CPP <40.

# Intracranial Pressure Monitoring Allows the Calculation of Cerebral Perfusion Pressure (CPP)

- CPP is calculated by subtracting ICP from mean arterial pressure (MAP).
- CPP represents the pressure gradient promoting cerebral blood flow.
- The optimal CPP for pediatric patients is likely between 50 and 65.

## Treatment of Increased ICP (figure 1)

If ICP remains above 20 or CPP <40 (not due to low MAP) for greater than 3 minutes, treatment should be implemented in a stepwise approach. The simplest steps involve ensuring that the patient is adequately sedated and that any irritating or noxious stimuli are not present. There are many options for sedating patients depending on the clinical indication; for prolonged sedation, the most common infusions are midazolam or morphine. If CPP is <40 and MAP is below normal for age, then appropriate fluid resuscitation should also be implemented as outlined above to restore CPP.

An increase in ICP may be due to:

- Hypercarbia
- Hypoxia
- Suctioning (pre-medication with lidocaine 1 mg/kg prior to suctioning may help blunt the increase in ICP, maximum dose is 6 mg/kg over 6 hours)
- Hyperthermia (temperature >38.5°C)
- Inadequate sedation/analgesia
- Technical problem with ICP monitor
- Decreased jugular venous drainage due to tight cervical spine collar or patient's HOB (head of bed) <30°

Once correcting for deviations in the above variables if ICP remains above 20 or CPP <40 further treatment must be initiated.

If ICP remains elevated despite further treatment, a repeat CT scan is recommended.

- If a ventriculostomy catheter is present, then one can drain CSF for 5 minutes as needed.

- Hyperosmolar therapy (either 3% NS or 25% mannitol): 3% NS may be given as a bolus (2–3 cc/kg over 10–15 minutes) or as an infusion 0.1–1.0 mL/kg/hour. Mannitol is given only as boluses 0.25–1.0 g/kg (due to risk of accumulation and reverse effect in injured brain areas). Serum osmolality must be kept below 320 mOsm/L with mannitol (due to risk of ATN as mannitol is excreted unchanged in urine); however, with 3% NS either alone or in combination with mannitol, a serum osmolality of 360 mOsm/L is acceptable.
- Neuromuscular blockade can be used to reduce ICP in severe TBI. Postulated mechanisms include reduction in airway and intrathoracic pressure increasing cerebral venous outflow, preventing shivering posturing as well as breathing against the ventilator. One must be careful to ensure that all members of the health care team are aware of the paralysis and are vigilant for potential risks including hypoxemia secondary to accidental extubation, unrecognized seizures, and increased risk of pneumonia as well as myopathy associated with steroid use. Appropriate sedation is paramount to avoid increased stress from conscious paralysis.

## Refractory Intracranial Hypertension

- Hyperventilation: Once a cornerstone of therapy for pediatric TBI, hyperventilation is now reserved for acute treatment of intracranial hypertension not responsive to sedation and analgesia, neuromuscular blockade, CSF drainage, and hyperosmolar therapy. Mild hyperventilation ($PaCO_2$ <35) may be used in the setting of refractory intracranial hypertension as defined above. Aggressive hyperventilation ($PaCO_2$ <30) is reserved for acute neurological deterioration secondary to tentorial or brain stem herniation. If prolonged hyperventilation is employed, then measurement of jugular venous saturation and/or cerebral blood flow and arterial jugular venous difference should be considered.
- If basal cisterns are open with no evidence of mass lesions, the addition of a lumbar drain may be considered.
- In patients with intractable intracranial hypertension and stable blood pressure, high dose barbiturate therapy may be considered. Although barbiturates have the advantage of decreasing resting cerebral metabolic rate and decreased cerebral blood flow, these benefits must be weighed against the risks of hypotension and the potential deleterious effects of prolonged inhibition of synaptic activity.

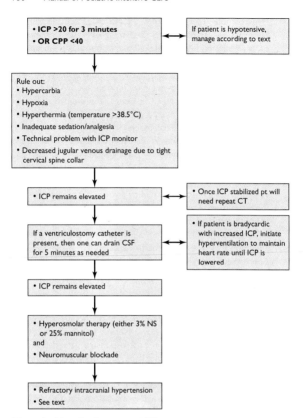

**Figure 1** Algorithm for increased ICP.

- For pentobarbital, a loading dose of 10/kg over 30 minutes, followed by 5 mg/kg q hourly times 3 doses, and then maintenance of 1 mg/kg/hour.
- For thiopental, a loading dose of 10–20 mg/kg followed by maintenance of 3–5 mg/kg/hour.
- Weaning is generally begun after 24 hours of good ICP control. It should be noted that there is no evidence to recommend one barbiturate over another.
- Hypothermia (core temperature less than 35°C) may be beneficial to decreasing refractory intracranial hypertension by decreasing cerebral metabolism, inflammation, cell death, and excitotoxicity; however, there have been no published studies

since 1973 evaluating the effect of hypothermia in children with severe TBI.

- Decompressive craniectomy either unilateral (frontal-temporal-parietal) in patients with unilateral cerebral swelling or bilateral frontal craniectomy for patient with bilateral cerebral swelling may be effective in the treatment of refractory intracranial hypertension. Suggested indications include patients within 48 hours of injury without episodes of sustained ICP elevation >40 mm Hg or persistent GCS of 3, secondary clinical deterioration, diffuse cerebral swelling of cranial CT imaging, evolving cerebral herniation syndrome.

# References

Davis RJ, Fan TW, Dean JM. Head and spinal cord injury. In: Rocer MC, ed Textbook of Pediatric Intensive Care, 2nd ed. Baltimore: Williams & Williams, 1992. p. 805.

Kokoska ER, Smith GS, Pittma T, et al. Early hypotension worsens neurological outcome in pediatric patients with moderately severe head trauma. J Pediatr Surg 1998;33:333–8.

Pigula FA, Wald SL, Shackford SR, et al. The effect of hypotension and hypoxia on children with severe head injuries. J Pediatr Surg 1993;28:310–316.

Emergency Paediatrics Section, Canadian Paediatric Society (CPS). Management of children with head trauma. CMAJ 1990;142:(9):949–52.

Advanced Trauma Life Support for Doctors. ATLS Student Manual, 8th ed. Chicago: American College of Surgeons, 2008.

Chesnut RM. Avoidance of hypotension: conditio sine qua non of successful severe head injury management. J Trauma 1997;42:S4–S9.

Chesnut RM, Marshall LF, Klauber MR, et al. The role of secondary brain injury in determining outcome form severe head injury. J Trauma 1993;34: 216–22.

Adelson PD, Bratton SL, Carney NA, et al. Guidelines for the acute medical management of severe traumatic brain injury in infants, children, and adolescents. Pediatr Crit Care Med 2003;4:S16.

Gausche M, Lewis RJ, Stratton SJ, et al. Effect of out of hospital pediatric endotracheal intubation on survival and neurological outcome: a controlled clinical trial. JAMA 2000;283:783–90.

Lewis RJ, Yee L, Inkelis SH, et al. Clinical predictors of post-traumatic seizures in children with head trauma. Ann Emerg Med 1993;22:1114–8.

Brain Injury Special Interest Group of the American Academy of Physical Medicine and Rehabilitation. Practice parameter: antiepileptic drug treatment of posttraumatic seizures. Arch Phys Med Rehabil 1998;79:594–7.

Young B, Rapp RP, Hack D, et al. Failure of prophylactically administered phenytoin to prevent post-traumatic seizures in children. Childs Brain 1983;10:185–92.

Downard C, Hulka F, Mullins RJ, et al. Relationship of cerebral perfusion pressure and survival in pediatric brain injured patients. J Trauma 2000;49:654–8.

Robertson CS, Valadka AB, Hannay HJ, et al. Prevention of secondary ischemic insults after severe head injury. Crit Care Med 1999;27:2086.

Brazilary Z, Augarten A, Sagy M, et al. Variables affecting outcome from severe brain injury in children. Intensive Care Med 1998;14:417–21.

HYPIT trial

# C. Assessment of Pediatric Cervical Spine Injury in Trauma

Jonathan Gilleland

Krishnapriya Anchala

## Key Principles

- C-spine injuries are rare but should be assumed in children presenting with multiple injuries.
- Young children are more prone to high (C1–4) c-spine injuries.
- Adolescents and teens are more prone to low (C5–7) injuries.
- CT or MRI should be used to evaluate high-risk patients.

## Introduction

Management of the pediatric trauma must include a low threshold for suspecting cervical spine injury. This is particularly true for significant blunt force, multi-system trauma bearing greater risk of cervical spine injury, or in the case of other painful injuries that may distract the examiner from recognizing C-spine injuries. A history of direct trauma to the head or neck is present in the majority of cervical spine injury. Falls and motor vehicle accidents are a more common cause of trauma in younger children vs sports injury and motor vehicle accidents in older children and adolescents.

Children under 8 years are at increased risk of cervical spine trauma compared to older children and adults secondary to anatomical differences:

- Younger children have proportionally larger heads.
- The fulcrum of cervical motion is at a higher position: C2–3 at birth; C5–6 >8 years to adolescence.
- Children have increased ligamentous laxity and underdeveloped cervical musculature.

- Horizontal orientation of facet joint articulation and wedge-shaped vertebral bodies allow for greater movement of cervical spine.
- Bony architecture of the spine allows for proportionally more distraction than the spinal cord in younger children predisposing to SCIWORA.

Pre-existing conditions may predispose a child to increased risk of cervical spine injury (eg, Down syndrome, Klippel-Feil syndrome, osteochondroplasias, mucopolysaccharidoses).

## Clinical Presentation

- Local symptoms may consist of pain, decreased range of motion, or spasm of surrounding musculature.
- Neurologic symptoms may range in severity from mild paresthesias or weakness to quadriplegia and may be transient in duration.
- A history of ambulation does not rule out the possibility of spinal injury.
- Suspected fracture to the mandible or posterior teeth may indicate transmission of force to the cervical spine.

## Physical Examination

Vital signs:

- Hypoventilation or apneustic breathing may be a sign of impaired diaphragmatic control (C3,C4,C5).
- Hypotension, bradycardia, and temperature instability suggest spinal shock.

Cervical examination:

- The cervical collar may be removed provided adequate midline stabilization of the cervical spine is to allow direct examination.
- Spinous processes and paraspinal musculature are palpated to identify any local tenderness, deformity, or muscle spasm.
- ** **Warning:** Most missed cases of cervical spine injury occur in the setting of a significant mechanism of injury and a *distracting injury*.

Neurologic evaluation:

- Perform a detailed examination of strength, tone, power, sensation, and reflexes.

- Features highly suggestive of cervical spine injury include:

  - flaccid muscle tone
  - isolated sensory deficit with possible sensory level localizing the injury
  - areflexia below level of injury is suggestive of spinal shock
  - absence of rectal tone (poor prognostic sign)
  - absence of bulbocavernous reflex also suggests spinal shock unless sacral involvement
  - \*\***<u>Warning:</u>** Reflex withdrawal movements may be present despite presence of spinal injury.

- **"The following three partial injury syndromes should warrant. . . ."** further radiologic evaluation if present despite absence of risk factors for cervical spine injury.
- **Central cord syndrome:** Upper limbs (particularly the hands) are paradoxically weaker than the lower limbs because of injury preferentially involving medial fibers of the cervical roots.
- **Brown-Sequard:** Representing "hemisection" of the spinal cord—motor loss on the ipsilateral side and pain/temperature impairment 1–2 levels below the lesion on the contralateral side.
- **Anterior spinal artery syndrome:** Interruption of main blood supply to the spinal cord with selective sparing of the dorsal columns (supplied by the posterior spinal arteries); patients are paralyzed with loss of pain and temperature but with preservation of vibration, light touch, and proprioception.

Radiologic assessment:

- In some children, clinical assessment alone may be all that is required to exclude cervical spine injury and safely avoid radiographic assessment. All of the following criteria must be met before this course of action is appropriate:

  - No neck pain, tenderness, or limitation to mobility
  - No focal neurologic deficit
  - Normal level of consciousness
  - No history of trauma to the cervical spine
  - No history suggesting significant mechanism of injury
  - No evidence of intoxication or sedation
  - No distracting injury
  - >8 yrs of age (insufficient literature to support application of criteria in younger children)

- Minimum evaluation includes three views of the cervical spine: cross-table lateral, AP, and open-mouth odontoid.

- Interpretation of C-spine X-rays in children (particularly <8 years) must incorporate recognition of **common pitfalls that represent normal variants** and not pathology:

  - Posterior arch of CI fuses by 3 years of age.
  - Anterior arch of CI remains unossified <I year of age and progressively ossifies between 6 and 9 years of age.
  - The basilar synchondrosis (epiphyseal plate at base of the odontoid) fuses with body of C2 by 6–7 years; a fusion line may remain as a normal variant into adolescence.
  - Cervical lordosis may be absent until adolescence.
  - Pseudosubluxation of C2 on C3 and C3 on C4 is a common finding in children <8 years.

A systematic approach to the interpretation of cervical spine radiographs may include the following:

| A | Alignment | malalignment, subluxation, distraction, lordotic curve |
|---|---|---|
| B | Bones | fractures, ossification centers, anterior and posterior vertebral columns |
| C | Cartilage | disc spaces, ossification centers |
| S | Soft tissue | prevertebral space, predental space |

Lateral view:

- All 7 cervical vertebrae must be visualized including the C7-TI interface; a swimmer's view may be utilized if the C7/TI articulation cannot be assessed.
- Alignment of 4 lines of contour maintained: anterior vertebral body line, posterior vertebral body line, spinolaminar line, and posterior spinous process line.
- **Pseudosubluxation** can be evaluated using the Swischuk line: the posterior cervical line between the anterior aspects of the CI and C3 spinous processes.

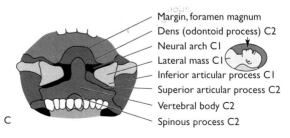

Margin, foramen magnum
Dens (odontoid process) C2
Neural arch CI
Lateral mass CI
Inferior articular process CI
Superior articular process C2
Vertebral body C2
Spinous process C2

C

- True subluxation or a **hangman's fracture** (traumatic Spondylolisthesis of C2) may be present if this line misses the anterior aspect of the C2 spinous process by ≥2 mm.

- **Atlantoaxial instability** can be detected using the atlas-dens interval (ADI).

  - Measured from the posterior margin of the anterior arch of C1 to the anterior margin of the dens; a normal value in children should not exceed 4.5 mm (normal adult value <3 mm) but may be normally increased in conditions such as Down syndrome.
  - In addition to detection of atlantoaxial instability and subluxation, widening of this space may indicate Jefferson fracture.

- The **prevertebral space** at the level of C3/C4 should not exceed 1/3 the AP diameter of the vertebrae.

  - Widening of the prevertebral space suggests hematoma, abscess, or fracture.
  - Accurate estimation of this space cannot be made in the presence of an endotracheal tube or NG tube that may create a falsely increased diameter.

AP view:

- May identify fractures in the lateral bony elements that cannot be visualized on the lateral view.

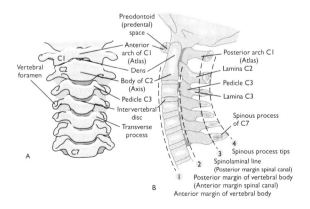

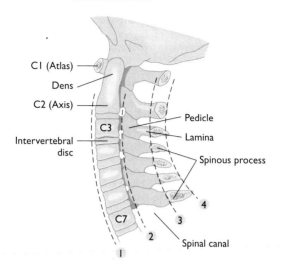

Odontoid view:

- Bilateral widening between the dens and lateral masses of the body of C2 suggest a Jefferson fracture (an unstable fracture of the C1 ring due to an axial loading injury to the head causing compression force to C1).
- **\*\*Warning:** Epiphyseal growth plate at the base of the odontoid process in younger children is sometimes confused with a true fracture.
- Waters' view may be required in children who cannot cooperate with an open-mouth odontoid view.

Flexion/extension views:

- Useful when AP, lateral, and odontoid views fail to identify a fracture despite the persistence of cervical pain or tenderness to palpation that may herald ligamentous injury.
- Should be obtained only in the setting of a patient who is capable of active range of motion of the neck and who can halt such movement if pain is elicited.
- Paraspinal musculature may splint the spine in the setting of ligamentous injury and prevent subluxation from occurring in the acute setting; follow-up X-rays are required in this setting approximately one week post-injury once acute muscle spasm has abated.

Computed tomography:

- More sensitive in assessment of bony structures and indicated in the setting of negative plain radiographic evaluation with persistence of high clinical suspicion of a cervical spine injury.
- Also plays a role in evaluating regions of the spine (particularly lower cervical spine) that cannot be adequately visualized using plain radiographs and in which the mechanism of injury is significant.
- May aid in evaluation of patients with altered mental status where clinical examination is not possible.
- Need to balance risk presented by increased radiation exposure compared to plain films.
- MRI should be considered if the reason for further diagnostic imaging is evaluation of spinal cord elements or soft tissue and ligamentous injury.

Magnetic resonance imaging:

- Superior to CT in evaluation of intervertebral discs, ligamentous injury, and spinal cord injury including hemorrhage, edema, and transection.
- Investigation of choice in the evaluation of children suspected of having SCIWORA.
- May not be as available as CT in certain centers.

In the critically ill intubated and ventilated patient with significant risk factors for cervical spine injury, C-spine precautions may be required for a prolonged duration until the cervical spine can be cleared clinically or by MRI evaluation.


## Initial Management

Maintenance of a patent airway that is sufficient for ventilation and oxygenation, adequate end-organ tissue perfusion, and control of hemorrhage are the primary goals during the initial management of any pediatric trauma. Care should be taken to ensure that the above goals are achieved without compromise to a potentially unstable cervical spine injury. Stable, midline immobilization of the cervical spine and appropriate maneuvers to gain access to the larynx for airway management should be implemented until the possibility of fracture is excluded.

- The lateral **C-spine X-ray** can be performed following the initial trauma assessment, particularly if significant injury to the cervical spine is suspected that may influence management.
- Remaining cervical spine X-rays should be performed in the radiology department once the patient has been stabilized adequately.

## Immobilization of the C-spine:

- Adequate immobilization includes a hard collar or tape and lightweight spacing devices with a full spine board.
- Saline or sandbags should not be used for C-spine immobilization.
- Elevation under the torso or a built-in depression in the spine board should be used for children under 8 years to accommodate for a proportionally larger occiput.
- Avoid rigid fixation of head-to-spine board in the uncooperative patient unless body securely strapped.

\*\***Warning:** Young children and infants too small for the spine board often require additional packing to ensure that they do not slide laterally and compromise the C-spine if log-rolled on the spine board.

- An appropriately sized cervical collar should rest firmly on the chest and clavicles with the chin snugly in the chin cup without causing airway compromise.
- If endotracheal intubation is required, the cervical collar is removed and another member of the trauma team maintains midline immobilization of the C-spine from a position below the head and neck; the forearms are placed on the torso while the hands are placed in a lateral position on the head.
- Cervical spine immobilization may be discontinued only when the patient has satisfied age-appropriate clinical and/or radiographic criteria.

## Clearing the C-spine:

- X-rays must be reviewed by personnel qualified to render an interpretation.
- The C-spine must be re-examined and all of the following criteria met:

  - No pain or tenderness to palpation along cervical spine
  - Absence of distracting injuries
  - Normal level of consciousness

- No focal neurologic deficits
- Normal *active* range of motion without pain or limitation

** **<u>Warning:</u>** The examiner should ask the patient to slowly move his or her head through flexion, extension, lateral flexion, and rotation; if at any point the patient cannot complete the full range of motion, or experiences pain or a motor-sensory deficit, midline immobilization should be immediately resumed and the collar reapplied. Passive range of motion is **never** used in the clearance of the C-spine. If the examiner is unable to clear the cervical spine by using the above criteria, consider referral to a neurosurgeon or orthopedic spine service.

## Critical Care Considerations

In the event of suspected spinal cord transection, immediate neurosurgical and orthopedic consultation should be obtained. Medical management should address appropriate inotropic support of spinal shock if present and consider administration of intravenous methylprednisolone if within 8 hours of spinal injury. The administration of glucocorticoids in the emergency treatment of spinal cord injury remains controversial and will vary between institutions. Intravenous fluid therapy should be used judiciously to minimize risk of cerebral edema, particularly if there is associated closed head injury.

# References

McDonald JW, Sadowsky C. Spinal cord injury. Lancet 2002, Feb 2;359:417–25.

Eleraky MA, Theodore N, Adams M, et al. Pediatric cervical spine-injuries: report of 102 cases and review of the literature. J Neurosurg 2000, Jan;92:12–7.

Herman MJ, Pizzutillo PD. Cervical spine disorders in children. Orthopedic Clinics of NA 1999, July;30(3):457–65.

Kriss VM, Kriss TC. SCIWORA in infants and children. Clin Pediatr 1996, Mar;119–24.

Caviness AC. Evaluation of cervical spine injuries in children. *UpToDate* 2003, Feb.

Woodward GA. Neck trauma. In: Fleisher GR, Ludwig S, eds. Textbook of Pediatric Emergency Medicine, 5th ed. Philadelphia: Lippincott, Williams & Wilkins; 2006. pp. 1389–1432.

# D. Acute Management of the Pediatric Burn

James Bain

Krishnapriya Anchala

## Key Principles

> - Initial assessment should always begin with airway, breathing, and circulation.
> - Circumferential burns, including those to the chest, are particularly concerning and may require escharotomy.
> - Most burns are preventable.

Burns and their related injuries are a leading cause of morbidity and mortality in children, ranking third among causes of injury-related deaths in children aged 1 to 9 years. Advancements in treatments of burns have allowed significant improvements in mortality, even for those with serious burns.

## Epidemiology

- In the United States—400,000 children are treated for burns annually

  - 3,000 deaths
  - 10,000–12,000 disability

- 50% are younger than 4 years old
- Younger children are more likely to have scalds
- 80% of burns are secondary to house fires
- 1–16% of burns are intentional
- Children with up to 95% of BSA burned can still survive

## Physiology

- Thermal injury to tissue: coagulation necrosis and cell death.
- Release of vasoactive mediators injures capillary endothelial cells resulting in capillary leak and edema (peaks at 24 hours and resolves in 3 to 5 days).

- Areas adjacent to burned tissue have sluggish circulation called the "zone of stasis." This area is susceptible to ischemia thereby extending the areas of necrosis.
- This is surrounded by the zone of hyperemia.

# Classification

Important: Classification must be assessed regularly, as the burn is dynamic.

- Superficial (first degree)

    - Erythema and pain with occasional minor blistering
    - Involves only the epidermis
    - Like a sunburn
    - Heals in 5–10 days with no residual scarring

- Partial thickness (second degree)

    - Epidermis and dermis
    - Moist and blister to white and dry that blanch with pressure and have reduced pain
    - Heal in 10–42 days, may have scarring
    - May progress to full thickness with infection, edema, inflammation, and ischemia
    - May require grafting

- Full thickness (third degree)

    - Necrosis through all layers into fat
    - Dry and charred to red and nonblanching with pressure
    - Not sensitive to touch
    - Requires grafting

- Fourth degree

    - Full thickness plus fat, fascia, muscle, or bone

## Estimating Body Surface Area

- Quick estimate: palm is 1%.
- Do not include superficial (first-degree) burns in total body surface area calculation.

## Location

- Assess for potential of disability.
- Beware of burns on face, eyes, ears, feet, perineum, hands, and joints.

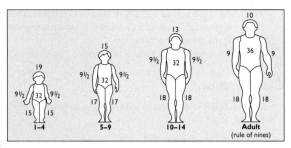

**Figure I**    Estimation of body surface area.

## Associated Injuries

- Smoke inhalation
- CO poisoning
- Fractures
- Trauma
- Non-accidental injury
- Underlying diseases

## Severity

### Minor

- BSA less than 5%
- No vital structures
- No full thickness
- No other complications

### Moderate

- 5–15% BSA
- Any full thickness
- Involves hands, feet, face, perineum
- Chemical or electrical

### Severe

- Greater than 15% BSA
- Full thickness greater than 5%
- Presence of smoke inhalation or CO poisoning

# Management

## BLS

- Remove all clothing.
- Flush with copious amounts of water for 20–30 minutes.

## ABC

A—Intubate if airway, respiratory, or neurologic compromise exists; if stridorous, intubate early with a smaller endotracheal tube.

- If history is consistent with inhalation injury, may need bronchoscopy.
- Intubate if deep facial burns or massive thoracic burns that decrease the compliance of the chest wall.

B—100% $O_2$

- May need hyperbaric oxygen if there is significant exposure to carbon monoxide (CO).

C—Large-bore IV catheters not through burned tissue, bolus 20 mL/kg isotonic fluid until fluid needs can be estimated using burn surface area.

- Weigh
- Catheterize
- NG

Assess for associated injuries, such as trauma or inhalation.

## Initial Wound Care

- Wait until stabilized.
- Try to be sterile.
- Irrigate with cool saline while avoiding hypothermia.
- Debride dead material while leaving blisters intact.
- Apply creams.
- Assess for tetanus status.

## Assess for Non-accidental Injury

- Developmental level of the child
- Consistency and plausibility of explanation
- Red flags

- Well-demarcated line in lower limb with no splash marks
- Accidental scalding with full-thickness burns
- Bruises or healed wounds
- Previous contact with Child Protective Services

## Involve Plastic Surgery Early

# When to Transfer to a Burn Center

- partial plus full greater than 10% BSA in <10 years
- partial plus full greater than 20% BSA in ≥10 years
- involvement of face, eyes, hands, feet, genitalia, perineum, and major joints
- full thickness greater than 5% BSA
- significant electrical burns including lightning
- significant chemical burns
- inhalation injury
- patients with pre-existing illness that could complicate management, prolong recovery, or affect mortality
- concomitant trauma that increases risk of morbidity or mortality and can be stabilized at trauma center before transfer to burn center
- patients requiring special rehabilitative, social, or long-term support including suspected non-accidental injury or neglect
- children with burns seen in hospitals without qualified personnel or equipment

Adapted from: Committee on Trauma, American College of Surgeons. Resources for optimal care of the injured patient. Chicago, IL: American College of Surgeons; 1999: p. 55.

# Fluids

## Day 1

- Parkland formula: 4 mL/kg/BSA% in ringer's lactate first half over 8 hours, then next half over 16 hours (calculated from time of injury).
- May need to add 5% dextrose in a young child.
- Add maintenance fluids on top in infants.
- Greater than 30% BSA consider central venous line (CVL) for ongoing fluid management.
- Target urine output greater than 1 cc/kg/hour calculated every 4 hours.

- No potassium as cells are leaky.
- Note that Parkland formula overestimates fluids in smaller BSA burns and underestimates fluid needs in larger BSA burns.

## Day 2

- IV at maintenance with glucose containing hypotonic fluid with potassium.
- Start oral feeds.

## Airway/Pulmonary

- Avoid non-depolarizing muscle relaxants for long periods of time post-burn (resistance and hyperkalemia).
- May need repeated laryngoscopy and bronchoscopy.
- Watch for ARDS and pulmonary edema (leaky capillaries).
- Inhalation injury: aggressive pulmonary toileting, elective intubation.

## Cardiovascular

- Cardiac output and oxygen consumption increase by 2–3 times.
- Hypovolemia may be due to interstitial leak.

## Hematological

- Anemia is secondary to erythrocyte damage and bone marrow suppression.

## Renal

- Watch for myoglobinuria.

## Pain

- Morphine, fentanyl, ketamine, and benzodiazepines.

## Infection

- Temperature will rise 1–2°C due to hypermetabolic state.
- Surveillance skin plating may be useful.
- Fungi and gram negatives are causes of infection due to the topical antibiotic regimen.

## Nutrition

- Extreme catabolic state.
- Requires maintenance of 1,800 kcal/m$^2$/day plus burn 2,200 kcal/m$^2$/day.
- Supplement with vitamin C and zinc.
- Try to feed enterally starting day 2.
- Restrict dietary fat to 15% (effect on immune function).
- H$_2$ blocker should be started within first 6 hours due to risk of ulcer.

## Ongoing Wound Care

- Pink and moist wounds (superficial partial-thickness burns) should be covered with a semi-occlusive dressing.
- Poor blanching areas or obvious full-thickness areas are treated with a topical antimicrobial agent.

    - 1% silver sulfadiazine

        - avoid if allergic to sulpha drugs
        - active against gram positive organisms

    - Neosporin® or bacitracin for facial areas (avoid large areas)

- Once to twice daily dressing changes with wound debridement and application of topical agents.
- Elevate a distal extremity to avoid edema.
- Watch circumferential burns for compartment syndrome.

## Rehabilitation

- Involve early.
- Involve child in dressings as opposed to distraction.

## Surgery

- Excision and grafting is indicated for areas of full thickness and areas of deep partial thickness.
- BSA greater than 50% should go to the OR soon.
- Scald burns should be observed for 2 weeks.

## Prevention

Scald burns are most common etiology for burn injuries requiring hospitalization in young children. All hot-water heaters should be set at less than 49°C (120°F).

- Water at 49°C (120°F) takes 10 minutes to produce same burn that at 55°C (131°F) would take only 30 seconds.
- Turn pot handles inward on stovetops.
- Do not leave hot liquid in cups or bowls unattended.

# Electrical Burns

In the Unites States, there are 1,500 deaths per year due to electrical burns.

- 2–3% of all admissions to hospital burn centers
- One-third are household burns
- Result from thermal energy produced as an electrical current passes through body

The extent of injury depends on:

- Resistance of skin, mucosa, and internal structures
- Type of current
- Frequency of current
- Duration of contact
- Intensity of current
- Pathway of current

Nerves, muscles, and blood vessels have low electrical resistance, so electricity causes severe damage to these structures. Flow through body usually takes one of three paths:
Hand to hand (most dangerous, with 60% mortality rate)

- Hand to hand
- Hand to foot
- Foot to foot

Cardiac effects of electrical burns are the most life-threatening.

- Dysrhythmias, most commonly ventricular fibrillation
- Myocardial damage

All patients with significant electrical injuries should have investigation:

- CBC
- Electrolytes
- BUN
- Creatinine
- UA with urine myoglobin
- ECG

- CXR
- Consider CK and cardiac enzymes

Management of medium- and high-voltage injuries (>200 volts):

- All patients with high-voltage injuries should be admitted.
- Observe children on cardiac monitor 24–72 hours due to risk of arrhythmias.
- If there is significant muscle damage, careful observation of fluid status is necessary due to risk of renal failure.
- Consider Foley catheter, alkalinization of urine.

Management of low voltage injuries:

- Consider observation for 4 hours on cardiac monitor, then discharge if no significant injuries found.

# References

Hansborough JF, Hansborough W. Pediatric burns. Pediatr Rev 1999;20:117–224.

Reed JL, Pomerantz WJ. Emergency management of pediatric burns. Ped Emerg Care 2005;21:118–29.

Tepas JJ, et al. Trauma. In: Fuchs S, Gausche-Hill M, Yamamoto Y, eds. APLS: The pediatric emergency medicine course, 4th ed. Sudbury: Jones and Bartlett; 2004. pp. 312–9.

# E. Emergent Presentations of Child Abuse

John Crossley
Anthony G Crocco

Child abuse is an important and unfortunately all too common reason for children to present to both the Emergency Department (ED) and the PICU. Despite numerous studies of its incidence, the differences in presentation types and significant underreporting (especially in middle class families) make it difficult to identify exact numbers. Some estimates put 10% of burns and fractures as being caused by abuse; others are much higher. US estimates are 500,000–4,000,000 incidences per year.

## Key Principles

- Abuse is more common than most practitioners think; the key is to always consider abuse.
- It is best managed by a multidisciplinary team, with focus on the child's best interest.
- Questioning must be open and non-judgmental.
- Documentation is critical.
- Most jurisdictions have a legal obligation to report abuse, but also protect physicians from legal action.

## Major Physiology/Pathophysiology

The dynamics of abuse are complex; abusive parents/caregivers are not always harmful to the child and the child may still have strong emotional ties to the parent/abuser. Abuse is usually brought on by multiple factors. Some of these factors are outlined in Table 1.

*Table I*
## Factors Linked to Abuse

| Family stress factors | Parent's psychological factors | Parenting factors | Child factors | Societal factors |
|---|---|---|---|---|
| Economic difficulty Poor housing Unemployment Illness Crowding | Impulse disorder Depression Drug/alcohol abuse Psychosis Developmental delay | Lack of preparation Poor role models Unrealistic expectations of child Use of corporal punishment Unsupportive spouse Inconsistent parenting | Provocative behavior Prolonged neonatal hospitalization Physical disabilities Developmental delay | Social isolation Distant or absent extended family High expectations for all parents Violence acceptable |

# Differential Diagnosis/Etiology

*Classification:* Abuse is generally broken into four groups, although many cases may involve more than one type. Emotional abuse in particular is almost always found in conjunction with other forms of abuse. The most commonly recognized categories are:

- Physical abuse
- Sexual abuse (misuse)
- Child neglect
- Emotional abuse

In terms of frequency of ED presentation, the following is an estimate.

- Physical 66%

  - Bruises and contusions 52%
  - Burns 13%
  - Skeletal 8%
  - Central nervous system 15%
  - Toxic ingestions 4%
  - Abdominal 2%
  - Misc 6%

- Sexual 7.4%
- Neglect 12.5%
- Multiple presentation 14%

## Physical Abuse

Traditionally, this area is the most commonly discovered and reported form, and is most likely to result in an ED visit for care. It is also the most easily identified in the ED, up to 10% of traumatic injuries brought to the ED are a result of abuse. Current Canadian statistics are that 49/1,000 children are physically abused.

Physical abuse is associated with the highest mortality of all abuse. Homicide is the leading cause of death of children 1–4 years, and the fourth leading cause for 5–14 years of age. Reports of patterns of injury vary, and as the ED population is selective, some minor injuries may not be brought there for treatment.

**Shaken Baby Syndrome**   Shaken baby syndrome (SBS) is a specific type of physical abuse. SBS was initially identified by Caffrey and consists of the combined finding of subarachnoid and subdural hemorrhages, metaphyseal fractures, and retinal hemorrhages.

The most commonly described mechanism of injury is shaking of the torso and sudden striking of the head against a hard surface. Rotational injury must also be a component of the force involved.

Almost all cases occur in children under 3, most under 1 year. Common symptoms include lethargy, irritability, seizures, increased or decreased tone, impaired consciousness, vomiting, poor feeding, breathing abnormalities, and apnea.

## Sexual Abuse

Most statistics demonstrate increasing frequency (10-fold over 10 years) probably due to greater acceptance of reporting and awareness than a true increase in incidence. Much less frequently presents to ED.

## Neglect

Neglect is probably the most common form of abuse, but also is the hardest to prove. It is rarely the presenting complaint to ED, although it may be the underlying cause of other presenting complaints (fatigue, weight loss, etc.). Neglect is generally divided into the following groups:

- Failure to meet the basic needs of the child
- Non-organic failure to thrive (ie, lack of food)
- Medical neglect
- Abandonment
- Truancy (lack of education)

## Emotional Abuse

Emotional abuse is difficult to define, and generally is not legally explored because of this. Primarily it consists of negative reinforcement either through directed actions or through lack of normal emotional support (although this overlaps with neglect). Most commonly found in conjunction with other forms, it would be unlikely to present to the ED except as emotional or behavioral complaints.

## Differential Diagnosis

It is important to realize that abuse is far more common than organic conditions that may mimic its appearance, such as congenital or acquired coagulopathies or bone disorders. However, these must be actively ruled out.

## Clinical Features/Evaluation

## Recognition of Physical Abuse

The key to identifying child abuse is accepting the high rate of occurrence and maintaining a high index of suspicion. Both history and physical examination are vital to diagnosis; one must evaluate history of injury as well as type. Patterns of injury may be different when inflicted versus accidental.

## Criteria for Evaluation

- History of injury:
  - How was injury inflicted? Plausible or not?
  - Absence of history (ie, unexplained)
  - Could the injury have been reasonably avoided with supervision?
  - Is there a changing or inconsistent history?

- History of repeated visits or hospitalization
- Was there delay in seeking medical care?
- Did caregiver/parent over-underestimate extent of injury?

- Medical history of prematurity, failure to thrive, not receiving adequate basic care (ie, immunizations)
- Child's age and developmental level
- Presence of other old or new injuries
- Interactions between parents and child
- Interactions between parents and ED staff

Remember to record all details, including the last two criteria.

## Sexual Abuse History

As previously mentioned, other forms of abuse may have less obvious physical evidence. In this category, there may be specific (ie, parental concerns, genital injuries) or nonspecific complaints. Table 2 outlines physical and behavioral problems that may be present in sexual abuse.

Interviewing the parent and child separately is essential. The child interview must both assess and provide emotional support to the child. Assess for:

- Language development
- Psychosexual development

*Table 2*
## Complaints in Sexual Abuse

| Specific complaints | | Non-specific complaints | |
| --- | --- | --- | --- |
| **Physical** | **Behavioral** | **Physical** | **Behavioral** |
| Genital bruising/ lacerations | Describes contact | Anorexia | Phobias, fears |
| Rectal lacerations | Inappropriate knowledge | Abdominal pain | Nightmares, refusal to sleep alone |
| STD | Compulsive masturbation | Enuresis | Runaways |
| Pregnancy | Sexual acting out | Dysuria | Aggressive behavior |
| | | Encopresis | Suicide attempts |
| | | Vaginal discharge | Abrupt behavior changes |
| | | Urethral discharge | |
| | | Rectal pain | |

- Potential to contaminate history by suggestion
- Child apprehensiveness
- Caregiver apprehension

## Physical Indicators

Physical examination for suspected sexual abuse often requires only external examination in pre-pubertal females; otherwise, it should be done as an examination under anesthesia (EUA).

- Does nature of injury match history?
- Pathognomonic markings (ie, cigarette burns)
- Multiple injuries
- Different stages of healing
- Multiple forms of injury (eg, burns AND fractures)
- Overall poor care
- Documented poisoning
- Failure to thrive
- Unexplainable findings

## Physical Examination

A complete physical examination of the child is necessary whenever abuse is suspected either by history or by presenting injury. The primary areas where physical abuse is recognized are the skin and musculoskeletal systems.

In some circumstances, neurologic injury can be considered pathognomonic of specific abuse types (see section on "Shaken Baby Syndrome").

### Skin

Most commonly identified area of injury, and generally found as bruises, abrasions, and burns. Although bruises can be accidental, accidental bruising is most common on the head and distal extremities (shins and forearms/elbows).

Suspicious patterns of bruising would include the following:

- Circular
- Linear
- Central/buttocks bruising

### Burns

Burns are less common as an accidental event, but do occur. Accidental burns generally are superficial on fingertips (brief contact/touching of hot object or a splash pattern on tipped fluids). Intentional burns are most commonly immersive, especially during toilet training. Other indicators of intentional burns:

- Delay in seeking treatment
- History of child being unsupervised during incident
- Child brought to ED by the parent who was not present at the time of injury
- Identifiable marks (shape of specific objects such as cigarettes)
- On areas normally covered by clothing (ie, under a diaper)
- Sparing of thicker skin (palms and soles)

## Hair

Hair changes/findings are much less common. One may see "traction alopecia," areas of hair removed by pulling. This is characterized by a normal scalp (ie, no lesions/redness) and patches of broken/shortened hair.

## Skeletal Injuries

There are many common accidental injuries (ie, clavicle or radial head dislocation). Others are much less common, such as femur and rib fractures. It is important to identify those features suggesting non-accidental in both types of fractures.

## Femur Fractures

Generally considered one of the most classic fractures for abuse, a study on consecutive femur fracture found 19/24 from abuse, in 2/3 of these cases the fracture was the only evidence. Another quoted only 3 identified causes:

- Major trauma [ie, motor vehicle crash (MVC)]
- Bone disorder (ie, osteogenesis imperfecta)
- Abuse (most common)

## Rib Fractures

Extremely uncommon accidentally in small children. Even in cases of CPR, broken ribs are rare. In the absence of major trauma, abuse is highly likely. In addition, the mean age for rib fractures differs greatly. The average age of a patient with rib fractures caused by abuse is 3 months. The average age of a patient with rib fractures due to an accidental cause is 8.5 years.

## Other Suspicious Fractures

- Clavicle fracture in children less than 2 years old other than those due to traumatic birth
- Vertebrae
- Sternum
- Pelvis
- Scapulae

Attempted dating of fractures is important to assess consistency of findings with history and presence of multiple episodes over time. Always involve a radiologist in this process. Table 3 outlines radiographic changes in fractures over time.

## Other Injuries

Although less common, any system can be involved in abuse. Gastrointestinal injury would include uncommon severe injuries to the liver or spleen, but mouth trauma is the most common (eg, tear of frenulum from jamming bottle to stop crying). Cardiopulmonary and genitourinary injuries also occur. Physical examination for suspected sexual abuse often requires only external examination in pre-pubertal females; otherwise it should be done as EUA.

**Ophthalmologic Evaluation** Part of the shaken baby syndrome (SBS) that is virtually diagnostic of abuse is the

*Table 3*
**Fracture Dating**

| 0–10 days | 10 days–8 weeks | 8 weeks and over |
|---|---|---|
| Soft-tissue edema | Periosteal new bone (layered) | Periosteal new bone matures and thickens |
| Joint fluid | Bone resorption making facture more visible | Callus denser and smoother |
| Visible fracture fragments | Callus (subtle then heavy) | Metaphyseal fragments incorporated into callus |
| Visible fracture lines | Metaphyseal fragments often more visible | Fracture lines disappear |
| | | Deformities and bumps may persist |

presence of retinal hemorrhages. The hemorrhages are found in 65–95% of patients with SBS and may be unilateral or bilateral, and with or without retinal detachments.

# Investigations

## Laboratory Investigations

Most commonly are limited to coagulation studies, CBC, INR/PTT, and urinalysis. Directed studies (ie, liver/pancreas in abdominal trauma) are more appropriate than broad screens as they are unlikely to identify additional useful information.

## Diagnostic Imaging

Skeletal survey looking for old and new fractures is a standard of care for suspected abuse, both because of availability and information details. Bone scans are not yet considered adequate as a sole investigation, although it is sometimes useful as an adjunct. You should consider arranging a skeletal survey for the following:

- Any child <1 year with a fracture
- Any child with severe or extensive fracture
- History of more than one fracture
- History of "soft bones" in child or family

# Management/Treatment and Eventual Disposition

## Management

A multidisciplinary team best manages evaluation and management of child abuse. The affected child often has multiple needs that cannot be met by the emergency department. Early involvement of social work and child protective services (CPS = CAS in Canada) is critical.

The key components of the emergency management are:

- Identify suspicious presentations.
- Collect historical and/or examination inconsistencies (as above).
- Complete relevant laboratory and radiographic evaluation.

## Documentation

Studies have shown that simple "checklists" improve detail and accuracy of documentation and improve legal outcomes. Use of diagrams, photos, or video is helpful. Documentation should be detailed but objective. For forensic purposes, one must also document the collection of evidence and maintain the "chain of evidence."

## Consultation

Most EDs and PICUs have social work teams that can liaise with CPS. Pediatric hospitals often have multidisciplinary teams that effectively manage cases and address follow up, which is often difficult to coordinate solely through the ED.

## Reporting Abuse

Most provinces/territories in Canada have mandatory reporting to Children's Aid Society when there are reasonable grounds to suspect that a child is or may be suffering or may have suffered abuse. Not reporting suspicion may result in successful prosecution of the physician, and could result in loss of licensure. All such jurisdictions have protection from liability for over-reporting, provided it is done "in good faith." It is essential that the first contact physician reports suspected abuse; don't leave it to others as the potential for "I thought someone else called" leaving children unprotected. Timely reporting is essential and may help ensure that siblings do not remain in an at-risk environment. After a report is made, ensure that the name of the intake worker and date/time of the report are included in the medical record.

## Informing Parents

Parents accompanying a child who has injuries suspicious for abuse must be informed if a report has been filed. Be prepared for an angry response, although some parents may respond with apparent indifference. It is generally best to inform the parents that you are legally obligated to report injuries that are suspicious for abuse and to convey that you share a common goal of looking out for the child's best interests. Try not to be accusatory, and be aware that you also must provide support to the parents.

## Disposition (Discharge)

Disposition should be decided in consultation with CPS/CAS or the internal consultation team if available. Admission should occur if injuries warrant, or if there is no safe environment outside of the hospital. Admission may also be warranted in cases of chronic medical problems in which abuse is suspected but not definitive (eg, Munchausen syndrome by proxy). Most common "safe discharge" scenarios would be:

- To non-abusive parent
- To removed relative (eg, grandparent)
- Directly to CAS/CPS (foster care)

Treatment of abuse is largely beyond the scope of the ED except to consider potential STD and/or HIV and pregnancy testing/counseling in sexual abuse.

## Summary

- Child abuse is much more common than most people think.
- The ED is a common site of first presentation for some forms.
- Failure to recognize injuries that are suspicious for abuse can have serious or life-threatening consequences for the child.
- Report suspected abuse yourself; don't leave it to others.

## References

American Academy of Pediatrics, Hymel KP, Committee on Child Abuse and Neglect, National Association of Medical Examiners. Distinguishing sudden infant death syndrome from child abuse fatalities. Pediatrics 2006;118:421–7.

Taitz J, Moran K, O'Meara M. Long bone fractures in children under 3 years of age: is abuse being missed in Emergency Department presentations? J Paediatr Child Health 2004;40:170–4.

Trocmé N, MacMillan H, Fallon B, De Marco R. Nature and severity of physical harm caused by child abuse and neglect: results from the Canadian Incidence Study. CMAJ 2003 Oct. 28;169(9):911–5.

MacMillan HL, Canadian Task Force on Preventive Health Care. Preventive health care, 2000 update: prevention of child maltreatment. CMAJ 2000 Nov 28;163(11):1451–8.

Newton AW, Vandeven AM. Unexplained infant and child death: a review of sudden infant death syndrome, sudden unexplained infant death, and child maltreatment fatalities including shaken baby syndrome. Curr Opin Pediatr 2006;18:196–200.

Keshavarz R, Kawashima R, Low C. Child abuse and neglect presentations to a pediatric emergency department. J Emerg Med 2002;23(4):341–5.

Duhaime AC, Christian CW, Rorke LB, Zimmerman RA. Non-accidental head injury in infants—The "shaken-baby syndrome." N Engl J Med 1998 Jun 18;338(25):1822–9.

King WJ, MacKay M, Sirnick A, Canadian Shaken Baby Study Group. Shaken baby syndrome in Canada: clinical characteristics and outcomes of hospital cases. CMAJ 2003 Jan 21;168(2):155–9.

Loo SK, Bala NMC, Clarke ME, Hornick JP. Child Abuse: Reporting and Classification in Health Care Settings, Health Canada, 1999.

Ludwig, S. Child abuse. In: Fleisher GR, Ludwig S, eds. Textbook of Pediatric Emergency Medicine, 5th ed. Philadelphia: Lippincott, Williams & Wilkins; 2006. pp. 1761–1801.

# Chapter 21

# End-of-Life Care

## A. Determination of Death

Lennox Huang

### Key Principles

- Death may be determined by either somatic (respiratory and circulatory) or neurologic (brain) criteria.
- Criteria for neurologic death vary across the world with no consensus.
- Declaration of death should be performed in the presence of parents or guardians when possible.
- Determination of death should include considerations of organ or tissue donation.
- Declaration of death should be done with empathy and clarity.

### Definition of Somatic Death

Somatic death is the irreversible cessation of cardiac and respiratory function.

1. Does not resume spontaneously.
2. Cannot be started with resuscitation.
3. Will not be restarted on morally justifiable grounds.

Declaration is generally performed by a physician when:

1. Patient is unresponsive.
2. Patient is apneic.
3. Patient has absent circulation.

- Convention is to examine a patient for 1 minute for the above criteria before declaring death.
- Complete neurologic exam is unnecessary.
- Testing for responsiveness to painful stimuli (sternal rub) is unnecessary.
- Auto-resuscitation has been reported in adult patients following up to 65 seconds of asystole.
- Duration of resuscitation required before declaring somatic death is controversial and varies according to clinical presentation. Refer to Chapter 5, "Resuscitation," for further details.
- There are evolving protocols for declaring somatic death in pediatric patients who are candidates for organ donation after cardio-circulatory death.
- Most existing protocols include rigorous monitoring and at least 2–10 minutes of absent cardiopulmonary function prior to declaration and initiation of organ procurement.

# Origins of Brain Death Concept

Modern considerations of isolated brain death arose in parallel with evolution of transplant medicine and ICU medicine. Neurologic determination of death allows for an ethical framework for organ donation.

- Pre-1960s, somatic death was the only accepted definition of death.
- 1968 Harvard ad hoc committee: Notion of brain death first defined.
- 1981 US Presidential commission recommendations led to the "Uniform Determination of Death Act (UDDA)," which distinguished between:

    (1)  irreversible cessation of circulatory and respiratory functions, or

    (2)  irreversible cessation of all functions of the entire brain, including the brain stem.

The Presidential commission recommendations excluded children under 5 years of age.

- 1987 US task force for determination of brain death in children was assembled, and guidelines published.
- 2003 Canadian Council for Donation and Transplantation published comprehensive report and recommendations for neurologic determination of death.

# Definition of Brain Death

Brain death is an irreversible cessation of brain function. There are three proposed formulations:

1. Whole brain = inclusive of brain stem (United States)
2. Higher brain = absent cortical function
3. Brain stem death = absent brain stem function (United Kingdom)

Effectively, whole brain definitions and criteria dominate current practice. There is no universally accepted definition of "brain death." Significant religious and cultural variation exists. No single consensus definition exists among medical professionals.

# Determination of Brain Death

There are three components in the determination of neurologic death.

1. History—absence of treatable or reversible conditions
2. Physical—coma, apnea, absent brainstem functions, time component
3. Confirmatory tests (not always required)—drug levels, EEG, cerebral blood flow (angiography/CT angiography)

- For highest certainty and to minimize parental doubt and potential legal complications, exam should be performed by two physicians with at least one physician not directly involved in the care of the patient.
- Physician declaring death should not be directly involved in the organ transplantation process.
- See Appendix 1 and Appendix 2 for Canadian consensus guidelines for determination of neurologic death.

# Mechanisms Leading to Brain Death

- >50% traumatic brain injury
- Stroke, intracranial hemorrhage
- Drowning
- Asphyxia
- Brain tumors

# Confounding Factors in the Determination of Brain Death

Consider potential reversible causes of coma. These include but are not limited to:

- Un-resuscitated shock
- Medications and intoxicants (eg, barbiturates, benzodiazepines, recent neuromuscular blockade, alcohols); if in doubt, quantitative testing should be performed
- Hypothermia

Brain death should *not* be declared without ancillary testing in the presence of confounding factors.

## Timing of Physical Examination

- Two evaluations separated by a period of time are often recommended for pediatric patients.
- Infants and neonates should have evaluations separated by a period of at least 24–48 hours, respectively.
- Time intervals separating evaluations in older children are more controversial and may not be necessary according to some protocols (Appendix 2).
- However, some time separation is often helpful for parents to digest the enormity of the situation.

## Components of Physical Exam

- Coma + apnea
- Absent brain stem reflexes:

  - Absent pupillary response
  - Absent cough + gag
  - Absent vestibulo-ocular response (doll's eye, cold calorics)

- Flaccid with no spontaneous movements or motor response (excluding spinal reflexes)

## Apnea Testing

See Figure 1.

**Apnea Test**

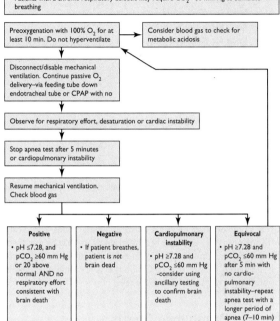

Figure 1

# Ancillary Testing

Angiography

- 4-vessel angiogram for cerebral blood flow is current gold standard
- Costly, invasive, requires technical expertise
- Rarely possible to perform at bedside

Radionuclide imaging

- Tc-99m with single photon emission computed tomography (SPECT) cerebral blood flow

- Costly
- Rarely possible to perform at bedside

## Electroencephalography (EEG)

- Most common supplementary test used
- Inexpensive, noninvasive
- Look for electrocerebral silence
- Tests superficial cortical function, not deep brain stem activity

## Transcranial Doppler

- Noninvasive, requires technical expertise
- Sensitive for absent perfusion

## CT angiography, MRI angiography, PET scanning

- In evolution, not enough evidence to support routine use

## Quantitative + qualitative drug level testing

- If specific confounding factors are suspected

Upon completion of physical exam including apnea test along with any necessary ancillary testing, brain death may be declared. Time of death should be documented as the time at which testing is initiated. Please refer to Chapter 21C for additional details regarding the organ donation process.

# How to Pronounce Death

Generally performed by physicians in a hospital setting.

*Prior to entering room:*

- Know the patient's name and age.
- Know the primary diagnosis and circumstances surrounding the death.
- Consider if case to be referred to the coroner.
- Notify local organ procurement organization.
- Consult with other medical team members: nurse, social worker, chaplain, etc.

*At the bedside:*

- Parents and their supports should be present.
- Introduce yourself and explain what you will be doing.

- Confirm somatic or neurologic death.
- Express empathy and allow grieving family time and space; balance privacy with staff availability.

*Minimum documentation in chart:*

- Name, identifying data
- Date, time
- Diagnosis
- Circumstances
- Additional forms vary with geographic location

# When to Refer to Coroner

- Individual criteria vary according to local laws and regulations.
- Less than 24 hours in the hospital.
- Sudden and unanticipated deaths.
- Deaths associated with potential criminal activity.
- Deaths associated with a procedure or operation.

# References

Canadian Council for Donation and Transplantation. Severe brain injury to neurologic determination of death: A Canadian forum. Report and Recommendations 2003.

Wijdicks EFM. Brain death worldwide, accepted fact but no global consensus in diagnostic criteria. Neurology 2002;58:20–25.

Ad Hoc Committee of the Harvard Medical School. A definition of irreversible coma. Report of the ad hoc committee of the Harvard Medical School to examine the definition of brain death. JAMA 1968 Aug 5;205(6):337–40.

Kohrman MH, Spivack BS. Brain death in infants: sensitivity and specificity of current criteria. Pediatr Neurol 1990 Jan–Feb;6(1): 47–50.

Outwater KM, Rockoff MA. Apnea testing to confirm brain death in children. Crit Care Med 1984 Apr;12(4):357–8.

President's Commission: Guidelines for the determination of death. JAMA 1981 Nov 13;246(19):2184–6.

Schwartz JA, Baxter J, Brill DR. Diagnosis of brain death in children by radionuclide cerebral imaging. Pediatrics 1984 Jan;73(1):14–8.

Task Force for the Determination of Brain Death in Children. Guidelines for the determination of brain death in children. Arch Neurol 1987 Jun;44(6):587–8.

Orlowski JP. Drowning, near-drowning, and ice-water submersions. Pediatr Clin North Am 1987 Feb;34(1):75–92.

**Checklist for Neurological Determination of Death (NDD) – Adults and Children age ≥ 1 year**

#### Section One: Minimum Clinical Criteria

a.  Deep unresponsive coma with the following established etiology: _____

b.  Confounding factors precluding the diagnosis?　　　　　　　　Yes☐　No☐

c.  Temperature (core) _____

d.  Brainstem Reflexes:

| | |
|---|---|
| Bilateral absence of motor responses: (excluding spinal reflexes) | Yes☐　No☐ |
| Absent cough: | Yes☐　No☐ |
| Absent gag: | Yes☐　No☐ |
| Bilateral absence of corneal responses: | Yes☐　No☐ |
| Bilateral absence of vestibulo-ocular responses: | Yes☐　No☐ |
| Bilateral absence of pupillary response to light: (pupils ≥ mid size) | Yes☐　No☐ |
| Apnea: | Yes☐　No☐ |

At completion of apnea test: pH_____  $PaCO_2$ _____mmHg

$PaCO_2$ ≥ 20 mmHg above the pre-apnea test level:　　　　　Yes☐　No☐

#### Section Two: Ancillary Tests

Ancillary tests, as defined by the absence of intracranial blood flow, should be performed when **any** of the minimum clinical criteria cannot be completed, **or** unresolved confounding factors exist.

Ancillary testing has been performed:　　　　　　　　　　　　Yes☐　No☐
Date: _____Time: _____

Absence of intracranial blood flow has been demonstrated by:
　Cerebral Radiocontrast Angiography　　　☐
　Radionuclide Angiography　　　　　☐
　Other _____

#### Section Three: Declaration and Documentation

The first and second physician's determinations may be performed concurrently. If performed at different points in time, a full clinical examination including the apnea test must be performed, without any fixed examination interval, regardless of the primary etiology.

**This patient fulfills the neurological determination of death:**

Physician:　Print name: _____　　Signature: _____

　　　　　Date: _____　　　　　　　　Time: _____

#### Section Four: Standard End-of-Life Care

| | |
|---|---|
| Is this patient medically eligible for organ and/or tissue donation? | Yes☐　No☐ |
| Has the option for organ or tissue donation been offered? | Yes☐　No☐ |
| Has consent been obtained for donation? | Yes☐　No☐ |

*Severe Brain Death to Neurological Determination of Death: A Canadian Forum*

<u>Checklist for Neurological Determination of Death–Adults and Children ≥ 1 Year</u>

<u>Age Definitions</u>
Children 1 – 18 years of age. (Infants < 1 year and Term Newborns – refer to separate checklist.)

<u>Overarching Principles</u>
**The legal time of death is marked by the first determination of death**. Existing law states that for the purposes of post-mortem donation, the fact of death shall be determined by two physicians. The first and second physician's determinations may be performed concurrently. If performed at different points in time, a full clinical examination including the apnea test must be performed, without any fixed examination interval, regardless of the primary etiology.

<u>Physicians Declaring Neurological Death</u>
Minimum level of physician qualifications to perform NDD is full and current licensure for independent medical practice in the relevant Canadian jurisdiction. This excludes physicians who are only on an educational register. The authority to perform NDD cannot be delegated. Physicians should have skill and knowledge in both the management of patients with severe brain injury and in determination of neurological death in the relevant age groups. For the purposes of post mortem donation, a physician who has had any association with the proposed transplant recipient that might influence the physician's judgment shall not take part in the declaration of death.

<u>Minimum Clinical Criteria</u>
**Established Etiology:** Absence of clinical neurological function with a known, proximate cause that is irreversible. There must be definite clinical and/or neuroimaging evidence of an acute central nervous system (CNS) event that is consistent with the irreversible loss of neurological function. NDD may occur as a consequence of intracranial hypertension and/or primary direct brainstem injury.

**Deep Unresponsive Coma:** A lack of spontaneous movements and absence of movement originating in the CNS such as: cranial nerve function, CNS mediated motor response to pain in any distribution, seizures, decorticate and decerebrate responses. **Spinal reflexes**, or motor responses confined to spinal distribution, may persist.

**Confounding Factors:**

1. Unresuscitated shock

2. Hypothermia (core temperature <34 degrees Celsius, by central blood, rectal or esophageal/gastric measurements)

3. Severe metabolic disorders capable of causing a potentially reversible coma. If the primary etiology does not fully explain the clinical picture, and if in the treating physician's judgment the metabolic abnormality may play a role, it should be corrected or an ancillary test should be performed.

4. Peripheral nerve or muscle dysfunction or neuromuscular blockade potentially accounting for unresponsiveness, or

5. Clinically significant drug intoxications (e.g. alcohol, barbiturates, sedatives); therapeutic levels and/or therapeutic dosing of anticonvulsants, sedatives and analgesics do not preclude the diagnosis.

    **Specific to Cardiac Arrest:** Neurological assessments may be unreliable in the acute post-resuscitation phase after cardiorespiratory arrest. In cases of acute hypoxic-ischemic brain injury, clinical evaluation for NDD should be delayed for 24 hours or an ancillary test could be performed.

    Examiners are cautioned to review confounding issues in the context of the primary etiology and examination. **Clinical judgment is the deciding factor.**

**Apnea Test:**
Optimal performance requires a period of preoxygenation followed by 100% $O_2$ delivered via the trachea upon disconnection from mechanical ventilation. The certifying physician must continuously observe the patient for respiratory effort. **Thresholds at completion of the apnea test: $PaCO_2$ ≥ 60 mmHg and ≥ 20 mmHg above the pre-apnea test level and pH ≤ 7.28 as determined by arterial blood gases.** Caution must be exercised in considering the validity in cases of chronic respiratory insufficiency or dependence on hypoxic respiratory drive.

<u>Ancillary Tests</u>
Demonstration of the global absence of intracranial blood flow is considered the standard for determination of death by ancillary testing. The following prerequisite conditions must be met prior to ancillary testing: i) established etiology, ii) deep unresponsive coma, iii) absence of unresuscitated shock and hypothermia. Currently validated techniques are 4-vessel cerebral angiogram or radionuclide cerebral blood flow imaging. EEG is no longer recommended. NDD can be confirmed by ancillary testing when minimum clinical criteria cannot be completed or confounding factors cannot be corrected.

*Severe Brain Death to Neurological Determination of Death: A Canadian Forum*

Checklist for Neurological Determination of Death (NDD) –
Infants age < 1year, Term Newborns > 36 weeks gestation

---

### Section One: Minimum Clinical Criteria

a.  Deep unresponsive coma with the following established etiology: _____

b.  Confounding factors precluding the diagnosis?                                                      Yes☐   No ☐

c.  Temperature (core) _____

d.  Brainstem Reflexes:

| | | |
|---|---|---|
| Bilateral absence of motor responses: (excluding spinal reflexes) | Yes☐   No ☐ | |
| Absent cough: | Yes☐   No ☐ | |
| Absent gag: | Yes☐   No ☐ | |
| Absent suck (newborns only): | Yes☐   No ☐   Not applicable ☐ | |
| Bilateral absence of corneal responses: | Yes☐   No ☐ | |
| Bilateral absence of vestibulo-ocular responses: | Yes☐   No ☐ | |
| Bilateral absence of oculo-cephalic responses: | Yes☐   No ☐ | |
| Bilateral absence of pupillary response to light: (pupils ≥ mid size) | Yes☐   No ☐ | |
| Apnea: | Yes☐   No ☐ | |

   At completion of apnea test: pH_____  PaCO$_2$ _____mmHg

   PaCO$_2$ ≥ 20 mmHg above the pre-apnea test level                          Yes☐   No ☐

### Section Two: Ancillary Tests

Ancillary tests, as defined by the absence of intracranial blood flow, should be performed when *any* of the minimum clinical criteria cannot be completed, **or** unresolved confounding factors exist.

Ancillary testing has been performed:                                                      Yes☐   No ☐
Date: _____ Time: _____

Absence of intracranial blood flow has been demonstrated by:

   Cerebral Radiocontrast Angiography        ☐
   Radionuclide Angiography                        ☐
   Other _____

### Section Three: Examination Interval, Declaration and Documentation

The first and second physician's determinations (a full clinical examination including the apnea test) should be performed at different points in time. For infants, there is no fixed examination interval. For newborns, the first exam should be delayed until 48 hours after birth and the interval between examinations should be ≥ 24 hours.

**This patient fulfills the criteria for neurological determination of death:**

| Physician | Print name: _____ | Signature: _____ |
|---|---|---|
| | Date: _____ | Time: _____ |

### Section Four: Standard End-of-Life Care

Is this patient medically eligible for organ and/or tissue donation?                Yes☐   No ☐
Has the option for organ and/or tissue donation been offered?                       Yes☐   No ☐
Has consent been obtained for donation?                                                    Yes☐   No ☐

*Severe Brain Injury to Neurological Determination of Death:  A Canadian Forum*

<u>Checklist for Neurological Determination of Death–Infants < 1 Year, Term Newborns > 36 Weeks Gestation</u>

### Age Definitions
Infants: ≥ 30 days, < 1 year (corrected for gestational age);
Term Newborns: >36 weeks gestation, age < 30 days (corrected for gestational age).

### Overarching Principles
**The legal time of death is marked by the first determination of death.**
Existing law states that for the purposes of post-mortem donation, the fact of death shall be determined by two physicians. For these age groups, the first and second physician's determinations, as defined by a full clinical examination including the apnea test, must be performed at two different points in time. For infants, there is no fixed interval regardless of the primary etiology. For term newborns, the first examination should be delayed 48 hours after birth and the interval should be ≥ 24 hours, regardless of primary etiology.

### Physicians Declaring Neurological Death
Minimum level of physician qualifications to perform NDD is full and current licensure for independent medical practice in the relevant Canadian jurisdiction. This excludes physicians who are only on an educational register. The authority to perform NDD cannot be delegated. Physicians should have skill and knowledge in both the management of patients with severe brain injury and in determination of neurological death in the relevant age groups. For the purposes of post-mortem donation, a physician who has had any association with the proposed transplant recipient that might influence the physician's judgment shall not take part in the declaration of death.

### Minimum Clinical Criteria
**Established Etiology:** Absence of clinical neurological function with a known, proximate cause that is irreversible. There must be definite clinical and/or neuroimaging evidence of an acute central nervous system (CNS) event that is consistent with the irreversible loss of neurological function. NDD may occur as a consequence of intracranial hypertension and/or primary direct brainstem injury.

**Deep Unresponsive Coma:** a lack of spontaneous movements and absence of movement originating in the CNS such as: cranial nerve function, CNS mediated motor response to pain in any distribution, seizures, decorticate and decerebrate responses. **Spinal reflexes**, or motor responses confined to spinal distribution, may persist.

#### Confounding Factors:
1. Unresuscitated shock

2. Hypothermia (core temperature <34 degrees Celsius for infants and < 36 degrees Celsius for newborns, by central blood, rectal, or esophageal/gastric measurements)

3. Severe metabolic disorders capable of causing a potentially reversible coma. If the primary etiology does not fully explain the clinical picture, and if in the treating physician's judgment the metabolic abnormality may play a role, it should be corrected or an ancillary test should be performed.

4. Peripheral nerve or muscle dysfunction or neuromuscular blockade potentially accounting for unresponsiveness, or

5. Clinically significant drug intoxications (e.g. alcohol, barbiturates, sedatives); therapeutic levels and/or therapeutic dosing of anticonvulsants, sedatives and analgesics do not preclude the diagnosis.

   **Specific to Cardiac Arrest:** Neurological assessments may be unreliable in the acute post-resuscitation phase after cardiorespiratory arrest. In cases of acute hypoxic-ischemic brain injury, clinical evaluation for NDD should be delayed for 24 hours or an ancillary test could be performed.

   Examiners are cautioned to review confounding issues in the context of the primary etiology and examination. **Clinical judgment is the deciding factor.**

### Apnea Test:
Optimal performance requires a period of preoxygenation followed by 100% $O_2$ delivered via the trachea upon disconnection from mechanical ventilation. The certifying physician must continuously observe the patient for respiratory effort. **Thresholds at completion of the apnea test: $PaCO_2 \geq$ 60 mmHg and $\geq$ 20 mmHg above the pre-apnea test level and pH $\leq$ 7.28 as determined by arterial blood gases.** Caution must be exercised in considering the validity in cases of chronic respiratory insufficiency or dependence on hypoxic respiratory drive.

### Ancillary Tests
Demonstration of the global absence of intracranial blood flow is considered the standard for determination of death by ancillary testing. The following prerequisite conditions must be met prior to ancillary testing: i) established etiology, ii) deep, unresponsive coma, iii) absence of unresuscitated shock and hypothermia. Currently validated techniques are 4-vessel cerebral angiogram or radionuclide cerebral blood flow imaging. EEG is no longer recommended. NDD can be confirmed by ancillary testing when minimum clinical criteria cannot be completed or confounding factors cannot be corrected.

*Severe Brain Injury to Neurological Determination of Death: A Canadian Forum*

# B. Withdrawal of Life-Sustaining Therapy

David Munson

Haresh Kirpalani

## Key Principles

- Convey empathy.
- Speak directly.
- Focus on compassion.
- Wait quietly.
- Review the goals.
- Guide parents through the process.
- Address spirituality.

## Introduction

Although this chapter largely deals with end-of-life care and withdrawal of life-sustaining therapy, the approach and principles are generalizable to any critically ill patient. Shared decision making and effective communication form the basis for family center care in the PICU. Supporting families is a duty shared by all team members in the PICU, including physicians, nurses, allied health staff, social workers, child life specialists, and spiritual counselors.

End-of-life decisions that may be made:

- Active withdrawal of full intensive care—this is usually read to mean withdrawal of artificial ventilation
- Non-escalation of therapy
- Decision not to re-institute intensive care if it is needed

Situations in which withdrawal of therapy may be considered:

- Brain death (See Chapter 21A.)
- Irreversible organ failure with no immediate possibility of organ transplantation
- Failed organ transplants
- No further medical hope in severe illnesses

- Decisions in which clear parental and/or child preference on grounds of quality of life have been made
- Repeated intensive care—the so-called "frequent flyer" with chronic disabling conditions

## Talking to Parents

In situations involving end-of-life care, parents are under tremendous burdens to do the best by their child, themselves, and their families. Parents experience a range of emotions: from anger to depression and from guilt to anxiety. At the same time, staff are put under extraordinary strain. Misunderstandings are frequent, and can result in distrust between parents and staff. Empirical work shows that parents vividly recall these discussions and times. At best, these memories can be of an honest and empowering situation where they helped their child through a period of suffering. At worst, these memories can be of a period where their voice was not heard. Some empiric knowledge of what happens in this setting is helpful.

In interviews with parents after the death of their child in these circumstances, Meert found that those expressing dissatisfaction of their care as "poor" were those who had had little time to prepare for this eventuality (suddenness of illness) and those who felt uninformed, and had little contact with the staff after the demise of the child in the recovery phase. In a time of crisis, honest, clear, and compassionate communication is the most important aspect of the caregiver/parent interaction. Appreciating parents' expectations and fears is the first step. Parental understanding of the complexities of a diagnosis or condition can decrease the anxiety associated with the unknown. Not only is it important to allow parents to tell their story, but it is also important that we listen.

### Shared Decision Making

Most parents wish to be involved in decision making around the end-of-life care, as expressed around care to their newborn. However, not all parents want the "responsibility" of having to "make the final decision." Physicians' and nurses' perceptions of parental involvement in decision making are often inaccurate, as is their ability to predict which patients wish to cede decision making. Parents rely more on physicians than friends and family to guide them in decision making. Finally, the style of delivery and how choices are described may unduly influence parent decisions. These following factors were found by Sharman to be important deciding factors for making decisions for their child: "their personal observations of their child's suffering, their perceptions of their child's will to survive, their need to protect and advocate for their child, and the family's financial resources and concerns regarding life-long care."

## Listening for "Sentinel" Key Phrases

Ensuring that parents are comfortable during emotionally laden discussions involves both the atmosphere of the discussion as well as the receptiveness of the caregiver. Parents may need to hear information more than once in clear simple language. Share information in a timely manner. The moment, content, and style of delivery affect understanding and acceptance. Truth-telling and professionalism should guide interactions but be tempered with a measure of compassion. Parents appreciate honest information on what is happening when problems arise, with clear prognoses and predictions of outcome, even when poor. However, they also wish to hold on to some hope, and one should avoid the temptation to argue with a family directly about their hope for recovery. Simply acknowledging their hope, and then directly addressing the concerns at hand can allow the conversation to progress without conflict. Balancing the "right amount of hope" continues to be a challenge for caregivers. Parents also require time to come to terms with the diagnosis and prognosis.

Be vigilant for both verbal and non-verbal expressions from the parents. The mother commenting below was indicating a point at which she could take little more: "There's been two episodes to where it took me over 4 minutes to resuscitate him, and the time before he came in the hospital, it took 10 minutes. He felt like rigor mortis. He felt really cold, and I thought that I was going to lose him, I really did. I cannot explain how I feel inside. It's hard to deal with the situation of watching your own child stop breathing on you, and you have to be the one to perform CPR. It wasn't so much what they told me. It was just what I'm going through with him myself."

Some Shortcuts to Effective Communication in These Settings:

A Communication Toolbox

- Convey empathy. Use "I wish things were different" instead of "I am sorry." Be open to a real connection with the family.
- Speak directly. Do not use euphemisms. Ask about a family's hopes and fears.
- Focus on compassion. The fundamental question is how best to love this patient.
- Wait quietly. Use the power of silence to convey empathy, reinforce your presence, and allow time for processing.
- Review the goals. Sometimes the two goals of medicine come into conflict, adding time versus adding quality. Be clear which medical interventions are consistent with stated goals.
- Guide parents through the process. Explore with them how they might participate in the care of their child. What will help them create meaning and memories?
- Address spirituality. Most families rely on spirituality for coping to some degree. Offer to assist in providing resources and support spiritual practices.

## The Process of Withdrawal

Although parents may feel frightened, those who stay over this period express gratitude, while those who do not express later regret. There are, however, some families who will choose not to be present, sometimes for cultural reasons, and their choice should be supported. Guiding parents through the process is important to do, whether this is by medical, nursing, clergy, or others. The time around removing ventilator support is profoundly personal and intimate. Every family has a different path toward grieving. Clinicians need to explore with the family the options they have to participate in the care of their child or baby and the opportunities for creating memories. The severity of illness may have prevented the parents from having the opportunity to hold their child. They may wish to hold her/him while still on the ventilator, before death. The parents may desire to climb into the bed for some final time of holding their child. A family may wish to give their infant a bath and dress him or her in baby clothes for the first time. In general, any opportunity to facilitate the parents being just that—parents—without having to focus on the monitors, tubes, and machines interfering should be made available. Help families understand what options they have to participate in the care of their child. Families need to be prepared for what they will see and hear. They need to know about color changes, gasping breaths, and the unpredictability of the time to death from the time of withdrawal of technological support.

*Table I*
## Selecting Medications

Goal: In general, when withdrawing mechanical ventilation, ensuring comfort requires sedation in addition to pain relief. The rule of double effect and recent clinical trials support our moral obligation to treat suffering at the end of life.

Narcotics:
- Morphine is the most commonly used analgesic. Dosing is 0.1–0.2 mg/kg for an opiate-naive patient, but should be titrated to effect with no real maximum.
- Hydromorphone is a semisynthetic narcotic that may be useful in older patients who have a morphine allergy.
- Fentanyl has a shorter half life, making it less ideal for use during end-of-life care.
- Meperidine should be avoided because of its centrally active metabolite.

Benzodiazepines:
- Midazolam is a short-acting sedative that can be effective in achieving sedation. Usual dosing is 0.1–0.2 mg/kg, but also should be titrated to effect. If multiple doses are expected, strongly consider starting an infusion.
- Lorazepam has a longer half life, but should not be used in neonates.

For patients who are difficult to sedate, plan ahead.
- Propofol has anesthetic and sedative properties and can be titrated to a specific level of sedation.
- Pentobarbital can also be effective in patients who are already resistant to benzodiazepines.

## Pain Control

The child should not experience pain or discomfort at the end of life. Medications to achieve adequate pain relief or sedation are appropriate. Narcotics, such as morphine, fentanyl, or hydromorphone, have good pain-relieving properties but often are not adequate on their own to deal with the symptoms of air hunger and respiratory distress. The goal should be to achieve moderate to deep sedation in the patient from whom mechanical ventilation is going to be withdrawn. Respiratory depression is a known side effect of narcotics and sedatives, but this is the cost of relief of pain. However, the medical team crosses into difficult ethical and legal territory if they choose such large doses of a medication that it is clear that their intent is to suppress respiratory drive and commit euthanasia.

## Withdrawing the Ventilator

There are two approaches: Firstly, "terminal extubation" describes removing the endotracheal tube without weaning ventilatory support. The advantage of extubation without adjustment in the ventilator rests mainly with the avoidance of prolonging the death. There may also be situations in which once a family has made a decision, delaying extubation only serves to heighten anxiety and anticipation in the family. The second approach is "terminal weaning," where the clinician gradually decreases ventilator support before extubating. In most cases, some combination of the two approaches is most appropriate.

Gradually weaning ventilator support has several advantages:

- Weaning the oxygen, pressures, and rate should provoke some signs of respiratory distress in the patient. This signal gives the clinician the opportunity to ensure that pharmacologic sedation is adequate.
- Second, while taking the time to titrate the medications as the ventilator support is decreased, the subsequent hypoxemia and hypercarbia may contribute to the level of sedation.

The clinicians should be meticulous in avoiding the concept that they are weaning the ventilator. The clinical use of the term weaning is fairly specific for improving status. When describing the plans to the family, simply explain that the amount of support given by the ventilator will be decreased so that the sedation can be titrated. There are also circumstances in which the mode of ventilation might be changed to facilitate time with the patient before withdrawal.

In the NICU especially it may be difficult or impossible to hold an infant while the baby is on the oscillator. Changing the baby to a conventional mode of ventilation may facilitate time holding the baby before he or she is extubated. Decreasing ventilatory support is best done over a short period of time in an effort to evaluate and adjust the level of sedation. Adequate time may be provided to titrate medications to treat symptoms without prolonging the dying process. Once it is ensured that adequate sedation has been achieved, extubation can be performed with minimal risk for increasing the patient's suffering.

## Steps to Consider When Withdrawing Care

- Obtain at least one independent second medical opinion; as best as possible, lay to rest any fundamental medical "uncertainties" that might make this step either controversial or difficult for the parents to thereafter live with.
- Ensure prior "directives" are not in conflict with decision if present.
- Ensure a full discussion with the family or guardians.
- Ensure as clear an understanding of the situation from the family's viewpoint as is possible. Have all relevant family or friends and relations been appraised?
- If raised by the family, consider potential for organ or tissue donation. (See "Organ and Tissue Donation" in Chapter 21.) Are there medical contraindications? (eg, Has there been significant hypoxia? Hypotension? etc?)
- Ensure a full and clear understanding among the medical, nursing, social work, physiotherapy, child care workers, and so on as to the reasons for embarking upon a withdrawal of technology.
- Ensure that adequate time has passed to allow a sense of "ease" that at least all that could be done has been done, and to ensure that there is no inconsistency between parents and caregivers.
- Ensure a clear documentation of all the relevant discussions and joint conclusions.
- Remember that decisions should be made on the basis of the child's best interest.

## Practical Matters to Discuss

When the substantive decision is made to withdraw care, ensure that the practical matters are clearly, simply, and compassionately reviewed:

- Who is going to be present? Parents-partners may behave quite differently. Do not force a situation on them, and respect their decision.
- Are other members of the family important to wait for? How will they be contacted?
- Discuss whether siblings should be involved and talk them through the pros and cons. (Pros: a memory; a clear sense of involvement; less "mystery." Cons: fear, child too young to understand and thus pros diminished, etc.)
- Who will remove care-giving apparatus? Surprisingly, some parents feel they wish to do so.
- Discuss how long it might take. Agonal breathing may occur, even despite formal brain death criteria having been met.
- Are any other cultural-religious matters required to be considered, such as involvement of clergy, or baptism?
- Will there be a postmortem?

## References

Williams C, Munson D, Zupancic J, Kirpalani H. Supporting bereaved parents: practical steps in providing compassionate perinatal and neonatal end-of-life care—A North American perspective. Semin Fetal Neonatal Med 2008 Oct;13(5):335–40.

Meert KL, Thurston CS, Sarnaik AP. End-of-life decision-making and satisfaction with care: parental perspectives. Pediatr Crit Care Med 2000;1:179–85.

Kavanaugh K, Savage T, Kilpatrick S, et al. Life support decisions for extremely premature infants: report of a pilot study. J Pediatr Nurs 2005;20(5):347–59.

Abe N, Catlin A, Mihara D. End of life in the NICU a study of ventilator withdrawal. MCN Am J Matern Child Nurs 2001;26(3):141–6.

Sharman M, Meert KL, Sarnaik AP. What influences parents' decisions to limit or withdraw life support? Pediatr Crit Care Med 2005 Sep;6(5):513–8.

Munson D. Withdrawal of mechanical ventilation in pediatric and neonatal intensive care units. Pediatr Clin North Am 2007;54(5):773–85.

Munson D, Leuthner SR. Palliative care for the family carrying a fetus with a life-limiting diagnosis. Pediatr Clin North Am 2007;54:787–98.

# C. Organ and Tissue Donation

Trisha Murthy
Nancy Hemrica
Lennox Huang

## Key Principles

- Disclosing death and discussing organ donation should be decoupled and ideally handled by separate health care professionals.
- Ideally, discussions with potential donor families should be handled by a professional trained in the organ procurement process.
- Discussions with the family must be empathetic and should not pressure the family toward a decision.
- The organ procurement/transplantation team must be separate from the critical care team caring for the patient.
- After declaration of neurologic death, the potential donor requires continued close management of physiologic variables to optimize organ perfusion.

## Organ Donation in the PICU

Consideration of organ donation and transplantation in the PICU is often a logical extension of caring for critically ill patients. Organ donation may be a controversial and/or emotionally laden topic for health care professionals and families. This chapter outlines some principles for considering organ donation, approaches for families, and care of the potential organ donor after declaration of neurologic death. For details around declaration of brain death, see Chapter 21A.

## Potential Patients

Any critically ill patient with the potential for progression to neurologic death should be considered for organ donation. These patients include but are not limited to the following:

- severe traumatic head injury
- spontaneous intracranial hemorrhage
- primary brain tumor
- metabolic disorders
- cerebral anoxia

## Donation after Cardiopulmonary Death

The discrepancy between organ supply and demand has led to increased interest in donation after cardiopulmonary death (DCD). The United Network for Organ Sharing (UNOS) database reported 683 organs retrieved from patients under 18 years of age via donation after cardiac death between 1993 and 2005. Although many pediatric hospitals are now implementing protocols for DCD, this is still a controversial area with little published pediatric experience.

## Requesting Donation and Notification of Organ Procurement Organizations

Many countries and jurisdictions have enacted routine notification legislation requiring the health care team to notify the local organ procurement organization (OPO) of candidates for organ or tissue donation. Well-established and well-resourced OPOs can aid in the organ donation process by supporting the health care team and/or directly participating in the donation discussions with the family. Decoupling the declaration of death and the discussion for organ donation allows for better family support and increased rates of organ donation.

## Approaching Families for Organ Donation: A Value-Based Approach

Rests on three premises:

- Most people, if given the opportunity to help someone or to save a life, will do so.
- The primary goal of donation is to improve the lives of others through transplantation.
- Organ donation is the right thing to do.

# Critical Components of Family Approach and Donation Discussion

1. Assessment of the staff, family, and situation

- Gather as much knowledge as possible about the patient and the family. Any unique dynamics or concerns should be addressed first.
- This information will help to formulate a communication plan that will ensure the family is approached in a timely and sensitive manner that is specific to their individual needs.
- There should be a detailed discussion of what the family has been told about brain death.

  - Has the patient been pronounced neurologically dead?
  - If so, what was the time?
  - Is the family aware, and do they fully understand what this means?
  - Ask the family to verbalize their understanding of brain death.

2. Establishment of a plan with all the members of the health care team

- Ensure that the donation discussion occurs at a separate time from the brain death discussion. "I understand this has been difficult news for you to hear. I would like to give you a moment to gather your thoughts and be together. I will come back and see you in a few moments and another member of our team will discuss with you some of the decisions that you will need to make."
- This allows for the introduction of the OPO or end-of-life specialist.
- Best practice evidence supports a collaborative and team approach in supporting and informing families.

3. Expression of condolences and acknowledgement of the loss

- Families will respond to and long remember genuinely conveyed empathy, an acknowledgement of the death and the loss the family has suffered.
- The person speaking with the family must have knowledge of the situation and what the family has suffered. You will not be accepted as part of the team if you don't know the situation.
- Seek first to understand, allow the family to set the pace, and ensure that they are supported throughout.

- Allow families to remember and talk about their loved one. This may be the time you help them to start thinking about the "legacy" they are leaving.
- Encourage families to talk about their loved one; this is part of the acceptance and healing process for the family. They are allowing you to be in a very personal and privileged place in their life.

4. The donation discussion:

- Begin this discussion **only** when it is determined that the family has full understanding of brain death and that they feel comfortable with the team that is sharing the information with them.
- Could use a segue like this: "Mr. and Mrs. Smith, because of the type of injury that Jim had, you and Jim have the unique and rare opportunity to save the lives of others through organ donation. I am going to explain to you what this means to those needing a life-saving transplant and what the process is."
- Whenever feasible, a person skilled in explaining donation options should lead the discussion once it has been initiated.
- Ensure that discussion occurs in a private location, away from the bedside if possible.
- Advise the family of time required to accomplish donation.
- Ensure that the family is aware of testing and procedures necessary to confirm suitability of organs/tissues.
- Allow family to request special religious or culture practices if of value to them.
- Advise the family on the impact on funeral arrangements.

5. Consent

Legal guidelines for consent for organ donation vary between jurisdictions. In Ontario, Canada, the legal age of consent for the purposes for donation is 16. The consent hierarchy according to the Trillium Gift of Life Act 2000 is in descending order of importance:

- Spouse or same sex partner
- Person's children
- Person's parents
- Person's siblings
- Any other next of kin
- Person in lawful possession of body

# Management of the Potential Organ Donor after Brain Death

## Background

- Following brain death, clinical management optimizes successful organ donation.
- Specific therapies are required to minimize the pathophysiologic changes in the brain dead donor.
- Overall goal is to increase the number of individual donors, organs transplanted per donor, graft function and survival, and recipient survival.

## Hypertension secondary to ICP

Pathophysiology:

- Increased ICP results in cerebral herniation and brainstem ischemia.
- Ischemia of the medulla oblongata results in a loss of vagal tone and unopposed sympathetic stimulation (lasts minutes to hours).
- Hypertension and severe vasoconstriction results in impaired end organ perfusion.
- Increased cardiac demand secondary to tachycardia and increased systemic vascular resistance results in myocardial ischemia.

Evidence:

- Animal studies support that sympathetic blockade prevents impaired end-organ perfusion and myocardial ischemia; however, this may only be effective if given prophylactically prior to the onset of unopposed sympathetic stimulation.

Indication:

- Treat arterial hypertension when blood pressure exceeds age-related norms:

- Newborns–3 months >90/60
- >3 months–1 year >110/70
- >1 year–12 years >130/80
- >12 years–18 years >140/90

Management:

1. Wean inotropes and vasopressors.
2. If hypertension persists, can start one of the following agents:
   – nitroprusside 0.5–5.0 μg/kg/min
   – esmolol 100–500 μg/kg bolus followed by 100–300 μg/kg/min
3. Obtain Serum lactate
4. Attempt to maintain central $MVO_2$ ≥60%

# Cardiovascular Management

Pathophysiology:

- Ischemia progresses to spinal sympathetic pathways resulting in decreases in heart rate, myocardial demand, and systemic vascular resistance.
- Cardiac output may increase, resulting in high output failure, decreased perfusion pressure, and further myocardial damage.
- Cardiovascular collapse eventually occurs if no intervention is initiated.

## A. Biochemical Perfusion Markers

Evidence:

- Adult studies of septic shock support that titrating therapy to central venous pressure central venous $O_2$ saturation, and blood pressure reduces morbidity and mortality.
- Pediatric studies of sepsis and pediatric cardiac surgery found lactate to be the best marker of perfusion to predict survivors and adverse events, respectively.

Recommendation:

- Monitor systemic perfusion by using mixed venous oxygen saturation, serum lactate, base deficit, and pH.
  - Rising serum lactate should prompt investigations into etiology.
- Central venous oximetry is commonly used in critically ill patients and is recommended for the pediatric donor for monitoring.
  - Adjust therapy to maintain central venous saturation ≥60%.

## B. Echocardiography

Evidence:

- Patients with brain death frequently have myocardial dysfunction, which is a risk factor for 30-day mortality in heart transplant recipients.
- Echocardiography with dobutamine stress may distinguish reversible myocardial dysfunction.
- The utility of serial echocardiography to assess myocardial dysfunction or predict graft survival has not been established.

Recommendation:

- 2D echocardiography to determine cardiac function for transplantation
- Serial echocardiography to re-evaluate myocardial function for transplantation and as a potential tool for hemodynamic therapy

## C. Pulmonary Arterial Catheterization

- Generally not used in PICU care
- Not routinely recommended but may be used to have a direct measure of cardiac function.

## Pharmacologic hemodynamic support

Pathophysiology:

- Hypotension results from volume depletion (secondary to fluid restriction, diuretics, third space losses, hemorrhage, and diabetes insipidus) and low systemic vascular resistance.

Evidence:

- In a Canadian study of pediatric donors, over 50% of donors had persistent hypotension and a third suffered cardiac arrest. Hypotension and cardiac arrest were more common in donors with low CVP and without antidiuretic hormone replacement.

- The theoretical risk that central and peripheral vasoconstriction with alpha-agonists could compromise transplantable organs has not been supported in studies with septic patients.

- Brain death and hypotension has been linked to vasopressin deficiency.
  - Arginine vasopressin (AVP) given to pediatric donors resulted in increased mean arterial pressures (MAP) and allowed for weaning of pressors.

Management:

- replace intravascular volume with crystalloid as necessary
- 1st line

  - Arginine vasopressin (AVP) 0.0003–0.0007 U/kg/min (0.3–0.7 mU/kg/min) to a maximum dose of 2.4 U/hour

- 2nd line

  - Norepinephrine, epinephrine, and phenylephrine titrated to clinical and biochemical effect (caution with doses >0.2 µg/kg/min)
  - Dopamine ≤10 µg/kg/min

## Glycemia and Nutrition

Pathophysiology:

- Hyperglycemia commonly occurs in brain dead donors

  - Result of insulin resistance, corticosteroid treatment and IV dextrose administration
  - Not reflective of pancreatic beta cell dysfunction and should not affect consideration of pancreatic islet cell transplantation
    - If indicated, clarify with HbA1C

Evidence:

- Glucose >11 mmol/L was observed in 60% of donors in one study.
- Glycemic control has not been studied with respect to improving graft survival.
- Glycemic control has been shown to improve survival with respect to septic deaths in critically ill patients.
- In children and adults with severe head injury, hyperglycemia is an independent risk factor for poor outcome.
- Animal studies support improved liver graft survival from enterally fed vs fasting donors.
- One human study exists which failed to demonstrate an effect of nutritional status on liver graft function.

Recommendation:

1. Continue intravenous (IV) dextrose infusions.
2. Start or maintain enteral feeding as tolerated.
3. Maintain parenteral nutrition if already initiated.
4. May start insulin infusion to maintain serum glucose 4–8 mmol/L.

# Diabetes Insipidus and Hypernatremia

Rationale:

- Posterior pituitary dysfunction is common in brain death secondary to compromised blood supply.
- Up to 75% of brain dead donors have undetectable antidiuretic hormone (ADH) levels and 87% had diabetes insipidus (DI).
- Hypernatremia is seen as a result of hyperosmolar therapy and poorly controlled diabetes insipidus.
- Donor hypernatremia >155 mmol/L is linked to hepatic dysfunction or graft loss after transplantation.

Evidence:

- Desmopressin (DDAVP®) has:

  - No adverse effect on early or late graft function after renal transplant.
  - Duration of action is 6–20 hours, so avoid giving close to organ procurement.

- AVP
  - Case series of pediatric and adult traumatic brain injuries demonstrated successful treatment of hypothalamic diabetes insipidus.
  - Concern of coronary, renal, and splanchnic vasoconstriction with high doses.
  - One study demonstrated poor function of transplanted kidneys in donors treated with AVP.
  - Cardiovascular and biochemical endpoints have demonstrated the safety of using DDAVP (antidiuretic effect) and AVP (vasopressor effect) concurrently.

- Hypernatremia

  - Correcting donor sodium (Na) to ≤155 mmol/L is associated with graft success equivalent to normonatremic donors.

Indications:

Diabetes insipidus is defined as:

1. Urine output >4 mL/kg/h accompanied by:

    a. Increasing serum Na ≥145 mmol/L
    b. Increasing serum osmolarity ≥300 mosM
    c. Dropping urine osmolarity ≤200 mosM

Recommendations:

1. Treat with continuous IV vasopressin infusion or intermittent IV DDAVP®

    a. Vasopressin in the following situations:

        i. Hemodynamic support needed.
        ii. Combination hormonal therapy started.

    b. DDAVP® can be used to supplement vasopressin.
    c. DDAVP® does not have to be discontinued prior to the operating room.

2. Treat serum Na >150 mmol/L

Management:

1. Titrate to urine output ≤3 mL/kg/h

    a. IV vasopressin infusion 0.0003–0.0007 U/kg/min (0.3–0.7 mU/kg/min) to a maximum of 2.4 U/h
    and/or
    b. Intermittent DDAVP® 0.25 to 1 µg IV q6h

2. Serum Na ≥ 130 ≤ 150 mmol/L
3. Urine output target 0.5–3 mL/kg/h

## Hormone Therapy

Pathophysiology:

- Thyroid hormone

  - Conversion of $T_4$ to active $T_3$ is inhibited after brain death.
  - Thyroid hormone improves cardiac output by increasing heart rate and contractility and decreasing afterload.

- Corticosteroid replacement

  - 50% of brain dead donors have a relative deficiency of ACTH.

- Donor lungs are thought to develop inflammation post brain death.
- Studies have shown an improvement in lung procurement rates in donors treated with methylprednisolone.

Evidence:

- United Network for Organ Sharing (UNOS) study of 18,726 brain dead donors showed increases in kidney, liver, and heart use from donors receiving three-drug hormonal therapy (thyroid hormone, vasopressin, corticosteroids).

  - $T_4$ used in 93% and $T_3$ in 6.9%, but numbers were not sufficient to determine a benefit of $T_3$ over $T_4$

Indications:

1a. 2D echo with ejection fraction ≤40%, or
1b. Hemodynamic instability (includes fluid resistant shock requiring vasopressor support
2. Consider using in all donors
3. Methylprednisone indicated for lung protection in all potential donors

Recommendation:

1. Tetra-iodothyronine ($T_4$) 20 µg IV bolus 10 µg/hour IV infusion (or 50–100 µg IV bolus then 25–50 µg IV bolus q12h)
2. Vasopressin 0.0003–0.0007 U/kg/min (0.3–0.7 mU/kg/min) to a maximum of 2.4 U/h.
3. Methylprednisolone 15 mg/kg (≤1 gm) IV q24h

## Transfusion Thresholds

Evidence:

- A large randomized control trial of adult critical care patients (TRICC) demonstrated equivalent survival at restricted transfusion threshold <70 g/L vs liberal transfusion threshold of 100 g/L (adult). Similarly LaCroix showed equivalent outcomes in a multi-center trial of children in a PICU.

Recommendation:

1. The optimal hemoglobin (Hb) targets for unstable donors is ≥90–100 g/L and the lowest acceptable is ≥70 g/L.

2. There are no predefined targets for platelets, INR, and PTT; bleeding patients should be transfused if clinically necessary.

3. Testing for donor serology and tissue typing should occur prior to transfusions to minimize cross-contamination.

## Invasive Bacterial Infections

Rationale:

- 5% of all donors are bacteremic at the time of organ procurement.
- In a study of 124 bacteremic donors, prophylactic treatment of recipients with broad-spectrum antibiotics (vancomycin, ceftazadime/cefotaxime) prevented transmission of bacterial infection in all.
- No evidence exists for the use of prophylactic antibiotics in organ donors.

Recommendations:

1. Pan-cultures daily (blood, urine, ETT)
2. Empiric antimicrobials for presumed or proven infection. No minimum duration of therapy prior to organ procurement is identified at present

## **Suggested Readings**

Dual Advocacy: A value-positive approach to obtaining Consent for Organ Donation. *Gift of Life Institute.* Philadelphia, PA (workshop series)

Mazor R, Baden HP. Trends in pediatric organ donation after cardiac death. Pediatrics 2007 Oct;120(4):e960–6.

Organ and Tissue Donation Manual 2005, Trillium Gift of Life Network.

Pediatric organ donation and transplantation policy statement: Organizational principles to guide and define the child health care system and/or improve the health of all children. Committee on Hospital Care and Section on Surgery. American Academy of Pediatrics. Pediatrics 2002 May;109:(5):982–4.

Trillium Gift of Life Network Act 2000

Shemie SD, Baker AJ, Knoll G, et al. National recommendations for donation after cardiocirculatory death in Canada: donation after cardiocirculatory death in Canada. CMAJ. 2006 Oct 10;175(8):S1.

Shemie SD, Ross H, Pagliarello J, et al. Organ donor management in Canada: recommendations of the forum on medical management to optimize donor organ potential. CMAJ 2006 Mar 14;174(6):S13–32.

# Chapter 22

# Procedures

Michael J. Michenko
Lennox Huang
Mark Walton

## General Approach to Procedures in the PICU

Procedures in the PICU may be performed for monitoring, diagnosis, or therapeutic reasons. Many modern PICUs have the ability to function as a limited operating room for emergency procedures if the patient is too unstable to be transported to an OR. Specific operations are beyond the scope of this chapter; however, there are some general principles which apply to all procedures regardless of complexity or invasiveness.

## Standard and Additional Precautions

- Practices previously described as universal precautions
- Precautions to prevent spread of infectious disease via blood and other bodily fluids and to protect both health care providers and patients
- Regulated by law in Canada and the United States
- Standard precautions applies to all bodily fluids except sweat
- See Table 1 for general principles

*Table 1*
**General Principles for Standard Precautions**

- Personal protective equipment
  - Gloves, gowns, goggles, shoe covers
- Engineering controls
  - Sharps disposal boxes, safety needles, needleless injection systems
- Work practice controls
  - Hand washing, proper handling of fluids/wastes
- Depending on the level of suspicion, individual patients may require higher levels of protective equipment
- Airborne precautions—negative pressure room, N95 fitted mask for caregivers
- Contact precautions—nonsterile gown, gloves, mask for close contact

## Clean Technique

1. Water +/− soap for grossly contaminated surfaces/wounds
2. Or sterile saline for irrigation
3. Or isopropyl alcohol wash/swabs/wipes
4. Standard precautions
5. Examples of procedures performed with clean technique

   - Peripheral intravenous (IV) lines
   - Minor laceration repair
   - Line/drain removal
   - Wound dressings

## Sterile or Aseptic Technique

Most invasive procedures performed in the ICU should follow sterile technique.

1. Preparation of the operator(s)

   - Surgical cap + gown
   - Wash + scrub hands, wear sterile gown, sterile gloves

2. Preparation of the patient

   - Clean patient of any gross contaminants (bodily fluids, dirt, etc)
   - Prep patient with sterile scrub (eg, providone-iodine, 2% chlorhexidine)
   - Conventionally, 3 concentric circle scrubs starting from procedure site and moving outwards

3. Preparation of sterile fields/barriers

- Fields should be as large as possible
- Unsterile persons should not reach over a sterile area
- Sterile persons should not reach over an unsterile area
- Check sterile packages for integrity, color tape indicator, expiration date

# Sedation/Analgesia

1. Ideally, with more complex procedures a separate person should be controlling the monitoring and administration of sedation
2. Local analgesia can be provided with lidocaine infiltration, regional blocks or topical analgesics
3. Care to avoid direct injection into vein or artery
4. Max dose for lidocaine infiltration 4 mg/kg, 7mg/kg if mixed with epinephrine

# Consent

- Whenever possible, informed consent should be obtained for all procedures, no matter how minor they may appear.
- Informed consent consists of a discussion of risks, benefits, and alternatives to the proposed treatment.
- Assent should be given by the child whenever possible.
- The process of formal documentation of consent varies between individual institutions.
- In emergencies when parents cannot be contacted, consent is presumed if the intervention is in the patient's best interest.

# Central Venous Lines

General indications:

- CVP monitoring
- Frequent blood draws
- Cardiac output monitoring via $SVO_2$
- Medication administration
- Parenteral nutrition
- Poor peripheral access
- Transvenous cardiac pacing device
- Renal replacement therapy (special catheter required, see Chapter 13, "Nephrology")

General contraindications

- Bleeding diathesis (relative contraindication)
- Overlying skin infection

Equipment

- Sterile gloves and drapes
- Sterile gown + mask also recommended for prevention of infection
- Providone-iodine or chlorhexidine
- Central venous catheter kit, appropriate gauge and length need a guide to size + length
- 1% lidocaine without epinephrine
- Pressure monitor (optional)
- Saline routine heparinization of lines not recommended
- Sterile gauze

General complications

- Inability to obtain access
- Hemorrhage
- Local or systemic infection

# Seldinger Technique

The Seldinger technique is a procedure initially developed to secure vascular access. It is named after Sven-Ivar Seldinger (1921–1998), a Swedish radiologist who introduced the procedure in 1953. The Seldinger technique is now used for vascular access, placement of pleural, peritoneal, cardiac, and enteral drains and tubes.

- There are several steps to the Seldinger technique (Figure 1):
    - Venipuncture is performed with a introducer needle, or a needle with a short catheter. (1, 2 in following diagram)
    - A soft-tipped guide wire is passed through the needle/short catheter and the needle/short catheter is removed. (Steps 3, 4)
    - Puncture site may need to be enlarged with a small nick from an 11-blade scalpel for larger catheters or tubes.
    - Depending on the size of line required, a dilator may be passed over the guide wire. For chest tube insertions, sequentially larger dilators may be used. (step 5)
    - Dilator is removed and catheter is passed over wire and wire is removed. (step 6)

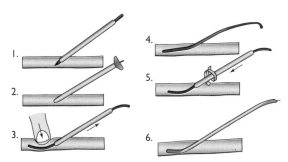

**Figure 1**    Seldinger technique.

To prevent embolization, the operator must always be able to visualize and or hold part of the wire at all times during the procedure.

Bedside ultrasound guidance may be used in several ways to aid in vessel catheterization:

1. General anatomy may be elucidated prior to venipuncture.
2. Continuous visualization of the vessel through the venipuncture and wire insertion process.
3. Confirmation of proper line placement within the vessel.

## Subclavian Catheterization using Seldinger Technique (Figure 2)

- Position patient supine in slight Trendelenburg (head down) position. May place a roll between scapulae. Identify insertion site. Prep, drape, and anesthetize the desired access site.
- The introducer needle is inserted at the junction of the medial and central thirds of the clavicle and "walked" down and under the clavicle, then aimed toward the sternal notch, parallel to chest wall and slowly advanced while aspirating back with the syringe. Free blood flow indicates vessel entry. (If bright red, pulsating blood return is encountered, withdraw and redirect the needle.)
- Remove the syringe and quickly place finger over hub to avoid air embolism. A free flow of blood confirms placement. The flexible guide wire is inserted through the needle and into the vein. Watch and listen to the ECG monitor as arrhythmias may occur if you advance the wire into the right atrium. Remove the needle over the guide wire, making sure the guide wire is securely held throughout removal of the needle.

  Optional: Enlarge the skin puncture site around the wire with an 11 scalpel blade to allow passage of the dilator and catheter.

- Slide the vein dilator onto the wire and advance it through the skin and into the vein. Be sure not to advance the guide wire. Remove vein dilator and slide the venous catheter over the wire and into the vein. Be sure to maintain guide wire in position.
- Remove guide wire, aspirate each lumen and attach saline filled hubs. Flush each lumen. Suture catheter into position or use alternative line-securing device and dress site with sterile gauze. Attach IV tubing.
- Obtain chest radiograph to check line placement and to rule out pneumothorax. Optimal placement of tip is at junction of SVC and RA; however, anywhere in SVC is adequate. Do not infuse if tip is in jugular vein, RA, or intracardiac.

Complications

1. Immediate
   - Pneumothorax
   - Hemothorax
   - Rarely air embolism, transient arrhythmias, cardiac tamponade

2. Delayed
   - Infection
   - Catheter tip embolus or thrombosis
   - Chylothorax
   - Cardiac perforation if tip left intracardiac

Right-sided subclavian catheterization is more difficult and associated with a higher risk of malpositioning.

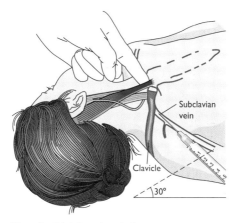

**Figure 2**   Subclavian catheterization.

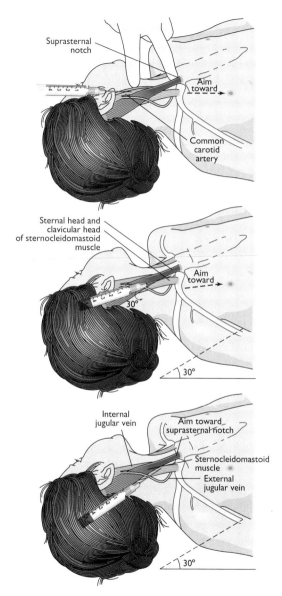

**Figure 3**    Internal jugular catheterization.

# Internal Jugular  (Figure 3)

- Position patient in mild Trendelenberg, head turned to opposite side of insertion.
- Insertion site is at apex of sternal and clavicular muscle bellies of the sternocleidomastoid.
- Aim needle at ipsilateral nipple, 30–45° angle to skin.
- Advance while aspirating.
- Place line with Seldinger technique (as in subclavian section).
- CXR for position, optimal is tip at junction of SVC and RA; however, anywhere in SVC is adequate.

Complications

1. Immediate
   - Carotid artery cannulation
   - Neck hematoma
   - Pneumothorax (lower risk than subclavian)

2. Delayed
   - Infection
   - Catheter tip embolus or thrombosis

# Femoral

- Position patient flat, with roll under hips, leg fully extended (not rotated or abducted at hip.) In infants, consider mild internal rotation at hip.
- Palpate femoral artery pulse just inferior (caudal) to inguinal ligament. Insertion site is inferior and medial to arterial pulsation (Figure 4).
- Aim needle towards umbilicus, at 15–30° angle to skin for infants, 45° angle to skin for larger children.
- Place line with Seldinger technique (as in subclavian section).
- X-ray to confirm placement unnecessary if flow is good and transduced pressure appropriate. If difficult insertion, and flow is poor, tip may be in ascending lumbar vein (line will be left of vertebra on A-P, when inserted in left groin will deviate posterior to vertebra on lateral X-ray.) Appropriate tip position on A-P is in IVC, right of vertebrae.

Complications

1. Immediate
   - Hematoma
   - Arterial cannulation and ischemic limb

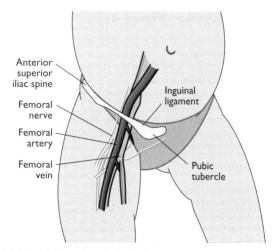

**Figure 4**   Femoral vascular landmarks.

2. Delayed
   - Infection
   - Catheter tip embolus or deep venous thrombosis

Femoral venous lines may have a slightly higher rate of thrombotic and infectious complications compared to subclavian and internal jugular lines. For all central lines, consider pressure measurement and blood gas analysis (as well as X-ray) to confirm placement in vein as opposed to artery, prior to initiating infusions.

Proper positioning is by far the most important step to ensure success and may require several assistants.

# Lumbar Puncture

Indications

- Investigation for CNS infection, metabolic disease
- Aid in diagnosis of subarachnoid hemorrhage
- Intrathecal medications
- Temporary alleviation of raised ICP
- Sampling of CSF for any other reason

Contraindications

- Abnormal focal neurologic exam without current neuroimaging
- Local infection at insertion site

- Elevated ICP (relative)
- Severe bleeding diathesis

Equipment

- Antiseptic solution
- Sterile gloves and drapes
- 1% lidocaine
- Appropriate sized LP needle with stylet
- Collecting vials × 4 for CSF
- Manometer with 3-way stopcock

Technique

In all cases, perform a careful neurologic exam to rule out a focal neurologic deficit.

In the standard positioning method, patient is placed on a firm surface in the lateral recumbent position, curled with knees drawn in towards the chest and lumbar and thoracic spine neck maximally flexed.

The lumbar region should be close to the edge of the bed, with the plane of the back and shoulders as perpendicular to the bed as possible. Patients who are stable from a cardiopulmonary perspective, may be positioned sitting, leaning over a pillow or table, with maximal lumbar and thoracic spine flexion. Proper positioning is by far the most important step to ensure success and may require several assistants (Figure 5).

The L4–L5 interspace is identified by drawing an imaginary line between the two posterior iliac crests. Using sterile technique, this area is cleaned, prepped, and draped.

Skin and deeper subcutaneous tissues are infiltrated with lidocaine.

The spinal needle with stylet is then passed into the L4–L5 interspace along the midline, bevel upward. Angle the needle slightly cephalad along an imaginary line between the site of entry and the umbilicus. As the needle is advanced, the stylet should be frequently withdrawn and replaced every 1–2 mm in order to identify the first drop of CSF (and avoid overpenetration).

Once CSF fluid is seen in the needle hub, the manometer is immediately attached to the needle via connecting tubing. Pressure measurement is normally done in the lateral recumbant position. Opening pressure should be measured promptly (do not wait more than 1 minute) with the patient's legs and hips extended. If the opening pressure is elevated (>180 mm CSF), try to eliminate factors that may cause false elevations.

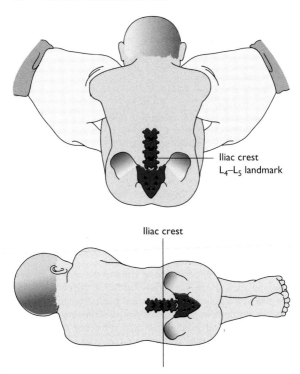

**Figure 5**   Lumbar puncture insertion sites.

Instruct patient to straighten his legs, breathe evenly, avoid Valsalva maneuvers, and relax his abdominal muscles. If the opening pressure remains markedly elevated, close the 3-way stopcock, collect only the CSF already in the manometer, disconnect all the tubing, reinsert stylet, and consider neurosurgical consultation.

If opening pressure is normal, CSF is then collected in tubes 1–4 in sequence. Manometer is reconnected afterward and a closing pressure recorded. Stylet is replaced and both needle and stylet removed together.

Patient should be instructed to lay flat for a few hours, to prevent post-LP (decompression) headache.

Complications
- Common complications:
  - Headache

- Serious complications are rare but include the following:
  - Cerebral herniation
  - Persistent CSF leak
  - Paralysis
  - Epidural hematoma
  - Subarachnoid epidural cyst

# Urinary Catheterization

An indwelling urinary catheter facilitates accurate and continuous determination of urine flow which is directly proportional to glomerular filtration rate and renal blood flow (thus tissue perfusion, also).

Indications

- Accurate measurement of urinary output
- Continuous core body temperature monitoring
- Neurogenic bladder, spinal cord injury
- Continuous or intermittent bladder irrigation
- Imaging of urinary tract
- Prevention of bladder rupture after mannitol administration

Contraindications

- Suspected urethral trauma, eg, blood at the urethral meatus
- Urethral stricture
- Congenital lower urinary tract abnormalities (relative contraindication)

Equipment

- Sterile gloves and drapes
- Antiseptic solution
- Sterile water and syringe
- Water-soluble lubricant
- An appropriately sized catheter
- Collection bag and tubing

Technique

- Cleanse with appropriate antiseptic:
- Male: Retract prepuce if uncircumcised (enough to see meatus), and swab penis to base
- Female: Separate labia and swab periurethral area
- Create a sterile field above and below urethra.
- Lubricate catheter.
- Insert catheter.

Male:
- Grasp penis, holding on sides and hold it erect; then insert catheter slowly into urethral meatus until urine is obtained.

Female:
- Separate labia and insert catheter into urethral meatus until urine is obtained.

Note: Urinary catheter sizes range from 6 to 14 French (Fr). A clear plastic No. 5 or 8 feeding tube may be used to catheterize infants and young children.

- Inflate balloon with sterile water if appropriate.
- Attach outlet end of catheter aseptically to a closed urine drainage system.

Bedside ultrasound has been used in pediatric emergency departments to confirm placement of catheters.

Complications

Urinary tract infection/colonization of the catheter. (See "Nosocomial Infections in the PICU" in Chapter 18.) Treatment of infection usually consists of empiric antimicrobials and catheter removal.

False tract/traumatic insertion, consult pediatric urology for these patients.

Urethral injury/tissue trauma.


# Nasogastric/Orogastric Tube Insertion

Indications

- To prevent or treat gastric distention when bowel sounds are absent, abdominal distention is present, or the patient requires mechanical ventilation.
- Allows for drainage and/or lavage in drug overdosage or poisoning.
- In trauma settings, NG tubes can be used to aid in the prevention of vomiting and aspiration, as well as for assessment of GI bleeding.
- NG tubes can also be used for enteral feeding initially.

Contraindications

- Blind nasogastric tube placement is contraindicated in the patient with serious facial or head trauma (caribiform plate disruption), because intracranial tube migration may result; an orogastric tube can usually be passed safely in these patients.

## Equipment

- NG/OG tube: 5F, 8F, 10F, 12F, 14F, 16F
- Syringe
- Water-soluble lubricant
- Adhesive tape
- Low-powered suction device OR drainage bag
- Stethoscope

## Technique

- Position patient with head elevated.
- Measure tube: from tip of nose to earlobe, then to a point between the xyphoid process and umbilicus for nasogastric insertion.
- From mouth to earlobe, then to a point between xyphoid process and umbilicus for orogastric insertion.
- Mark tube at measured level with tape.
- Lubricate tube.
- Insert tube.
- **Nasogastric:** Inspect nostril and begin inserting tube into nostril at a slight downward angle. Nose may be pressed slightly upward. Do not force.
- **Orogastric:** Hold infant's mouth open and direct tube to back of mouth. Insert gently, with a downward angle. Insert to designated mark.
- Observe for signs of distress during insertion. Ask child to swallow during insertion, if age appropriate.

Check for proper position with air insertion. Instill air into tube with a syringe. Premature infants receive 0.5 cc; full-term infants receive 1–2 cc. Use 3 cc for toddlers and older children. Listen to the epigastric area of the abdomen with a stethoscope for "whoosh."

Secure tube with tape taking care not to create pressure on the nares, as this may cause necrosis.

## Complications

- Aspiration
- Tissue trauma
- Placement of the catheter can induce gagging or vomiting; therefore, suction should always be ready to use in the case of this happening.

# Intraosseous (IO) Access

Intraosseous infusion can provide a very rapid and dependable route of vascular access in children of all ages (where vascular access is likely to be difficult in settings where it is most urgent).

Almost any infusate can be instilled at a rapid rate through an intraosseous line, including blood and blood products, glucose, crystalloids, pressor agents including epinephrine, dopamine and dobutamine, and atropine. Battery powered IO devices are used in some institutions. There is currently no data available comparing these newer devices with manual insertion.

Indications

- Emergency fluid and drug infusion, especially in setting of circulatory collapse where rapid IV access is essential
- Difficult IV access
- Burn or other injury preventing access to the venous system at other sites

**Contraindications** (all relative in the setting of emergent resuscitation)

- Overlying cellulitis
- Bony lesion at site
- Osteomyelitis
- Fracture of bone  (absolute contraindication)
- Previous intraosseus attempts on same bone

Equipment

- Antiseptic solution
- 1% lidocaine if local anesthesia is appropriate (optional in the moribund patient)
- 3-ml syringe with 25-gauge needle for infiltration of local anesthetic
- Sterile gloves and drape
- IV infusion set
- 18- or 20-gauge short spinal needle or bone marrow needle
- Syringe
- Flush solution (saline or sterile water)
- Gauze pads and tape (optional)

Technique

- Position leg with towel behind knee, leg extended, moderate external rotation at hip.

- Identify landmarks and prepare the insertion site with iodine or alcohol solution. Sites for insertion (Figure 6):

1. Proximal tibia 2 to 5 cm below the tibial tuberosity in the midline in children.
2. Distal femur anterolateral surface, approximately 3 cm above lateral condyle.
3. Distal tibia may also be acceptable especially in older children.
4. Iliac crest.

Infiltrate the overlying skin to the periosteum if the patient is sensitive to pain.

For insertion into the proximal end of the tibia, the spinal needle is directed perpendicular to long axis of bone (or directed slightly inferior) and perpendicular to anteromedial surface of bone. The goal is to angle away from the region of the growth plate.

For insertion in distal femur select site on anterolateral area and angle away from the knee (directed slightly superior).

Advance needle (with stylet in place) through skin, subcutaneous tissue, and cortex of bone into the marrow space using a rotary "screwing" motion until bony cortex has been penetrated.

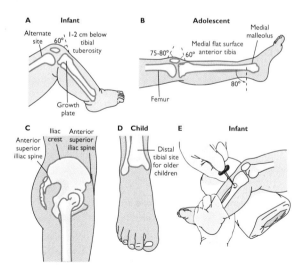

**Figure 6**  Intraosseous insertion sites.

Expect moderate resistance. Entrance into the medullary cavity will be heralded by a "pop" or a sudden loss of resistance. Only 2–4 mm insertion depth into medulla is necessary.

Manually stabilize needle. Before removing stylet aspirate first and if marrow obtained it can be sent for cross match. Attempt to flush with normal saline. There is often some resistance, but if fluid flushes reasonably easily without evidence of swelling, the needle can be considered properly placed.

Detach syringe and connect IV tubing to begin infusion. Secure in position with tape.

If initial attempt fails, may make one additional attempt on other tibia or femur, using new needle.

Complications

- Local abscess or cellulitis
- Osteomyelitis
- Injury to growth plate has not been identified as a complication that occurs with any significant frequency
- Fluid/drug extravasation
- Consider prophylactic antibiotics if not performed with sterile technique
- Should try to obtain definitive venous access and remove IO within several hours of insertion

# Arterial Line

Indications

- Real time, continuous measurement of arterial blood pressure
- Sampling of arterial blood (ie, multiple ABG sampling)
- Pressor agents being infused
- CPP monitoring for MAP

Contraindications

- Severe bleeding diathesis
- Compromised perfusion beyond proposed site

Equipment
- Use standard #22–18 gauge over-the-needle intravenous catheter (#24 gauge may rarely be necessary in tiny infants, though most infants are most easily cannulated with #22 gauge)
- Antiseptic solution and alcohol swabs

- Tapes for securing
- Pressure set, tubing, transducer

# Technique

## Insertion Sites

1. Radial artery

   - start at proximal wrist crease, directly over pulsation
   - perform Allen test to confirm good ulnar flow
   - position with wrist in flexion, tape thumb down and in line with radius
   - consider cardiac anatomy (eg, do not insert on ipsilateral side of Blalock Taussig shunt)

2. Dorsalis pedis

   - at point of maximal pulsation

3. Posterior tibial

   - position with ankle in full dorsi flexion
   - tart at point of maximal pulsation

4. Femoral artery

   - last resort as risk of limb ischemia/femoral artery clot
   - start at point of maximal pulsation
   - consider placing long 3 Fr single lumen catheter in larger children as standard intravenous catheters tend to become dislodged
   - Clean site.
   - May "nick" skin at desired site with #18 gauge needle to decrease skin resistance.
   - Palpate pulse with fingers of one hand, and hold stylet/catheter in other.
   - Standard technique: start aiming for center of pulsation, angled at approx. 30' to skin. Insert slowly until flow ("flashback") is seen in catheter hub. Without removing stylet, advance catheter forward into artery (as in standard peripheral IV insertion technique).
   - The "through and through" technique may be used, but is often less successful in children due to the small caliber of the artery: Insert until "flashback" is seen and advance further to perforate back wall of artery. Remove stylet, then slowly withdraw catheter until pulsatile flow is seen. Advance catheter forward into artery lumen.

- Attach pressure tubing and ensure adequate waveform.
- Stabilize with tape $(+/-$ suture) and armboard.

Complications

- Arterial thrombosis; risk increases with decreasing wrist circumference
- Occult bleeding
- Cerebral embolization; occurs with vigorous flushing of radial catheters
- Catheter related septicemia
- Ischemic necrosis of digits (rare)

# Pericardiocentesis

Indications

For emergency relief of pericardial tamponade with severe hemodynamic compromise or shock state refractory to fluid loading or pharmacological intervention.

If the patient is hemodynamically stable, the procedure is best performed by a pediatric cardiologist with echocardiographic/fluroscopic guidance.

Equipment

- Pericardiocentesis tray and other equipment should include the following:

  - Local anesthetic
  - Antiseptic solution
  - Sterile drapes and gloves
  - Mask
  - Syringe and needle (for local anesthetic)
  - 20 to 60 mL syringes

- Needle for procedure

  - Infant: I inch (2.5 cm), 20-gauge needle
  - Older child: 1.5 to 2 inch (3 to 5 cm), 20-gauge needle
  - Adolescent: 3 inch (7.5 cm), 18- to 20-gauge needle

- Alligator clip attached to a precordial lead

Technique (Figure 7)

- Administer sedation and monitor patient if time and patient's clinical condition permit.

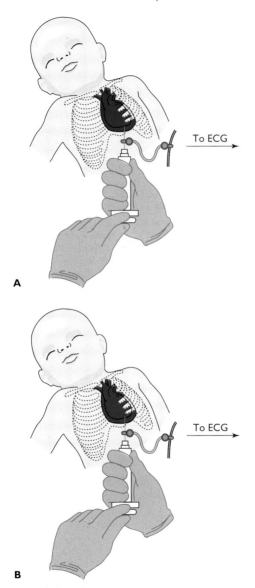

**Figure 7** Pericardiocentesis.

- Apply antiseptic solution to the precordial area.
- Apply sterile drapes.
- Administer local anesthetic.
- If possible, place patient slightly in reverse Trendelenburg.
- Attach needle to syringe and attach alligator clip to proximal portion of the needle. Procedure can be performed using anatomic landmarks alone.
- Insert needle under left costal margin, just lateral to xyphoid, at a 45° angle to skin, aiming toward left shoulder.
- Advance, constantly aspirating, until fluid or blood appears in syringe.
- If fluid is obtained, the pericardial space should be drained as much as possible.
- If an ECG lead has been attached to the needle, ECG changes will be observed when contact with the ventricular wall is made, (ie, ST segment changes, QRS widening, or PVC.) If any of these are observed the needle should be withdrawn slightly until the ECG change disappears. Remove needle if the ECG tracing does not normalize.
- If no ECG lead is used, the ECG monitor should be observed by another team member for changes in rhythm.
- Accurate needle placement can be aided by ultrasonography/ echocardiology, if available.

Complications

Pericardiocentesis is an invasive procedure and therefore has associated risks. However, the risks of the procedure are outweighed by its potential benefits. Complications have become less common due to guided imaging techniques. Possible risks include:

- Puncture of the myocardium.
- Puncture of a coronary artery.
- Myocardial infarction.
- Needle induced arrhythmias.
- Pneumopericardium.
- Pericarditis.
- Accidental puncture of the stomach, lung, or liver.

In cases of recurrent pericardial effusion, a pericardial catheter may also be placed with ultrasound guidance using a modified Seldinger technique.

# Thoracentesis

Indications

- Pleural effusion
- Tension pneumothorax

Contraindications

- An uncorrectable coagulopathy
- Respiratory insufficiency or instability (unless therapeutic thoracentesis is being performed to correct it)

Equipment

- Antiseptic solution
- Sterile drapes and gloves
- 14- to 22-gauge angiocath
- 10- to 20-ml syringes
- Three-way stop cock (optional)

Technique

Consider ultrasonography guided thoracentesis, if available.

For a **tension pneumothorax** the standard approach is with a 14-gauge angiocath (a smaller catheter or a butterfly needle may be used in infants). After prepping and draping, the needle is inserted through the second intercostal space mid-clavicular line and the air is aspirated. The plastic angiocath can be left in place open to the air until a chest tube is inserted through the mid or anterior axillary line 5th intercostal space. If no air is obtained, however, one must consider inserting a chest tube as the lung may have been damaged during insertion of the needle.

For a needle thoracentesis for **pleural effusion** the approach can be with the patient supine and the thoracentesis done in the midaxillary line (Figure 8). In co-operative patients a needle thoracentesis can also be done with the child sitting leaning over a bedside table. Either guided by ultrasound or by dullness on percussion the area of the chest wall is prepped. The selected area is anesthetized with a 25-, 27-, or 30-gauge needle. The presence of fluid can be confirmed by aspirating the chest with this small gauge needle. An angiocath attached to a syringe is inserted through the skin and passed into the chest by passing just over the rib. Once fluid is aspirated remove the needle and thread the plastic angiocath further into the chest

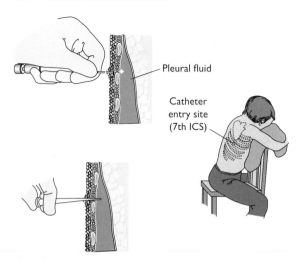

Pleural fluid

Catheter entry site (7th ICS)

**Figure 8**    Thoracentesis for pleural effusion.

and adjust accordingly to enable aspiration of fluid. A three-way stop cock will enable aspiration of fluid without letting air enter the chest.

This may be repeated; however, if repeated, thoracentesis are required, then one must consider inserting a chest tube.

Complications

- Pneumothorax due to air leaking through the needle or due to trauma to underlying lung hemorrhage into the pleural space or chest wall due to needle damage to the subcostal vessels.
  - Vasovagal or simple syncope
  - Air embolism (rare but catastrophic)
  - Introduction of infection
  - Puncture of the spleen or liver due to low or unusually deep needle insertion

# Tube Thoracostomy

Indications
- Pneumothorax
- Hemothorax
- Drainage of pleural effusion, empyema, or chylothorax

Contraindications

There are no contraindications to chest tube placement in patients symptomatic from the above-listed indications. However, care should be used in patients with a potential for serious bleeding.

Commercially available chest tube insertion kits that utilize the Seldinger technique are available. Some centers use these exclusively. Benefits of this approach include:

- Less traumatic
- Better tolerated by patient
- May be used for air or serous fluid
- Permits tight seal at chest wall

Disadvantages:

- Use discouraged if  possibility that lung is adhered to chest wall (insertion wire may pierce lung)
- Open technique recommended for blood, pus, or thick fluid
- Open method still recommended for trauma

Selection of chest tube size:

- Selection of chest tube size and type is dependent on the indication. In general, pneumothoracies may be treated with a smaller sized chest tube including pig-tailed catheters or central venous catheters. Pleural effusions and especially empyemas should be drained with larger chest tubes. A general guide for chest tubes placed for fluid drainage is given in the table below:

| | |
|---|---|
| Neonate | 10–14 Fr |
| Child | 18 Fr |
| Older child/teen | 28 Fr |
| Adult | 28–32 Fr |

**Equipment** (much of this should be in a procedure tray for chest tube placement)

- Antiseptic solution
- Sterile drapes and gloves
- No. 11 scalpel blade and handle
- Curved Kelly clamp
- Suture (size 2–0 or 0) and suture scissors
- Needle holder
- Sterile petrolatum-impregnated gauze
- Sterile gauze and tape
- Suction apparatus

- Chest tube of appropriate size (size 10 Fr for neonates and infants and up to 28 Fr for teenagers): One should consider inserting a larger chest tube in trauma because of the high probability of blood being present
- 1% lidocaine with epinephrine, 10 ml syringe, 25- and 22-gauge needles
- Water-sealed chest drainage system

## Technique (Figure 9)

- Position patient supine.
- Insertion site is usually at the anterior axillary line just behind the lateral edge of the pectoralis major at the level of the nipple (5th intercostal space).
- Prep and drape exposed lateral aspect of the chest wall around the insertion site. Generously anesthetize the insertion site along the insertion tract to the pleura. Appropriate position can be checked by aspiration through the needle used for instilling the local anesthetic.
- The skin should be incised directly over the body of the rib, with the incision length being 1 1/2 times the diameter of the chest tube to be used.
- The Kelly clamp is then used to bluntly dissect superiorly over the superior margin of the next higher rib. The clamp is then pushed through the parietal pleura with tips closed and with slow steady pressure. Once the pleura has been penetrated, the clamps are opened wide to enlarge the insertion tract and remove. Operator's index finger can also be inserted along the tract in older children to further enlarge the opening if needed.
- The chest tube is grasped near the end to be inserted with the Kelly clamp (jaws of the clamp parallel to the length of the tube) and advanced into the pleural space. Do not use a trochar that comes with some chest tubes. These can cause serious injury to intrathoracic structures. Once the tube is inserted so that all drainage ports are inside the thoracic cavity, the tube is connected to the chest drainage system and sutured in place with a suture by closure of the skin edges of the incision around the tube and tying the suture ends up around the tube. The area should be dressed with sterile petrolatum-impregnated gauze and sterile gauze sponges. Chest radiograph should be obtained to confirm proper placement.
- Removal is accomplished by having the patient inhale fully, hold his or her breath, and pulling the tube out swiftly. Cover with air-tight dressing.

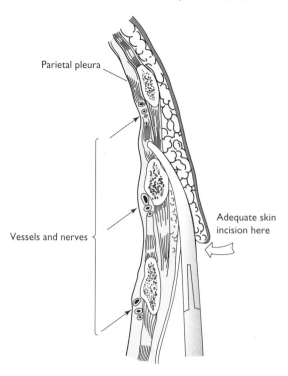

Parietal pleura

Vessels and nerves

Adequate skin incision here

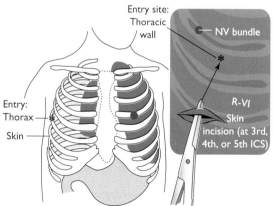

Entry site: Thoracic wall

NV bundle

Entry: Thorax

Skin

R-VI
Skin incision (at 3rd, 4th, or 5th ICS)

**Figure 9**   Tube thoracostomy.

Complications

- Hemorrhage at the site of insertion
- Infection
- Hematoma
- Lung laceration leading to pneumothorax or bronchopleural fistula
- Injury to heart, great vessels or other intrathoracic structures
- Laceration of intra-abdominal organs if tube is inadvertently inserted into the abdominal cavity
- False tract with persistence of initial indication for chest tube placement

# Paracentesis

Ultrasound guidance may be useful to determine the best area on the abdominal wall.

Indications

Diagnostic

- To allow categorization of transudate vs. exudate, neoplastic vs. non-neoplastic, infectious vs. non-infectious

Therapeutic

- Inability to achieve ventilatory goals in an intubated patient
- Severe respiratory distress
- Patient discomfort
- Abdominal compartment syndrome

**Contraindications** (relative)

- Previous abdominal surgery
- Large abdominal mass
- Bowel obstruction

Equipment

- Sterile gloves and drapes, prep, etc.
- Procedure tray
- I percent lidocaine without epinephrine
- 10-cc syringe plus 60-cc syringe if large volume of ascitic fluid
- 16- to 22-gauge angiocath depending on the size of the child
- Sterile gauze

Technique

- Patient position supine
- Possible insertions sites

  - Right mid or left mid abdomen
  - Avoid enlarged liver and bowel
  - Consider a Foley catheter and nasogastric tube to drain bladder and stomach, respectively

Prep, drape, and anesthetize the selected insertions sites. With the small gauge (25-gauge) needle for lidocaine injection confirm the presence of ascitic fluid and gauge the depth of peritoneal cavity. Attach angiocath (18- or 20-gauge most commonly) to a 10-cc syringe and insert perpendicular to this skin applying negative pressure to the syringe. Once fluid is aspirated advance the angiocath catheter over the needle and removing the needle. Observe nature of fluid and take samples for culture and biochemical analysis. If large volume of fluid is to be removed use 60-cc syringe. If large volume of fluid is removed be wary of fluid shifts and monitor the patient closely. Consider if fluid replacement with albumin.

# Venous Cutdowns

These are time-consuming and should be resorted to after unsuccessful peripheral IV insertion, interosseous insertion, percutaneous, and central venous access.

The simplest technique involves using the site anterior to the medial malleolus. This is like a peripheral IV and is a very temporary venous access technique. Other sites, that can be selected and can be performed at the bedside in the pediatric intensive care unit, are the saphenous vein at the top of the leg or the antecubital fossa. If the catheter can be threaded centrally they often can be used for more long-term use. More formal techniques such as insertion of long-term catheters like Hickman or Broviac catheters use the external or internal jugular veins or the subclavian veins and are done in the operating room usually and will not be discussed here.

Indications

Inability to obtain venous access
The need for central venous access which is reliable for pressors or long-term antibiotic use

Contraindications

Standard venous access is available
Infection at cutdown site
Trauma to groin or abdomen
Orthopedic or vascular injury proximal to cutdown site

Equipment

The details here are much same for all these procedures.
Silastic® cutdown catheters are needed in sizes 2, 3, 4 Fr.
Antiseptic solution
Local anesthetic
Syringes, needles
Scalpels
Suture material
IV extension tubing, saline flush

## Technique

1. Medial malleolus
   - The area is prepped and draped.
   - 1% lidocaine without epinephrine is infiltrated.
   - Transverse incision made anterior to the medial malleolus.
   - Using a snap spreading longitudinally the vein is usually isolated close to the bone.
   - A suitable size angiocath can then be inserted into the vein and secured with suture or steristrips.

2. Saphenous vein in the groin
   - The lower abdomen, groin and leg to the knee is prepped and draped.
   - Local anesthetic is infiltrated.
   - Transverse incision made at the top of the leg below the groin crease.
   - Dissection through this incision will show the vein.
   - The vein is dissected free and isolated between two ties of absorbable suture.
   - Silastic® catheter (size 2, 3, or 4 Fr) is selected and trimmed so that no catheter remains out of the skin at the insertion site.
   - A venotomy is made and catheter inserted.
   - The catheter is secured with either sutures or steristrips and the incision closed.
   - The catheter can be tunneled after instilling local anesthetic from inferior and lateral on the leg, prior to insertion in the vein in order to avoid diaper area.

- An abdominal X-ray AP and lateral shoot through is done to confirm position in the inferior vena cava not in the ascending lumbar vein.

# Antecubital Fossa Cut Down

- The arm is restrained and prepped and draped in the usual manner.
- Local anesthetic is infiltrated.
- Transverse incision is made more medially in the antecubital fossa; dissection through this incision will show the vein.
- The vein is dissected free and isolated between two ties of absorbable suture.
- Silastic® catheter (size 2, 3, or 4 French ) is selected and trimmed after measuring the distance from the incision to the angle of Louis on the chest wall so that no catheter remains out of the skin at the insertion site.
- A venotomy is made and catheter inserted.
- The catheter is secured with either sutures or steristrips and the incision closed.
- Chest x-ray is done to confirm position of the tip of the line.

Complications

- Infection
- Hematoma formation
- Thrombophlebitis
- Hemorrhage
- Unsuccessful cannulation

# Suggested Readings

2005 American Heart Association Guidelines for Cardiopulmonary Resuscitation and Emergency Cardiovascular Care: Part 12: Pediatric Advanced Life Support. Circulation 2005 Dec;112:IV–167–IV–187.

Fleischer G, Ludwig S, et al. Editors. Textbook of pediatric emergency medicine, 5th edition. Philadelphia: Lippincott Williams & Wilkins. 2005.

Gausche-Hill M, Fuchs S, Yamamoto L. Editors. APLS: The pediatric emergency medicine resource, 4th ed. American Academy of Pediatrics. American College of Emergency Physicians. Jones and Bartlett. 2004.

PALS Provider Manual. American Academy of Pediatrics. American Heart Association. 2002.

# Chapter 23

# Pharmacology

## A. Pharmacologic Considerations for the PICU

Mark Duffett

Drug therapy in the PICU presents unique challenges due to the broad range of ages, sizes, and developmental stages of the patients, their unstable clinical condition, and the limited nature of medication studies in this population. Making decisions about medication use and dosing the PICU often requires extrapolation from other populations, neonates, non-critically ill children and adults, and critically ill adults. This relies on knowledge of the characteristics of the medications, of the patients and prudent clinical judgment. We recommend the use of specialized references for specific situations, but some important considerations are:

### Dosing Recommendations and Calculations

- When based on the age of the patient, our divisions (such as infants, children, and adults) are quite arbitrary and may not be clinically or physiologically sensible in individual patients. For example the physiology of a 1-year-old may be quite different than that of post-pubertal teenager.
- Most dosing recommendations are based on the patient's weight. The dose calculated using the weight should generally not exceed the maximum dose recommended for adults. Weight-based doses may need to be re-evaluated in patients with abnormal body composition such as obesity, cachexia, or significant volume overload.

- It is usually helpful to round doses to a convenient volume or use whole vials or pre-prepared doses. This may simplify the medication administration process.

## Developmental and Age-Related Differences

- The pediatric population encompasses a broad range of patients with differing absorption, distribution, metabolism, and excretion. While a detailed discussion of developmental pharmacokinetics and pharmacodynamics is beyond the scope of this book, it is important to recognize and consider these factors when individualizing drug therapy.

## Pharmacokinetic Considerations in the Critically Ill Patient

Critically ill children are a heterogeneous group, and alterations in pharmacokinetics will vary widely depending on the nature and severity of the patient's condition and the characteristics of the drugs in question. Some general pharmakinetic considerations in the critically ill patient are:

- Absorption: As with other types of patients who require medication formulations suitable for administration via feeding tubes and the interactions enteral feeds. In addition, critically ill patients often have delayed gastric emptying and impaired intestinal transit as a consequence of surgery, impaired perfusion, or due to medications (especially opiates). Absorption can also be decreased by inadequate perfusion of gastrointestinal tract and by mucosal atrophy and denudation. Intramuscular and subcutaneous absorption may also be reduced, particularly in patients with poor perfusion due to hypotension, vasoconstriction, or significant edema.
- Distribution: The distribution of drugs may also be affected in the critically ill patients, primarily due to changes in body composition and changes in plasma protein levels (especially hypoalbuminemia). While in the acute setting the volume of distribution for some drugs may be changed by fluid administration and shifts often resulting in increased total body water and increased extracellular water, other factors such as loss of muscle mass may also become important. For drugs that are highly protein bound, decreased levels of plasma proteins will result in a higher concentration of free drug, which may lead to toxicity.

- Metabolism: In addition to the differences among patients due to developmental or age-related changes in drug metabolism.
- Excretion: Many critically ill patients will have reduced capacity to eliminate many drugs primarily, but not exclusively, due to reduced renal function. Many drugs are at least partially dependant on renal function for excretion, and dose adjustment to avoid toxicity may be required in patients with renal dysfunction. All of the methods for estimating GFR and creatinine clearance using serum creatinine assume stable renal function which may not be a realistic assumption in critically ill patients. Other factors need to be considered when dosing drugs in unstable patients:

  - patient response and clinical signs and symptoms of efficacy and toxicity. Decreased clearance may lead to accumulation of drugs or metabolites, commonly resulting in excessive or prolonged effects.
  - drug levels where possible and practical.
  - rate and direction of change of serum creatinine.
  - urine output (Consider 24 hour urine collection for creatinine clearance calculation. Shorter periods of urine collection may be appropriate in select patients.)
  - choose drugs which are not dependant on renal clearance if possible.
  - avoid drugs with the potential for nephrotoxicity if possible.
  - extra-corporeal elimination of drugs via peritoneal dialysis, hemodialysis, CRRT, and ECMO may be significant and should be considered when making dosing decisions.

# Drug Interactions

Recognizing and managing the risk of drug interactions in a patient receiving multiple medications is a challenging task. The following, although not exhaustive, is a list of drugs that are frequently implicated in clinically relevant interactions. Specialized resources should be consulted for more information.

| | |
|---|---|
| Anti-infectives | rifampin |
| | fluconazole, voriconazole |
| | erythromycin, clarithromycin |
| | anti-retrovirals |
| Immunosupressants | cyclosporin |
| | tacrolimus |
| | sirolimus |

| Cardiovascular drugs | warfarin |
| | digoxin |
| | amiodarone |
| Anticonvulsants | phenytoin |
| | phenobarbital |
| | carbamazepine |
| | valproic acid |
| | lamotrigine |
| Other drugs | aminophylline/theophylline |
| | midazolam |

# Drug Levels

For effective ordering and interpreting of drug levels it is important to consider:

- What is the clinical indication for measuring the level? Is the concern toxicity or efficacy?
- What is the appropriate time to measure the level with respect to the dose? Whether a trough, peak, or random level more appropriate will depend on the drug and the indication for the level.
- Most levels should be measured once the drug has had time to reach steady state which is usually reached after three to five half-lives of the drug. This may not always be realistic due to the clinical situation of the patient, fluctuating renal function and the use of loading doses. When not measured at steady state levels should be interpreted in the light of the clinical situation and if the steady state level is likely to be higher or lower than the currently measured one.

# Tips for Safer Order Writing

The Institute for Safe Medication Practices (ISMP) provides some guidelines, but each institution should develop its own processes and standards.

## General Principles

- Date and time all orders.
- Use generic drug names only.
- Drug names must be written in full; do not use abbreviations for drug names (examples: levo, $MSO_4$, $MgSO_4$, HCTZ).

- Write "once daily" or "q24h" instead of "QD" or "OD."
- Write out the word "microgram" or use mcg, do not use μg.
- Write out the word "unit," the letter U has been misinterpreted as a 0, resulting in a 10-fold overdose.
- Write the patients weight on each order.
- Include the intended dose per kilogram on each order.
- Specify dose (in mg or mcg, units, etc.) not volume when ordering medications.
- Always place a zero in front of a decimal point (eg, .2 mg should be 0.2 mg) and never place a decimal and a zero after a whole number (eg, 4.0 mg should be 4 mg).
- In addition to the above, all orders for parenteral electrolytes should include the volume and type of diluent and the rate or duration for infusion. Each hospital should standardize the units used for ordering electrolytes such as calcium, magnesium, and phosphate.
- All orders for medications to be given by continuous infusion must include:

    - patient's weight
    - amount of drug (in mg, mcg, units etc., NOT mL)
    - type of diluent
    - total volume of infusion solution
    - dose
    - *if* order includes the provision for titration, specific parameters and a maximum dose must be given

        Example: Wt = 30 kg, add 90 mg of dopamine to a total volume of 50 mL NS, run at 5 microgram/kg/min, titrate to keep MAP greater than 70 mm Hg. Maximum 20 mcg/kg/min.

Hospitals should have systems and tools in place to reduce the need for calculations and the potential for error. Examples include "smart" IV pumps, dose calculators, patient specific dosing charts, and standardized infusion mixtures.

# References

Kearns GL, Abdel-Rahman SM, Alander SW, et al. Developmental pharmacology—Drug disposition, action, and therapy in infants and children. N Engl J Med 2003 Sep 18;349(12):1157–67.

Levine SR, Cohen MR, Blanchard NR, et al. Guidelines for preventing medication errors in pediatrics. J Pediatr Pharmacol Ther 2001;6:426–42.

# B. Toxicology

Anthony G. Crocco
John Crossley

## Introduction

Although the vast majority of poisonings are related to ingestion, we will use the term poisoning to also include iatrogenic overdose medications.

Additional texts may be required for further details on other intoxications. Local poison control centers can help with additional information. Most guidelines are based on expert consensus.

## Epidemiology

The distribution of poisonings throughout childhood varies greatly. Children <6 years have seven times the poisonings than children 13 to 19. But adolescents experience four times the mortality compared to their younger counterparts, as they are more likely to intentionally ingest more dangerous medications. The most common poisonings by age group are given in Table 1.

Some substances produce significant mortality, such as analgesics. These ingestions are so common that significant mortality occurs. Table 2 outlines the common causes of poisoning-related mortality.

*Table 1*

**Top Five Categories of Poisonings for Age Groups Younger than 6 and Older than 19**

|  | **Less than 6 Years** | **Over 19 Years** |
|---|---|---|
| Top 5 poisonings | • Cosmetics, personal care products | • Analgesics |
|  | • Cleanings substances | • Sedatives, hypnotics, anti-psychotics |
|  | • Analgesics | • Cleaning substances |
|  | • Foreign bodies | • Antidepressants |
|  | • Topical poisons | • Bites/envenomation |

*Table 2*
## The Most Common Causes of Poisoning-Related Mortality—All Ages

Analgesics
Sedatives, hypnotics, anti-psychotics
Antidepressants
Stimulants, street drugs
Cardiovascular drugs

## "One Pill Kills"

There are a few toxic exposures which, even given a limited exposure, pose a significant risk of mortality in children. These are summarized in Table 3.

*Table 3*
## Common Toxic Substances That Can Kill with Limited Exposure

| Substance | Notes |
|-----------|-------|
| Antimalarial medications | • Chloroquine potentially lethal dose: 20 mg/kg |
| | • Hydroxychloroquine potentially lethal dose: 20 mg/kg |
| | • Cardiotoxic effects include conduction delays |
| | • CNS effects include depression of level of consciousness and seizures |
| Camphor | • Potentially lethal dose: 100 mg/kg |
| | • CNS effects include agitation, apnea, depression of level of consciousness, seizures |
| Clonidine | • Potentially lethal dose: 0.01 mg/kg |
| | • Cardiovascular effects include transient hypertension, hypotension, bradycardia |

| Substance | Notes |
|---|---|
|  | • Other effects include miosis, hypotonia, depression of level of consciousness, and respiratory drive |
| Methyl salicylates | • Potentially lethal dose: 150 mg/kg |
|  | • Respiratory alkalosis and metabolic acidosis predominate |
|  | • CNS effects include depression of level of consciousness and seizures |
| Sulfonylureas | • Potentially lethal dose (glyburide): 0.1 mg/kg |
|  | • Be prepared to treat severe hypoglycemia |
| Calcium channel antagonists | • Cardiovascular effects include hypotension, bradycardia, reflex tachycardia, heart block, cardiac arrest |
| Cyclic antidepressants | • CNS effects include depression of level of consciousness and seizures |
|  | • Cardiovascular effects include conduction abnormalities, arrhythmias, hypotension |
|  | • Look for anticholinergic toxidrome |
| Opioids/opiates including Lomotil | • CNS effects include depression of level of consciousness and respiratory depression |
|  | • Miosis |
|  | • Lomotil may also produce an anticholinergic toxidrome |
| Toxic alcohols | • CNS effects include depression of level of consciousness, respiratory repression, visual disturbance |
|  | • Metabolic effects include increased anion gap metabolic acidosis and osmolar gap |
|  | • Renal failure and ECG changes may be noted late in the course of ingestion |

## Non-toxic Exposures

Many ingestions require simple identification to determine toxicity, often through a poison control center.

Identification of all possible substances or ingredients:

- Single product involved in exposure
- Unintentional expose, (ie, not suicidal)
- "CAUTION," "WARNING," "DANGER" do not appear on product label
- Reliable approximation of quantity and route of exposure possible
- Patient is asymptomatic
- Follow-up (n) or repeat assessment is possible

## Initial Emergency Management

Use the **ABCDE** approach below. This is done in conjunction with an "**AMPLE**" history. (See Table 4.)

Relevant details of the events surrounding the poisoning are needed. (See Table 5.)

*Table 4*
**The AMPLE History**

| |
|---|
| A—Allergies |
| M—Medications |
| P—Past medical history |
| L—Last meal |
| E—Events surrounding poisoning |

*Table 5*
**Information to Obtain Regarding Events Surrounding Poisoning**

| Who | |
|---|---|
| | • Past medical history of the patient |
| | • Clinical changes noted in the patient since poisoning including change in level of consciousness, respiratory function, etc. |

| | |
|---|---|
| | • Patient weight needs to be accurately documented to establish dose per kilogram |
| What | • Specific product name including concentration |
| | • Maximum potential exposure |
| | • Other potential exposures including other medications in the house |
| Where | • Location of poisoning |
| | • Any intervention that was taken prior to presentation to your center |
| When | • Time of poisoning |
| | • Time over which patient was exposed |
| Why | • Unintentional versus intentional |
| | • Potential for other exposed victims |
| How | • Route of poisoning |

## Primary Survey: ABCDE

### A—Airway

- Firstly, any medication that alters the level of consciousness (eg, benzodiazepines and psychoactive substances) can decrease airway protective reflexes.
- Secondly, some poisonings result in airway edema (eg, caustics and smoke inhalation).
- Other indications for taking control of the airway include route of administration for medication and protection of airway prior to charcoal administration.
- Manage airway problems as previously described in the book.

## B—Breathing

- Many ingestions can depress respiratory drive.
- Many poisonings can result in bronchorrhea and bronchospasm.
- Manage respiratory problems as previously described in the book.

## C—Circulation

- Toxic effects range from hypotension to hypertension as well as rhythm changes.
- An ECG should be considered.
- Manage circulation problems as previously described in the book.

## D—Disability

- Assess level of consciousness, pupillary size, and response and possible seizure activity.
- Manage neurological changes including seizures as previously described in the book.

## E—Environment/Exposure

- In topical exposure, remove clothing soiled with exposure substance, completely undress child, wash if needed, and keep dry and warm.
- In cases of intentional or inflicted poisonings, specific care should be taken to ensure the patient is safe from him/herself and others.

## "ABCs" of Toxicology

A-B-C is similar to those of the primary survey.

### D—Decontamination   The goal is to prevent systemic absorption.

- For ocular or dermal exposures, topical lavage is best.
- For ingestions, the choices are to remove the unabsorbed medication from the stomach, prevent its absorption, or improve its passage through the gastrointestinal tract.

### Serum of Ipecac

- Not used routinely because: limited proven efficacy; delays in administration of charcoal, whole bowel irrigation, or oral antidotes; risk of aspiration.

- *Ipecac should be given only on the advice of a toxicologist.* Indications may include presentation of a life-threatening ingestion within 60 minutes in an alert, conscious patient.
- Contraindications include loss of airway protection, corrosive or hydrocarbon ingestion, ingestion of substance that may lead to airway compromise within 60 minutes.
- Dose: 6–12 mo = 5–10 mL + 120–240 mL water; 1–12 yrs = 15 mL + 240 mL water; adolescent = 15–30 mL + 240 mL water. Repeat once if necessary.

## Gastric Lavage

- Not routinely used because: limited efficacy shortly after ingestion; requires large-bore nasogastric (NG) tube.
- Indications include presentation of a life-threatening ingestion within 60 minutes in a patient with a stable or secured airway.
- Contraindications include loss of airway protection, corrosive or hydrocarbon ingestion, patients at risk of intestinal perforation.
- Child is usually positioned in the left lateral position. Lavage is performed by administering 10 mL/kg (maximum 300 mL) of warmed normal saline via NG tube. The same volume is removed. This process can be repeated.

## Single Dose Activated Charcoal

- Commonly used, relatively safe. Administration within 1 hour of ingestion produces best results. Administration after 1 hour may be beneficial in certain ingestions including sustained release medications.
- Indications: ingestion of a potentially toxic amount of absorbable substance, especially for those toxins without a safe, generally available antidote.
- Contraindications: unprotected or unstable airway, perforation of gastrointestinal tract, caustic or hydrocarbon ingestion. Aspiration of charcoal can be a life-threatening event.
- Dose: child <1 year = 1 g/kg; child 1–12 = 25–50 g; adolescent 25–100 g.
- Not useful for alcohols, acids, alkali, essential oils, hydrocarbons. Limited use with metals including iron, lithium, and all elemental toxins.

## Cathartics

- Increases gastrointestinal motility. Improves the taste of charcoal. Risks with repeated use include electrolyte abnormalities.

- Indications for use include with the first dose of charcoal.
- Contraindications: recent abdominal surgery or trauma, obstruction or perforation of gastrointestinal tract, absent bowel sounds, corrosive ingestion, hypovolemia, or electrolyte abnormality. Avoid magnesium-containing cathartics in patients with renal disease or heart block.
- Relative contraindications: age <1 year due to risk of significant fluid shifts and electrolyte changes.
- Dose: Sorbitol = 1–2 g/kg single dose. 10% magnesium citrate = 4 mL/kg.

## Whole Bowel Irrigation with Non-absorbable Polyethylene Glycol

- Administered via NG tube until stools are clear, thereby clearing the gastrointestinal track of toxic substances.
- Indications: ingestion of sustained-release or enteric-coated medications. May also be useful for ingestion of drug packets or ingestion of substances not well absorbed by charcoal, such as iron.
- Contraindications: obstruction, perforation, or hemorrhage of the gastrointestinal track, hemodynamic instability, unstable uncontrolled airway, and uncontrollable vomiting.
- Dose via NG tube: 9 mo–6 yrs = 500 mL/h; 6–12 yrs = 1,000 mL/h; adolescents = 1,500–2,000 mL/h (or until clear).

**E—Elimination Strategies**    The goal is to improve the removal of the poison and its metabolites from the body after absorption has taken place.

## Multiple Dose Activated Charcoal

- Improves elimination of toxins already absorbed by interfering with entero-entero, entero-hepatic, and entero-gastric circulation.
- Indications: life-threatening ingestion of carbamazepine, dapsone, phenobarbital, quinine, or theophylline. Multiple dose activated charcoal may help with life-threatening ingestions of amitriptyline, dextropropoxyphene, digitoxin, digoxin, disopyramide, nadolol, phenylbutazone, phenytoin, piroxicam, salycilates, and sodolol.
- Absolute contraindications: an unprotected airway, intestinal obstruction, and a damaged gastrointestinal tract. Evidence of decreased peristalsis is a relative contraindication.
- Dose: initial dose as for "single dose activated charcoal" above. Half of the initial dose is then administered every 2 hours.

# Bicarbonate Administration Including Alkalinization of Urine

- Proposed benefits include the prevention of movement of ionized drugs into tissues, increasing urinary excretion of drugs, increasing sodium gradient, reversing acidosis, treating hyperkalemia, and treating myoglobinuria.
- Use in poisonings with tricyclic antidepressants and salicylates.
- For alkalinization of urine, 50–100 mEq of sodium bicarbonate in 1 L of D5 ½ normal saline run at 2–3 mL/kg/hour. Close monitoring of urinary pH is required, keeping levels between 7 and 8.
- For correction of acidosis, 0.5–1 mEq/kg boluses are used.
- Monitor fluid status, electrolytes, and pH.

## Hemodialysis/Hemoperfusion

- May help to eliminate toxic substances from the serum. Less useful for substances that have a large volume of distribution. Ensure patient is hemodynamically stable.
- Hemodialysis is useful for smaller, water-soluble compounds that are loosely bound to protein. Allows for restoration of electrolyte balance and volume status.
- Hemoperfusion is useful for larger, lipid-soluble compounds that are protein bound. Careful monitoring of thrombocytopenia is required.
- Specific intoxications that may require hemodialysis or hemoperfusion include low molecular-weight alcohols, theophylline, lithium, and salicylates.

**F—Find an Antidote** Many different antidotes are available, but not all are beneficial. For example, consider the flumazenil antidote for benzodiazepine overdoses. Because flumazenil lowers the seizure threshold, it may result in intractable seizures, whereas most benzodiazepine overdoses can be managed with supportive care. A partial list of antidotes to some of the more common intoxications is presented in Table 6.

## Toxidromes

Definition: a constellation of signs and symptoms typically found with a specific intoxication.

Table 7 outlines several common toxidromes. The most useful features to examine include the vital signs, the level of

*Table 6*
**Antidotes to Common Intoxications\***

| Toxin | Antidote |
|---|---|
| Benzodiazepines | Flumazenil |
| Carbon monoxide | Oxygen |
| Digoxin | Digoxin antibodies |
| Iron | Desferrioxamine |
| Methaemoglobinaemia | Methyolene blue |
| Methanol & ethylene glycol | Ethanol, fomepizole (alcohol dehydrogenase inhibitor) |
| Opiates | Naloxone |
| Organophosphate insecticides | Atropine, pralidoxime |

Modified from Riordan et al. (2002)

\*Care must be taken in administering antidotes, as side effects of antidotes may create clinical problems. Do not use the list in isolation to manage patients.

consciousness, the ocular reaction, presence of bowel sounds, and the skin.

## Ancillary Tests

Various tests not only help with identification of an intoxication, but also help to characterize the effects. These tests can be divided into those sent to the laboratory, ECG, and imaging (Table 8, 9).

## Management of Common Ingestions

**Acetaminophen**    Mechanism of toxicity: The metabolites of acetaminophen include N-acetly-p-benzoquinone imine (NAPQI), known to be hepatotoxic-causing cellular necrosis. NAPQI is normally readily detoxified by glutathione in the liver prior to excretion in the urine or bile. When the amounts of NAPQI overwhelm the available glutathione, hepatic injury occurs.

A single acute dose greater than 150 mg/kg is believed to be the minimum dose required to produce hepatotoxicity. This threshold may be lower if the ingestion is chronic, if the patient is fasting or malnourished, has a history of liver disease, has a co-ingestion, is

*Table 7*
**Common Clinical Toxidromes**

| Toxin | Clinical Features | Examples |
|-------|-------------------|----------|
| Anticholinergic | • Increased temperature | • Atropine |
| | • Delirium, mumbling speech | • Antihistamines |
| | • Tachycardia | • Plants: belladonna, jimson weed |
| | • Skin and mucus membranes: dry, flushed | |
| | • Urinary retention | |
| | • Decreased bowel sounds | |
| | • Mydriasis and blurred vision | |
| | • Possible seizures and coma | |
| Sympathomimetic | • Hypertension, tachycardia | • Cocaine |
| | • Increased temperature | • Amphetamines |
| | • Diaphoresis | • Theophylline |
| | • Agitation, excessive speech | • Caffeine |
| | • Altered sleep | • Ephedrine |
| | • Increased bowel sounds | • Pseudoephedrine |
| | • Possible seizures and arrhythmias | • $B_2$ agonists |

*(continued)*

| Toxin | Clinical Features | Examples |
|-------|-------------------|----------|
| Opiod | • Depressed level of consciousness | • Morphine |
| | • Respiratory depression | • Heroin |
| | • Miosis | • Oxycodone |
| | • Bradycardia, hypotension | • Hydromorphone |
| | • Decreased temperature | • Meperidene |
| | • Hyporeflexia | • Dextromethorphan |
| | | • Clonidine and other Alpha-2 receptor agonists |
| Anticholinesterase (Cholinergic) | • Defecation increased | • Organophosphates (insecticides) |
| | • Urination increased | • Carbamates |
| | • Miosis | • Physostigmine |
| | • Bronchorrhea, bronchospasm | • Neostigmine |
| | • Emesis | • Edrophonium |
| | • Lacrimation | |
| | • Salivation | |
| Sedative-Hypnotic | • Hypotension | • Barbiturates |
| | • Decreased respiration | • Benzodiazepines |
| | • Decreased temperature | • Paraldehyde |
| | • Depressed level of consciousness, slurred speech | • Chloral hydrate |
| | • Ataxia | • Ethanol |
| | • Hyporeflexia | • Neuroleptics |

*Table 8*
**Useful Laboratory Tests in Intoxications**

| | |
|---|---|
| CBC | • A low hemoglobin may signify hemorrhagic shock |
| | • Elevated white cell count may be seen in iron overdoses |
| Glucose | • Hypoglycemia can be found with ingestions of oral hypoglycemics and insulin excess |
| | • Hyperglycemia can be found in iron overdoses |
| Electrolytes | • Potassium |
| | • Sodium |
| Anion gap | • $[Na]—[Cl]—[HCO_3]$ |
| | • Normal 8–12 |
| | • Increased in: MUDPILES |
| | • Methanol, uremia, diabetic ketoacidosis, paraldehyde, iron, INH, lactic acidosis, ethanol, ethylene glycol, carbon monoxide, cyanide, ASA, toluene |
| Blood gas | • Establish acidosis or alkalosis |
| | • Check co-oximitry for evidence of carboxyhemoglobin |
| Measured osmolality | • Helps to establish osmolal gap |
| Calculated osmolality | • $2[Na] + [glucose] + [BUN]$ |
| Osmolar gap | • Measured osmolality—calculated osmolality |
| | • Normal between 0–5 |

*(continued)*

|  | |
|---|---|
|  | • Increased in: acetone, alcohols, ethylene glycol, magnesium, mannitol, IV contrast, renal failure, elevated ketones, lactic acidosis |
| Drug levels | • Helpful for acetaminophen and salicylate intoxication |
|  | • Rarely helpful for other poisonings in the acute setting, as acute management is unchanged |
|  | • Can be helpful in ruling out intoxication as a cause of disturbed behavior |
| Liver function tests | • Useful acutely as a baseline |
| Renal function tests | • Useful acutely as a baseline |
| bHCG | • Pregnancy can be a precipitant to intoxication or suicide |
|  | • Good to know if you've got two patients instead of one! |

*Table 9*

## Significance of ECG Changes in Poisoned Patient

| ECG Change | Significance |
|---|---|
| Wide QRS (> 0.1 second) | • Consider ingestion of type 1a antidysrhythmic: ie, TCA, procainamide, quinidine |
|  | • Consider cocaine |
| Bradycardia | • Consider cholinergic exposure, B blockers, Ca channel blocker, opiates |
| Ischemia, infarction | • Cocaine, sympathomemetics |

In addition, occasionally imaging studies may help. This is the case when ingestion of radio-opaque substances is questioned or when there has been ingestion of packets of drugs. Chest radiology can be helpful in cases of inhalation or aspiration.

diabetic, or is on other medications that use the liver for metabolism. The Rumack-Matthew nomogram is used to estimate the risk of toxicity for a single acute ingestion (see Figure 1).

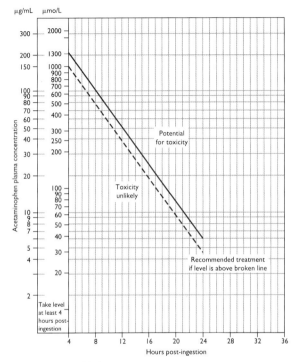

**Figure 1** Rumack-Matthew nomogram.

Table 10 outlines the four stages of acetaminophen toxicity. Absence of clinical features should not be reassuring. Life-threatening intoxications may present symptom-free.

**Approach**   Initial approach is ABCs. Administer activated charcoal as soon as possible. Maximum effect is seen if given in the first 1–2 hours; although administration as late as 6–8 hours may be indicated if there was a co-ingestion or ingestion was of a delayed-release preparation.

*Table 10*
**Clinical Stages of Untreated Acetaminophen Toxicity**

| Stage | Time Following Ingestion | Clinical Characteristics |
| --- | --- | --- |
| I | 30 min to 24 hours | Anorexia, nausea, vomiting, malaise, pallor, diaphoresis |
| II | 24 to 48 hours | Resolution of the above symptoms; right upper quadrant abdominal pain and tenderness; elevated bilirubin, prothrombin time, hepatic enzymes; oliguria |
| III | 72 to 96 hours | Peak liver function abnormalities; anorexia, nausea, vomiting, malaise may reappear |
| IV | 4 days to 2 weeks | Resolution of hepatic dysfunction or death from hepatic failure |

Initial investigations at 4 hours post-ingestion should include acetaminophen level, liver function tests, glucose, renal function tests, electrolytes, and tests for co-ingestions, especially salicylates. Although these tests are done no earlier than 4 hours post-ingestion, charcoal therapy should start as soon as the child arrives. (See contraindications above.)

**Level of acetaminophen is above the threshold on the Rumack-Matthew nomogram:**

- If the level is above the threshold then hospitalization is required for IV administration of NAC or for monitoring of acetaminophen levels and liver function tests.
- N-acetylcysteine (NAC), the antidote for acetaminophen toxicity, should be used. NAC works by increasing the available

glutathione and improving detoxification of NAPQI. There are several strategies for NAC administration and little evidence to support one dosing compared to another (Table 11).

## In fulminant hepatic failure, liver transplantation should be considered. Level of acetaminophen is below the threshold on the Rumack-Matthew nomogram:

- If time of ingestion is accurate, and if child is otherwise clinically stable and safe with no co-ingestion, he/she can be sent home.
- If there is doubt about the timing of the dose or whether there may be delayed absorption, NAC should be started.

*Table 11*
## Three Different Strategies for Administration of N-acetylcysteine

| Duration of NAC | Route | Method |
|---|---|---|
| 24 hrs | IV | • Loading dose: 150 mg/kg over 15 min<br>• 2nd infusion: 50 mg/kg over 4 hours<br>• 3rd infusion: 100 mg/kg over 16 hours |
| 48 hrs | IV | • Loading dose: 70 mg/kg<br>• Maintenance dose: 70 mg/kg every 4 hours<br>• Continue maintenance doses 17 times or until acetaminophen level is non-toxic |
| 78 hrs | Oral | • Loading dose: 140 mg/kg<br>• Maintenance dose: 70 mg/kg every 4 hours<br>• Continue maintenance doses 17 times or until acetaminophen level is non-toxic |

- Monitor liver function tests.
- If evidence of hepatic failure, early consultation should be made to a gastroenterologist to consider liver transplantation.
- Further acetaminophen levels after NAC has been started do not alter management.

**Salicylate**    Mechanism of toxicity: Clinically relevant effects are on acid-base metabolism. Salicylates stimulate the respiratory center leading to respiratory alkalosis. In addition, salicylates interfere with the citric acid cycle (Krebs cycle) promoting lactate and ketoacid production and resulting in a wide anion gap metabolic acidosis. This acidosis often results in a secondary respiratory alkalosis. Thus, salicylates produce a mixed acid-base picture: respiratory alkalosis and metabolic acidosis. Other effects include development of non-cardiogenic pulmonary edema and ototoxicity.

Salicylates are found not only in over-the-counter antipyretics and pain medications, but also in oil of wintergreen and topical anti-wart preparations. Acute ingestions greater than 120 mg/kg are considered toxic. Concretions of pills, enteric coated preparations, and delayed release preparations may have peak levels beyond 12 hours.

**Approach**    Initial approach is ABCs. Supportive care includes oxygen delivery and management of seizures. Obtain intravenous access for fluid administration and access for medication. Features of severe poisoning include coma, seizures, renal failure, or pulmonary edema. In these, consider early dialysis (13D–Renal Replacement Therapy).

Laboratory investigations: urinalysis, urine pH, electrolytes, renal function tests, coagulation studies, blood gas, and salicylate level. Initial levels are drawn at 4 hours. The Done nomogram is no longer used to follow salicylate ingestion toxicity, as its predictive value is poor. Rather, clinical parameters, as well as results from repeat urine and serum exams, should be followed closely.

Early decontamination is important; do not wait for laboratory confirmation of ingestion. If ingestion is greater than 500 mg/kg and presents within an hour of ingestion, perform gastric lavage. Start activated charcoal as early as possible and every 3–4 hours until the salicylate level begins to drop. Fluid support should be used to maintain hydration and urine output.

Start sodium bicarbonate infusion to maintain a normal pH as well as to alkalinize the urine to a pH greater than 7.5.

Indications for dialysis include serum salicylate level greater than 700 mg/L, ongoing acidosis despite bicarbonate, seizures, coma, renal failure, pulmonary edema, or clinical deterioration.

Ongoing monitoring is critical. The patient should be kept in a monitored area and blood gas, serum salicylate levels, electrolytes, and urine pH should be repeated at least every 3 hours.

**Alcohols**    Mechanism of toxicity: Ethanol intoxication is most common, but be aware of other potential toxic alcohols. Table 12 describes the differences between the common toxic alcohols. Metabolism of alcohols usually involves two separate enzymes: alcohol dehydrogenase and aldehyde dehydrogenase. Ethanol and isopropanol (isopropyl alcohol) cause toxicity directly. With methanol and ethylene glycol, it is the metabolites produced by the enzyme alcohol dehydrogenase that causes toxicity, specifically glycolic acid, oxalic acid, formaldehyde, and formic acid.

Intoxication with alcohols produces a characteristic depression in the level of consciousness with alterations in mentation, speech, and gait. Respiratory and hemodynamic depression may be seen. The osmolar gap is often elevated.

Isopropyl alcohol is metabolized to acetone, which may further depress the level of consciousness and can often be picked up clinically. Both methanol and ethylene glycol produce metabolites that cause a significant metabolic acidosis with increased anion gap. Respiratory compensation may be seen.

**Approach**    Initial approach is ABCs. Decontamination is not effective due to the rapid absorption of alcohols. Gastric lavage may be effective if performed within 1 hour. Charcoal does not bind alcohols well, but may be indicated if there is a co-ingestion.

For ethanol and isopropyl alcohol ingestions, supportive care is required. Hemodialysis can effectively eliminate these two alcohols, but is rarely required.

For methanol and ethylene glycol ingestions, three levels of therapy need to be considered. Firstly, supportive care is required. Secondly, the accumulation of the toxic metabolites of both methanol and ethylene glycol can be minimized by

*Table 12*
## Alcohols Commonly Used for Intoxication

| Alcohol | Common Sources | Toxic Metabolite | Toxic Ingested Dose | Clinical Features |
|---------|----------------|------------------|---------------------|-------------------|
| Ethanol | Beer, wine, liquor | No | 0.7 g/kg of pure ethanol | Depressed CNS, gastrointestinal irritation |
| Isopropyl alcohol | Rubbing alcohol Cleaning solutions Antifreeze | No | 0.5 mL/kg of 70% isopropyl alcohol | Depressed CNS, gastrointestinal irritation, acetone breath, mild metabolic acidosis |
| Methanol | Windshield wiper fluid Paint remover Varnish Solvents Gasoline Antifreeze | Yes | 100 mg/kg | Depressed CNS, gastrointestinal irritation, metabolic acidosis, blindness, seizures, death |
| Ethylene glycol | Radiator fluid Antifreeze Windshield wiper fluid Adhesives Solvents | Yes | 1.5 mL/kg of 95% ethylene glycol | Depressed CNS, gastrointestinal irritation, metabolic acidosis, seizures, coma, cardiac dysrhythmias, renal failure, pulmonary and cerebral edema, death |

inhibiting their binding to alcohol dehydrogenase. This is accomplished with either ethanol or fomepizole. Last is the consideration of dialysis.

*Table 13*

**Indications for Administration of Ethanol or Fomepizole after Methanol or Ethylene Glycol Ingestion**

- Serum concentration of methanol or ethylene glycol >20 mg/dL

OR

- History of ingestion of methanol or ethylene glycol AND osmolal gap >10 mOsm/kg $H_2O$

OR

- Strong suspicion of ingestion of methanol or ethylene glycol AND at least two of the following:
  - Arterial pH <7.3
  - Serum bicarbonate <20 mmol/L
  - Osmala gap >10 mOsm/kg $H_2O$
  - Urinary oxylate crystals (ethylene glycol only)

Table 14 compares the use of ethanol and fomepizole. Severe metabolic acidosis can be corrected by administration of sodium bicarbonate.

Although administering ethanol or fomepizole can delay metabolism of the toxic alcohol, they do not assist with elimination. For this reason, in all cases where ethanol or fomepizole is required, consideration should be made regarding dialysis. Consultation with a toxicologist or a nephrologist may be necessary.

**Caustics**   Mechanism of injury: Caustics, whether acid or alkali, can cause both short- and long-term injury. Although both cause direct tissue necrosis, alkali exposures tend to cause more injury with worse prognosis. Tissues involved may include skin, eyes, mouth, pharynx, esophagus, gastrointestinal tract, trachea, and respiratory tract.

**Approach**   General approach is ABCs. Early assessment and monitoring of the airway is crucial. Remove all contaminated clothing early. Decontamination with charcoal is not effective. If caregivers use gastric lavage, care must be taken as gastroesophageal erosion may perforate with NG tube insertion.

Table 14

**Comparison of Ethanol and Fomepizole for the Treatment of Methanol and Ethylene Glycol Ingestions**

|  | **Ethanol** | **Fomepizole** |
|---|---|---|
| Dose | Loading dose: 750 mg/kg IV | Loading dose: 15 mg/kg IV (max 1 g) given over 30 minutes |
|  | Maintenance: 100–150 mg/kg/hour until serum concentration of methanol/ethylene glycol is less than 20 mg/dL | Maintenance doses: 10 mg/kg q12h IV for 4 doses, then 15 mg/kg q12h until serum concentration of methanol/ethylene glycol is less than 20 mg/dL |
|  | Maintenance dose increases to 175–250 mg/kg/hour during hemodialysis | Dose frequency changes to q4h during hemodialysis |
| Monitoring | Keep ethanol level around 100 mg/dL (20 mmol/L) | Glucose levels |
| Benefits | Inexpensive | Does not alter level of consciousness |
|  |  | Not a continuous infusion |
| Limitations | Continuous infusion Difficult to titrate dose Avoid if altered level of consciousness | Hypoglycemia |

Additionally, vomiting may result with NG insertion, causing further injury and increasing the risk of aspiration.

Exposures that are dermal or ocular should have copious irrigation with sterile water or normal saline. Any affected clothing should be removed. Topical pH can be measured with litmus paper. Once the pH has been normalized, a burn dressing should be applied. Do not attempt to neutralize the exposure, as an exothermic reaction will occur causing a thermal burn.

Consultation should be sought with ophthalmology or plastic surgery as appropriate. Respiratory burns, whether topical in the upper airway or inhalational, require urgent intervention as local edema, may rapidly progress, leading to airway obstruction. Therefore, early control of the airway should be established. Ingestion of caustic substances may result in erosive injury of the esophagus. These patients are at risk of short-term perforation and long-term strictures. Consultation with gastroenterology is required for endoscopy consideration.

**Carbon Monoxide**    Mechanism of toxicity: Carbon monoxide (CO) is produced from the combustion of hydrocarbon fuel and is a common poisoning in house fires. CO binds to hemoglobin with greater than 200 times the affinity of oxygen, thus decreasing the oxygen-carrying capacity of the blood and resulting in tissue hypoxia. CO has been described as the silent killer because it is a non-irritating, odorless, and colorless gas.

Co-oximitry is used to calculate the concentration of carboxyhemoglobin in the blood. General guidelines relating symptoms to specific levels do not correlate well. However, patients with less than 5% carboxyhemoglobin are often asymptomatic. At between 5 and 10%, the patient may begin to complain of shortness of breath and headaches. As the level climbs between 10 and 30%, the symptoms increase to include nausea, vomiting, and changes in level of consciousness. Patients with greater than 30% carboxyhemoglobin may present comatose, seizing, or with absent vital signs. The classic description of cherry-red lips seen with CO poisoning is common.

**Approach**    General approach is ABCs. In all cases of suspected CO poisoning, 100% oxygen via re-breather mask needs to be administered. The half-life of CO is greater than 4 hours on room air. This half-life is dropped to around 60 minutes with 100% oxygen. The elimination can be further enhanced with hyperbaric oxygen, although the use of this modality is limited by its availability. Hyperbaric oxygen has been shown to improve cognitive outcome following a CO exposure and should also be considered in high-risk patients such as small children and pregnant women. The local poison control center can assist further decision making regarding hyperbaric oxygen.

In all cases of CO poisoning, care should be taken to find any other potentially exposed victims.

## Cyclic Antidepressants

Mechanism of toxicity: Cyclic antidepressants inhibit neurotransmitter reuptake, leading to multiple clinical effects. Adrenergic excess leads to increased heart rate and blood pressure. Secondary catecholamine depletion can lead to a decrease in blood pressure with compensatory tachycardia. Blockade of fast sodium channels in the myocardium can lead to hypotension and conduction disturbances. Anticholinergic effects may heighten the hypotension and tachycardia as well as delay gastric transit. ECG changes may include sinus tachycardia, AV block, prolonged QRS, prolonged QT, and increased R wave in AVR.

Clinical features may include central nervous system depression including coma and seizures. In addition, an anticholinergic toxidrome may also be seen.

## Approach

Severity of ingestion cannot be predicted by early clinical findings and all ingestions should be taken seriously. Initial approach is ABCs. Routine ECGs should be done, and if prolongation of the QRS is noted, sodium bicarbonate should be administered.

## Narcotics and Benzodiazepines

Mechanism of toxicity: Narcotic and benzodiazepine overdoses are relatively common due to their common outpatient and inpatient use. Diagnosis is often based on history of exposure as well as clinical toxidrome. The predominant effects are depression of level of consciousness, depression of respiratory function, loss of airway protective reflexes, and cardiovascular depression.

## Approach

Initial approach is ABCs. Carefully evaluate the airway protective reflexes, the respiratory effort, and the circulation. The cornerstone of management is supportive care. The airway may require noninvasive support such as nasopharyngeal airway (nasal trumpet) or oral airway. In some cases, if there is inadequate airway protection, an endotracheal tube may be required. Inadequate respiratory effort can be supported with assisted ventilation. Inadequate circulation usually responds to volume resuscitation.

For narcotic intoxications, the antidote naloxone should be given. Remember that the half-life of naloxone is often shorter than the narcotic, and therefore the patient needs adequate monitoring and further naloxone doses may be required. The benzodiazepine antidote, flumazenil, is rarely used as it can precipitate seizures.

**Lead**   Mechanism of toxicity: Chronic lead intoxication in children, although less commonplace, still results from exposure to such environmental sources as peeling paint and contaminated dirt. A full discussion of chronic lead exposure is beyond the scope of this chapter. Acute exposure to lead, usually through the oral route, is potentially life threatening. Symptoms of an acute exposure may include signs of encephalitis, irritability, headache, ataxia, seizures, altered level of consciousness, hypertension, constipation, and vomiting. Laboratory investigation may reveal anemia, evidence of nephropathy, or evidence of hepatitis.

**Approach**   Initial approach is ABCs. Supportive care for altered level of consciousness and seizures may be required. Initial investigations should include serum lead, zinc protoporphyrin, complete blood count with smear as well as hepatic and renal function tests. Radiographs may reveal radio-opaque ingested lead. Serum lead levels above 10 mcg/dL indicate lead poisoning. Lead is not well absorbed by charcoal. Gastric lavage can be used to decontaminate acute intoxications. Whole bowel irrigation is indicated if there is concern about any remaining lead in the gastrointestinal tract. Chelation agents such as dimercaprol and DMSA can be used to enhance elimination. These agents should be given with the assistance of a poison control center.

**Iron**   Mechanism of toxicity: Pediatric exposures to iron are potentially life threatening. Gastrointestinal ingestion of iron causes significant mucosal erosion leading to hemorrhage and shock. Iron interferes with mitochondrial activity, leading to metabolic acidosis. Additionally, capillary permeability is affected, leading to third spacing of fluid, and propagating shock. Elevated serum iron can lead to myocardial injury, hepatic necrosis, as well as injury to the lungs, pancreas, and kidneys. The four clinical stages of acute iron toxicity are outlined in Table 15. Ingestions of less than 20 mg/kg have a low risk of toxicity. Ingestions between 20 and 60 mg/kg pose a moderate risk and ingestions greater than 60 mg/kg have a high risk of toxicity.

**Approach**    Initial evaluation of ABCs is crucial. Treatment of shock and supportive care are the cornerstone. Initial investigations should include CBC, serum iron, baseline liver and renal function tests, coagulation studies, blood gas, electrolytes, and glucose. Serum iron levels greater than 350 mcg/dL correlate with toxicity. Radiographs of the abdomen may reveal iron tablets.

Decontamination via gastric lavage with a large-bore NG tube is best done within an hour of ingestion. There is some evidence that activated charcoal may be beneficial. Further decontamination with whole bowel irrigation is indicated in the absence of contraindications. Elimination

Table 15
**The Clinical Stages of Iron Toxicity**

| Stage | Timing | Clinical Features |
|-------|--------|-------------------|
| 1 | 0–3 hours | • Gastrointestinal injury |
| | | • Nausea, vomiting (+/- blood), diarrhea (+/- blood), abdominal pain |
| | | • Bleeding may result in shock |
| 2 | 12 hours | • Temporary clinical improvement |
| 3 | 24–48 hours | • Systemic toxicity |
| | | • Altered level of consciousness, seizures, shock, metabolic acidosis, hepatic and renal injury |
| 4 | >2 weeks | • Gastrointestinal scarring with possible strictures |

strategies include the use of chelating agents such as deferoxamine. Consultation with a local poison control center is indicated.

**Cocaine** Mechanism of toxicity: Cocaine can be taken by several routes including inhalation (smoked), intra-nasal mucosa (snorted), intravenous, and intramuscular. The systemic effects of cocaine can be increased by ethanol. The effects of cocaine are multiple. Tachycardia, hypertension, and hyperthermia are common. Cardiac effects can include cardiac ischemia, dysrhythmias, myocarditis, coronary artery spasm, and sudden death. Pulmonary complications include bronchoconstriction, airway injury, pneumothorax, pulmonary hemorrhage or infarct, non-cardiogenic pulmonary edema, pneumonitis, and respiratory depression. Central nervous system effects include euphoria, agitation, delerium, seizures, and stroke. Gastrointestinal effects include decreased motility, gastrointestinal ischemia, and ulceration. Other effects include thrombus formation, aortic dissection, and splenic infarction.

**Approach** Patients who may have cocaine intoxication require a careful assessment of ABCs. Cardiorespiratory monitoring is required. An electrocardiogram is required to assess for ischemic changes or dysrhythmias. Supportive care is essential as the child may develop altered level of consciousness, seizures, and cardiac changes. Initial management of hypertension or agitation is best achieved with benzodiazepines. There has been some discussion about the role of beta-blockers for the treatment of hypertension secondary to cocaine use. These should be administered only in consultation with a poison control center as alpha-blocking agents may be indicated.

## Disposition

As for any clinical presentation, questions arise as to when it is safe to send a child home or out of the PICU. Although it is not possible to describe discharge criteria for all toxic exposures, several guidelines for consideration prior to discharge will be described. Table 16 outlines three specific areas to consider. Additional specific recommendations can be obtained from the local poison control center.

Table 16
## Issues to Consider Prior to Discharge

| Toxic Exposure | Patient | Social Situation |
|---|---|---|
| • Substance<br>• Amount of exposure<br>• Half-life<br>• Peak effect<br>• Immediate clinical manifestations<br>• Delayed clinical manifestations | • Age<br>• Signs and symptoms of exposure<br>• Concurrent medical issues<br>• Interactions with other medications taken | • Ability of family to monitor patient at home<br>• Safety of home environment<br>• For intentional exposures, consideration of psychiatric referral<br>• Social work referral<br>• Children's aid/ equivalent agency |

Table 17
## Important Points and Common Pitfalls

Always assume the worst case scenario in terms of amount of exposure (mg/kg).

Never forget the possibility of head trauma in a patient who presents with altered level of consciousness. Confirmation of intoxication does not rule out intracranial injury, but increases the risk!

Monitor and reassess frequently.

Be careful if inserting a gastric tube in caustic ingestions. You may convert a partial thickness esophageal erosion to full thickness!

Don't wait until you have the results of a 4- or 6-hour drug level before starting decontamination. Charcoal works best when given early!

Body packers can present with multiple well-wrapped packets of drugs. They have often "packed for a trip." Body stuffers can present with less amounts taken, but wrapped improperly. They have often stuffed to hide evidence.

The effects of chronic intoxications may be significant at lower serum levels than acute intoxications.

Some medications may have more than one active ingredient. Always look up the composition of any substance (ie, over-the-counter decongestants).

Watch out for long-acting or sustained-release medications. Their effects may be seen later than expected.

Be careful when a patient has no bowel sounds. There may be delayed absorption!

Be wary of giving antidotes that may precipitate seizures or withdrawal.

Watch out for "one pill kills" intoxications.

# References

Goldfrank L, Flomenbaum N, Lewin N, et al. Toxicologic emergencies, 8th edition. McGraw-Hill: New York, 2006.

Krenzelok EP, McGuigan M, Lheur P. Position statement: ipecac syrup. American Academy of Clinical Toxicology; European Association of Poisons Centres and Clinical Toxicologists. J Toxicol Clin Toxicol 1997;35:699–709.

Vale JA. Position statement: gastric lavage. American Academy of Clinical Toxicology; European Association of Poisons Centres and Clinical Toxicologists. J Toxicol Clin Toxicol 2004;42(7):933–43.

Chyka PA, Seger D. Position statement: single-dose activated charcoal. American Academy of Clinical Toxicology; European Association of Poisons Centres and Clinical Toxicologists. J Toxicol Clin Toxicol 1997;35:721–41.

Barceloux D, McGuigan M, Hartigan-Go K. Position statement: cathartics. American Academy of Clinical Toxicology; European Association of Poisons Centres and Clinical Toxicologists. J Toxicol Clin Toxicol 1997;35:743–52.

Tenenbein M. Position statement: whole bowel irrigation. American Academy of Clinical Toxicology; European Association of Poisons Centres and Clinical Toxicologists. J Toxicol Clin Toxicol 1997;35:753–62.

Vale JA, Krenzelok EP, Barceloux. Position statement and practice guidelines on the use of multi-dose activated charcoal in the treatment of acute poisoning. J Toxicol Clin Toxicol 1999;37:731–51.

Olson KR editor. Poisoning & drug overdose, 3rd edition. Stamford: Appleton & Lange. 1999, pp. 345–46.

Borkan SC. Extracorporeal therapies for acute intoxications. Crit Care Clin 2002;18: 393–420.

American Academy of Pediatrics, Committee on Drugs. Acetaminophen toxicity in children. Pediatrics 2001;108:1020–4.

Brok J, Buckley N, Gluud C. Interventions for paracetamol (acetaminophen) overdoses (Cochrane Review). In: The Cochrane Library, Issue 4, 2002. Oxford: Update Software.

Dargan PI, Wallace CI, Jones AL. An evidence based flowchart to guide the management of acute salicylate (aspirin) overdose. Emerg Med J 2002;19: 206–9.

Riordan M, Rylance G, Berry K. Poisoning in children 2: painkillers. Arch Dis Child 2002;87:397–9.

Mokhlesi B, Leikin JB, Murray P, Corbridge TC. Adult toxicology in critical care. Part II: specific poisonings. Chest 2003;123:897–922.

Weaver LK, et al. Hyperbaric oxygen for acute carbon monoxide poisoning. NEJM 2002;347(14):1057–67.

Harrigan RA, Brady WJ. ECG abnormalities in trycyclic antidepressant ingestion. Am J Emerg Med 1999;17:387–93.

Papanikolaou NC et al. Lead toxicity update. A brief review. Med Sci Monit 2005;11(10):RA329–36.

VanArsdale JL, et al. Lead poisoning from a toy necklace. Pediatrics 2004;114:1096–9.

Baranwal AK, Singhi SC. Acute iron poisoning: management guidelines. Indian Pediatrics 2003;40:534–40.

Shanti CM, Lucas CE. Cocaine and the critical care challenge. Crit Care Med 2003;31:1851–9.

Litovitz TL. 2001 Annual report of the American Association of Poison Control Centers Toxic Exposure Surveillance System. Am J Emerg Med 2002; 2 (5):391–452.

Matteucci MJ. One pill can kill: assessing the potential for fatal poisonings in children. Pediatric Annals 2005;34:964–8.

Michael JB, Sztajnkrycer MD. Deadly pediatric poisons: nine common agents that kill at low doses. Emerg Med Clin North Am 2004;22:1019–50.

Riordan M, Rylance G, Berry K. Poisoning in children 1: general management. Arch Dis Child 2002;87:392–6.

Ford MD, Delaney KA, Ling LJ, Erickson T. Clinical Toxicology. Philadelphia: W.B. Saunders Company; 2001, pp. 31–2.

Poisoning & Drug Overdose, 3rd edition. Olson KR, ed. Stamford: Appleton & Lange; 1999, p. 31.

Clinical policy for the initial approach to patients presenting with acute toxic ingestion or dermal or inhalation exposure. American College of Emergency Physicians: Clinical policy for the initial approach to patients presenting with acute toxic ingestion or dermal or inhalation exposure. Ann Emerg Med June 1999;33:735–61.

Linden CH, Rumack BH. Acetaminophen overdose. Emerg Med Clin North Am 1984;2:103–19.

Poisoning & Drug Overdose, 3rd ed. Olson KR, ed. Stamford: Appleton & Lange; 1999, p. 335.

CPS: Compendium of pharmaceuticals and specialties, 36th ed. Canadian Pharmacists Association. 2001:980–82.

Poisoning & Drug Overdose, 3rd ed. Olson KR, ed. Stamford: Appleton & Lange; 1999, pp. 162, 166, 197, 219.

Tenenbein M. Recent advancements in pediatric toxicology. Pediatr Clin North Am 1999;46:1179–88.

Barceloux DG, Krenzelok EP, Olson K, Watson W. American Academy of Clinical Toxicology practice guidelines on the treatment of ethylene glycol poisoning. J Toxicol Clin Toxicol 1999;37:537–60.

Barceloux DG, Bond GR, Krenzelok EP, et al. The American Academy of Clinical Toxicology ad hoc committee on the treatment guidelines for methanol poisoning: American Academy of Clinical Toxicology practice guidelines on the treatment of methanol poisoning. J Toxicol Clin Toxicol 2002;40:415–46.

Poisoning & Drug Overdose, 3rd ed. Olson KR, ed. Stamford: Appleton & Lange; 1999, pp. 367–71.

Tenenbein M. Recent advancements in pediatric toxicology. Pediatr Clin North Am 1999;46:1179–88.

# C. Formulary

## Mark Duffett

## Comparative Drug Charts

*Table I*
**Medications for Intubation**

| | Drug | Dose | Onset of Action | Comments |
|---|---|---|---|---|
| Sedatives | midazolam | 0.1–0.25 mg/kg | 1–2 min | ↓BP if hypovolemic, minimal effect on ICP |
| | propofol | 1–2 mg/kg | < 1 min | ↓ICP, ↓BP |
| | thiopental | 2–5 mg/kg | < 1 min | ↓ICP, ↓BP |
| | etomidate | 0.2–0.4 mg/kg | 1 min | ↓ICP, minimal effect on BP |
| Analgesics | morphine | 0.2 mg/kg | 2–5 min | Minimal effect on ICP, may ↓BP |
| | fentanyl | 2–5 microgram/kg | 1 min | Minimal effect on ICP and BP |
| | remifentanil | 2–4 microgram/kg | < 1 min | Duration of action 3–10 min |
| Sedative/ Analgesic | ketamine | 1–2 mg/kg | 1–2 min | bronchodilation, ↑ICP, little effect on BP |
| Paralytics | rocuronium | 1 mg/kg | 45–90 sec | Duration of action: 30–60 min |
| | vecuronium | 0.2 mg/kg | 0.5–2 min | Duration of action: 30–60 min |
| | succinylcholine | 1–2 mg/kg | 45–60 sec | Duration of action: < 10 min |
| Adjuvants | atropine | 0.02 mg/kg | 1–2 min | minimum 0.1, maximum 1 mg |
| | lidocaine | 2 mg/kg | 5 min | |

*Table 2*
## Comparison of Inotropes and Vasopressors

| | Receptor Specificity | | | | SVR | Inotropic Effects | Heart Rate |
|---|---|---|---|---|---|---|---|
| | $\alpha$ | $\beta_1$ | $\beta_2$ | $V_1$* | | | |
| Dopamine | high dose | +++ | + | − | ↑ (high dose) | ++ | ↑↑ |
| Dobutamine | + | +++ | ++ | − | ↓ | +++ | ↑ |
| Epinephrine | +++ | +++ | + | − | ↑ | ++ | ↑↑ |
| Milrinone** | − | − | − | − | ↓ | +++ | - |
| Norepinephrine | +++ | ++ | − | − | ↑↑ | + | ↑ |
| Phenylephrine | +++ | − | − | − | ↑↑ | − | - |
| Vasopressin | − | − | − | +++ | ↑↑ | − | - |

*Vasopressin receptor type 1.

**Milrinone is a phosphodiesterase inhibitor.

*Table 3*
## Approximate Equivalent Doses of Opioid Analgesics

| | Oral Dose | Parenteral Dose |
|---|---|---|
| Codeine | 200 mg | 120 mg |
| Fentanyl | N/A | 100 micrograms |
| Hydromorphone | 4 mg | 2 mg |
| Meperidine | 300 mg | 75 mg |
| Morphine | 20 mg | 10 mg |

*Table 4*
## Approximate Equivalent Doses of Corticosteroids

| | Equivalent Dose (mg) |
|---|---|
| Dexamethasone | 0.75 |
| Hydrocortisone | 20 |
| Methylprednisolone | 4 |
| Prednisone | 5 |
| Prednisolone | 5 |

*Table 5*
## Comparison of IV Solutions

| IV Solution | Sodium (mEq/L) | Dextrose (g/L) | Osmolarity (mOsm/L) |
|---|---|---|---|
| Sodium chloride 0.45% | 77 | 0 | 154 |
| Sodium chloride 0.9% | 154 | 0 | 308 |
| Sodium chloride 3% | 513 | 0 | 1030 |
| Dextrose 5% | 0 | 50 | 250 |
| Dextrose 5% sodium chloride 0.2% | 39 | 50 | 320 |
| Dextrose 5% sodium chloride 0.45% | 77 | 50 | 405 |
| Dextrose 5% sodium chloride 0.9% | 154 | 50 | 560 |
| Dextrose 10% | 0 | 100 | 505 |
| Dextrose 10% sodium chloride 0.2% | 39 | 100 | 575 |
| Dextrose 10% sodium chloride 0.45 | 77 | 100 | 660 |
| Dextrose 10% sodium chloride 0.9% | 154 | 100 | 813 |
| Dextrose 3.3% sodium chloride 0.3% | 51 | 33 | 273 |
| Lactated Ringer's[†] | 130 | 0 | 273 |

[†]Also contains calcium 1.5 mmol/L, potassium 4 mEq/L, and lactate 28 mmol/L

## Medications

### Acetaminophen

Analgesic and antipyretic
PO/PR: 40–60 mg/kg/DAY ÷ q4–6h (maximum 60 mg/kg or 4 g/DAY).

A single dose greater than 150 mg/kg is generally considered to be toxic, but toxicity has been reported at lower doses (90–120 mg/kg/DAY). Rectal absorption may be erratic.

| Weight (kg) | Single Dose (mg) |
|---|---|
| 2.5–3.9 | 40 |
| 4.0–5.4 | 60 |
| 5.5–7.9 | 80 |
| 8.0–10.9 | 120 |
| 11.0–15.9 | 160 |
| 16.0–21.9 | 240 |
| 22.0–26.9 | 320 |
| 27.0–31.9 | 400 |
| 32.0–43.9 | 480 |
| 44–over | 650 |

## Acetazolamide

Carbonic anhydrase inhibitor diuretic.
Diuretic:

PO: 5–10 mg/kg/DAY ÷ q8–24h (maximum 1 g/DAY).
    Increases urinary bicarbonate loss and alkalinizes urine.

## Acetylcysteine

Antidote for acetaminophen overdose:

IV: Total dose 300 mg/kg IV over 21 hours:
    150 mg/kg over 15–60 minutes, then:
    50 mg/kg over 4 hours (12.5 mg/kg/h), then:
    100 mg/kg over 16 hours (6.25 mg/kg/h)
    Alternative regimens include:
    140 mg/kg followed by 70 mg/kg q4h for 12 doses
PO: 140 mg/kg, then 70 mg/kg q4h for 17 doses. Repeat dose if
emesis occurs within 1 hour.
Mucolytic:

INH: Infants: 1–2 mL of 20% solution nebulized q6–8h
    Children: 3–5 mL of 20% solution nebulized q6–8h
    Adolescents: 5–10 mL of 20% solution nebulized q6–8h

    Longer courses of therapy may be indicated if there is
delayed presentation or slow resolution of liver function

abnormalities. If symptoms of histamine release and brochospasm occur, hold infusion, give antihistamines +/− corticosteroids and brochodilators, and then restart infusion. Pretreatment with a bronchodilator is usually recommended prior to inhaled therapy.

## Acetylsalicylic Acid

Antiplatelet:

PO: 5 mg/kg/DOSE q24h. Minimum 20 mg, usual maximum 80 or 325 mg.

Kawasaki disease:

PO: 80–100 mg/kg/DAY ÷ q6h; reduce dose to 3–5 mg/kg q24h once fever resolves.
   Supplied as 80-mg chewable tablets and 325 and 650 mg tablets.

## ACTH

See Cosyntropin.

## Activated Charcoal

See Charcoal.

## Acyclovir

Antiviral.
Herpes simplex encephalitis:

IV: 45 mg/kg/DAY ÷ q8h (60 mg/kg/DAY has been used in infants).

Other herpes simplex infections:

IV: 15–30 mg/kg/DAY ÷ q8h

Varicella (severe) or in immunocompromised hosts:

IV: 30–45 mg/kg/DAY ÷ q8h, switch to PO when lesions crusted.
PO: 80 mg/kg/DAY ÷ qid (maximum 800 mg/DOSE).
   Ensure adequate urine output. Adjust dosing interval in renal impairment.

## Adenosine

Antiarrhythmic.

Treatment of SVT:

IV: 0.1 mg/kg bolus (maximum 6 mg); if no response in 2 minutes: 0.2 mg/kg bolus (maximum 12 mg).

Not effective for atrial fibrillation/flutter or ventricular fibrillation. Adverse effects such as dyspnea, arrhythmias, bradycardia, flushing, and sinus and AV block are very common but are usually transient due to short (10 seconds) half-life of drug. Give rapid IV bolus followed by rapid NS flush.

## Albuterol

See Salbutamol.

## Alprostadil

Prostaglandin $E_1$.

Maintenance of flow through patent ductus arteriosus:

IV: Initially 0.05 microgram/kg/min; use lowest effective dose; 0.01–0.1 microgram/kg/min has been used.

May cause apnea; be prepared to intubate. Most effective in infants less than 96 hours of age.

## Alteplase

Thrombolytic.

Unblocking of occluded catheters:

Intracatheter: Instill 1 mg/mL solution into occluded lumen. Maximum volume equal to the internal volume of catheter lumen, to maximum of 2 mL. Leave in place for 30 min to 2 h; then aspirate solution.

Do not infuse. May repeat once if ineffective.

## Amiloride

Potassium-sparing diuretic.
PO: 0.625 mg/kg q24h (usual maximum 10 mg/DOSE)

# Amikacin

Aminoglycoside antibiotic.
IV: 15–20 mg/kg/DAY ÷ q12–24h.

Adjust dosing interval in renal impairment. Ototoxicity and nephrotoxicity may occur; consider monitoring trough levels (<5–10 mg/L) in patients at risk for nephrotoxicity, septic shock, concurrent nephrotoxins, fluctuating renal function, or extended treatment courses. May potentiate muscle weakness with neuromuscular blockers. Reserved for gram negative organisms with documented resistance to other aminoglycosides.

# Aminocaproic Acid

Fibrinolysis inhibitor.

Treatment of excessive bleeding due to hyperfibrinolysis:

IV: 50–100 mg/kg, then 30–50 mg/kg/h until bleeding stops (maximum 1 g/h).

Rapid IV injection may cause hypotension, bradycardia, arrhythmias. Give loading dose over 1 hour.

# Aminophylline

Bronchodilator.

Acute bronchospasm:

IV: 6 mg/kg, then infusion (based on ideal body weight):

| | |
|---|---|
| 2–6 months: | 0.4–0.5 mg/kg/h |
| 6–11 months: | 0.6–0.7 mg/kg/h |
| 1–12 years: | 0.8–1 mg/kg/h |
| >12 years | 0.7 mg/kg/h |

No longer first line for treatment of asthma, high dose inhaled/IV $\beta_2$ agonists and corticosteroids are preferred. Dose adjustments are required in CHF, liver dysfunction, multisystem organ failure, shock, and in smokers. Aminophylline has many drug interactions, including ciprofloxacin, clarithromycin, erythromycin, check specialized references before use. Draw level 30 minutes after end of bolus infusion and 12–24 hours after initiation of continuous infusion.

Target serum level is 10–15 mg/L (55–83 micromol/mL).

## Amiodarone

Antiarrhythmic.
IV: 5 mg/kg loading dose, then 5–15 microgram/kg/min.

Give loading dose over 20–60 minutes for perfusing rhythms or rapid bolus for VF. Rapid IV boluses are limited to the treatment of VF because of the associated hypotension, which may respond to reducing the infusion rate. Heart block requiring pacing has occurred. Do not use in cardiogenic shock, severe sinus node dysfunction, sinus bradycardia, 2nd- and 3rd-degree AV block. Central line required for concentrations >2 mg/mL.

## Amlodipine

Calcium channel blocker antihypertensive.
PO: 0.1–0.3 mg/kg q24h (usual maximum 10 mg/DAY)

## Amoxicillin

Penicillin derivative oral antibiotic.
PO: 25–50 mg/kg/DAY ÷ q8h (maximum 1 g/DOSE).

For severe infections and for suspected penicillin resistant *S. pneumoniae* doses of up to 100 mg/kg/DAY have been tolerated (maximum 1 g/DOSE). Use ampicillin if IV therapy is required.

## Amoxicillin/Clavulanic Acid

Penicillin derivative antibiotic and beta-lactamase inhibitor.
PO: 25–40 mg/kg/DAY of amoxicillin component ÷ q8h (maximum 500 mg/DOSE).

Active against gram positive, gram negative, and anaerobic organisms.

## Amphotericin B

(Amphotericin B Deoxycholate, Conventional
Amphotericin B)
Antifungal.
IV: 0.6–1 mg/kg/DOSE q24h.

For *Candida species* use 0.6–0.8 mg/kg/DAY and 1 mg/kg/DAY for *Aspergillus species*. Traditionally give ½ dose on first day and increase to full dose over 1–2 days, but may give full dose on first day. Consider hydration (10 mL/kg of normal saline) pre-amphotericin to reduce the risk of nephrotoxicity. Commonly causes nephrotoxicity, hypokalemia, and hypomagnesemia. Not compatible with any saline solutions, dilute to 0.1 mg/mL or less in dextrose solutions and infuse over 2–6 hours.

## Amphotericin B Lipid Complex (Abelcet®)

Liposomal Amphotericin B (AmBisome®)
Antifungal (lipid formulations of amphotericin B).
IV: 3–5 mg/kg q24h.

Consider using these in renal insufficiency, if nephrotoxicity develops while on standard Amphotericin B or with clinical failure with alternate agents. These lipid formulations are better tolerated but are very costly.

## Ampicillin

Penicillin derivative antibiotic.

Meningitis:

IV: 200 mg/kg/DAY ÷ q6h (maximum 2 g/DOSE).

Other infections:

IV: 100–200 mg/kg/DAY ÷ q6h (maximum 2 g/DOSE).

Doses of 400 mg/kg/DAY have been used for meningitis. Adjust dosing interval in renal impairment. Use amoxicillin if oral therapy is required.

## Arginine

Treatment of urea cycle disorders.

OTC or CPS deficiency:

IV: 0.2 g/kg as a loading dose; then 0.2 g/kg/DAY as a continuous infusion.

ASL or ASS deficiency:

IV: 0.6 g/kg as a loading dose; then 0.6 g/kg/DAY as a continuous infusion.

## ASA, Aspirin

See Acetylsalicylic acid.

## Atracurium

Non-depolarizing neuromuscular blocking agent.

IV: 0.4 mg/kg q30min prn or 0.4 mg/kg; then 2–15 microgram/kg/min.

Does not require dosage modification in renal or hepatic impairment. Regular sedation, analgesia, and ocular lubrication required. Monitor depth of paralysis using peripheral nerve stimulation when using infusions (target 1–2 twitches out of 4). Onset of action is within 2 minutes, duration of action is 30–40 minutes. Prolonged weakness may occur, especially when corticosteroids are used concurrently with non-depolarizing neuromuscular blocking agents.

## Atropine

Vagolytic.

Bradycardia:

IV: 0.02 mg/kg/DOSE, minimum dose: 0.1 mg, maximum dose: 0.5 mg for child, 1 mg for adolescent.

If giving via ETT, increase IV dose 2–10 fold and dilute to 3–5 mL with NS. Follow with several positive pressure breaths.

## Azathioprine

Immunosupressant.

Dose varies with indication and the individual protocol, but usually:

PO/IV: 1–5 mg/kg/DOSE q24h.

Dose adjustment required in renal dysfunction.

## Azithromycin

Azolide antibiotic (related to the macrolides).
PO/IV: 10 mg/kg (maximum 500 mg) once; then 5 mg/kg (maximum 250 mg) q24h × 4. For serious infections may give 10 mg/kg q24h.

Chlamydial infection (non-gonococcal urethritis or cervicitis):

PO: 1 g once (minimum weight 45 kg).

## Budesonide

Inhaled corticosteroid.
NEB: 0.25–1 mg bid via nebulizer

## Caffeine

Respiratory stimulant.

Apnea of prematurity:

PO/IV: 10–20 mg/kg of caffeine citrate (equivalent to 5–10 mg/kg of caffeine base) as a loading dose then: 5 mg/kg of caffeine citrate (2.5 mg/kg of caffeine base) q24h.

## Calcium

Electrolyte.
Treatment of hypocalcemia, hyperkalemia, hypermagnesemia, and calcium channel antagonist overdose. These doses are suggested starting doses; increase and repeat as required.

Calcium gluconate:

IV: 50–100 mg of calcium gluconate/kg/DOSE (0.5–1 mL/kg/DOSE)

or

IV: Add 1 g of calcium gluconate to a total of 50 mL NS (0.046 mmol/mL) and give 0.05-0.1 mmol/kg/h (1–2 mL/kg/h), adjust rate q4h

Calcium chloride:

IV: 10–20 mg of calcium chloride/kg/DOSE (0.1–0.2 mL/kg/DOSE)

## Calcium Polystyrene Sulfonate

See Cation Exchange Resins.

|  | **Elemental Calcium** | | |
|---|---|---|---|
| Calcium gluconate 10% (100 mg/mL) | 9 mg/mL | 0.45 mEq/mL | 0.23 mmol/mL |
| Calcium chloride 10% (100 mg/mL) | 27.2 mg/mL | 1.4 mEq/mL | 0.7 mmol/mL |

If treating asymptomatic hypocalcemia, infuse dose over at least 1 hour.

# Calcium Resonium

See Cation Exchange Resins.

# Calfactant

Bovine lung surfactant.
Pediatric ALI/ARDS
Intratracheal: $\geq$10 kg: 80 mg/m$^2$/DOSE
<10 kg: 3 mL/kg/DOSE
Dose may be repeated in 12 hours if oxygenation does not improve.

# Captopril

Angiotensin converting enzyme inhibitor.
PO: 0.1–0.3 mg/kg/DOSE q8h initially, increase dose based on response (usual maximum 6 mg/kg/DAY or 200 mg/DAY).

Monitor blood pressure closely after first dose: may cause profound hypotension.

# Carbamazepine

Anticonvulsant.
PO: 10–20 mg/kg/DAY initially, usual maintenance dose is 20–30 mg/kg/DAY; divide daily dose ÷ q8–12h.

Serum trough concentration target is 17–51 micromol/L (4–12 microgram/mL).

# Carnitine

Treatment of carnitine deficiency:

Maintenance:

PO/IV: 50–100 mg/kg/DAY ÷ q6–12h (maximum 300 mg/kg/DAY).

Metabolic crisis:

PO/IV: Loading dose of 50–100 mg/kg (maximum 300 mg/kg); then 50–100 mg/kg/DAY (maximum 300 mg/kg/DAY) as a continuous infusion or ÷ q4–6h.

# Caspofungin

Antifungal.

IV: 70 mg/m$^2$ (maximum 70 mg); then 50 mg/m$^2$ (maximum 50 mg) q24h
    Dosage adjustment may be required hepatic impairment. Caspofungin has many drug interactions including cyclosporine, carbamazepine, dexamethasone, and phenytoin; check specialized references before use.

## Cation Exchange Resins

Treatment for non-acute hyperkalemia.

Sodium or calcium polystyrene sulfonate:

PO/PR: 0.5–1 g/kg/DOSE may be repeated q4–6h prn (usual maximum 30–60 g/DOSE)
    Give in orally water or juice; do mix with fruit juices with high potassium content such as orange juice. Mix in water for rectal administration and retain in colon for up to several hours, and for a minimum of 30–60 minutes.

## Cefazolin

First generation cephalosporin.
IV: 75–150 mg/kg/DAY ÷ q8h (maximum 6 g/DAY).
    Adjust dosing interval in renal impairment.

## Cefepime

Fourth generation cephalosporin.
IV: 150 mg/kg/DAY ÷ q8h (maximum 6 g/DAY).
    Adjust dosing interval in renal impairment. Active against *Pseudomonas aeruginosa*.

## Cefixime

Oral third generation cephalosporin.
PO: 8 mg/kg/DAY ÷ q12–24h (maximum 400 mg/DAY)

Uncomplicated cervical/urethral gonorrhea:

PO: 400 mg once (minimum weight 45 kg).
    Adjust dose in renal impairment. Not active against *Pseudomonas aeruginosa* or *Staphylococcus aureus*.

## Cefotaxime

Third generation cephalosporin.

Meningitis:

IV: 200 mg/kg/DAY ÷ q6h (maximum 8 g/DAY).

Other infections:

IV: 100–200 mg/kg/DAY ÷ q8h (maximum 6 g/DAY).
     Adjust dosing interval in renal impairment. Not active against *Pseudomonas aeruginosa*.

## Cefotetan

Second generation cephalosporin.
IV: 60 mg/kg/DAY ÷ q12h (maximum 6 g/DAY).
     Adjust dosing interval in renal impairment. Active against anaerobic organisms.

## Cefoxitin

Second generation cephalosporin.
IV: 80–160 mg/kg/DAY ÷ q8h (maximum 8 g/DAY).
     Adjust dosing interval in renal impairment. Active against anaerobic organisms.

## Cefprozil

Oral second generation cephalosporin.
PO: 30 mg/kg/DAY ÷ q12h (maximum 1 g/DAY).
     Adjust dose in severe renal impairment.

## Ceftazidime

Third generation cephalosporin.
IV: 75–150 mg/kg/DAY ÷ q8h (maximum 6 g/DAY).
     Adjust dosing interval in renal impairment. Active against *Pseudomonas aeruginosa*.

## Ceftriaxone

Third generation cephalosporin.

Meningitis:

IV/IM: 50 mg/kg/DOSE q12h (maximum 2 g/DOSE).

Other infections:

IV/IM: 50–75 mg/kg q24h (maximum 2 g/DAY).
     No dosage adjustment required in renal impairment. Not active against *Pseudomonas aeruginosa*.

## Cefuroxime

Second generation cephalosporin.

Epiglottitis/facial cellulitis:

IV: 150 mg/kg/DAY ÷ q8h (maximum 1.5 g/DOSE).

Other infections:

IV: 75–150 mg/kg/DAY ÷ q8h (usual maximum dose is 750 mg/DOSE).
PO: 20–30 mg/kg/DAY ÷ bid (maximum 1 g/DAY).
  Adjust dosing interval in renal impairment.

## Cephalexin

First generation cephalosporin.
PO: 25–50 mg/kg/DAY ÷ qid, for severe infections can give 100 mg/kg/DAY (maximum 4 g/DAY).
  Adjust dosing interval in renal impairment.

## Charcoal

Adsorbent used in toxic ingestions.
PO: 1–2 g/kg once.
PO: Multiple dose therapy 0.5 g/kg q4–6h.
  Give via NG if necessary, consider antiemetics.

## Chloral Hydrate

Sedative and hypnotic.

Procedural Sedation:

PO/PR: 80 mg/kg, may repeat half dose if no effect in 30 min (maximum 2 g/DOSE).

Sedation:

PO/PR: 25–50 mg/kg/DOSE (maximum 500 mg q6h or 1 g hs).
  Avoid in liver dysfunction. Tolerance develops and withdrawal may occur after long-term use. For PR use dilute syrup with water.

## Chlorothiazide

Thiazide diuretic
PO: 20 mg/kg/DAY ÷ q12h (maximum 1 g/DAY)
IV: 4 mg/kg/DAY ÷ q12h.

# Ciprofloxacin

Quinolone antibiotic.
IV/PO: 20–30 mg/kg/DAY ÷ q12h (maximum 400 mg/DOSE IV or 750 mg/DOSE PO).

Excellent oral absorption, use IV only if PO contraindicated. Feeds, formula, calcium, magnesium, iron, antacids and sulcralfate reduce absorption, hold feeds for 1 hour before and 2 hours after dose. Adjust dosing interval in renal impairment. Quinolones are not generally considered to be first line drugs in pediatrics, but ciprofloxacin has been used safely in children. Active against *Pseudomonas aeruginosa*.

# Cisatracurium

Non-depolarizing neuromuscular blocking agent.
IV: 0.1 mg/kg then 0.03 mg/kg prn or 0.1 mg/kg then 1–3 microgram/kg/min (range 0.5–10 microgram/kg/min).

Does not require dosage modification in renal or hepatic impairment. Regular sedation, analgesia and ocular lubrication required. Monitor depth of paralysis using peripheral nerve stimulation when using infusions (target 1–2 twitches out of 4). Onset of action within 2–3 min, duration of action is 30–40 min. Prolonged weakness may occur, especially when corticosteroids are used concurrently with non-depolarizing neuromuscular blocking agents.

# Clarithromycin

Macrolide antibiotic.
PO: 15 mg/kg/DAY ÷ q12h (maximum 1 g/DAY).

Drug interactions include theophylline, carbamazepine, cisapride, digoxin, cyclosporine, tacrolimus, check specialized references before use. Adjust dose in severe renal impairment.

# Clindamycin

Antibiotic.
IV: 30–40 mg/kg/DAY ÷ q8h (maximum 900 mg/DOSE).
PO: 10–20 mg/kg/DAY ÷ q6–8h (maximum 450 mg/DOSE).

May potentate muscle weakness with neuromuscular blockers. Oral suspension is very poorly tolerated, avoid if possible, use 150 mg capsules or an alternative antibiotic. Active against gram positive and anaerobic organisms.

## Clonidine

Antihypertensive.
PO: 2–4 microgram/kg/DOSE q4–6h, may be increased to maximum 25 microgram/kg/DAY.

Do not discontinue clonidine abruptly to prevent rebound hypertension.

## Cloxacillin

Beta-lactamase-resistant penicillin.
IV: 100–200 mg/kg/DAY ÷ q6h (maximum 8 g/DAY).
PO: 25–50 mg/kg/DAY ÷ q6h (maximum 500 mg/DOSE).

Higher oral doses are poorly tolerated, usually use cephalexin instead. Primarily used in Staphylococcal infections.

## Codeine

Opioid analgesic used to treat mild-moderate pain.
PO/IM/SC: 0.5–1 mg/kg q4h prn (maximum 60 mg/DOSE).

Not for IV use due to significant histamine release and possible cardiovascular side effects. Not commonly used in ICU setting.

## Cosyntropin

Adrenal function testing agent.

Standard dose:

IV: 15 microgram/kg (maximum 250 mcg). Measure cortisol at baseline and 60 min post cosyntropin injection.

Low dose:

IV: Low dose: 1 microgram. Measure cortisol at baseline and 30 min post cosyntropin injection.

## Co-trimoxazole (Trimethoprim/ Sulfamethoxazole)

Sulfa derivative antibiotic.

Bacterial infections:

PO/IV: 8 mg/kg/DAY (of trimethoprim component) ÷ q12h.

Pneumocystis carinii pneumonia (PCP):

PO/IV: 20 mg/kg/DAY (of trimethoprim component) ÷ q6h.

Excellent oral absorption, use IV only if PO contraindicated. Maintain good fluid intake and urine output. Adjust dosing interval in renal impairment. Monitor CBC and LFTs. Do not use in patients with G-6-PD deficiency. If PCP is severe (ie, hypoxia), consider adding methylprednisolone 1 mg/kg q24h.

Order in mL of suspension or injection or number of tablets:

Suspension: 8 mg trimethoprim and 40 mg sulfamethoxazole/mL.

Injection: 16 mg trimethoprim and 80 mg sulfamethoxazole/mL.
Tablet: 80 mg trimethoprim and 400 mg sulfamethoxazole.
DS tablet: 160 mg trimethoprim and 800 mg sulfamethoxazole.

## Cyclosporine

Immunosuppressant.

IV dose is approximately 30–50% of oral dose. Dose and target serum levels vary widely with indication and the individual protocol, but usually:
IV: 3–6 mg/kg/DAY ÷ q12h.
PO: 5–10 mg/kg/DAY ÷ q12h.

Requires dose reduction in liver or renal dysfunction. Cyclosporine interacts with many medications, including fluconazole, erythromycin, tacrolimus, diltiazem, methylprednisolone, grapefruit juice, phenytoin, phenobarbital, carbamazepine, trimethoprim, check specialized references before use. Trough levels usually 100–300 microgram/L but varies with the indication.

## Dantrolene

Malignant hyperthermia treatment:
IV: 1 mg/kg, repeat as needed to maximum of 10 mg/kg. Regimen may be repeated if symptoms recur.

## Desmopressin (DDAVP)

Analogue of vasopressin.

Diabetes Insipidus:

PO: 25–100 microgam/DOSE q12–24h.
Nasal: 2.5–10 microgram/DOSE q12–24h.
IV/IM/SC: 0.25–1 microgram/DOSE q12–24h (maximum 4 microgram/DOSE).

Coagulopathy:

IV/SC: 0.3 microgram/kg/DOSE (maximum 20 microgram/DOSE).

Used as replacement therapy in diabetes insipidus, treatment of prolonged bleeding times and mild bleeding associated with some types of hemophilia. Parenteral dose is approximately 10% of intranasal dose and 1% of the oral dose. In the treatment of diabetes insipidus check urine output, volume status, serum and urine electrolytes prior to each dose.

Nasal spray = 10 microgram/puff, nasal solution = 100 microgram/mL.

## Dexamethasone

Corticosteroid.

Croup:

IV/IM/PO: 0.6 mg/kg once.

Meningitis:

IV: 0.15 mg/kg/DOSE q6h for 4 days. Begin with first antibiotic dose.

Prevention of post-extubation stridor:

IV: 0.25–0.5 mg/kg/DOSE (maximum 10 mg/DOSE) q6h × 6 doses. Begin 24 hours pre-extubation if possible.

Increased ICP due to space occupying lesion:

IV/PO:0.2–0.4 mg/kg initially followed by 0.3 mg/kg/DAY ÷ q6h.

Discontinuation of therapy >14 days requires gradual tapering. Consider supplemental steroids at times of stress if patient has received long-term or frequent bursts of steroid therapy. Prolonged weakness may occur when corticosteroids are used concurrently with non-depolarizing neuromuscular blocking agents.

## Dextrose

Treatment of hypoglycemia:

IV: 0.5–1 g/kg/DOSE:
1–2 mL/kg of 50% dextrose
5–10 mL/kg of 10% dextrose
1 mmol of dextrose (0.2 g of dextrose) provides 2.8 kJ (0.67 kcal).

# Dexmedetomidine

Alpha-2 adrenergic agonist.

Sedation and analgesia in intubated/ventilated patients:

IV: 10 mcg/kg over 10 min then 0.2–0.7 mcg/kg/h.
  May cause hypotension and bradycardia, but causes minimal respiratory depression.

# Diazepam

Benzodiazepine sedative, anxiolytic, and amnestic.

Status epilepticus:

IV: 0.25 mg/kg/DOSE (maximum 5 mg, 10 mg for older children).
PR: 0.5 mg/kg/DOSE (maximum 20 mg/DOSE).

ICU sedation:

IV: 0.1–0.3 mg/kg q1h prn.
  Fast onset and short duration of action with single doses, duration of action prolonged with continued use. Not first line drug for ICU sedation due to short duration of action and the potential for accumulation. Withdrawal may occur if discontinued abruptly after prolonged use. Not recommended for continuous infusion due to poor solubility. Can give parenteral preparation rectally, diluted with water.

# Digoxin

| **Total** Digitalization Dose (maximum 1 mg) | Maintenance Dose (usual maximum 250 microgram/DAY) |
|---|---|
| **Divide dose** q6h × 3 doses | Begin 12 h after last loading dose |

Usually divide daily maintenance dose q12h if less than 10 years of age, otherwise give dose once daily. Doses based on ideal body weight, decrease dose for patients with renal impairment. Digoxin has many drug interactions including nifedipine, verapamil, amiodarone, erythromycin, cisapride and sucralfate, check specialized references before use. IV dose is approximately 80%

|  | PO | IV | PO | IV |
|---|---|---|---|---|
| 37 weeks –2 years | 50 microgram/ kg | 35 microgram/ kg | 10 microgram/ kg/DAY | 8 microgram/ kg/DAY |
| >2 years | 40 microgram/ kg | 30 microgram/ kg | 8 microgram/ kg/DAY | 6 microgram/ kg/DAY |

of PO dose. Monitor trough levels (0.5–2 microgram/L or 1–2.6 micromol/L).

## Dimenhydrinate

Antihistamine used to treat nausea and vomiting.
IV/IM/PO: 1 mg/kg/DOSE q4–6h (maximum 50 mg/DOSE).

## Diphenhydramine

Antihistamine used primarily to treat urticaria.
IV/IM/PO: 0.5–1 mg/kg/DOSE q6h (maximum 50 mg/DOSE).

## Divalproex

See Valproic Acid and Derivatives.

## Dobutamine

Inotrope.
IV: 2–20 microgram/kg/min.
    Correct hypovolemia first to prevent hypotension. Give via central line if possible.

## Domperidone

Prokinetic agent.
PO: 1.2–2.4 mg/kg/DAY ÷ q6h (maximum 80 mg/DAY).

## Dopamine

Vasopressor and inotrope.

Hypotension and shock:

IV: 2–20 microgram/kg/min.

Correct hypovolemia first. Consider changing to, or adding another drug at 15–20 microgram/kg/min or if tachycardia occurs. Give via central line if possible.

## Enalapril, Enalaprilat

Angiotensin converting enzyme inhibitor.

Hypertension, CHF:

PO: 0.1 mg/kg/DAY ÷ q12–24h, increase as required (maximum 0.5 mg/kg/DAY or 40 mg/DAY).
IV: 5–10 microgram/kg/DOSE q6–12h, titrated to clinical effect (usual maximum 30 microgram/kg/DOSE or 5 mg/DOSE).

Monitor blood pressure and renal function. There is limited experience with the use of IV enalaprilat in pediatrics. Enalaprilat is the IV formulation of enalapril.

## Enoxaparin

Anticoagulant, low-molecular weight heparin.
Treatment:
SC: <2 months of age: 1.5 mg/kg/DOSE q12h.
>2 months of age: 1 mg/kg/DOSE q12h.
Prophylaxis:
SC: <2 months of age: 0.75 mg/kg/DOSE q12h.
>2 months of age: 0.5 mg/kg/DOSE q12h.

Monitor platelets and hemoglobin. Avoid in severe renal dysfunction. Anti-factor Xa level drawn 4 hours post SC injection should be 0.5–1 unit/mL for treatment and 0.2–0.4 unit/mL for prophylaxis.

## Epinephrine

Vasopressor and inotrope.

Symptomatic bradycardia or pulseless arrest:

IV: 0.01 mg/kg/DOSE (0.1 mL/kg of 1:10,000 solution).
ETT: 0.1 mg/kg/DOSE (0.1 mL/kg of 1:1,000 solution).

Refractory hypotension/shock:

IV: 0.1–1 microgram/kg/min (doses of 0.01–1 microgram/kg/min have been used).

Post-extubation stridor/croup:

NEB: 2.5–5 mg/DOSE (2.5–5 mL of 1:1,000 solution) prn.
1:10,000 solution = 0.1 mg/mL and 1:1,000 solution = 1 mg/mL.

## Epinephrine (Racemic)

Post-extubation stridor/croup:

NEB: 0.25–0.5 mL of 2.25% solution via nebulizer prn.

## Epoprostenol

Prostaglandin I2.
Pulmonary Hypertension:

IV: 2–20 nanogram/kg/min.
    Epoprostenol should only be diluted in the supplied diluent and is stable at room temperature for only short periods of time. If possible the infusion should not be interrupted.

## Erythromycin

Macrolide antibiotic.
IV: 25–50 mg/kg/DAY ÷ q6h (maximum 4 g/DAY).
PO: 20–40 mg/kg/DAY ÷ q6h (maximum 2 g/DAY).
    Has many drug interactions, may increase levels of midazolam, carbamazepine, theophylline, cyclosporine, phenytoin, check specialized references before use. GI adverse effects common, even with IV use. Thrombophlebitis common.

## Esmolol

Short acting β blocking agent.

Atrial fibrillation/atrial flutter/SVT/hypertension:

IV: 100–500 microgram/kg then 50–300 microgram/kg/min. Titrate by 50–100 microgram/kg/min q5–10 min. High doses of 500–1,000 micrograms/kg/min have been rarely required.
    Short-term use only, consider bolus dose with each increase in infusion. Change to longer acting agent once desired effect is achieved. Duration of action is approximately 10 min.

## Ethacrynic Acid

Loop diuretic.
IV: 0.5–1 mg/kg/DOSE.

Use only if poor response to appropriate doses of furosemide. Repeat doses are not usually recommended but have been given q8–12h.

# Ethanol

Treatment of methanol or ethylene glycol overdose:

IV: Give ethanol 10% in D5W:

|  | **Dose** | **Volume of 10% Ethanol** |
|---|---|---|
| Loading dose: | 600 mg/kg | 7.6 mL/kg |
| Maintenance dose: | 66 mg/kg/h | 0.8 mL/kg/h |
| Hemodialysis: | 118 mg/kg/h | 1.5 mL/kg/h |

These doses are suggested starting doses for non-drinkers, higher rates will be required for drinkers. Titrate to keep ethanol level >22 mmol/L. Expect intoxication and CNS depression and hypoglycemia in children.

# Etomidate

Sedative.

Endotracheal intubation:

IV: 0.2–0.4 mg/kg.
Onset of action is within 1 min, minimal hemodynamic effects.

# Famotidine

$H_2$ receptor antagonist.

Reduction of gastric acid secretion:

IV: 1 mg/kg/DAY ÷ q12h (usual maximum 40 mg/DAY).
PO: 2 mg/kg/DAY ÷ q12h (usual maximum 80 mg/DAY).
IV dose is approximately 50% of oral dose. Modify dosage interval for patients with renal impairment.

# Fentanyl

Short-acting narcotic analgesic.

Procedural sedation, non-ventilated patients:

IV: 0.5–1 microgram/kg/DOSE, repeated prn.

Sedation/analgesia of ventilated ICU patients:

IV: 1–2 microgram/kg then 1–5 (usual maximum 10) microgram/kg/h and/or 1–2 microgram/kg/DOSE q1–2h prn.

   Reduce dose if used in combination with benzodiazepines. Use with caution in non-ventilated patients due to potential for respiratory depression. Rapid IV administration may cause chest wall rigidity with subsequent difficulty with ventilation (give naloxone or paralysis). Withdrawal may occur if discontinued abruptly after prolonged use.

## Ferrous Sulfate

See Iron.

## Filgrastim

Granulocyte colony stimulating factor.
Prevention or treatment of chemotherapy induced neutropenia.
SC/IV: 5 mcg/kg/DOSE q24h.

   Dose may be increased to 10 mcg/kg/DOSE q24h if inadequate response.

## Fluconazole

Antifungal.

Oropharyngeal candidiasis:

IV/PO: 3 mg/kg q24h.

Esophageal candidiasis:

IV/PO: 6 mg/kg q24h (maximum 400 mg/DAY).

Candidemia:

IV/PO: 12 mg/kg once (maximum 800 mg) then 6 mg/kg/DAY (usual maximum 400 mg/DAY, but higher doses have been used).

   Excellent oral absorption, use IV only if PO contraindicated. Adjust dosing interval in renal impairment. May increase serum levels of cyclosporine, midazolam, cisapride, phenytoin. *Aspergillus* species and *Candida krusei* are intrinsically resistant; *Candida glabrata* may respond to higher doses.

## Flumazenil

Benzodiazepine antagonist.
IV: 0.01 mg/kg/DOSE (maximum 0.2 mg/DOSE), q1–3 min prn (maximum total dose is 0.05 mg/kg or 1 mg ).

Reverses sedation but may not reliably reverse respiratory depression. Monitor for recurring sedation, as repeat doses may be required. May precipitate seizures and/or benzodiazepine withdrawal. Not recommended for routine use in the PICU or in suspected overdoses.

## Fluticasone

Inhaled corticosteroid.
INH: 125–500 microgram q12h.

Higher doses may be required if administered through a ventilator due to loss of drug in the circuit.

## Fomepizole

Treatment of methanol or ethylene glycol overdose:

IV: 15 mg/kg then 10 mg/kg q12h until levels are below toxic range. Doses may require adjustment during hemodialysis or if therapy is required for longer than 48h.

## Furosemide

Loop diuretic.
PO: 1–2 mg/kg/DOSE, adjust dose/frequency prn, usually q6–24h.
IV: 0.5–2 mg/kg/DOSE, adjust dose/frequency prn, usually q6–24h or begin at 0.1 mg/kg/hour and titrate to clinical effect (maximum 0.5 mg/kg/h).

## Gabapentin

Anticonvulsant.
PO: 10–30 mg/kg/DAY ÷ q8h increased as tolerated. Usual maintenance dose: 20–50 mg/kg/DAY (usual maximum 3,600 mg/DAY).

## G-CSF

See Filgrastim.

## Gentamicin

Aminoglycoside antibiotic.
IV: 5–6 mg/kg/DOSE **q24h** or 2.5 mg/kg/DOSE **q8h**.

Once daily dosing should be used for all patients >1 month of age, except in the treatment of endocarditis and in patients with extensive burns. Adjust dosing interval in renal impairment. Ototoxicity and nephrotoxicity may occur, consider monitoring trough levels (target <2 mg/L) in patients at risk for nephrotoxicity; septic shock, concurrent nephrotoxins, fluctuating renal function or extended treatment courses. May potentiate muscle weakness with neuromuscular blockers.

## Glucagon

Treatment of hypoglycemia:

IV/IM/SC: 0.025–0.1 mg/kg/DOSE (maximum 1 mg/DOSE) or <20 kg give 0.5 mg, >20 kg give 1 mg. May need to repeat dose and/or give glucose due to short duration of action.

Hypotension and bradycardia caused by β blocker overdose:

IV: 0.05–0.15 mg/kg then 1–5 mg/h (maximum 15 mg/h), titrate to heart rate and blood pressure.

## Glycopyrrolate

Anticholinergic

Reduction of secretions:

IV: 4–10 microgram/kg/DOSE q6h.
PO: 40–100 microgram/kg/DOSE q6h.

Note difference in IV and PO doses due to reduced bioavailability.

## Heparin

Anticoagulant.
IV: 75 units/kg bolus then:

<1 year of age: 28 units/kg/hour.
>1 year of age: 20 units/kg/hour.

Measure APTT 4 hours after loading dose and adjust heparin to maintain APTT at 60–85 s. Monitor platelets and hemoglobin.

| APTT (s) | Bolus (units/kg) | Hold (min) | Rate Change (units/kg/h) | Repeat APTT (h) |
|---|---|---|---|---|
| <50 | 50 | 0 | ↑20% | 4 |
| 50–59 | 0 | 0 | ↑10% | 4 |
| 60–85 | 0 | 0 | 0 | 24 |
| 86–95 | 0 | 0 | ↓10% | 4 |
| 96–120 | 0 | 30 | ↓10% | 4 |
| >120 | 0 | 60 | ↓15% | 4 |

## Hydralazine

Antihypertensive, vasodilator.
IV: 0.1–0.5 mg/kg/DOSE q4–6h (usual maximum 20 mg/DOSE).
PO: 0.75 mg/kg/DAY ÷ q6h, increase as required and tolerated (maximum of 5 mg/kg/DAY).

May cause reflex tachycardia. Onset of action within 15 min after IV administration.

## Hydrochlorothiazide

Thiazide diuretic.
PO: 2–4 mg/kg/DAY ÷ q12h.

## Hydrocortisone

Corticosteroid.

Acute asthma:

IV: 5 mg/kg/DOSE ÷ q6h for 24–48 hours then reassess.

Anaphylaxis:

IV: 5–10 mg/kg/DOSE.

Anti-inflammatory:

IV: 2.5–10 mg/kg/DAY ÷ q6–8h.

Acute adrenal crisis:

IV: 1–2 mg/kg then:

| Infants: | 25–150 mg/DAY ÷ q6h. |
| Older children: | 150–300 mg/DAY ÷ q6h. |

Discontinuation of therapy >14 days requires gradual tapering. Consider supplemental steroids at times of stress if patient has received long-term or frequent bursts of steroid therapy. Prolonged weakness may occur when corticosteroids are used concurrently with non-depolarizing neuromuscular blocking agents.

## Hydromorphone

Narcotic analgesic.

Sedation/analgesia:

IV: 10–20 microgram/kg/DOSE q2–4h and increase as required or 20 microgram/kg then 2–10 microgram/kg/h.
For breakthrough, use 1–1.5 times the hourly dose +/− increase the infusion.
Reduced doses may be required if used in combination with benzodiazepines. Use with caution in non-ventilated patients due to potential for respiratory depression. There is no upper dose limit if increased gradually. To prevent withdrawal, avoid abrupt cessation following high doses or long duration of therapy (>5 days). Common adverse effects are pruritis, nausea and constipation, which may be overlooked in PICU patients.

## Ibuprofen

Analgesic and anti-inflammatory (NSAID).
PO: 5–10 mg/kg/DOSE q6–8h (maximum 2,400 mg/DAY).
Adverse effects include renal dysfunction, GI irritation, and ulceration.

| Weight (kg) | Single Dose (mg) |
|---|---|
| 2.5–3.9 | 20 |
| 4.0–5.4 | 30 |
| 5.5–7.9 | 40 |
| 8.0–10.9 | 60 |
| 11.0–15.9 | 100 |
| 16.0–21.9 | 150 |
| 22.0–26.9 | 200 |
| 27.0–31.9 | 250 |
| 32.0–43.9 | 300 |
| 44-over | 400 |

## Imipenem

Broad spectrum antibiotic.

IV: 60–100 mg/kg/DAY ÷ q6h (maximum 4 g/DAY).
  Increase dosing interval for patients with renal impairment. Allergic reactions may occur in patients with penicillin hypersensitivities.

## Insulin

Recombinant human insulin.

Diabetic ketoacidosis:

IV: 0.05–0.1 units/kg/h initially. **For IV administration MUST use regular insulin.**

Hyperkalemia:

IV: 0.1 units/kg AND dextrose 0.5 g/kg.

Diabetes mellitus:

SC: 0.3–0.5 unit/kg/DAY in divided doses (as a combination of short and long acting insulins). Adjust as required based on blood glucose measurements, usually 0.5–1 unit/kg/DAY.
  With continuous infusions measure blood glucose q1h initially, adjust dose as required based on blood glucose measurements.

## Ipratropium

Inhaled anticholinergic bronchodilator.

Severe asthma:

NEB: 125–250 microgram (0.5–1 mL) q4–6h.
INH: 2–4 puffs q4–6h.
   Higher doses may be required if administered through a ventilator due to loss of drug in the circuit.

## Iron

Treatment of iron deficiency anemia:

PO: 4–6 mg/kg/DAY (of elemental iron) ÷ q8–24h.

Prevention of iron deficiency anemia:

PO: 2–3 mg/kg/DAY (of elemental iron) q24h.
Give with food if GI upset occurs.

## Isoproterenol

β adrenergic agonist.

Temporary management of bradycardia:

IV: 0.025–1 microgram/kg/min (maximum 2 microgram/kg/min).
   Used for the treatment of atropine resistant bradyarrhythmias, ventricular arrhythmias due to A-V block. Increases risk of arrhythmias.

## Kayexalate®

See Cation Exchange Resins.

## Ketamine

Dissociative anesthetic and analgesic.

Procedural sedation/intubation:

IV: 0.5–2 mg/kg/DOSE.
IM: 3–5 mg/kg/DOSE.

Sedation in intubated patients (rarely used):

IV: 5–20 microgram/kg/min.

Ketamine has little respiratory or cardiovascular depressant effects. Useful for short painful procedures. Avoid in the presence of increased ICP or intraocular pressure. Emergence reactions such as vivid dreams or hallucinations may be treated with benzodiazepines.

## Ketorolac

Analgesic and anti-inflammatory (NSAID).
IV/IM: 0.5 mg/kg/DOSE (maximum 15–30 mg) q6h.
PO: 10 mg q6h (minimum weight 45 kg).

For oral use give ibuprofen or naproxen for younger children. There is limited experience with multiple dose ketorolac in pediatric patients. Adverse effects include renal dysfunction, GI irritation, and ulceration.

## Labetalol

Antihypertensive, $\alpha$ and $\beta$ receptor blocker.

Hypertensive urgencies/emergencies:

IV: 0.2–0.5 mg/kg/DOSE (maximum 20 mg) q15–20 min until desired response is obtained or 0.5–3 mg/kg/h.

Start low and titrate based on response.

## Lactulose

Osmotic laxative.

PO: infants:  2.5–5 mL q8–24h.


children:  5–10 mL q8–24h.

adolescents:  15–30 mL q8–24h.

## Lansoprazole

Inhibitor of gastric acid secretion (proton pump inhibitor).
PO: 0.5–1.6 mg/kg q24h (maximum 15 or 30 mg/DOSE).

## Levalbuterol

Bronchodilator, $\beta_2$ agonist.
NEB: 0.31, 0.63 or 1.25 mg/DOSE.
INH: 90 mcg (2 puffs) q8h, dose and frequency may be increased in the treatment of acute asthma.

Titrate dose to effect and/or adverse effects (tachycardia, tremor, and hypokalemia). For most patients metered dose inhalers with a spacer device are the preferred method of drug delivery. Wet nebulization is less efficient and more costly.

## Levofloxacin

Quinolone antibiotic.
IV/PO: There is limited experience with levofloxain in pediatrics. Some centers use 10 mg/kg/DOSE q24h (maximum 500 mg/DOSE).

Excellent oral absorption, use IV only if PO contraindicated. Feeds, formula, calcium, magnesium, iron, antacids and sulcralfate reduce absorption, hold feeds for 1 hour before and 2 hours after dose. Adjust dosing interval in renal impairment. Quinolones are not generally considered to be first line drugs in pediatrics.

## Lidocaine

Antiarrhythmic:

IV: 1 mg/kg/DOSE, repeat prn to a maximum of 3 mg/kg then 20–50 microgram/kg/min.

Prevention of increased ICP with intubation or suctioning:

IV: 1–2 mg/kg/DOSE.

Use the lower end of the dosing range for patients in shock or with CHF due to reduced lidocaine clearance. Initial dose may be given via ETT, increase IV dose 2–10-fold and dilute to 3–5 mL with NS. Follow with several positive pressure breaths.

## Linezolid

Antibiotic.
IV/PO: 10 mg/kg/DOSE (maximum 600 mg) q12h.

Q8h dosing has been used in younger children. Excellent oral absorption, use IV only if PO contraindicated. Linezolid has many drug interactions, including serotonergic agents (eg, SSRIs and tricyclic antidepressants), meperidine, dextromethophan, check specialized references before use.

## Lorazepam

Benzodiazepine sedative, anxiolytic and amnestic.

Status epilepticus:

IV: 0.1 mg/kg/DOSE (usual maximum 4 mg/DOSE).
PR: 0.2 mg/kg/DOSE.

ICU sedation:

IV/PO: 0.05–0.1 mg/kg/DOSE q1h prn +/− scheduled doses (may increase to 0.2 mg/kg/DOSE).

Intermediate duration of action and no active metabolites. Withdrawal may occur if discontinued abruptly after prolonged use. Not recommended for continuous infusion due to poor solubility. May give parenteral preparation rectally, diluted with water.

## Magnesium Sulfate

Electrolyte.

Hypomagnesemia:

IV: 25–100 mg/kg of magnesium sulfate (maximum 5 g). Usual maximum rate is 20 mg/kg of magnesium sulfate/h.

Severe asthma:

IV: 25–75 mg/kg (maximum 2 g) of magnesium sulfate once over 20 min.

Torsades des pointes:

IV: 25–50 mg/kg of magnesium sulfate (maximum 2 g) rapid infusion.

Watch for hypotension with faster infusion rates. Usual dilution for infusion is 10 mg of magnesium sulfate/mL. Order in mg or g of magnesium sulfate to reduce the potential for error. 1 g of magnesium sulfate = 4 mmol of magnesium = 8 mEq of magnesium = 100 mg of elemental magnesium.

## Mannitol

Osmotic diuretic.

Reduction of intracranial pressure:

IV: 0.25–1 g/kg (1.25–5 mL/kg of 20% solution) over 15–30 min q4–6h prn.

Contraindicated in anuric patients. Monitor serum osmolality if frequent doses are required.

## Meperidine

Narcotic analgesic.

IV: 1–2 mg/kg/DOSE q3–4h.

Not recommended for routine use in the ICU. Avoid in renal impairment due to the accumulation of metabolites, which may cause seizures. Oral use not usually recommended due to poor absorption and lack of pediatric formulations.

## Meropenem

Broad spectrum antibiotic.

Meningitis:

IV: 120 mg/kg/DAY ÷ q8h (maximum 6 g/DAY).

Other infections:

IV: 60 mg/kg/DAY ÷ q6–8h (usual maximum 500 mg IV q6h, or 1 g IV q8h).

Cystic fibrosis:

IV: 75 mg/kg/DAY ÷ q8h (usual maximum 6 g/DAY).

Spectrum of activity similar to that of imipenem. Increase dosing interval for patients with renal impairment. Allergic reactions may occur in patients with penicillin hypersensitivities.

## Methylene Blue

Treatment of drug induced methemoglobinemia:

IV: 1–2 mg/kg/DOSE, may repeat in 1 hour prn.

## Methylprednisolone

Corticosteroid.

Acute asthma:

IV: 1 mg/kg q24h. Higher doses of 1–2 mg/kg/DOSE q6h have been used initially until improvement seen (usually 24–48 hours) then q24h or switch or oral prednisone.

Anti-inflammatory:

IV: 1–2 mg/kg q24h.

High dose/pulse therapy:

IV: 10–30 mg/kg q24h × 1–3 doses.

Spinal cord injury:

IV: 30 mg/kg IV over 15 min then 5.4 mg/kg/h beginning 45 min later and continuing for 23 or 48 h.

Discontinuation of therapy >14 days requires gradual tapering. Consider supplemental steroids at times of stress if patient has received long-term or frequent bursts of steroid therapy. Prolonged weakness may occur when corticosteroids are used concurrently with non-depolarizing neuromuscular blocking agents.

## Metoclopramide

Antiemetic, gastrointestinal prokinetic agent.
IV/PO: 0.4–0.8 mg/kg/DAY ÷ q6h (usual maximum 40 mg/DAY).

Extrapyramidal reactions occur more commonly in children and may be treated with diphenhydramine.

## Metolazone

Thiazide diuretic.
PO: 0.2–0.4 mg/kg/DAY ÷ q12–24h (usual maximum 10 mg/DOSE).

## Metronidazole

Anti anaerobic antibiotic.

Anaerobic infections:

IV/PO: 20–30 mg/kg/DAY ÷ q12h (maximum 1 g/DAY).

C. difficile:

IV/PO: 30 mg/kg/DAY ÷ q6–8h (maximum 1.5 g/DAY).

Excellent oral absorption, use IV only if PO contraindicated or not tolerated. Enteral administration preferred for colitis caused by C. difficile, but IV can be used.

## Midazolam

Benzodiazepine sedative, anxiolytic, and amnestic.

Procedural sedation:

IV: 0.05–0.1 mg/kg/DOSE, repeat prn to desired level of sedation.

Refractory status epilepticus:

IV: 0.2 mg/kg then 1 microgram/kg/min, increased q15 min prn, most cases require less than 5 microgram/kg/min.

ICU sedation:

IV: 0.05–0.1 mg/kg/DOSE q1–2h prn or 1–3 microgram/kg/min and 0.05–0.1 mg/kg q1h prn (usual maximum 6 microgram/kg/min).

   Midazolam has a short duration of action after single doses, but may have an extended duration of action after repeated dosing due to accumulation. Continuous infusions of benzodiazepines for ICU sedation are recommended only if intermittent boluses are ineffective. Always order a breakthrough dose to treat acute agitation if using a continuous infusion. Withdrawal may occur if discontinued abruptly after prolonged use.

## Milrinone

Inotrope and vasodilator.
IV: 50 microgram/kg over 15 min then 0.25–0.75 microgram/kg/min.

   Used for short-term treatment of refractory CHF. Hemodynamic effects are similar to dobutamine, watch for hypotension, especially with the loading dose.

## Morphine

Narcotic analgesic.

Sedation/analgesia:

IV: 0.05–0.1 mg/kg/DOSE q2–4h and increase as required or 0.1 mg/kg then 10–40 (usual maximum 100) microgram/kg/h and 0.1 mg/kg/DOSE q1–2h prn.

   Reduced doses may be required if used in combination with benzodiazepines. Use with caution in non-ventilated patients due to potential for respiratory depression. There is no upper dose limit if increased gradually. To prevent withdrawal, avoid abrupt cessation following high doses or long duration of therapy (>5 days). Common adverse effects are pruritis, nausea and constipation, which may be overlooked in PICU patients.

## Mycophenolate

Immunosupressant.
Dose and target serum levels vary widely with indication and the individual protocol, but usually:
PO/IV: 600 mg/m$^2$/DOSE q12h (maximum 2 g/DAY).
 Dose adjustment required in renal dysfunction.

## Nafcillin

Beta-lactamase-resistant penicillin.
IV: 100–200 mg/kg/DAY ÷ q6h (maximum 8 g/DAY).
 Primarily used in Staphylococcal infections.

## Naloxone

Narcotic antagonist used to reverse opioid induced respiratory depression.

Opioid overdose/respiratory arrest:

IV/IM/SC: 0.1 mg/kg q1–2 min prn (maximum of 2 mg/DOSE).

 Partial reversal of opioid induced respiratory depression:

IV/IM/SC: 0.01 mg/kg q1–2 min prn until desired effect.

Treatment of opioid induced pruritis:

IV: 0.25–2 microgram/kg/h.
 May precipitate withdrawal in narcotic dependent patients. Will also reverse analgesia. If giving via ETT, increase IV dose 2–10-fold and dilute to 3–5 mL with NS. Follow with several positive pressure breaths.

## Neostigmine

Reversal of non-depolarizing neuromuscular blocking agents:

IV: 0.025–0.1 mg/kg/DOSE (usual maximum dose 0.5–2 mg/DOSE, to a total dose of 5 mg).
 Will not reverse the effects of succinylcholine. Give with atropine to prevent bradycardia and other cholinergic effects. Complete reversal may take several minutes and repeat doses may be required.

## Nifedipine

Antihypertensive, calcium channel blocker.

Hypertensive urgencies:

PO: 0.25–0.5 mg/kg/DOSE, usual maximum 10 mg/DOSE. Try to use 5 or 10 mg/DOSE.

Hypertension:

PO: 0.5–1 mg/kg/DAY.

May cause rapid and profound hypotension. Bite and swallow capsule for rapid (<5 min) effect. Available as 5 and 10 mg short acting capsules (dose q6–8h) and 10 and 20 mg long acting tablets (dose q12h) and 20, 30, and 60 mg extended release tablets (dose q24h).

## Nitroglycerin

Antihypertensive, vasodilator.
IV: 0.5–5 (maximum 10) microgram/kg/min.

Titrate to effect, tolerance may develop, requiring dosage adjustment.

## Nitroprusside

Antihypertensive, vasodilator.
IV: 0.5–3 (maximum 5) microgram/kg/min

Titrate to response, doses greater than 4 microgram/kg/min are rarely required. Monitor for cyanide toxicity (check cyanide and thiocyanate levels) in patients with renal insufficiency, with high doses or prolonged infusions.

## Norepinephrine

Vasopressor with $\alpha$ and $\beta$ activity.
IV: 0.05–1 microgram/kg/min.

Give via central line.

## Nystatin

Topical antifungal.

Oral candadiasis:

| | |
|---|---|
| PO: infants: | 100,000 units swish and swallow q6h. |
| children: | 250,000 units swish and swallow q6h. |
| adolescents: | 500,000 units swish and swallow q6h. |

## Octreotide

Synthetic analogue of somatostatin.

GI bleeding:

IV: 1 microgram/kg then 1 microgram/kg/h (usual maximum 50 microgram/h).

## Omeprazole

Inhibitor of gastric acid secretion (proton pump inhibitor).
PO: 0.7–1.4 mg/kg/DAY ÷ q12–24h (maximum 40 mg/DAY).

Do not give crushed tablets without sodium bicarbonate solution. An oral solution is available for doses other than 10 and 20 mg but is very unpalatable and should be given via feeding tube.

## Ondansetron

Antiemetic.
IV/PO: 0.15 mg/kg/DOSE q8h (maximum 8 mg/DOSE).

## Oxacillin

Beta-lactamase-resistant penicillin.
IV: 100–200 mg/kg/DAY ÷ q6h (maximum 8 g/DAY).
Primarily used in Staphylococcal infections.

## Oxcarbazepine

Anticonvulsant.
PO: 10 mg/kg/DAY ÷ q12h initially, increased as tolerated to usual maximum of 30 mg/kg/DAY.

Oxcarbazepine has many drug interactions, consult a specialized reference before use.

## Pancuronium

Non-depolarizing neuromuscular blocking agent.
IV: 0.1 mg/kg/DOSE q1h prn.

Regular analgesia, sedation, and ocular lubrication required. Duration of action may be prolonged for patients with renal impairment. May cause tachycardia. Duration of action prolonged in renal dysfunction. Prolonged weakness may occur, especially when corticosteroids are used concurrently with non-depolarizing neuromuscular blocking agents.

## Pantoprazole

Inhibitor of gastric acid secretion (proton pump inhibitor).
There is limited experience with pantoprazole in pediatric patients.
PO/IV: Adult dose: 40 mg q24h (maximum q12h), 1 mg/kg q24h has been used in pediatric patients.

Major gastrointestinal hemorrhage:

IV: Adult dose: 80 mg loading dose then 8 mg/h.
    There is more data with the use of oral omeprazole in pediatric patients. Intravenous and oral pantoprazole provide equivalent acid suppression. Do not crush tablets.

## Paraldehyde

Anticonvulsant.
IV: 100–200 mg/kg over 20 min to 2 h, may follow with 20–50 mg/kg/h, titrated to response.
PR: 200–400 mg/kg/DOSE.
    Give rectally diluted with an equal amount of saline or oil (mineral or olive). Solutions must be mixed in glass and protected from light. Paraldehyde has largely been supplanted by other less toxic and easier to administer agents.

## Penicillin G

Antibiotic.

Moderate to severe infections:

IV: 100,000–400,000 units/kg/DAY ÷ q4–6h (maximum 24 million units/DAY).

Meningitis:

IV: 400,000 units/kg/DAY ÷ q4h (maximum 24 million units/DAY).
    Increase dosing interval for patients with renal impairment.

## Pentobarbital

Barbiturate sedative and anticonvulsant.

Procedural sedation:

IV: 1–3 mg/kg, repeat doses of 1–2 mg/kg may be given q5–10 min until adequate sedation (usual maximum 6 mg/kg or 200 mg total dose).

Refractory status epilepticus/uncontrolled intracranial hypertension:

IV: 3–5 mg/kg over 20 min then 1–3 mg/kg/hour, higher doses may be required.

Hypotension is common, especially with rapid infusion, treat promptly with fluids and vasopressors. Avoid extravasation, central line preferred. Respiratory depression is common. Coma usually occurs at 20–40 mg/L (88–177 micromol/L), but higher levels may be required. Has no analgesic properties.

## Phenobarbital

Barbiturate anticonvulsant.

Status epilepticus:

IV: 15–20 mg/kg over 20–30 min.

Maintenance:

IV/PO: 3–5 mg/kg/DAY ÷ q12–24h.

Usual serum level for seizure control: 65–172 micromol/L (15–40 mg/L).

## Phentolamine

α receptor blocker.

Treatment of α agonist drug extravasation:

SC: Infiltrate area of extravasation, dilute 5 mg in 10 mL of NS and do not exceed 0.1–0.2 mg/kg or 5 mg total dose.

Use within 12 hours of extravasation. Effective in extravasations of dopamine, epinephrine, norepinephrine, and phenylephrine.

## Phenylephrine

Vasopressor, α receptor agonist.

Refractory hypotension and shock:

IV: 0.1–2 microgram/kg/min (usual maximum 4 microgram/kg/min).

For tetralogy of Fallot/hypercyanotic spells may give bolus of 5–10 microgram/kg before beginning infusion. Give via central line.

## Phenytoin

Anticonvulsant, antiarrhythmic.

Status epilepticus:

IV: 15–20 mg/kg over 20 min.

Maintenance:

IV/PO: 5 mg/kg/DAY (range 3–10 mg/kg/DAY) ÷ q8–12h.

Anti-arrhythmic:

IV: 1.25 mg/kg q5min until arrhythmia suppressed (maximum of 15 mg/kg total dose), or 15 mg/kg over 20 min.

May require higher doses for patients with head injuries. Must be diluted in saline only and requires in-line filter (0.22 micron). Hold feeds before and after enteral administration as continuous feeds and formula may decrease bioavailability of oral products. Significantly increased free fraction in patients with hypoalbuminemia may result in underestimation of effective drug concentration and difficulty in interpretation of drug levels and toxicity may occur at "therapeutic" serum levels. Therapeutic level: 40–80 micromol/L (10–20 microgram/mL).

## Phosphate

Electrolyte.
IV: 0.15–0.6 mmol/kg of phosphate/DOSE as either potassium or sodium phosphate.

Correct deficit slowly and check serum phosphate and potassium after each dose. Maximum rate of administration is 0.3 mmol of phosphate/kg/h (to maximum of 15 mmol/h). Potassium phosphate supplies approximately 1.5 mEq of potassium for each mmol of phosphorus and carries the risk of arrhythmias and cardiac arrest with rapid IV administration.

## Phytonadione

See Vitamin K.

## Piperacillin

Broad spectrum penicillin.
IV: 200–300 mg/kg/DAY ÷ q6h (maximum 16 g/DAY).

Adjust dose interval in severe renal impairment. Active against *Pseudomonas aeruginosa*.

## Piperacillin/Tazobactam

Broad spectrum penicillin with beta-lactamase inhibitor.
IV: 200–300 mg/kg/DAY (of piperacillin component) ÷ q6–8h. Maximum dose is 4.5 g (4 g piperacillin + 0.5 g tazobactam) q6–8h.

Order in mg or g of piperacillin, for example, give piperacillin/tazobactam (as x mg of piperacillin component) IV q8h. Adjust dosage interval for patients with severe renal impairment. Active against gram positive (including *S. aureus*), gram negative, and anaerobic organisms.

## Potassium Chloride

Electrolyte.

Treatment of hypokalemia:

PO: 1–2 mEq/kg/DAY ÷ q6–12h.
IV: 0.25–1 mEq/kg/DOSE.

**Risk of arrhythmias and cardiac arrest with rapid IV administration.** Dose recommendations assume normal renal function. Maximum rate of administration in PICU is 0.5 mEq/kg/h (maximum 20 mEq/h). Use 0.1 mEq/mL for peripheral use, 0.2 mEq/mL for central lines. For maintenance fluids the usual maximum concentration for a peripheral IV is 40 mEq/L.

## Potassium Phosphate

See Phosphate.

## Prednisone, Prednisolone

Corticosteroid.

Acute asthma:

PO: 1–2 mg/kg q24h.

Anti-inflammatory or immunosuppressive:

PO: Usually 0.5–2 mg/kg 24h, dose may be tapered as tolerated.

1 mg prednisone = 1 mg prednisolone. Discontinuation of therapy >14 days requires gradual tapering. Consider supplemental steroids at times of stress if patient has received long-term or frequent bursts of steroid therapy. Prolonged weakness may occur when corticosteroids are used concurrently with non-depolarizing neuromuscular blocking agents.

## Procainamide

Antiarrhythmic.

IV: Loading dose:

15 mg/kg over 30–60 min or 3–5 mg/kg over 5 min q5–10 min until arrhythmia is suppressed (maximum 1 g total dose).
Infusion: 20–80 microgram/kg/min.

Discontinue if QRS increases to >50 of baseline or hypotension develops. Do not use with other drugs that prolong the QT interval such as amiodarone.

## Prochlorperazine

Antiemetic.
IV/PO: 0.1–0.15 mg/kg/DOSE q6–8h (maximum 10 mg/DOSE).

Not usually used in children due to increased risk of extrapyramidal reactions, but may be used in older children and adolescents. Extrapyramidal reactions can be treated with diphenhydramine.

## Propofol

General anesthetic.

Procedural sedation and intubation:

IV: 1–3 mg/kg.

ICU sedation:

IV: 0.5–4 mg/kg/h.

High dose and prolonged use in children is not recommended because of a suggested risk of fatal metabolic acidosis. May cause hypotension, local pain with infusion, and infection (lipid vehicle is an excellent medium for microbial growth).

## Propranolol

Non-selective β receptor blocker.

Arrhythmias:

IV: 0.01–0.15 mg/kg/DOSE (maximum 3 mg/DOSE). May repeat q6–8h prn.
PO: 0.5–4 mg/kg/DAY ÷ q6–8h (usual maximum 320 mg/DAY).
Tetralogy Spells:
IV: 0.05–0.1 mg/kg/DOSE over 10 min (usual maximum 0.25 mg/kg/DOSE or 3 mg/DOSE).
PO: 1–6 mg/kg/DAY ÷ q6–8h (usual maximum 320 mg/DAY).
  Note difference between IV and PO doses. Use is contraindicated in bradycardia, heart block, and asthma.

## Protamine

Heparin antidote.
IV: Dose of protamine is based on the amount of heparin received and the time since last heparin dose:

| Time since Last Heparin Dose | Protamine Dose (Maximum 50 mg) |
| --- | --- |
| <30 min | 1 mg per 100 units heparin |
| 30–60 min | 0.5–0.75 mg per 100 units heparin |
| 60–120 min | 0.375–0.5 mg per 100 units heparin |
| >120 min | 0.25–0.375 mg per 100 units heparin |

  Can also give 1 mg for each 100 units of heparin given within the previous 2 h, to a maximum of 50 mg/DOSE. Give over at least 10 min. Use with caution in patients with known reactions to fish. Check APTT 15 minutes after administration of protamine. May need repeat doses if heparin was given by SC injection due to slower absorption. Protamine will not reliably neutralize low molecular weight heparins, but with life-threatening bleeding can try 1 mg protamine for every 1 mg or 100 units of low molecular weight heparin.

## Racemic Epinephrine

See Epinephrine.

## Ranitidine

$H_2$ receptor antagonist.

Reduction of gastric acid secretion:

IV: 2–6 mg/kg/DAY ÷ q6–12h (usual maximum 50 mg q6–8h).
PO: 4–10 mg/kg/DAY ÷ q8–12h (usual maximum 300 mg/DAY).
IV dose is approximately 50% of oral dose. Modify dosage interval for patients with renal impairment. May add daily dose to TPN or give as a continuous infusion.

## Remifentanil

Opioid anesthetic and analgesic.

Rapid sequence induction:

IV: 2–4 microgram/kg.

Short-term sedation:

IV: 0.05–0.3 microgram/kg/min.
    Rapid onset of action, very short duration of action (3–10 min). Other agents preferred for continuing sedation and analgesia. Has no amnestic activity, the addition of propofol or benzodiazepines should be considered.

## Resonium Calcium®

See Cation Exchange Resins.

## Rocuronium

Non-depolarizing neuromuscular blocking agent.

Endotracheal intubation:

IV: 0.6–1.2 mg/kg/DOSE (usual maximum 50 mg/DOSE).
    Rapid onset of action (<1 min), duration of action is approximately 30–60 min.

## Salbutamol

Bronchodilator, $\beta_2$ agonist.

Acute asthma:

MDI: Start at 2–4 puffs q20–60min prn. Higher doses may be required if administered through a ventilator due to loss of drug in the circuit.
NEB: 0.01–0.03 mL/kg/DOSE (5 mg/mL solution, maximum 1 mL) in 2–3 mL NS q½–4h, may give continuously if required.
IV: 15 microgram/kg over 10 min or 1 microgram/kg/min, increase q15 min prn to maximum of 10 microgram/kg/min.

Maintenance therapy:

MDI: 1–2 puffs q4h prn.

Acute treatment of hyperkalemia:

IV: 4 microgram/kg over 20 min.
    Titrate dose to effect and/or adverse effects (tachycardia, tremor, and hypokalemia). For most patients metered dose inhalers with a spacer device are the preferred method of drug delivery. Wet nebulization is less efficient and more costly. Monitor serum potassium, especially with IV. Cardiac monitoring required for IV use. Salbutamol is also known as albuterol in the United States.

## Senna

Stimulant laxative.

| PO: infants: | 1 or 2.5 mL (1.7 or 4.25 mg) q24h. |
| children: | 2.5 or 5 mL (4.25 or 8.5 mg) q24h. |
| adolescents: | 5 or 10 mL (8.5 or 17 mg) q24h. |

    Some patients, particularly those receiving opioids, may require higher doses and/or more frequent administration. Also supplied as 8.6 mg tablets.

## Septra®

See Co-trimoxazole.

## Sodium Bicarbonate

Alkalinizing agent.

Cardiopulmonary resuscitation/metabolic acidosis:

IV: 1 mEq/kg/DOSE.

Urinary alkalization:

IV: 0.6 mEq/kg q4h.

Avoid extravasation, tissue necrosis can occur. Incompatible with many drugs including calcium, atropine, and epinephrine. For bolus doses use 4.2% (0.5 mEq/mL) in neonates, otherwise use 8.4% (1 mEq/mL). For continuous infusions use 100 mEq/L or 150 mEq/L in D5W if via peripheral line or undiluted 1 mEq/mL if via central line.

## Sodium Benzoate

Treatment of urea cycle disorders:
IV: 250–500 mg/kg/DAY as a continuous infusion or divided q6h

(250 mg/kg loading dose may be given). For adolescents may use 5 g/m$^2$/DAY.

## Sodium Benzoate/Sodium Phenylacetate

Treatment of urea cycle disorders:
IV: 250–500 mg/kg/DAY of each component as a continuous infusion or divided q6h (250 mg/kg loading dose may be given). For adolescents may use 5 g/m$^2$/DAY.

Solution contains 100 mg/mL of each component.

## Sodium Chloride 3% (0.513 mmol/mL)

Electrolyte.

Reduction of raised intracranial pressure:

IV: 2–5 mL/kg/DOSE.

Correction of hyponatremia:

(Correct long-standing hyponatremia slowly, serum sodium should rise no faster than 0.5 mmol/L/h unless symptomatic or if seizures occur.)
IV: usual maximum rate of administration: 2 mL/kg/h of NaCl 3% or replace estimated sodium deficit, mEq of sodium $\times$ 0.6 $\times$ wt (kg) $\times$ (target plasma sodium − present plasma sodium).

Central line recommended for solutions >0.9%. Rapid correction of long-standing hyponatremia has been associated with central pontine myelinolysis. Follow serum sodium and osmolality frequently.

## Sodium Phosphate

See Phosphate.

## Sotalol

Antiarrhythmic.
PO: 2–5 mg/kg/DAY ÷ q12h (usual maximum 320–480 mg/DAY).
Infants tend to require lower doses than older children. Monitor heart rate, QTc interval.

## Spironolactone

Potassium sparing diuretic.
PO: 1–3 mg/kg/DAY ÷ q12–24h.

## Succinylcholine

Depolarizing neuromuscular blocking agent.
IV: 1–2 mg/kg/DOSE (maximum 150 mg).
IM: 2.5–4 mg/kg/DOSE.
　　Onset of action within 30–60 seconds, duration of action less than 5–10 min. Contraindicated in hyperkalemia, increased intraocular pressure, extensive burns, crush injuries, and rhabdomyolysis. Bradycardia may be reduced by pre-treatment with atropine and should be routinely given in children less than 5–8 years of age. Repeat doses of succinylcholine increase risk of bradycardia and asystole and should generally be avoided.

## Sucralfate

GI mucosal protection.
PO: 40–80 mg/kg/DAY ÷ q6h (maximum 1 g/dose).
　　Sucralfate has many drug interactions, decreasing the absorption of enterally administered medications, check specialized references before use.

## Tacrolimus

Immunosupressant.
Dose and target serum levels vary with indication and the individual protocol, but usually:
PO: 0.15–0.4 mg/kg/DAY ÷ q12h.
IV: 0.01–0.15 mg/kg/DAY as a continuous infusion.

Tacrolimus has many drug interactions, check specialized references before use. Trough levels 5–15 mcg/L.

## Terbutaline

INH: 0.5 mg (1 puff) prn.
IV: 20 mcg/kg then 0.4 mcg/kg/min. Increase infusion q30 min as needed to maximum 3 mcg/kg/min. Loading dose may be repeated prior to each dose increase.

## THAM

See Tromethamine.

## Theophylline

See Aminophylline.

## Thiopental

Barbiturate anticonvulsant and anesthetic.

Induction:

IV: 3–5 mg/kg/DOSE, may repeat prn.

Status epilepticus/refractory increased intracranial pressure:

IV: 3–5 mg/kg over 2–5 min, may repeat if required, then 1.5–5 mg/kg/h initially, higher doses have been required. Hypotension is common, especially with rapid IV injection, treat promptly with fluids and vasopressors. Avoid extravasation, central line preferred. Respiratory depression is common. Coma usually occurs at 30–130 mg/L (124–536 micromol/L) but very high levels may be required. Has no analgesic properties.

## Tobramycin

Aminoglycoside antibiotic.
IV: 5–6 mg/kg/DOSE **q24h** or 2.5 mg/kg/DOSE **q8h**.
INH: multiple regimens exist, most commonly: 40–80 mg q8h or 300 mg q12h.

Once daily dosing should be used for all patients >1 month of age, except in the treatment of endocarditis and in patients with extensive burns. Adjust dosing interval in renal impairment. Ototoxicity and nephrotoxicity may occur, consider monitoring trough levels (target <2 mg/L) in patients at risk for nephrotoxicity; septic shock, concurrent nephrotoxins, fluctuating renal function, or extended treatment courses. May potentiate muscle weakness with neuromuscular blockers. Reserved for documented or suspected resistance to gentamicin.

## Tranexamic Acid

Fibrinolysis inhibitor.

Treatment of excessive bleeding due to hyperfibrinolysis:

PO: 25 mg/kg q6–12h (usual maximum 1.5 g/DOSE).
IV: 10 mg/kg/DOSE q6–8h (usual maximum 1 g/DOSE).
        There is limited experience with using tranexamic acid in children.

## Tromethamine (THAM)

Alkalinizing agent.
IV: Dose depends on severity of acidosis. Usual dose is 1–2 mEq/kg.
        Give each dose over at least 1 hour via central line. Sodium bicarbonate is preferred unless patient is hypernatremic. Lower doses may be required in renal dysfunction. 1 mEq of tromethamine = 3.3 mL of solution.

## Valproic Acid and Derivatives

Anticonvulsant.
PO: 15–20 mg/kg/DAY increased to a maximum of 30–60 mg/kg/DAY ÷ q6–12h.
IV: Divide total daily maintenance q6h.
        Desired therapeutic range: 350–690 micromol/L (50–100 microgram/mL). Dosing is equivalent for valproic acid, divalproex, and sodium valproate.

## Vancomycin

Antibiotic.

Meningitis:

IV: 60 mg/kg/DAY ÷ q6h (maximum 4 g/DAY).

Other infections:

IV: 40 mg/kg/DAY ÷ q6–12h (maximum 2 g/DAY).

Pseudomembranous colitis refractory to metronidazole:

PO: 50 mg/kg/DAY ÷ q6h (maximum 500 mg/DAY).

Reserved for the treatment of infections caused MRSA or coagulase negative Staphylococci. Infuse over at least I hour to avoid red man syndrome, increase infusion duration if reaction occurs. Adjust dosage interval for patients with renal impairment. Consider monitoring trough levels in patients with septic shock, concurrent nephrotoxins, fluctuating renal function, or extended treatment courses. Trough levels should be 5–12 mg/L, but higher levels may be appropriate in some clinical situations.

## Vasopressin

Antidiuretic hormone, vasoconstrictor.

Diabetes insipidus:

IV: 0.0005–0.01 unit/kg/h (0.5–10 milliunits/kg/h), requirements are highly variable, desmopressin is usually preferred.
Refractory septic shock:
IV: 0.3–1 milliunit/kg/min to usual maximum of 2 units/h. There is little experience with using vasopressin in pediatric septic shock. Usual maximum dose is 2 unit/h.

In refractory septic shock, add vasopressin to allow dosage reduction of conventional vasopressors, keep titration of vasopressin to a minimum and use the lowest effective dose. In the treatment of diabetes insipidus follow urine output, volume status, serum, and urine electrolytes frequently.

## Vecuronium

Non-depolarizing neuromuscular blocking agent.
IV: 0.1 mg/kg q30min prn or 1–2 microgram/kg/min.
Intermittent boluses preferred. Monitor depth of paralysis using peripheral nerve stimulation with infusions (target 1–2 twitches out of 4). Onset of action is within 1–2 min, duration of action is approximately 30–60 min and may be prolonged in patients with renal and hepatic dysfunction. Prolonged weakness may occur, especially when corticosteroids are used concurrently with non-depolarizing neuromuscular blocking agents.

## Verapamil

Calcium channel antagoinist antiarrhythmic.

Supraventricular tachydysrhythmias (>1 year of age):

IV:  0.1 mg/kg/DOSE (maximum 5 mg/DOSE), may repeat once in 30 min if needed.

Do not use for SVT in patients less than 1 year due to reports of refractory hypotension and cardiac arrest. Give IV under ECG monitoring. Have IV calcium chloride available. Adverse effects include severe hypotension and AV block. Can precipitate congestive heart failure and/or heart block if given with β-blockers.

## Vitamin K

Reversal of prolonged clotting times or warfarin induced anticoagulation:

IV/PO: 0.5–10 mg/DOSE.

Use lower doses if there is no significant bleeding and patient will require warfarin in the future. May repeat in 6–8 hours. Injection may be given by mouth, undiluted or in juice or water.

## Voriconazole

Antifungal.
IV/PO: 6 mg/kg/DOSE q12h for 2 doses then 4 mg/kg/DOSE q12h.

Dose adjustment required in hepatic dysfunction. The use of the IV formulation is not recommended in severe renal dysfunction due to accumulation of a component of the IV solution. Voriconazole has many drug interactions, check specialized references before use.

# Blood Products

## Albumin

Colloid plasma volume expander (human plasma protein).
IV: 0.5–1 g/kg/DOSE:
5% solution (50 mg/mL): 10–20 mL/kg/DOSE.
25% solution (250 mg/mL): 2–4 mL/kg/DOSE.

Use 5% solution for fluid resuscitation and volume expansion, 25% albumin is very viscous and hyperosmolar, use with caution.

## Cryoprecipitate

Contains factor VII and fibrinogen.
IV: 1 unit/5 kg–1 unit/10 kg.

## Factor VIIa (recombinant)

Recombinant clotting factor.
IV: 90 mcg/kg/DOSE. Repeat doses may be required.

## Fresh Frozen Plasma

Contains all coagulation factors.
IV: 10 mL/kg

## Immune Globulin, Intravenous (IgG, IVIg)

Pooled human immune globulins.

ITP:

IV: 0.8–1 g/kg q24h for 1–2 doses.

Kawasaki disease:

IV: 2 g/kg once.

Guillain-Barré syndrome:

IV: 1 g/kg q24h for 2 days or 0.4 g/kg q24h for 4 days.

Streptococcal toxic shock:

IV: 1 g/kg q24h for 1–2 doses.

Hypogammaglobulinemia:

IV: 0.4–0.6 g/kg q3–4 weeks.
     Most adverse reactions, fever and hypotension are related to the rate of infusion. Anaphylaxis can occur. For most products begin at 0.5 mL/kg/h and increase q15min if tolerated to maximum of 4 mL/kg/h or 250 mL/h.

## Red Cell Concentrate

IV: 10 mL/kg.

## Platelet Concentrate

IV: 1 unit/5 kg–1 unit/10 kg.

## Tetanus Immune Globulin

IM: 4 units/kg (maximum 250 units).

## Varicella-Zoster Immune Globulin

IM: 125 units/10 kg (maximum 625 units).

# Normal and Reference Values

"Normals" for the following tables were derived by using the following approach:

- If there is a single source, it is cited.
- More often, there are several sources; these are averaged.
- Where variations across sources are substantial, a range is given.
- Some figures were rounded-off and adjusted to fit age distributions.

Pause when results are "out of range," as this may not represent a problem needing a "fix." Consider the following:

- Is this due to lab or sampling error?
- Is the patient symptomatic?
- What is the evidence that correction would be of benefit?
- Is there a risk to correcting an abnormal result?

Finally, these values are representative only. Always check against your own laboratory ranges if these are available, as values are also dependent on the test methodology used.

SI units (Standard International Units/Systeme International d'Unites) based on the metric system are used in Canada and many parts of the world. Traditional/Conventional Units are used in most laboratories in the United States.

*Table 1*
## Standard Prefixes

| | | |
|---|---|---|
| pico | $10^{-12}$ | p |
| nano | $10^{-9}$ | n |
| micro | $10^{-6}$ | μ |
| milli | $10^{-3}$ | m |
| centi | $10^{-2}$ | c |
| deci | $10^{-1}$ | d |

*Table 2*
## Serum Electrolytes

| | Conventional Units | SI Units |
|---|---|---|
| **Sodium** | | |
| Newborn | 134–145 mmol/L | 134–145 mmol/L |
| Infant (1 mo–1 yr) | 134–142 mmol/L | 134–145 mmol/L |
| Child (1 yr–10 yrs) | 135–142 mmol/L | 134–145 mmol/L |
| 10 yrs to adult | 135–142 mmol/L | 134–145 mmol/L |
| **Potassium** | | |
| Newborn | 4.0–6.5 mmol/L | 4.0–6.5 mmol/L |
| Infant (1 mo–1 yr) | 3.7–5.3 mmol/L | 3.7–5.3 mmol/L |
| Child (1 yr–10 yrs) | 3.5–5.2 mmol/L | 3.5–5.2 mmol/L |
| 10 yrs to adult | 3.5–5.2 mmol/L | 3.5–5.2 mmol/L |
| **Chloride** | | |
| Newborn | 97–110 mmol/L | 98–106 mmol/L |
| Infant (1 mo–1 yr) | 98–106 mmol/L | 98–106 mmol/L |
| Child (1 yr–10 yrs) | 98–106 mmol/L | 98–106 mmol/L |
| 10 yrs to adult | 98–106 mmol/L | 98–106 mmol/L |
| **Calcium** | | |
| Newborn | 7.0–11.0 mg/dL | 1.75–2.75 mmol/L |
| Infant (1 mo–1 yr) | 9.0–11.0 mg/dL | 2.25–2.75 mmol/L |
| Child (1 yr–10 yrs) | 8.8–10.8 mg/dL | 2.2–2.7 mmol/L |
| 10 yrs to adult | 8.6–10 mg/dL | 2.2–2.5 mmol/L |

| **Ionized Calcium** | | |
|---|---|---|
| Newborn | 4.20–5.68 mmol/L | 1.05–1.4 mmol/L |
| Infant (1 mo–1 yr) | 4.20–5.68 mmol/L | 1.05–1.4 mmol/L |
| Child (1 yr–10 yrs) | 4.80–5.52 mmol/L | 1.1–1.38 mmol/L |
| 10 yrs to adult | 4.64–5.28 mmol/L | 1.16–1.32 mmol/L |
| **Magnesium** | | |
| Newborn | 1.4–2.0 mmol/L | 0.7–1.0 mmol/L |
| Infant (1 mo–1 yr) | 1.5–2.6 mmol/L | 0.6–1.05 mmol/L |
| Child (1 yr–10 yrs) | 1.5–2.6 mmol/L | 0.6–1.05 mmol/L |
| 10 yrs to adult | 1.5–2.6 mmol/L | 0.6–1.05 mmol/L |
| **Phosphate** | | |
| Newborn | 4.5–9.0 mg/dL | 1.45–2.91 mmol/L |
| Infant (1 mo–1 yr) | 4.5–6.7 mg/dL | 1.45–2.16 mmol/L |
| Child (1 yr–10 yrs) | 3.7–5.6 mg/dL | 1.2–1.8 mmol/L |
| 10 yrs to adult | 2.7–4.5 mg/dL | 0.87–1.45 mmol/L |

*Table 3*
**Serum Chemistries**

| | **Conventional Units** | **SI Units** |
|---|---|---|
| **Fasting Glucose** | | |
| Newborn | 45–99 mg/dL | 2.5–5.6 mmol/L |
| Infant (1 mo–1 yr) | 45–99 mg/dL | 2.5–5.6 mmol/L |
| Child (1 yr–10 yrs) | 60–100 mg/dL | 3.3–5.6 mmol/L |
| 10 yrs to adult | 74–106 mg/dL | 4.1–5.9 mmol/L |
| **AST** | | |
| Newborn | 25–140 U/L | 25–140 U/L |
| Infant (1 mo–1 yr) | 15–66 U/L | 15–66 U/L |
| Child (1 yr–10 yrs) | 15–60 U/L | 15–60 U/L |
| 10 yrs to adult | 5–45 U/L | 5–45 U/L |
| **ALT** | | |
| Newborn | 6–50 U/L | 6–50 U/L |
| Infant (1 mo–1 yr) | – | – |
| Child (1 yr–10 yrs) | 5–45 U/L | 5–45 U/L |
| 10 yrs to adult | 5–45 U/L | 5–45 U/L |

|  | **Conventional Units** | **SI Units** |
|---|---|---|
| **GGT** | | |
| Newborn | 0–147 U/L | 0–147 U/L |
| Infant (1 mo–1 yr) | 4–120 U/L | 4–120 U/L |
| Child (1 yr–10 yrs) | 5–65 U/L | 5–65 U/L |
| 10 yrs to adult | 0–5 U/L | 0–5 U/L |
| **LDH** | | |
| Newborn | 290–2000 U/L | 290–2000 U/L |
| Infant (1 mo–1 yr) | 180–500 U/L | 180–500 U/L |
| Child (1 yr–10 yrs) | 150–500 U/L | 150–500 U/L |
| 10 yrs to adult | 100–330 U/L | 100–330 U/L |
| **Ferritin** | | |
| Newborn | 25–200 ng/mL | 25–200 U/L |
| Infant (1 mo–1 yr) | 50–600 ng/mL | 50–600 U/L |
| Child (1 yr–10 yrs) | 7–140 ng/mL | 7–140 U/L |
| 10 yrs to adult | 10–250 ng/mL | 10–250 U/L |
| **Iron** | | |
| Newborn | 22–184 µg/dL | 4–33 µmol/L |
| Infant (1 mo–1 yr) | 22–184 µg/dL | 4–33 µmol/L |
| Child (1 yr–10 yrs) | 22–184 µg/dL | 4–33 µmol/L |
| 10 yrs to adult | 22–184 µg/dL | 4–33 µmol/L |
| **Amylase** | | |
| Newborn | 5–65 U/L | 5–65 U/L |
| Infant (1 mo–1 yr) | – | – |
| Child (1 yr–10 yrs) | 30–131 U/L | 30–131 U/L |
| 10 yrs to adult | 30–131 U/L | 30–131 U/L |
| **Lipase** | | |
| Newborn | 10–85 U/L | 10–85 U/L |
| Infant (1 mo–1 yr) | 9–128 U/L | 9–128 U/L |
| Child (1 yr–10 yrs) | 10–150 U/L | 10–150 U/L |
| 10 yrs to adult | 10–220 U/L | 10–220 U/L |

## Total Bilirubin

| | | |
|---|---|---|
| Newborn | *varies according to age – see Figure 1 | |
| Infant (1 mo–1 yr) | <1.2 mg/dL | <21 µmol/L |
| Child (1 yr–10 yrs) | 0.3–1.3 mg/dL | 5–21 µmol/L |
| 10 yrs to adult | 0.3–1.3 mg/dL | 5–21 µmol/L |

## Creatine Kinase

| | | |
|---|---|---|
| Newborn | 10–700 U/L | 10–700 U/L |
| Infant (1 mo–1 yr) | 5–130 U/L | 5–130 U/L |
| Child (1 yr–10 yrs) | 5–130 U/L | 5–130 U/L |
| 10 yrs to adult | 5–130 U/L | 5–130 U/L |

## Albumin

| | | |
|---|---|---|
| Newborn | 2.5–5.5 g/dL | 25–55 g/L |
| Infant (1 mo–1 yr) | 2.1–5.7 g/dL | 21–57 g/L |
| Child (1 yr–10 yrs) | 2.0–5.8 g/dL | 20–58 g/L |
| 10 yrs to adult | 3.1–5.4 g/dL | 31–54 g/L |

## Prealbumin

| | | |
|---|---|---|
| Newborn | 7–39 mg/dL | 70–390 mg/L |
| Infant (1 mo–1 yr) | 8–34 mg/dL | 80–340 mg/L |
| Child (1 yr–10 yrs) | 12–30 mg/dL | 120–300 mg/L |
| 10 yrs to adult | 18–45 mg/dL | 180–450 mg/L |

## Lactate (arterial)

| | | |
|---|---|---|
| Newborn | <27 mg/dL | 0.0–3.0 mmol/L |
| Infant (1 mo–1 yr) | 5–14 mg/dL | 0.5–1.6 mmol/L |
| Child (1 yr–10 yrs) | 5–14 mg/dL | 0.5–1.6 mmol/L |
| 10 yrs to adult | 5–14 mg/dL | 0.5–1.6 mmol/L |

## Urea (BUN)

| | | |
|---|---|---|
| Newborn | 4–12 mg/dL | 1.4–4.3 mmol/L |
| Infant (1 mo–1 yr) | 5–18 mg/dL | 1.8–6.4 mmol/L |
| Child (1 yr–10 yrs) | 5–18 mg/dL | 1.8–6.4 mmol/L |
| 10 yrs to adult | 6–20 mg/dL | 2.1–7.1 mmol/L |

*(continued)*

|  | Conventional Units | SI Units |
|---|---|---|
| **Creatinine** | | |
| Newborn | 0.3–1.0 mg/dL | 27–88 µmol/L |
| Infant (1 mo–1 yr) | 0.2–0.4 mg/dL | 18–35 µmol/L |
| Child (1 yr–10 yrs) | 0.3–0.7 mg/dL | 27–62 µmol/L |
| 10 yrs to adult | 0.5–1.3 mg/dL | 44–115 µmol/L |
| **Ammonia** | | |
| Newborn | 90–150 µmol/L | 64–107 µmol/L |
| Infant (1 mo–1 yr) | 79–129 µmol/L | 56–92 µmol/L |
| Child (1 yr–10 yrs) | 29–70 µmol/L | 21–50 µmol/L |
| 10 yrs to adult | 0–50 µmol/L | 0–35.7 µmol/L |
| **Osmolality** | | |
| Newborn | 275–295 mOsm/kg $H_2O$ | 275–295 mOsm/kg $H_2O$ |
| Infant (1 mo–1 yr) | 275–295 mOsm/kg $H_2O$ | 275–295 mOsm/kg $H_2O$ |
| Child (1 yr–10 yrs) | 275–295 mOsm/kg $H_2O$ | 275–295 mOsm/kg $H_2O$ |
| 10 yrs to adult | 275–295 mOsm/kg $H_2O$ | 275–295 mOsm/kg $H_2O$ |
| **C–reactive Protein** | | |
| Newborn | 0–0.8 mg/dL | 0–8.0 mg/L |
| Infant (1 mo–1 yr) | 0–0.8 mg/dL | 0–8.0 mg/L |
| Child (1 yr–10 yrs) | 0–0.8 mg/dL | 0–8.0 mg/L |
| 10 yrs to adult | 0–0.8 mg/dL | 0–8.0 mg/L |
| **TSH** | | |
| Newborn | 0.5–16.0 mU/L | 0.5–16.0 mU/L |
| Infant (1 mo–1 yr) | 0.5–7.0 mU/L | 0.5–7.0 mU/L |
| Child (1 yr–10 yrs) | 0.5–6.0 mU/L | 0.5–6.0 mU/L |
| 10 yrs to adult | 0.5–5.0 mU/L | 0.5–5.0 mU/L |

| **Thyroxine T4** | | |
| --- | --- | --- |
| Newborn | 7.7–19.5 µg/dL | 100–250 nmol/L |
| Infant (1 mo–1 yr) | 5.1–15.6 µg/dL | 65–200 nmol/L |
| Child (1 yr–10 yrs) | 5.1–12.8 µg/dL | 65–165 nmol/L |
| 10 yrs to adult | 3.9–12.1 µg/dL | 50–155 nmol/L |
| **Free T4** | | |
| Newborn | 0.8–2.78 ng/dL | 10–36 pmol/L |
| Infant (1 mo–1 yr) | 0.76–2.00 ng/dL | 10–26 pmol/L |
| Child (1 yr–10 yrs) | 0.81–1.72 ng/dL | 10–22 pmol/L |
| 10 yrs to adult | 0.79–1.57 ng/dL | 10–20 pmol/L |

For term infants with bilirubin levels at or above the high zone, further testing or treatment is required.

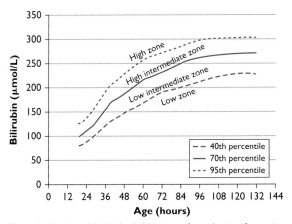

**Figure 1**   Newborn bilirubin levels. Nomogram for evaluation of screening total serum bilirubin (TSB) concentration in term and later preterm infants, according to the TSB concentration obtained at a known postnatal age in hours. Plot the TSB on this figure, then refer to Table 4 for action to be taken.

*Table 4*
## Hematologic Values

|  | Conventional Units | SI Units |
|---|---|---|
| **Hemoglobin (Hb)** | | |
| Newborn | 12.7–18.6 g/dL | 127–186 g/L |
| Infant (1 mo–1 yr) | 10.3–12.5 g/dL | 103–125 g/L |
| Child (1 yr–10 yrs) | 10.5–12.7 g/dL | 105–127 g/L |
| 10 yrs to adult | 10.7–15 g/dL | 107–150 g/L |
| **Leukocyte Count (WBC)** | | |
| Newborn | 5–30 × $10^9$/L | 5–30 × $10^9$/L |
| Infant (1 mo–1 yr) | 5–15 × $10^9$/L | 5–15 × $10^9$/L |
| Child (1 yr–10 yrs) | 5–11.5 × $10^9$/L | 5–11.5 × $10^9$/L |
| 10 yrs to adult | 4.5–10 × $10^9$/L | 4.5–10 × $10^9$/L |
| **Platelet Count** | | |
| Newborn | 150 × $10^9$/L | 400 × $10^9$/L |
| Infant (1 mo–1 yr) | 150 × $10^9$/L | 400 × $10^9$/L |
| Child (1 yr–10 yrs) | 150 × $10^9$/L | 400 × $10^9$/L |
| 10 yrs to adult | 150 × $10^9$/L | 400 × $10^9$/L |
| **Absolute Reticulocyte Count** | | |
| Newborn | 200–300 × $10^9$ | 200–300 × $10^9$ |
| Infant (1 mo–1 yr) | 5–250 × $10^9$ | 5–250 × $10^9$ |
| Child (1 yr–10 yrs) | 10–100 × $10^9$ | 10–100 × $10^9$ |
| 10 yrs to adult | 10–100 × $10^9$ | 10–100 × $10^9$ |
| **PT** | | |
| Newborn | 12–23 sec | 12–23 sec |
| Infant (1 mo–1 yr) | 10–12 sec | 10–12 sec |
| Child (1 yr–10 yrs) | 10–12 sec | 10–12 sec |
| 10 yrs to adult | 10–15 sec | 10–15 sec |

**APTT**

| | | |
|---|---|---|
| Newborn | 35–52 sec | 35–52 sec |
| Infant (1 mo–1 yr) | 24–36 sec | 24–36 sec |
| Child (1 yr–10 yrs) | 26–36 sec | 26–36 sec |
| 10 yrs to adult | 27–40 sec | 27–40 sec |

**D–Dimer**

| | | |
|---|---|---|
| Newborn | 0.88–2.74 μg/mL | 0.88–2.74 μg/mL |
| Infant (1 mo–1 yr) | 0.10–0.42 μg/mL | 0.10–0.42 μg/mL |
| Child (1 yr–10 yrs) | 0.10–0.56 μg/mL | 0.10–0.56 μg/mL |
| 10 yrs to adult | 0.05–0.42 μg/mL | 0.05–0.42 μg/mL |

*Table 5*
**Cerebrospinal Fluid Values for Healthy Term Infants**

| Age | 0–24 h | 1 d | 7 d |
|---|---|---|---|
| Polymorphs/mm³ | 3 (0–70) | 7 (0–26) | 3 (0–48) |
| Lymphocytes/mm³ | 2 (0–20) | 5 (0–16) | 1 (0–4) |
| Protein g/L | 0.63 (0.32–2.40) | 0.73 (0.40–1.48) | 0.47 (0.27–0.65) |
| Glucose mmol/L* | 2.8 (1.8–4.3) | 2.7 (2.1–3.6) | 3.1 (2.7–3.4) |

*Value must be compared with blood sugar concentration; mean ratio is about 0.8.

*Table 6*
## CSF Values for Children and Infants Over 7 Days

|  | Conventional Units | SI Units |
|---|---|---|
| Glucose* | 38–65 mg/dL | 2.1–3.6 mmol/L |
| Lactate | <25 mg/dL | <2.5 mmol/L |
| Pyruvate | 0.3–0.9 mg/dL | 0.03–0.08 mmol/L |
| Protein | 15–45 mg/dL | 0.15–0.45 g/L |
| CSF IgG | <0.1 of total CSF protein | <0.1 of total CSF protein |

*Usually 60–80% of serum glucose level.

# Suggested Reading

Cheng A, Williams B, Sivrarjan V. The HSC Handbook of Pediatrics, 10th ed. Elsevier Canada; 2003.

Fisher DA. Thyroid disorders in childhood and adolescence. In Sperling MA, ed. Pediatric Endocrinology, 2nd ed. Philadelphia: Saunders; 2002.

Gunn V, Nechyba C, Barone M. Harriet Lane Handbook: A Manual for Pediatric House Officers. Philadelphia: C.V. Mosby; 16th ed. (June 15, 2002).

Heckmann M, Wudy SA, Haack D, Pohlandt F. Reference ranges for serum cortisol in well preterm infants. Arch Dis Child Neonatal Ed 1999;81:F171–F174.

Monagle P, Chan A, deVeber G, Massicotte P. Andrew's Pediatric Thromboembolism and Stroke, 3rd ed. Location: BC Decker; 2006.

Naidoo BT. The cerebrospinal fluid in the healthy newborn infant. S Afr Med J 1968;42:933.

Perrone S, et al. Nucleated red blood cell count in term and preterm newborns: reference values at birth. Arch Dis Child Fetal Neonatal Ed 2005;90:F174–175.

Rosenthal P. Assessing liver function and hyperbilirubinemia in the newborn. National Academy of Clinical Biochemistry. Clin Chem. 1997 Jan;43(1):228–34.

Soldin SJ, Brugnara C, Wong C. Pediatric Reference Intervals, 5th ed. Washington, DC: American Association of Clinical Chemistry (AACC) Press; 2005.

# Index